THE ROUTLEDGE HANDBOOK OF HEALTH COMMUNICATION AND POPULAR CULTURE

The Routledge Handbook of Health Communication and Popular Culture offers rich insights into the ways in which communication about health through popular culture can become a part of healing, wellness, and health-related decisions.

This Handbook allows readers to understand and consider messages that inform and influence health-related choices through pop culture in the public sphere. Written in an accessible narrative style and including interdisciplinary, global, and diverse perspectives, a vast team of contributing authors from the field explores the intersections between health communication and popular culture. The Handbook is divided into five parts: Framing of Health-Related Issues in Popular Culture; Exploring Popular Culture Influences on Health Behaviors and Beliefs; Considering Pro-Social Public Health Interventions in Popular Culture; Understanding Health Issues in Popular Culture from Diverse Perspectives; and Pop Culture and Health Communication: Looks to the Future.

The Handbook will be of interest to students and scholars in the fields of Communication Studies, Health Communication, Public Health Policy, Media Literacy, and Cultural Studies.

Christina S. Beck is a Professor in the School of Communication Studies at Ohio University (USA) and Past-President of the National Communication Association and Central States Communication Association.

ROUTLEDGE HANDBOOKS IN COMMUNICATION STUDIES

THE ROUTLEDGE HANDBOOK OF CORPORATE SOCIAL RESPONSIBILITY COMMUNICATION
Edited By Amy O'Connor

THE ROUTLEDGE INTERNATIONAL HANDBOOK OF RESEARCH ON WRITING, 2ND EDITION
Edited By Rosalind Horowitz

THE ROUTLEDGE HANDBOOK OF PRIVACY AND SOCIAL MEDIA
Edited By Sabine Trepte and Philipp Masur

THE ROUTLEDGE HANDBOOK OF ETHNICITY AND RACE IN COMMUNICATION
Edited By Bernadette Marie Calafell and Shinsuke Eguchi

THE ROUTLEDGE HANDBOOK OF PUBLIC SPEAKING RESEARCH AND THEORY
Edited By Stevie M. Munz, Tim McKenna-Buchanan and Anna M. Wright

THE ROUTLEDGE HANDBOOK OF RHETORIC AND POWER
Edited by Nathan Crick

THE ROUTLEDGE HANDBOOK OF CONTEMPORARY FEMINIST RHETORIC
Edited by Jacqueline Rhodes and Suban Nur Cooley

THE ROUTLEDGE HANDBOOK OF HEALTH COMMUNICATION AND POPULAR CULTURE
Edited by Christina S. Beck

For additional information on this series please visit https://www.routledge.com/Routledge-Handbooks-in-Communication-Studies/book-series/RHCS, and for information on other Routledge titles visit www.routledge.com.

THE ROUTLEDGE HANDBOOK OF HEALTH COMMUNICATION AND POPULAR CULTURE

Edited by Christina S. Beck

Routledge
Taylor & Francis Group
NEW YORK AND LONDON

Designed cover image: Getty Images | PeopleImages

First published 2025
by Routledge
605 Third Avenue, New York, NY 10158

and by Routledge
4 Park Square, Milton Park, Abingdon, Oxon, OX14 4RN

Routledge is an imprint of the Taylor & Francis Group, an informa business

ISBN: 978-1-032-56618-4 (hbk)
ISBN: 978-1-032-56619-1 (pbk)
ISBN: 978-1-003-43640-9 (ebk)

DOI: 10.4324/9781003436409

Typeset in Times New Roman
by Deanta Global Publishing Services, Chennai, India

CONTENTS

CONTRIBUTORS

Suraj Arshanapally (MPH, Yale School of Public Health) is a Health Communication Specialist at the Centers for Disease Control and Prevention. He is also the Managing Editor for the CDC Yellow Book, a travel medicine publication. Suraj is passionate about the use of communication and storytelling for public health impact and social change. He has presented at conferences such as the National Conference on Health Communication, Marketing, and Media and has published in journals such as the *Journal of Medical Internet Research* and *Perspectives in Public Health*.

Rokeshia Renné Ashley-McNamee (Ph.D., University of Missouri-Columbia) is an Associate Professor of Communication at Florida International University and entrepreneur. She is a highly productive scholar whose research on Black women's bodies and Black maternal health has been published in several books and journals, such as *Communication, Culture & Critique*; *The Howard Journal of Communications*; *Health Communication*; and *Journal of Black Studies*. Dr. Ashley's research has been featured by *The Washington Post*, *Psychology Today*,*The Miami Times*, *National Public Radio's Academic Minute*, *The Conversation*, *Yahoo! News*, *Black Enterprise*, *Tavis Smiley's* KBLA 1580 am, Areva Martin's *The Special Report*, *Allure* magazine and more; collectively over 60 million readers across varying platforms. To broaden the impact of her work, Dr. Ashley published the children's book *SunFlower Child* in 2020.

Jennifer Stevens Aubrey (Ph.D., University of Michigan, 2004) is a Professor at the University of Arizona (USA). She takes classes on media, mass communication theory, and child and adolescent development in the Department of Communication at the University of Arizona. With an emphasis on gender and child/adolescent development, her research focuses on media effects on emotional, mental, and physical health in young people. Topically, her research tends to center on issues related to sexuality and body image. Her research has been published in such top-tier journals as *Health Communication*, *Media Psychology*, and *Journal of Communication*.

Erica Weintraub Austin (Ph.D., Stanford University) is dedicated to collaborative efforts that help people use media to make decisions that are best for themselves and to help their communities. She is a Professor and the Founding Director of the Edward R. Murrow Center for Media and Health Promotion Research in the Edward R. Murrow College of Communication at Washington State University. A fellow in the International Communication Association, she is ranked among the World's Top 1% Scientists for "Lifetime Impact" in Communication and Media Studies, Public Health according to Elsevier's Data Repository. Austin focuses her research on how strengthening media literacy can facilitate healthier decision-making and engagement in health, science, and civics among children, adolescents, and adults.

Jay Baglia (Ph.D., University of South Florida) is an Associate Professor in the College of Communication with a focus on health communication, gender communication, and performance studies. In 2005, Baglia published *The Viagra Ad Venture: Masculinity, Media, & the Performance of Sexual Health* with Peter Lang Publishing. Along with co-editor Rachel E. Silverman, Dr. Baglia published a volume of pregnancy loss narratives, *Communicating Pregnancy Loss: Narrative as a Method for Change*, in Peter Lang's Health Communication Series in 2015. Both *The Viagra Ad Venture* and *Communicating Pregnancy Loss* won the OSCLG Outstanding Book Award (in 2006 and 2015, respectively). In addition, he has book chapters, book reviews, and essays in journals such as *Health Communication, Family Medicine, Cultural Studies <> Critical Methodologies, Text & Performance Quarterly, Women & Language*, and the *Journal of Dramatic Theory & Criticism.*

Christina S. Beck (Ph.D., University of Oklahoma) is a Professor in the School of Communication Studies at Ohio University (USA) and Past-President of the National Communication Association and Central States Communication Association. Beck has produced 11 books and numerous book chapters, journal articles, and conference presentations. Beck's 2015 co-authored book, *Celebrity Health Narratives and the Public Health*, and her 2022 single-authored book, *Celebrity in the Time of Covid: Fandom and the Influence of Pandemic Messaging*, bridge her work in health communication, popular culture, fandom, and media audiences.

Heather J. Carmack (Ph.D., Ohio University) is a Professor of Health Services Research and Senior Associate Consultant at Mayo Clinic. She is also a communication scholar interested in health communication, organizational communication, patient safety, thanatology, and research methods. Her research focuses on communication produced by and surrounding health organizations, examining the different ways in which health is organized and practiced. She focuses on communication produced by hospitals, practitioners, and patients in order to understand how different publics communicate about medical errors, patient safety, and death and dying.

Elisia L. Cohen (Ph.D., University of Southern California Annenberg School for Communication and Journalism) is a Professor and Director of the Hubbard School of Journalism and Mass Communication at the University of Minnesota. Dr. Cohen began her career at Saint Louis University, rising through the ranks as she developed innovative media and community-based outreach strategies to improve cancer prevention and detection behaviors in underserved communities. At the University of Kentucky, she was awarded the campus Sarah Bennett Holmes Award in recognition of her leadership, research, and service. She also was recognized with the American Public Health Association's 2016 Mayhew Derryberry Award. Her research has been supported by the Centers for Disease Control and Prevention, National Institutes of Health, and private industry. Her research on media reporting and public understanding of disease has appeared in journals such as *Health Communication, Health Education and Behavior, Journal of Applied Communication Research, Journal of Broadcasting and Electronic Media, Journal of Communication, Journal of Communication in Healthcare, Journal of Health Communication, Qualitative Health Research*, and *Prometheus*. She has edited four volumes of *Communication Yearbook.*

Alan D. DeSantis (Ph.D., Indiana University) is a Professor in the Department of Communication at the University of Kentucky (USA). His research has focused on masculinity and fraternity life, cigar smoking, and the illicit use of ADHD stimulants on American college campuses. Currently, his teaching and research interests are focused on English-speaking film history and criticism.

Diane B. Francis (Ph.D., University of North Carolina at Chapel Hill) is an Associate Professor of Communication Studies at Northeastern University with a joint appointment in Applied Psychology. She is a communication and health equity scholar – she conducts applied research at the intersections of communication, race, and health. Her academic research is centered on how communication strategies – both traditional and digital – can best be harnessed to mitigate health disparities, primarily among Black populations. Her work is funded by grants from the National Institutes of Health and the Substance Abuse and Mental Health Services Administration and has been published in leading journals across communication, public health, and medicine, including *Health Communication*, *Journal of Health Communication*, *Social Science & Medicine*, and *Preventive Medicine*.

Heather Gahler (Ph.D. candidate at the University of Arizona, USA) is a Media Effects Scholar, working on the effects of social media on body image among diverse populations. She is interested in understanding how social media influences perceptions of body image among different racial/ethnic groups, gender minorities, and within the LGBTQ+ community. In recent years, her research has focused on how Instagram influences body image differently depending on one's racial/ethnic group and the racial/ethnic group of one's followers. Her recent publications have appeared in *Body Image*, *Computers in Human Behavior*, and *Psychology of Popular Media*. She has taught classes on children and media, the history of media effects, research methods, and public speaking, among others.

Leandra H. Hernández (Ph.D., Texas A&M University) is an Assistant Professor in the Department of Communication at the University of Utah (USA). She enjoys teaching health communication, gender studies, and media studies courses. She utilizes Chicana feminist and qualitative approaches to explore Latina/o/x cultural health experiences, Latina/o/x journalism and media representations, and reproductive justice and gendered violence contexts. Her teaching philosophy is informed by social justice approaches, and she is passionate about mentoring undergraduate students through diverse and inclusive research projects. She is the co-author of one monograph and co-editor of six co-edited volumes. Further, her research is published in several books, as well as in *Health Communication*, *Frontiers in Communication*, *Women's Studies in Communication*, *Journal of Media and Religion*, *Communication Research*, *QED: A Journal in GLBTQ Worldmaking*, and *Departures in Critical Qualitative Research*.

Yan Huang (Ph.D., The Pennsylvania State University) is an Assistant Professor of integrated strategic communication in the Jack J. Valenti School of Communication at the University of Houston. Her research investigates how content features and technological aspects of media campaigns shape audience responses to health and prosocial messages. Her work has appeared in such journals as *Health Communication*, *Information, Communication & Society*, *International Journal of Advertising*, *Journal of Communication*, *Journal of Health Communication*, *Journal of Public Relations Research*, and *Science Communication*, among others. She received an AEJMC Emerging Scholar Award in 2021 and a Faculty Research Award from the AEJMC Mass Communication and Society Division in 2022.

Michael Hviid Jacobsen (Ph.D., Aalborg University) is a Professor of Sociology at Aalborg University, Denmark. He is the editor of *The Poetics of Crime* and *Postmortal Society* and co-editor of *Death in Contemporary Popular Culture*, *The Sociology of Zygmunt Bauman*, *Encountering the Everyday*, *The Transformation of Modernity*, *Utopia: Social Theory and the Future*, *Liquid Criminology*, *Emotions and Crime: Towards a Criminology of the Emotions*, *Exploring Grief: Towards a Sociology of Sorrow*, and *Imaginative Methodologies: The Poetic Imagination in the Social Sciences*.

Marian Jaitto-Jeffrey is a media and communication professional currently pursuing a doctoral program in health communication in the Department of Communication at the University of Kentucky

(USA). Her research focus is on persuasive message design to facilitate health behavior change as it relates to risk behavior prevention and health promotion across various media platforms. Marian's research interests include narrative communication, behavioral and mental health, patient–provider interactions, and health campaigns. She has attended and presented at several conferences including the National Communication Association, Central States Communication Association, World Communication Association, and the Kentucky Conference on Health Communication.

Evie Kendal (Ph.D., Monash University) is an emerging technology bioethicist and public health scientist whose work focuses on reproductive biotechnologies, health communication and media, and space ethics. She is a Lecturer in Health Promotion at Swinburne University of Technology's Department of Health Sciences and Biostatistics. Evie's research interests include artificial womb technology, ethical issues in aerospace medicine, planetary defense, and public health education. Evie heads the Ethical, Legal, and Social Implications of Emerging Technologies (ELSIET) research group, housed at the Iverson Health Innovation Research Institute. Her publications include a journal article about bioethics and science fiction as well as the co-edited book, *Teaching Medicine and Medical Ethics Using Popular Culture*.

Kimberly N. Kline (Ph.D., University of Georgia) is a Professor at the University of Texas at San Antonio (USA). She uses traditional and contemporary communication theory and methods from rhetoric, mass media, cultural studies, psychology, and sociology to explore the social management of health issues. Her empirical research employs both qualitative and quantitative methodologies to address topics such as health and illness representations in popular media (i.e., entertainment, journalistic, advertising), socially constructed understandings associated with pregnancy/childbirth and intersex, and the cultural sensitivity for African-American audiences and persuasive potential of breast cancer early detection interventions. She collaborates with public health professionals to develop and implement diabetes and HPV vaccine health education interventions for Hispanic audiences. Her research can be found in such journals as *Health Communication, Journal of Health Communication, Social Science and Medicine, The Journal of Adolescent Health, Patient Preference and Adherence, Women & Languageand* in edited volumes including *Communication Yearbook, The Handbook of Health Communication, Evaluating Women's Health Messages,* and *Constructing Our Health: The Implications of Narrative for Enacting Illness and Wellness.*

Sarah S. LeBlanc (Ph.D., University of Missouri) is an Associate Professor of Interpersonal Communication at Purdue University, Fort Wayne. She enjoys teaching health communication and the dark side of relationships. Her research is heavily embedded in her engagement with her local community, specifically working to address menstrual stigma and period poverty, especially among high-poverty ZIP codes. She has examined postpartum communication and mother-scholar identities. Her most current work appears in *Women's Health*, the *Southern Journal of Communication*, and the *Atlantic Journal of Communication.*

Amanda R. Martinez (Ph.D., Texas A&M University) is an Associate Professor and Chair of the Communication Studies Department at Davidson College. She studies media effects, gender, race, ethnicity, and intergroup communication with a focus on underrepresented populations, identity, intersectionality, race-based media stereotyping, humorous communication in entertainment contexts, and health communication. Her publications appear in several peer-reviewed journals, including *Mass Communication & Society, the Howard Journal of Communications, Southern Communication Journal, Health Communication,* and *Women's Studies in Communication*. Her work appears in several edited books, and she is co-editor of the Cultural Media Studies book series (Peter Lang Publishing). As a Chicana feminist, her Latina/o/x communication studies research angle aims to elevate the complexities of cultural roots and experiences by shattering monoliths prevalent across important realms of societal representation, especially health, education, and mass media. Recently, she has co-authored publications with her students on social media topics, and she has published about mentorship and undergraduate thesis writing.

Michaela D. E. Meyer (Ph.D., Ohio University) is a Professor of Communication at Christopher Newport University. She is a critical identity scholar who has published extensively on media representation and popular culture. Her work has appeared in numerous journals including *The Review of Communication, Communication Studies, Sexuality & Culture, Health Communication, The Popular Culture Studies Journal*, and *The Journal of Autoethnography*. In addition to her co-edited collection *Adventures in Shondaland* with Rutgers University Press, she has also contributed to a number of academic collections including *Women, Feminism and Pop Politics, Contemporary Studies of Sexuality and Communication*, and *Communicating Pregnancy Loss*.

Stevie M. Munz (Ph.D., Ohio University) is an Associate Professor at Utah Valley University in Orem, Utah. As a scholar, she is invested in a line of inquiry-engaging questions about how human beings understand and communicate their relational, political, and social identity experiences. Through critical ethnographic and narrative methods, her published research reflects her commitment to understanding and archiving the stories from women, LGBTQ+ students and teachers, and historically minoritized voices. Her teaching philosophy is centered on engaging students through equitable and performative learning opportunities, which includes servicing learning and community-engaged research projects.

Alane L. Presswood (Ph.D., Ohio University) is a Lecturer and the Public Speaking Course Coordinator in the Communication and Media Studies Department at Pace University in New York City. She researches the ways in which historically marginalized rhetors use social media and popular culture to gain increased access to the public sphere. Her 2020 book, *Food Blogs, Postfeminism, and the Communication of Expertise*, describes the relationships between individual brands, reader communities, and sociocultural trends to demonstrate how digital platforms both enable and constrain women as public communicators.

Farren Rodrigues is a Ph.D. student in the Department of Health, Behavior and Society at the Johns Hopkins University Bloomberg School of Public Health. Her research interests center on global health, health communication, and social and behavior change.

Jimmy Sanderson (Ph.D., Arizona State University) is an Associate Professor in the Department of Kinesiology and Sport Management at Texas Tech University. His research interests center on social media and sport, along with sport and health.

Raffi Sarkissian (Ph.D., University of Southern California) is an Assistant Professor of Communication Studies at Christopher Newport University. His research encompasses LGBT media representation, queer film festivals, and industry award shows. He has published articles in the *International Journal of Communication* and *Spectator* as well as chapters in *Popular Culture and the Civic Imagination and Queer Youth Media Cultures*.

Suruchi Sood (Ph.D., University of New Mexico) is the Director of Communication Science at the Johns Hopkins Center for Communication Programs and a Senior Scientist at the Department of Health, Behavior, and Society in the Bloomberg School of Public Health. As a multidisciplinary health communication scholar, Dr Sood has managed capacity-building and research projects covering five continents in over 30 low- and middle-income countries. Additionally, she has over 12 years of graduate-level teaching experience, much of it at the Dornsife School of Public Health at Drexel University, Philadelphia. She has established a substantial research and teaching/mentoring program throughout her academic and professional career. She recently co-authored a textbook, *Fundamentals* *of Health Communication: Planning, Implementing and Evaluating Public Health Communication.* She was awarded the American Public Health Association (APHA), Public Health Education and Health Promotion (PHEHP) Section's 2019 Everett M. Rogers Award, which honors outstanding contributions to advancing the study and/or practice of public health communication.

Heather Stuart (Ph.D., University of Calgary) is the Bell Canada Chair in Mental Health and Anti-stigma Research, the first ever in Canada, as well as a Professor in the Department of Public Health Sciences and the Department of Psychiatry and Rehabilitation Therapy. Dr Stuart is also the Senior Consultant to the Mental Health Commission of Canada's Opening Minds, Anti-stigma initiative and the past and founding Chair of the World Psychiatric Association's Stigma and Mental Health Scientific Section. She has worked in both hospital and community-based mental health treatment systems and with international agencies such as the World Health Organization, the Pan American Health Organization, and the World Psychiatric Association. In 2018, Dr Stuart was named to the Order of Canada and inducted as a Fellow in the Royal Society of Canada.

Andrew D. Sutherland (M.A., West Virginia University) is currently a Ph.D. student at the Edward R. Murrow College of Communication at Washington State University. Andrew's research focuses on media literacy, psychophysiology, and the intersections of health and political communication. Specifically, his interest focuses on the cognitive and emotional dimensions of information processing and how those dimensions can enhance or hinder media literacy skills and their application to decision-making.

Adriana Teodorescu (Ph.D., Babeş-Bolyai University) is a Ph.D. Lecturer in the Department of Social Work, Babeş-Bolyai University, Cluj-Napoca, Romania. She is the ambassador for Romania of The Association for the Study of Death and Society; co-editor of *Death in Contemporary Popular Culture* (Routledge, 2020). Her research interests include death studies, social gerontology, cultural studies, and digital sociology.

Sathyaraj Venkatesan (Ph.D., IIT Kanpur, India) is a Professor of English in the Department of Humanities and Social Sciences at the National Institute of Technology, Tiruchirappalli (India), where he specializes in health humanities and comics studies, with an emphasis on graphic medicine. He is the author/co-author/editor/co-editor of nine books, including *Pandemics and Epidemics in Cultural Representation* (Singapore: Springer, 2022), *Infertility Comics and Graphic Medicine* (New York/London: Routledge, 2021), *India Retold* (New York: Bloomsbury, 2021), *Mental Disorders and Graphic Medicine* (New York/London: Routledge, 2021), and *Gender, Eating Disorders and Graphic Medicine* (New York/London: Routledge, 2020). He has published more than a hundred research articles in journals such as *Medical Humanities, Perspectives in Biology and Medicine, Journal of Medical Humanities, American Medical Association Journal of Ethics (AMA), Health, Concentric, Journal of Graphic Novels and Comics, and World Literature Today,* among others. Currently, he is working on his tenth book tentatively titled *COVID-19 and Graphic Medicine,* contracted with Palgrave Macmillan/Springer Nature.

Jennifer Walton (Ph.D., Bowling Green State University) is a Professor and School Director at Radford University (USA). Her research focuses on public scholarship and has been featured in *USA Today, The Columbus Dispatch, The Tennessean* among many others. She published a scholarly book entitled *A Rhetorical Analysis of Six Hollywood Films about Politics: Presenting the Candidate as a Movie Star* and had two book chapters appear in *Teaching Communication Creatively: Practical Ideas to Enhance Student Learning.* She is currently working on a book highlighting the health and social issues portrayed in soap operas.

Weirui Wang (Ph.D., The Pennsylvania State University) is an Associate Professor in the Department of Communication at Florida International University. Dr. Wang's research focuses on information processing and persuasion, with a special emphasis on understanding narrative persuasion, stigmatization/destigmatization, and misinformation correction in communicating health, science, and risk. Her work has been published in *Public Understanding of Science*, *Science Communication*, *Information, Communication and Society*, *Computers in Human Behavior*, *Media Psychology*, and *Health Communication*, among others. Dr. Wang currently serves as an Associate Editor for the *Asian Journal of Communication*.

Amy L. Yoder is an independent scholar. Her work focuses on copy and content writing for a variety of organizations, with a heavy emphasis on internal communications in a healthcare setting. She is also skilled in knowledge translation, copy editing, and project management.

Brianna R. Yoder (Ph.D., University of Georgia) is an Assistant Professor of Instruction in the Multidisciplinary Studies Program at the University of Texas at San Antonio. Her scholarship focuses on nonprofit organizations, where she has used qualitative discourse analysis to examine gendered discourse in sexual harassment and parental leave policy documents. Additionally, she has worked to build capacity in nonprofit organizations to increase program effectiveness, enhance leadership, and engage community members.

Jiaqi Zeng (M.A., Georgetown University, 2020) is a PhD student in communication at the University of Arizona. Her research focuses on media effects on people's psychological health and behavior.

ACKNOWLEDGMENTS

I am incredibly grateful for the opportunity to edit the *Routledge Handbook of Health Communication and Popular Culture*. Back in the mid-1980s, I was trying to figure out the topic for my MA thesis, and I met with my advisor, Dr. Jim Wilcox, at Bowling Green State University. I told him that I didn't have any great ideas for a thesis topic. He asked, "Well, what do you like?" Having just come from watching an episode of *Guiding Light*, I chuckled and replied, "Well, I like soap operas, but I can't write about that!" He looked at me very seriously and posed a question that would change the trajectory of my career: "Why not?" I'm grateful to Dr. Wilcox for his encouragement, and I wish that he were still with us to witness the impact of his question and support on my scholarly journey.

I'm also very appreciative of Dr. Sandra Ragan, my dissertation advisor at the University of Oklahoma, for inviting me to help her with transcribing data for a project that she was doing on communication in a women's health setting. Without that project, I'm not sure that I would have been drawn to Health Communication. That invitation also comprised a powerful turning point for me and my career. I'm truly forever thankful for her role in helping me to launch a program of research in Health Communication.

In 1999, I was working on another book project when I stumbled upon a way to bridge my interests in popular culture and Health Communication. I wrote a small section of that book on celebrity health narratives, and this work has been rewarding because I truly believe that this discourse powerfully shapes public conversations about health and wellness. I have also enjoyed exploring the intersections between my two strands of scholarship.

Working on the *Routledge Handbook of Health Communication and Popular Culture* has been a true joy and a gift. I would like to thank Alexandra deBrauw, Commissioning Editor at Routledge, for this incredible opportunity to be part of this project. I am also grateful to all the contributors for their work. This book features the work of a terrific team of authors, and I thank them for their insightful and compelling contributions.

I close by thanking my family. When I originally committed to this project, I was supposed to be on sabbatical during Spring 2024. Due to a need in our department, I agreed to defer my sabbatical, but I remained committed to finishing this project on time. Balancing this editorial work along with my other responsibilities as Associate Director for Graduate Studies, instructor, advisor, committee member, etc. has been challenging, requiring many late nights. I'm incredibly thankful to my husband, Roger Aden, for everything that he has done with and for our family when I've been busy with editing and writing.

Finally, I'd like to thank our daughters, Brittany Nicole, Chelsea Meagan, Emmy Grace, and Ellie-Kate. As I get ready to hit "send" on this document, please know that you won't have to hear me say that I'm "working on a manuscript" again – at least not for the immediate future. I'm so glad that we share a love of Disney, sports, and pop culture, and I look forward to the adventures that await. I love each of you!

1

CONSEQUENTIALITY OF POPULAR CULTURE FOR CONTEMPORARY HEALTH COMMUNICATION

Christina S. Beck

Memories can be a funny thing … As I interact now with my 11-month-old granddaughter, I sometimes wonder what she's thinking (i.e., "I have the silliest Grammy!") and what, if anything, she might remember from otherwise mundane moments (e.g., Disney's *Bear in the Big Blue House* on loop as she bangs on her musical toys or cuddles with her stuffed Minnie Mouse). As I try to reclaim now long-ago snippets from my own childhood, flashes of *Captain Kangaroo* on our small black-and-white television come to mind. I recall my mom watching "her stories" (*The Guiding Light* and *As the World Turns*) on that same tiny television as she ironed, and I sat nearby. I remember that I was a bit older (maybe five or six?) when I watched my dad wave his arms fervently at a slightly larger TV set, yelling at the refs of a Chicago Bears game for "robbing" "his" team of a victory.

From what I'm told, I could have had some other pretty cool moments that would seemingly be more likely "core memories" (see Disney's *Inside Out*). For example, from the time that I was an infant, apparently, I got to ride on a horse with my dad a lot, and I know that I welcomed a baby sister when I was six. However, as much as I press my brain to recall any images from those moments in my first six years of life, I get *Captain Kangaroo*, soap operas, and a football game.

Even five-and-a-half decades later, those memories linger from a simple black-and-white television set with "rabbit ears" and three networks. In the years that have followed, much has changed for me – I'm now the mom of four and a "Grammy," not the little kid staring with wide eyes at images on a small screen (and watching adults entertained by a daily drama or irritated by a sports outcome). However, more importantly, for the purposes of this book, popular culture has changed. As I talk with my students at Ohio University, most have never known a time when cords connected telephones to walls. Most can't recall a time before computers or the internet. I honestly don't feel that old, but, sometimes, I feel like a dinosaur in their midst. Soon, those of us with memories of pre-cell phone, pre-internet, pre-social media, pre-streaming times will be just as extinct as a brontosaurus. However, whether as someone who can close her eyes and recall a different, simpler time or someone who only knows a world in which information can be accessed on a device in the palm of her hand, few of us can (or choose to) get away from popular culture as easily as those days of flipping the "off" switch on the only "device" in our house – that old black-and-white television set with the rabbit ears.

As both a fan and a scholar who has written about interpretive communities and television viewing, I have long been convinced that popular culture comprises an important part of our everyday lives (see, e.g., Beck, 2012). My husband likes to do Wordle every morning; I enjoy working out

DOI: 10.4324/9781003436409-1

every day while watching *General Hospital*. (I still haven't stopped watching soap operas after those early days of co-viewing with my mom.) In my case, though, tuning in every day isn't just a casual habit. I'm a fan of the genre and the show. As I wrote in my article about intersecting narratives between the sagas on soap operas and the lives of long-time viewers, I grieved the loss of *Guiding Light* and *As the World Turns* when they got pulled from the air – I literally felt like I'd had a death in the family (for related work on parasocial connections, see, e.g., Forster, 2023; Frost, 2023).

However, as much as I love soap operas and "my stories," my fandom pales in comparison to others who participate actively in online communities, attend fan events, and write and post fan fiction (for related work on participatory fandom in this era of postmodernism and transmedia, see, e.g., Ang, 1996; Barton & Lampley, 2014; Booth, 2015; Click & Scott, 2018; Gray et al., 2017; Hills, 2002; Jenkins, 2013; Stein, 2015). Other fans create YouTube montages of favorite scenes and write (and then post) fan fiction about shows no longer on the air, using a host of social media platforms. When I happen to scroll on Facebook or Twitter (now "X"), I end up lurking on soap opera-related pages and reading posts filled with fan speculation and gossip about "what's next" when we "tune in tomorrow." I wish that I had more time to listen to soap opera-related podcasts or YouTube series, or to watch online soap operas, or to read autobiographies from soap opera actors who have portrayed their roles for decades. When I put my phone down after a few minutes of "playing" on social media, I always feel that I'm missing more "out there" about the characters or actors or shows, but I don't have nearly enough time to pursue or consume all that awaits online.

I suggest that the sheer enormity and ubiquity of contemporary popular culture make it increasingly consequential for how individuals encounter the world. For many, popular culture no longer "just" encompasses buying an album of a favorite musical artist, for example. We follow the musician on various mediated platforms, watch videos of performances on YouTube, re-post related photos and articles on our own social media platforms, and, of course, go-to concerts and share our selfies from those neat in-person experiences.

My two older daughters grew up with Taylor Swift's music, and they excitedly purchased tickets for her "Eras Tour" concert in Cincinnati as soon as they became available. Spilde (2024, para. 6) described:

> [t]he tour, an amalgamation of each of Swift's album cycles—complete with a micro-revival of each record's specific aesthetics and visual themes—[as] a dream come true for Swifties. It was a celebration of their love for their favorite artist.

My daughters bought special outfits to wear to the concert, acquired t-shirts at the concert venue, and splattered their own social media accounts with images from the concert. As "Swifties," they weren't alone. According to Millman (2023), Taylor Swift's Eras Tour "is the highest grossing tour of all time … with the tour becoming the first ever to gross at least $1 billion" (para. 1). Spilde noted:

> The Eras Tour wasn't just a massive success; it was its own subculture. Fans made and traded friendship bracelets for the shows, speculated over which secret songs Swift would perform each night with their Swiftie-exclusive mathematical algorithms, and planned their lives out months in advance, in accordance with each stop.
>
> *(para. 5)*

Released on Disney+ in March 2024, "Swift fans watched 16.2 million hours of the blockbuster 3.5 hour concert in just three days" (Mastrangelo, 2024, para. 2). Swift's high-profile relationship with Travis Kelce, a professional football player with the Kansas Chiefs, put her "on stage" at NFL games too, as she cheered prominently from his family's box. When the Chiefs advanced to the Super Bowl and Swift was scheduled to perform in Tokyo, a media frenzy ensued about whether she would make it back in time for the big game, and even the Japanese Embassy chimed in to assure fans that they would help to make it happen (see, e.g., Bailey, 2024; Li, 2024; Squires, 2024). (Yes, she arrived in time for the game, and the Chiefs won.)

Even as I chuckle a bit about the extent to which the tour and those Kansas City football games dominated traditional and social media outlets for much of 2023 and early 2024, it illustrates the hypermediated nature of contemporary popular culture – a context with implications more far-reaching than "just" liking a particular musical artist or sports team. Our experiences with popular culture provide lenses (plural intended) through which we process information and make choices, including important (and potentially life-altering) decisions about health, wellness, and well-being. Whether we are engaging with a genre every day, interacting with communities online, watching films, listening to music, following a celebrity, or reading certain newspapers or magazines, that content becomes part of how we come to understand what constitutes a "risky" versus "safe" choice, a "healthy" relationship versus a "toxic" one, a "prudent" decision regarding preventive care or a "waste of time or money." Further, as I detail in this chapter, this hypermediated landscape overflows with conflicting, confusing, and confounding images and alternate viewpoints, belying simple, straightforward decision-making based on clear, definitive information.

In this book, we explore the consequentiality of popular culture in this postmodern era for grappling with messages and decisions about health. In this introductory chapter, I begin by defining popular culture and describing the technological advances that have fueled its ubiquity in contemporary society. I then discuss COVID-19 as an exemplar for understanding the powerful role that popular culture has played in shaping perspectives about illnesses, treatments, and preventive measures. I close by highlighting key themes in this book and previewing the chapters in this collection.

Popular Culture in This Postmodern Era

As I invited potential contributors for this book, I received the same question multiple times – "How, exactly, are we defining 'popular culture'?" I had to pause on that one. My first response encompassed both surprise at the question – we all just *know* pop culture, right? – as well as hesitation – how, exactly, *am* I defining popular culture?

As my early childhood memories (and lack thereof) illustrate, I've always been drawn to popular culture. I named my first childhood dog, "Samantha," after the main character in the hit 1960s television show, *Bewitched.* (My Samantha was "bewitching," I informed my mom at the time.) One of our current dogs got the name, "Trixie," after the title character of the book series (*Trixie Belden*) that I read again and again as a pre-teen. I wrote my MA thesis on the relational communication patterns of young soap opera couples (see Beck, 1992). I'm a travel softball mom, an avid sports fan (like my dad), and a researcher with a current interest in celebrity health narratives (see, e.g., Beck, 2022; Beck et al., 2014, 2015). Surely, a definition of "popular culture" should have come easily to me, but it didn't.

I'm comforted a bit by Storey's (2024, p. 1) acknowledgment that "to study popular culture we must first confront the difficulty posed by the term itself." For example, Hall (2018) noted the challenges in defining popular culture in terms of its origin – i.e., "springing up from the authentic wellsprings of the masses" or by "looking at inventories of form" (p. 931). Williams (2018) added that "[i]f you add the difficult word 'popular,' then you are immediately in difficulties" (p. 904).

Tracing the history of popular culture theorizing extends beyond the scope of this chapter, but I direct readers to how Storey (2024) chronicled those theoretical traditions. He concluded with a nod to the complexities of this contemporary hypermediated era. Storey argued that "[p]erhaps the most significant thing about postmodernism for the student of popular culture is the dawning recognition that there is no absolute categorical difference between high and popular culture" (p. 223). Indeed, Powers (2022) suggested that "for the most part, it is safe to say that these days, a movie, a TikTok video, a tweet, and a song are as much 'culture' as a novel or a painting. Cultural forms may be widely loved or reviled, expensive or not" (pp. 468–469). Powers concluded by answering "[w]hat does 'popular' mean, then? I have argued that popular culture should be reserved for instances of popularizing practices. That means meaning, community, and connection" (p. 469).

Extending from Powers, this book envisions *popular culture* broadly, with those "popularizing practices" encompassing the gamut of contemporary mediated platforms (television, film, radio, podcasts, music, social media) as well as literature, art, newspapers, sports, etc. Through each of these forms (and others that might exist around the globe that I might not know), people co-orient to their world as well as reflexively, collectively co-shape emergent meanings of events, relationships, and their own positionalities (see related work by Gergen, 1991, 1994).

In his 1991 book, *The Saturated Self*, Gergen discussed the consequentiality of technological advances for our enactment of self, relationships, and communities. In passing, he mentioned the development of video rental services as just one example. Now, over 30 years later, technology continues to evolve at an ever-escalating pace (see, e.g., Hoehe, 2020). Surely, just as video rentals became prevalent as a convenient way to watch movies at home in the 1990s and then declined with the emergence of streaming services in the 2000s (see, e.g., Olito & Britter, 2023; Zawislak, 2024), relatively new developments (such as podcasts and social media) and specific examples of popular culture artifacts noted in this book will soon be dated by what will, inevitably, come next. However, regardless of what technological developments (and concurrent forms of popular culture) occur in the future, Gergen's reflections on this era of postmodernism hold value for the conversations in this book about popular culture and Health Communication.

To begin, Gergen (1991) pointed to the relational implications of increasing technology, arguing that "[t]he technological achievements of the past century have produced a radical shift in our exposure to each other" (p. xi). Of course, technology continues to shift and redirect the nature of our connections with others. We can message or "follow" people around the planet in addition to (and sometimes instead of) participating in face-to-face exchanges. Millions have worked their minds with Wordle or played interactive games with friends on their cell phones (see, e.g., Mueller, 2024; Shabbir, 2024), not to mention the myriad mediated options and opportunities for entertainment alone. Hoehe (2020, p. 93) asserted:

> We can constantly interact, and connect, with each other by use of digital devices and social media. Coping with the daily demands of life as well as pursuing pleasure in recreational activities appears inconceivable without the use of smartphones, tablets, computers, and access to Internet platforms.

As Gergen (1991, p. xi) noted, "Small and enduring communities, with a limited cast of significant others, are being replaced by a vast and ever-expanding array of relationships." Rather than being restricted to physical contexts and in-person interactions, we can dabble in a host of online spaces as our interests expand and evolve, granting us freedom and flexibility but also, necessarily, resulting in splintered selves with multiple concurrent identities and fragmented, not singular communities. Moreover, as I will discuss further in the next section, this postmodern playfulness, reconceptualization of "roots" and commitment, and remnants from the COVID-19 pandemic have sprouted alternate lifestyles and work/life models, such as #vanlife and preferences for remote work (see, e.g., Smite et al., 2023; Trujillo, 2023), with direct and indirect implications for health and wellness.

One of those implications involves the processing of health-related information. This hypermediated, chaotic technological landscape – coupled with economic and political uncertainties and some corresponding relational tensions, at least in the United States – has muddied clarity on what constitutes "truth," "reality," and "facts." According to Gergen (1991, p. 7), "The postmodern condition more generally is marked by a plurality of voices vying for the right to reality—to be accepted as legitimate expressions of the true and the good." Gergen continued to note that "[a]s we absorb multiple voices, we find that each 'truth' is relativized by our simultaneous consciousness of compelling alternatives" (p. 16).

In contemporary society, we might converse with family members (who have their own concurrent, diverse circles of influence). We might talk with friends and acquaintances, both in person as well as those we have met during other times in our lives or encountered online. We watch television and YouTube videos, see ads, listen to podcasts or the radio while driving, glance at a magazine article in the supermarket check-out line, follow celebrities on social media, exchange messages in chat rooms or other online groups, read articles, attend public events (such as theater productions, sports competitions, or political rallies), and visit spaces designed for entertainment and/or education, including museums, art galleries, and amusement parks. In so doing, we encounter perspectives about an array of issues, including ones that could pertain to perspectives on and/or decision-making about health, well-being, fitness, etc. If faced with conflicting messages from various communities in our lives, the challenge becomes sorting out what to believe. Gergen (1991, p. 119) explained:

> If the traditional categories are collapsing, and genres continuously blurring, blending, and re-forming, what are we to make of common claims to knowledge? Everyone, from family members to physicians and government leaders, confidently informs us of "what is the case." When the "objects of knowledge" acquire a puttylike character, how are such "reports," "factual descriptions," or "insights" to be regarded? ... That is, words are not mirrorlike reflections of reality, but expressions of group convention.

Back in the 1960s and 1970s, legendary CBS Nightly News anchor Walter Cronkite calmly and confidently concluded his nightly newscast with "And that's the way it is" (McCall, 2021, para. 1), asserting a singular, factual nature of what had been communicated. People believed him. Bowman (2009) cited a survey that "labeled Cronkite [as] the most trusted man in America" (para. 6), and audiences tuned in for his reporting of the news. According to McCall, Cronkite's audience amounted to an "estimated 27–29 million viewers per night, when the nation's population was just over 200 million ... more than the combined audiences now for the evening broadcasts of CBS, NBC, and ABC, with the nation's population now exceeding 320 million" (para. 6). McCall credited Cronkite with strict adherence to journalistic integrity, and he also reminded us that "[t]he media landscape was much different in the time of Cronkite. There were fewer competitors for the national news audience. The average news consumer never saw social media, partisan websites, or cable news" (para. 8). Without the roar of other competing voices and the lure of alternative platforms, accepting Cronkite's take on the world in the 1960s and 1970s proved far less complicated for audience members than the conundrums that envelop us in the 2020s, especially given that this decade began with our first global pandemic in the era of social and mass media. As I argue in the next section, popular culture, as it has emerged in this postmodern, hypermediated era, played an integral role in how many experienced and responded to COVID-19.

COVID-19 as Exemplar and Consequential Historical Moment

As I write this chapter, health officials wrestle with whether to categorize COVID-19 now as a "pandemic" or simply "endemic," like the flu or other viruses that continue to cause hospitalizations and deaths but do not overwhelm medical facilities and resources (see Ducharme, 2024). As Ducharme noted, "The SARS-CoV-2 virus still kills thousands of people around the world each month, saddles still more with chronic symptoms known as Long COVID, and continues to evolve ... But are we still in a pandemic? No one seems to know for sure" (para. 3–4).

Certainly, just as the virus lingers, so do the societal, emotional, physical, relational, and economic ramifications and lessons of living through the pandemic (see, e.g., Alizadeh et al., 2023; Evans et al., 2023; Panchal et al., 2023; Pedrosa et al., 2020; The British Academy, 2021). Indeed, The British Academy (para. 2) asserted that "[w]e are in a COVID decade: the social, economic and cultural effects of the pandemic will cast a long shadow into the future." For example, going through COVID-19 both illuminated and exacerbated pervasive societal issues, such as racial inequities and socioeconomic divides (see, e.g., Jacobson et al., 2021; Lopez et al., 2021; Paul et al., 2021; Wen et al., 2023) as well as spotlighted the importance of prioritizing mental health – both in the short-term, as individuals struggled with social isolation, grief, fear, uncertainty, etc. during the pandemic – and in the long-term, as individuals adjust to new normals and work toward ongoing mental well-being in these years since the peak of COVID-19 (see, e.g., Gramlich, 2023; Nealon, 2021). Of course, exploring all effects of the pandemic in depth extends beyond the space available in this chapter. Instead, here I focus on two aspects of the pandemic that underscore the ever-increasing consequentiality of popular culture for messages about health – the fracturing of institutional connections and the reliance on an array of sources beyond traditional health-related experts.

Fracturing of Institutional Connections

As I reflect on those early months of COVID-19 in 2020, I remember "sheltering at home" with my husband and youngest daughter, who was in the 6th grade at the time. Our oldest daughter lived about two miles from our house with her husband, but we didn't see them in person for weeks. Our second-oldest daughter worked in New York City then, and I recall watching the news and feeling so frightened for her. Blessedly, her employer allowed employees to work remotely, so she remained in a small apartment, along with three other friends who agreed not to venture out either. Our third-oldest daughter was in her sophomore year of college. She came home during Spring Break and did not return to campus until the following fall. We were all incredibly fortunate to retain jobs that did not require us to leave our homes. Especially in retrospect, I am so grateful that we were able to stay safe and not have to worry about finances or putting our health at risk. We had enough to eat and adequate internet for all that we needed and wanted to do online.

However, even from that definite position of privilege, I can't say that COVID-19 didn't change some things for our family. Social isolation from friends and teammates was the hardest for our youngest (student-athlete) daughter. Although she reconnected with travel softball teammates two months later, she continued learning online during all of 7th grade, and she only saw most local peers on a computer screen for over a year. As college-level educators, my husband and I witnessed the stress and loneliness of our own students as we taught our classes via Zoom for two-and-a-half semesters.

Yet, even after the need for social distancing eventually faded, the introduction of Zoom and Teams has continued to alter the educational landscape for students, faculty, and administrators. Students in my daughter's high school still need to navigate at least two different online platforms for submitting work and accessing material, even while now being taught in person. Four years after we first heard the word "COVID-19," our academic department persists in utilizing alternative formats for what would have been face-to-face interactions before COVID-19 (see, e.g., Benito et al., 2021; Bombardieri, 2021). The hallways in my office space tend to be far quieter than before, and our student organizations have yet to return to their pre-COVID-19 vitality. That taste of remote work has impacted other industries beyond academia as well (see, e.g., Shanbhogue, 2023; Vyas, 2022). In fact, our second-oldest daughter realized that she enjoyed working from home so much that she has opted to do so post-COVID-19.

Although, of course, initiated by necessity to save lives at the outset of the pandemic, these sorts of shifts in how (and where) we accomplish our jobs and tasks have further fractured connections to institutions. For example, Sharp and Spencer (2022) found that some of their respondents adjusted their priorities, especially with a reduced emphasis on work and jobs. Indeed, the pandemic prompted reflections about what mattered most, where to invest time and energy, and, as I detail in the next section, who and what to trust.

Reliance on Sources Beyond Traditional Health-Related Sources

At a time when most individuals had to be homebound … when many needed to remain physically disconnected from co-workers or classmates as well as extended family members and friends … when even going to the doctor seemed risky, given the possibility of contracting the virus if not already infected … when people wrestled with uncertainties surrounding a novel virus … they also had to discern what sources could (should) be deemed credible. Of course, some lacked technological options as the pandemic exposed the problem of inadequate internet access for rural areas or families who couldn't afford internet in their homes (e.g., Janse et al., 2021; Jiang & Breen, 2023). However, those with internet access increasingly turned to online communities for entertainment, news, and support during those days when we were asked to remain home (see, e.g., Neely et al., 2021).

As I think back on March of 2020, I remember wondering what to make of this new health threat, and I recall feeling shocked as I read about actors Tom Hanks and Rita Wilson's disclosure on Instagram that they were hospitalized with COVID-19 in Australia. As Freeman (2020, para. 12) noted, Hanks isn't just any actor – "Hanks is regularly referred to as 'America's Dad' and is so revered his face will probably be carved into Mount Rushmore." If prominent individuals such as Hanks and Wilson could contract it, given the preventive measures that their production team had likely taken, I wondered how much of a threat it could be for my family. I wasn't alone.

In a study conducted within 24 hours after the disclosure, Myrick and Willoughby (2022) found that 587 of 682 participants had already heard the news. According to Myrick and Willoughby, "People reported that Hanks' diagnosis highlighted the reality of COVID-19, broadening their understanding of the severity of the illness and their own susceptibility" (p. 828), and " approximately half (47.8%) of the sample indicated some change in response to Hanks' illness disclosure" (p. 830). Notably, "[s]ome participants reported no change because they felt the situation was being exaggerated … Others reported experiencing no change because they were already highly engaged in preventative measures, such as increased social distancing" (p. 830).

That divide exemplified what emerged as opposing orientations to messages about the pandemic, ultimately splitting many in the United States into one of two general campsthose who grasped the threat of the pandemic and tried to mitigate its spread, and those who disputed its severity and, in some cases, even its existence (Beck, 2022). As I explained in a book about celebrity and COVID-19, "So many voices entered the public sphere to share their perspectives on Covid-19" (p. 147).

Although sports organizations canceled major events (including the annual March Madness for Division 1 college basketball) and weeks of games, celebrities, traditional media, streaming services, and social media activity filled that void and then some. In my book (Beck, 2022), I described the influx of celebrities beyond just Tom Hanks and Rita Wilson who posted about their personal experiences with (and perspectives about) COVID-19. Some hosted specials on television that raised money for those who needed food and support amid significant job losses (Spector, 2020). John Krasinski created and hosted a short YouTube series, *Some Good News*, in which he highlighted short "feel good" pieces (Paskin, 2020). Other celebrities reconnected with past co-workers by arranging YouTube reunions and inviting fans to watch (Welk, 2020; see also www.thelocherroom.com/). Moreover, according to Kafka (2020), streaming service Netflix boomed during COVID-19, adding 16 million subscribers in the first quarter of 2020 and 10 more million in the second, as binge-watching shows helped people to pass the time at home.

Amid the nostalgic flurry of online reunions and hours spent viewing episode after episode of sitcoms or dramas, government officials and public health officers tried to share important information through special press conferences with updates on the spread of the disease and the rate of hospitalizations among other mediated efforts (see Beck, 2022). However, even those official attempts to communicate potentially life-saving guidance got complicated by former President Trump's own press conferences – events that exacerbated the chaos by sometimes affirming and sometimes countering the recommendations of his own staff members – occasionally during the very same appearance (see, e.g., Cillizza, 2020). Meanwhile, social media platforms buzzed with information and, on some, conspiracy theories (see, e.g., Kuzelewska & Tomasuk, 2022), coinciding with rhetoric on conservative talk radio and Fox News that downplayed the virus as well as questioned preventative measures such as mask-wearing, social distancing, and vaccinations (see, e.g., Rosenwald, 2021).

Importantly, I argue that those who commented on social media, television, and talk radio, and who wrote in newspapers and magazines, and who appeared publicly at large-scale gatherings, and who communicated decisions (whether about getting a vaccination, refusing to wear a mask, or canceling a sporting event), implicitly and rhetorically "co-constructed the meaning of COVID-19, foregrounding the sources, stories, and statistics that made sense to them and framing emergent narratives for others who read their posts, watched their interviews or shows, and believed them to be credible and convincing" (Beck, 2022, p. 147).

Harkening back to Gergen (1991), this situation epitomized a postmodern fragmentation of perspectives on what could and should be believed. Although two general sets of positions became distinct, individual decision-making about what constituted "facts" or should be considered as "good practice" was much more nuanced as individuals sorted through an array of vastly different competing viewpoints, sources, and health and lifestyle choices circulating on the internet, through the unique lens of their own personal experiences, insights, community identifications, what their communities communicated about the pandemic, etc.

The shifting public health guidelines (as additional information became available about the novel virus) also hindered clear understanding about what to do and believe. Tyson and Funk (2022) reported:

> confusion … [as] the most common reaction to shifts in public health guidance [with] 60% of U.S. adults say[ing] they've felt confused as a result of changes to public health officials' recommendations on how to slow the spread of the coronavirus.
>
> *(para. 2)*

Moreover, Neely et al. (2021) found that 63% of social media users "were unlikely to fact-check what they see on the internet with a health professional, despite the high levels of mistrust in the accuracy of COVID-19–related information on social media" (para. 4). Indeed, confidence in U.S. public health officials and health care professionals declined during the pandemic, although largely dependent on political affiliation (see, e.g., Stolzenberg et al., 2023; Tyson & Funk, 2022); yet, notably, trust in public health and health care increased in some other parts of the world (see, e.g., Skirbekk et al., 2023).

Weighing Health Information

The COVID-19 pandemic provides a compelling example of the power and persuasiveness of popular culture on health-related perspectives and decision-making. Certainly, the pandemic comprises a unique case, at least in the United States, given that it occurred at a particular historical moment, concurrent with an especially divisive political context, coupled with prominent cases of racial injustice that received wide-ranging media coverage and online engagement (see, e.g., Chavez, 2020; Jackson, 2022; Roberts, 2021).

However, I suggest that the pervasiveness of popular culture and mediated platforms during the pandemic fueled not only media consumers' ability to attain information (albeit potentially conflicting). Those outlets also served as a springboard for anyone with a social media account who wanted to produce and share their own content, enabling them to launch an array of assertions (including conspiracy theories about COVID-19) and intensely question (and sometimes attack) those in what were previously considered to be established, credible positions of authority. That hypermediated landscape, coupled with fractured physical and emotional connections to institutions and in-person communities, continues to serve as the context in which people need to weigh information about health and wellness and well-being.

In his work on narrative theorizing, Fisher (1989) asserted that "humans are ... storytellers" (p. 5), and he identified narrative rationality and fidelity as essential to a compelling story. As he put it, "We naturally and without formal instruction ask about any account of any sort whatever whether or not it 'holds together' and adds up to a reliable claim to reality" (p. 194). He noted that "[w]e identify with stories or accounts when we find that they offer 'good reasons' for being accepted" (p. 194). Narratives need to "ring true with the stories they know to be true in their lives" (p. 5).

As people in everyday life, we reflect on what "rings true" to us, given our values, beliefs, traditions, experiences, communities, and, yes, even fandoms. Cloud (2018) explained that "[n]ot only are knowledges matters of perspective, they are also historically variant and specific" (p. 24). With so many constantly shifting and emerging messages as part of "popularizing practices" (Powers, 2022, p. 469), finding "coherence" (Fisher, 1989, p. 5) can be challenging but internally necessary "in order for us to live life in a process of continual re-creation" (p. 5). However, what ends up "ringing true" to us can be highly consequential in terms of our health and what we opt to believe (or choose not to believe) about health messages.

Brumfiel (2022) told the story of a woman named Stephanie and her family. Brumfiel noted that "[i]n the years leading up to her death, Stephanie had become embroiled in conspiracy theories" (para. 3), garnered through videos that she had watched on the internet. According to Brumfiel, "When the COVID vaccines came along, Stephanie absolutely refused to get one because she falsely thought the shots contained tiny microchips" (para. 27). When she eventually contracted the disease and became gravely ill, her daughter insisted on taking her to the hospital, but she refused some treatments, and she "claim[ed] the drug was actually being used to kill COVID patients" (para. 49). A doctor asked, "'Why didn't you take any of the treatments Stephanie?' She found every little piece of energy in her and yelled back at him, 'BECAUSE IT'LL KILL ME!'" (para. 50, emphasis original). Stephanie passed away a few days later.

While public health information, readily available through mainstream and social media, obviously countered those conspiracy theories, Stephanie's daughter attributed her mom's death to misinformation (Brumfiel, 2022). To be clear, Brumfiel painted an impression of a person with convictions drawn not from something that she casually read in passing on the internet but rather from what she adamantly held to be true, based on her immersion into and consumption of that form of popular culture.

Although admittedly an extreme case, it underscores the potential of popular culture to comprise a factor in how people think about health – as well as the potential for people to disregard health information from official sources or to treat that guidance as not as credible as other material from their own sources. With the myriad messages in popular culture available to conflict with or counter public health messages, the intersection of popular culture and Health Communication has become a serious and important one for Health Communication scholars and practitioners, public health officials, medical professionals, etc. COVID-19 certainly illustrated the ways in which the contemporary hypermediated landscape and postmodern loss of connection have clouded clear and consistent messaging about health from a Health Communication perspective.

Overview of This Collection

I would like to begin this overview by thanking and applauding the contributors to this volume. In their respective chapters, they provide valuable references to important literature while also integrating powerful examples from popular culture. Together, they highlight diverse examples from a wide range of popular culture sources. Although each chapter certainly stands alone, each chapter also includes references to other chapters in the book, as appropriate, so that the reader can cross-reference related work across the collection.

This book offers a comprehensive examination of the intersection between contemporary popular culture and messages about an array of health-related topics, including mental illness, sexual health, body image, food, risky behaviors, medical errors, and pro-health choices. Drawing from a wide range of popular culture forms (e.g., television, film, books, social media, graphic novels, newspapers, video games, memes, sports, social influencers, and celebrity discourse), the book as a whole, the collection reflects on the role(s) that popular culture plays in how we come to learn about and understand health, wellness, and well-being. Together, these chapters offer a comprehensive examination of not only varied forms of popular culture but also key issues such as misinformation, media literacy, medical ethics, educational possibilities, and diverse perspectives. As a collection, the book provides a valuable foundation for understanding the challenges that await those in Health Communication and Public Health as well as health care professionals as they strive to disseminate health recommendations and information, counter misconceptions, and encourage adherence to best practices for health, wellness, and well-being.

I hope that this book serves as a catalyst for further work that will equip health care providers to better respond to questions and concerns arising from health care seekers' viewpoints (whether from what they saw on a television show, read on a celebrity post, or learned from "Dr. Google"). Moreover, because I don't believe that the "genie" of social media or the internet will ever be put back "in the bottle," I encourage partnerships between experts in popular culture and Health Communication beyond the strategic and intentional use of popular culture for message dissemination. How can what we know about popular culture enable us to better share information amid the myriad concurrent messages on the hypermediated landscape?

References

Alizadeh, H., Sharifi, A., Damanbagh, S., & Nazarnia, M. (2023). Impacts of the COVID-19 pandemic on the social sphere and lessons for crisis management: A review. *Natural Hazards*, *117*, 2139–2164.

Ang, I. (1996). *Living room wars: Rethinking media audiences for a postmodern world*. Routledge.

Bailey, A. (2024, February 11). Taylor Swift traveled from Tokyo to Los Angeles for the Super Bowl. *Elle*. https://www.elle.com/culture/celebrities/a46569506/can-taylor-swift-make-super-bowl-with-travis-kelce/

Barton, K. M., & Lampley, J. M. (Eds.). (2014). *Fan culture: Essays on participatory fandom in the 21st century*. McFarland.

Beck, C. S. (1992). An analysis of relational communication patterns between young soap opera couples. *Florida Communication Journal*, *20*(1), 16–77.

Beck, C. S. (2012). Intersecting narratives: Enjoying daytime drama as viewers (and actors) experience the days of their lives. *Communication Studies*, *63*, 152–171.

Beck, C. S., Aubuchon, S. M., McKenna, T. P., Ruhl, S., & Simmons, N. (2014). Blurring personal health and public priorities: An analysis of celebrity health narratives in the public sphere. *Health Communication, 29*(3), 244–256. https://doi.org/10.1080/10410236.2012.741668

Beck, C. S., Aubuchon, S., Ruhl, S., Simmons, N., & Tenzek, K. (2015). *Celebrity health narratives and the public health*. McFarland.

Beck, C. S. (2022). *Celebrity in the time of Covid: Fandom and the influence of pandemic messaging*. McFarland.

Benito, A., Yenisey, K. D., Khanna, K., Masis, M. F., Monge, R. M., Tugtan, M. A., Arava, L. D., & Vig, R. (2021). Changes that should remain in higher education post COVID-19: A mixed-methods analysis of the experiences at three universities. *Higher Learning Research Communications*, 11. https://doi.org/10.18870/hlrc.v11i0.1195

Bombardieri, M. (2021, April 15). COVID-19 changed education in America—permanently. *Politico*. https://www.politico.com/news/2021/04/15/covid-changed-education-permanently-479317

Booth, P. (2015). *Playing fans: Negotiating fandom and media in the digital age*. University of Iowa Press.

Bowman, K. (2009, July 27). The decline of the major networks. *Forbes*. https://www.forbes.com/07/25/media-network-news-audience-opinions-columnists-walter-cronkite.html?sh=6a480c147a5f

Brumfiel, G. (2022, April 24). Their mom died of COVID: They say conspiracy theories are what really killed her. *NPR*. https://www.npr.org/sections/health-shots/2022/04/24/1089786147/covid-conspiracy-theories

Chavez, N. (2020). 2020: The year America confronted racism. *CNN*. https://www.cnn.com/interactive/2020/12/us/america-racism-2020/

Cilliza, C. (2020, August 11). The 34 wildest lines from Donald Trump's wildly inaccurate coronavirus press conference. *CNN*. https://www.cnn.com/2020/08/11/politics/donald-trump-press-conference-coronavirus/index.html

Click, M. A., & Scott, S. (Eds.). (2018). *The Routledge companion to media fandom*. Routledge.

Cloud, D. (2018). *Reality bites: Rhetoric and the circulation of truth claims in U.S. political culture*. Ohio State University Press.

Ducharme, J. (2024, March 11). Experts can't agree if we are still in a pandemic. *Time*. https://time.com/6898943/is-covid-19-still-pandemic-2024/

Evans, S. L., Jones, R., Alkan, E., Sichman, J. S., Haque, A., de Oliveira, F. B. S., & Mougouei, D. (2023). The emotional impact of COVID-19 news reporting: A longitudinal study using natural language processing. *Human Behavior and Emerging Technologies*, Article ID 7283166. https://doi.org/10.1155/2023/7283166

Fisher, W. (1989). *Human communication as narration: Toward a philosophy of reason, value, and action*. University of South Carolina Press.

Forster, R. T. (Ed.). (2023). *The Oxford handbook of parasocial experiences*. Oxford University Press.

Freeman, H. (2020, July 6). Tom Hanks on surviving coronavirus. *The Guardian*. https://www.theguardian.com/film/2020/jul/06/tom-hanks-on-surviving-coronavirus-i-had-crippling-body-aches-fatigue-and-couldnt-concentrate

Frost, K. (2023). *The power of parasocial interaction: Exploring the psychology, media, and technology behind celebrities, influencers, and our unseen relationships*. Book Bound Studios.

Gergen, K. J. (1991). *The saturated self*. BasicBooks.

Gergen, K. J. (1994). *Realities and relationships: Soundings in social construction*. Harvard University Press.

Gramlich, J. (2023, March 2). *Mental health and the pandemic: What U.S. surveys have found*. Pew Research Center. https://www.pewresearch.org/short-reads/2023/03/02/mental-health-and-the-pandemic-what-u-s-surveys-have-found/

Gray, J., Sandvoss, C., & Harrington, C. L. (2017). *Fandom: Identities and communities in a mediated world* (2nd ed.). New York University Press.

Hall, S. (2018). Popular culture, politics, and history. *Cultural Studies*, *32*(6), 929–952.

Hills, M. (2002). *Fan cultures*. Routledge.

Hoehe, M. R. (2020). Going digital: How technology use may influence human brains and behavior. *Dialogues in Clinical Neuroscience*, *22*(2), 93–97. https://doi.org/10.31887/DCNS.2020.22.2/mhoehe

Jackson, T. (2022, January 24). Racism in America. *PBS*. https://www.pbs.org/articles/racism-in-america

Jacobson, M., Chang, T., Shah, M., Pramanik, R., & Shah, S. (2021). Racial and ethnic disparities in SARS-CoV-2 testing and COVID-19 outcomes in a Medicaid managed care cohort. *American Journal of Preventive Medicine*, *61*(5), 644–651.

Janse, A. M., Isaakson, A., & Chang, A. (2021, November 22). Life without reliable internet remains a daily struggle for millions of Americans. *NPR*. https://www.npr.org/2021/11/22/1037941547/life-without-reliable-broadband-internet-remains-a-daily-struggle-in-nevada

Jenkins, H. (2013). *Textual poachers: Television fans and participatory culture* (20th anniversary ed.). Routledge.

Jiang, W., & Breen, K. (2023, June 8). U.S. investing billions to expand high-speed internet access to rural areas: "Broadband isn't a luxury anymore." *CBS News*. https://www.cbsnews.com/news/high-speed-internet-rural-areas-broadband-isnt-a-luxury-anymore-us-investing-billions/

Kafka, P. (2020, July 16). The pandemic has been great for Netflix. *Vox*. https://www.vox.com/recode/2020/7/16/21327451/netflix-covid-earnings-subscribers-q2

Kuzelewska, E., & Tomasuk, M. (2022). Rise of conspiracy theories in the pandemic times. *International Journal for the Semiotics of Law*, *35*, 2373–2389.

Li, D. K. (2024, January 29). Fans all want to know: Will Taylor Swift make it to the Super Bowl? *NBC News*. https://www.nbcnews.com/pop-culture/pop-culture-news/taylor-swift-super-bowl-arrive-in-time-kelce-rcna136242

Lopez, L., Hart, L. H., & Katz, M. H. (2021). Racial and ethnic health disparities related to COVID-19. *Journal of the American Medical Association, 325*(8), 719–720.

Mastrangelo, D. (2024, March 19). Taylor Swift Eras Tour film notches 4.6 million views on Disney+. *The Hill.* https://thehill.com/homenews/media/4542358-taylor-swift-eras-tour-film-views-disney-plus/

McCall, J. (2021). Cronkite signed off 40 years ago; it seems like an eon in news standards. *The Hill.* https://thehill.com/opinion/technology/541882-cronkite-signed-off-40-years-ago-it-seems-like-an-eon-in-news-standards/

Millman, E. (2023, December 8). Taylor Swift's Eras tour is the highest-grossing of all time and first-ever to hit $1 billion. *Rolling Stone.* https://www.rollingstone.com/music/music-news/taylor-swift-eras-tour-highest-grossing-all-time-1-billion-1234921647/

Mueller, S. (2024, March 14). Millions have played Wordle, but there's more to the game that you'd expect. *CNN.* https://www.cnn.com/2024/03/14/us/wordle-new-york-times-cec/index.html

Myrick, J. G., & Willoughby, J. F. (2022). A mixed methods inquiry into the role of Tom Hanks' COVID-19 social media disclosure in shaping willingness to engage in prevention behaviors. *Health Communication, 37*(7), 824–832.

Nealon, M. (2021, October 9). The pandemic accelerant: How COVID-19 advanced our mental health priorities. *United Nations.* https://www.un.org/en/un-chronicle/pandemic-accelerant-how-covid-19-advanced-our-mental-health-priorities

Neely, S., Eldredge, C., & Sanders, R. (2021). Health information seeking behaviors on social media during the COVID-19 pandemic among American social networking site users. Survey study. *Journal of Medical Internet Research, 23*(6), e29802. https://doi.org/10.2196/29802

Olito, F., & Britter, A. (2023, April 24). Blockbuster: The rise and fall of the movie rental store, and what happened to the brand. *Business Insider.* https://www.businessinsider.com/rise- and-fall-of-blockbuster

Panchal, N., Saunders, H., Rudowitz, R., & Cox, C. (2023). The implications of COVID-19 for mental health and substance abuse. *KFF.* https://www.kff.org/mental-health/issue-brief/the-implications-of-covid-19-for-mental-health-and-substance-use/

Paskin, W. (2020, April 28). How John Krasinski became America's new dad. *Slate.* https://slate.com/culture/2020/04/john-krasinski-some-good-news-americas-new-dad.html

Paul, A., Englert, P., & Varga, M. (2021). Socio-economic disparities and COVID-19 in the USA. *Journal of Physics: Complexity, 2*(3), 035017. https://doi.org/10.1088/2632-072X/ac0fc7

Pedrosa, A. L., Bitencourt, L., Fróes, A. C. F., Cazumbá, M. L. B., Campos, R. G. B., de Brito, S. B. C. S., & Silva, A. C. S. (2020, October). Emotional, behavioral, and psychological impact of the COVID-19 pandemic. *Frontiers in Psychology, 11,* 566212. https://doi.org/10.3389/fpsyg.2020.566212

Powers, D. (2022). The problem of popular culture. *Communication Theory, 4*, 461–470.

Roberts, J. D. (2021, June 9). Pandemics and protests: America has experienced racism like this before. *Brookings.* https://www.brookings.edu/articles/pandemics-and-protests-america-has-experienced-racism-like-this-before/

Rosenwald, B. (2021, September 13). Talk radio's death trend a metastasization of conservative media culture. *NBC News.* https://www.nbcnews.com/think/opinion/talk-radio-s-covid-death-trend-metastasization-conservative-media-culture-ncna1279023

Shabbir, U. (2024, July 21). The 7 best sports games for iOS and Android. *Make Use Of.* https://www.makeuseof.com/the-best-sports-games-for-ios-and-android/

Shanbhogue, R. (2023, November 13). The fight over remote working will heat up in 2024. *The Economist.* https://www.economist.com/the-world-ahead/2023/11/13/the-fight-over-remote-working-will-heat-up-in-2024

Sharp, M., & Spencer, A. (2022, August 18). Many Americans say they have shifted their priorities around health and social activities during COVID-19. *Pew Research Center.* https://www.pewresearch.org/short-reads/2022/08/18/many-americans-say-they-have-shifted-their-priorities-around-health-and-social-activities-during-covid-19/

Skirbekk, H., Magelssen, M., & Conradsen, S. (2023). Trust in healthcare before and after the COVID-19 pandemic. *BMC Public Health, 23*(1), 863. https://doi.org/10.1186/s12889-023-15716-6

Smite, D., Moe, N. B., Hildrum, J., Gonzalez-Huerta, J., & Mendez, D. (2023, January). Work-from-home is here to stay: Call for flexibility in post-pandemic work policies. *Journal of Systems and Software, 195.* https://doi.org/10.1016/j.jss.2022.111552

Spector, E. (2020, April 9). How 18 celebrities have mobilized to fight the Coronavirus pandemic. *Vogue.* https://www.vogue.com/article/celebrities-donating-fundraising-coronavirus-relief

Spilde, C. (2024, January 1). 2023 was the year Taylor Swift became insufferable. *The Daily Beast.* https://www.thedailybeast.com/obsessed/2023-was-the-year-taylor-swift-became-insufferable

Squires, B. (2024, February 11). Yes, Taylor Swift made it to the Super Bowl. *Vulture.* https://www.vulture.com/2024/02/will-taylor-swift-go-to-the-super-bowl.html

Stein, L. E. (2015). *Millennial fandom: Television audiences in the transmedia age.* University of Iowa Press.

Stolzenberg, L., Huang, A., Usman, M., & MacGregor, G. (2023). A descriptive survey investigating the impact of the COVID-19 pandemic on the public's perception of healthcare professionals. *Cureus*, *15*(7), e41703. https://doi.org/10.7759/cureus.41703

Storey, J. (2024). *Cultural theory and popular culture: An introduction* (10th ed.). Routledge.

The British Academy. (2021). The COVID decade: Understanding the long-term societal impacts of COVID-19. https://www.thebritishacademy.ac.uk/publications/covid-decade-understanding-the-long-term-societal-impacts-of-covid-19/

Trujillo, S. (2023, January 31). They changed everything and adopted #vanlife: Here's what they learned. *The Guardian*. https://www.theguardian.com/lifeandstyle/2023/jan/31/vanlife-nomad-living-us-families

Tyson, A., & Funk, C. (2022, February 9). Increasing public criticism, confusion over COVID-19 response in U.S. *Pew Research*. https://www.pewresearch.org/science/2022/02/09/increasing-public-criticism-confusion-over-covid-19-response-in-u-s/

Welk, B. (2020, May 11). 19 movie and TV casts that reunited remotely during coronavirus, from 'The Goonies' to 'Full House.' *The Wrap*. https://www.thewrap.com/movie-and-tv-casts-that-reunited-remotely-during-coronavirus-from-the-goonies-to-full-house-photos/

Wen, M., Shi, L., Li, Y., Chen, Z., Chen, B., Zhang, L., Li, H., Li, J., Han, X., & Su, D. (2023). Racial-ethnic disparities in psychological distress during the COVID-19 pandemic in the United States: The role of experienced discrimination and perceived racial bias. *BMC Public Health*, *23*, 957. https://doi.org/10.1186/s12889-023-15912-4

Williams, R. (2018). Popular culture: History and theory. *Cultural Studies*, *32*(6), 903–928.

Vyas, L. (2022). "New normal" at work in a post-COVID world: Work-life balance and labor markets. *Policy and Society*, *41*(1), 155–167.

Zawislak, G. (2024, January 28). Evolution of streaming services has shaped society. *The Pony Express*. https://sahsponyexpress.com/122539/focus/evolution-of-streaming-platforms-has-shaped-society/

PART I

Framing of Health-Related Issues in Popular Culture

2
POPULAR CULTURE AND HEALTH INFORMATION

Kimberly N. Kline, Amy L. Yoder, and Brianna R. Yoder

"Hi, Barbie!!!" my daughter and her wife effusively chimed in as I (Kim) came down the stairs in my hot-pink T-shirt with matching super sparkly earrings. I understood the assignment, and I enthusiastically replied, looking at my firstborn, Brianna, "Hi, Barbie!!!" and then Amy, "Hi, Barbie!!!" (the extra exclamation points are intentional). The three of us – two Millennials and me, a GenXer – were totally pumped to see the new *Barbie* movie, with no youngsters in tow as an excuse. This movie is not another animated movie where Barbie played a character like Rapunzel or the flower fairy Elina – it is live action, with Barbie speaking as a person in her own right. Also, we had heard it put feminist social commentary about gender relations and expectations center-screen. We saw the movie in the summer of 2023, when Taylor Swift's Eras and Beyonce's Renaissance concert tours took the world by storm, grossing billions of dollars each (Conkline, 2023). Their powerful fanbases gathered at every tour stop, where Swifties swapped friendship bracelets, and the BeyHive held hands while Beyonce said, "Everybody on mute!" It was a summer of shared sisterhood, and *Barbie* theaters were full of women and girls dressed in pink, calling out, "Hi, Barbie!" The movie promised to be another opportunity for female empowerment through camaraderie.

For me, the irony of this moment was inescapable. I had been adamantly opposed to kindergarten-aged Brianna having Barbie dolls when her interest piqued in the mid-'90s. Somehow, I had cottoned onto the idea that Barbie was not good for young girls, and I used the opportunity to talk to my then-six-year-old about unobtainable beauty standards, the hyper-sexualization and objectification of women, and the preservation of traditional binary gender roles. (Brianna confirms I used exactly those words.) Oh, and I made it a point to buy her "action figures" – the girls from the *Mighty Morphin Power Rangers* and *Sailor Moon*. Her grandmother thwarted my anti-Barbie efforts, blithely saying "yes" to all her granddaughter's requests, and Brianna amassed an impressive collection of the dolls along with those action figures. Despite the Barbies, Brianna is now doing fine. She's been married to a woman for over a decade, subverting many of those traditional gender roles, and she's good with the fact that she'll never be able to walk around looking like an airbrushed celebrity. For all of her grandmother's efforts, Sailor Moon turned out to be Brianna's most influential media figure. So, a win for me?

It turns out, though, I wasn't wrong to be concerned about Barbie. Plenty of evidence suggests that toys really matter when it comes to health and well-being. The book *Gender Typing of Children's Toys: How Early Play Experiences Impact Development* devoted numerous chapters to exploring the complex causes and consequences of gendered toy play (Weisgram & Dinella, 2018); in one chap-

DOI: 10.4324/9781003436409-3

ter, Leaper and Bigler (2018) noted that "toys that sexualize girls and women, such as female dolls dressed in mini-skirts, midriff-baring shirts, and high heels ... may contribute to girls' concerns with physical attractiveness and *undermine body image*" (p. 295, our emphasis). In turn, researchers linked negative body image with disordered eating beliefs and behaviors (Grabe et al., 2008; Spettigue & Henderson, 2004), which can lead to a number of mental and physical problems (Walsh-Childers, 2017). In her book, *When Medicine Goes Awry: Case Studies in Medically Caused Suffering and Death*, Clarke (2022) detailed the deaths of two teenage girls who took prescribed medications – drugs given off-label and not for their intended purpose. The drugs killed them, but Clarke didn't just blame the pharmaceuticals. Rather, she maintained that "the conditions for which the medications that caused their deaths were being prescribed were socially constructed conditions reflecting oppressive gender-based beauty norms" (p. 118).

However, Barbie isn't entirely to blame for the systemic and sexist socialization of our children from a young age. Barbie comprises just one part of the popular culture ecosystem – and the popular *media* ecosystem within it – that enlivens her. These ecosystems flow into each other, overlapping and sometimes existing fully within one another. Here, we have purposely flipped the metaphor from the commonly used but somewhat static term "environment," which basically refers to one's surroundings, to the more dynamic term "ecosystem," which acknowledges the interconnectedness of mediated forms of popular culture and the interaction of people with their media biome. The popular media ecosystem plays a significant role in how individuals grow to understand themselves and their place in the world. In other words, popular media, in particular, serves as an ecosystem that fertilizes and sustains individuals' understanding of themselves and their place in the world. Consider, for example, the "thin ideal" and the ways in which it is sustained by:

> familiar representations of women and girls of all ages via hyper-sexualization and unattainable portrayals of female beauty; glorification of especially thin models and actresses as "sexy" and "glamorous"; and presenting thinness as an expression of self-control and success" and "may be a form of gender inequality and a significant impediment to girls' health and well-being."
>
> *(Lemish, 2015, p. 123)*

Popular culture bombards young women with images of "skinny" models, celebrities, characters in movies and TV shows, ads, magazines, animated cartoons, music videos, video games, and even news stories that uphold the thin ideal (Betz & Ramsey, 2017). With the advent of social media (e.g., Instagram, TikTok, YouTube, Facebook), peers and "everyday" people perpetuate the thin ideal through personal photos and videos (Huang et al., 2021). The popular media ecosystem shames, stereotypes, and stigmatizes fatness, and young women absorb these messages and project them onto their own bodies. Gisselli Rodriguez (2018) posted on a website for those affected by eating disorders that she "was frequently exposed to Barbie, Victoria's Secret advertisements and novellas—all of which repeatedly perpetuated the same beauty ideal" (para. 1). Gisselli was miserable in high school, battled with self-confidence issues, and begged for breast implants for her 18th birthday. While she eventually "rewire[d] past thoughts" to lead a life where she advocates for healthy body image and fair representation in media, not everyone escapes the ecosystem unscathed – or at all (para. 6; see also Chapter 5, this volume).

Popular media informs our individual and social understandings of health and, in turn, influences health-related human activities, thus making popular media a vital area of study for scholars of Health Communication. Several books and chapters provide scoping reviews of the health-related empirical research related to health (Kline, 2017), and the chapters in this Handbook promise to bring these up to date. Generally, popular media research relevant to the concerns of Health Communication scholars has been informed by two traditions: media effects and critical cultural studies, also referred to as social-scientific and humanities approaches (Vorderer et al., 2020). In her reviews of popular media research, Kim acknowledged contributions from both traditions, describing health challenges related to illness, conditions, lifestyles, wellness, the political/sociocultural context (Kline, 2006), informational value, and ideological hegemony (Kline, 2011). In other reviews, she foregrounded theoretical (Kline, 2017) and methodological (Kline, 2003) approaches in health-related pop media inquiry, in both cases recognizing both traditional media effects and critical cultural approaches.

Fundamentally, scholars from both traditions are attempting to understand how various popular media artifacts participate in personal, public, and sociocultural negotiations. Vorderer et al. (2020), while primarily tracing the history of media effects research, discussed how scholars siloed these two traditions. They concluded that "now that the field and questions that it raises have grown well beyond the traditional boundaries, it might be time to also find explanations by crossing such well-known boundaries of our field" (p. 12). With this work, we seek to add to that conversation. Ultimately, scholars concerned with popular media as it relates to health, illness, and wellness want to improve individual and social health outcomes. Thus, rather than comparing and contrasting, in this chapter, we un-silo these traditions so that we can benefit from the strengths of each.

Levels of Media Influence on Knowledge/Understanding

Looking at the broad landscape of popular media research related to health, illness, wellness, etc., we recognize levels of media influence that resonate with an ecological model which "begins with individuals at the core, moving out to the wider socio-economic, cultural and environmental factors that influence health for individuals, communities, and whole societies" (Lewis & Lewis, 2015, p. 8). Neuendorf (1990) observed that media encompasses one part of a constellation of influences that *individuals* are exposed to regarding health. Brown and Walsh-Childers (1994) also noted the primacy of the "personal" or individual level as they extended their typology of media influence to include implications for *public level* (i.e., public policy) understandings and negotiations (see also Brown & Walsh-Childers, 2002; Walsh-Childers, 2017; Walsh-Childers & Brown, 2009). One can extend these levels to further include the sociocultural level that emphasizes how one's lived experience of health is influenced by social, political, and cultural forces. While it is easier to describe and understand each of these "levels" as partitioned from one another, we feel that it is more productive to note their interconnection. Thus, studying today's media ecosystem necessitates recognition that each of the levels works in tandem with one another – each being influenced by the others and influencing in turn. Below, we discuss each of these levels in more depth as they relate to popular media.

Personal Level

When Health Communication debuted as a formal discipline in the early 1980s (Kreps & Thornton, 1984), two primary branches of inquiry emerged (Kreps et al., 1998). One trajectory focused on health care delivery, which concentrated on interpersonal and group communication (e.g., provider/consumer relationships, health care teams, and social support). Alternatively, the health promotion path focused on persuasive Health Communication campaigns, including the *intentional and strategic* use of mass media to educate people. Given their attention to the implications of mass media, scholars in this line of research quickly realized mass media messages could also *unintentionally* help or hinder health promotion efforts. That is, the "success or failure of educational and informational campaigns depends largely on the broader cultural context into which they are injected" (Gerbner et al., 1982, p. 291).

The Health Communication discipline also has roots in cognitive-behavioral science, social psychology (Zoller & Kline, 2008), and social-scientific theories "where the locus of choice is the individual," such as the Theory of Reasoned Action, the Health Belief Model, and the Extended Parallel Process Model (Dutta-Bergman, 2005, p. 106). Thus, the lion's share of popular media research has been concerned with how news, entertainment, advertising, and now "new" media representations might alter audience members' knowledge, attitudes, and beliefs in ways that are presumed to influence individual health behaviors. The question remains how media informs knowledge and understanding in ways that impact the choices that we, as individuals, can make with regard to our health.

The impetus for much of the individual-level media research involves the expectation that we could alleviate chronic illnesses like diabetes, cancer, cardiovascular disease, and HIV/AIDS if only individuals would assume responsibility for their risky lifestyle behaviors, such as smoking cigarettes, dipping tobacco, using illicit drugs, drinking alcohol, and having unsafe sex; it would also help if they would engage in preventive behaviors like eating right and exercising (Signorielli, 1993; Walsh-Childers, 2017). Extended literature reviews such as Signorielli's groundbreaking book *Mass Media Images and Impact on Health: A Sourcebook* and Walsh-Childer's more recent *Mass Media and Health: Examining Media Impact on Individuals and the Health Environment* demonstrate how scholars who pursue this line of research consider media a barrier or (sometimes) facilitator to individuals making the choice to engage in these healthier lifestyle behaviors, assuming people would be positioned to act on the information provided and make so-called good choices if popular media representations provided appropriate information (see also Chapter 10, this volume).

For example, when TV shows came back from a production hiatus caused by the 2020 COVID-19 pandemic lockdown and quarantines, many included pandemic-related storylines and featured characters wearing masks (e.g., Cambra-Badii et al., 2022, on medical dramas). The first episode of the 22nd season of *Law & Order: SVU* was situated in the new pandemic reality, and characters often wore masks (Easton, 2020). Yet, viewers of this episode might also notice that characters did not follow best practices in their mask-wearing, typically pulling the mask down to deliver their lines. On the other hand, in the first two episodes of *Grey's Anatomy* season 17, every character, including patients, bystanders, police officers, and doctors, wore some kind of Personal Protective Equipment (PPE) and, notably, did not remove masks when speaking (James, 2021). Viewers could, however, see the characters speaking because the doctors frequently wore helmet-like masks that had a full-face transparent barrier, and the storylines featured never-aired flashback scenes. Even if the choice to include pandemic safety measures in these fictional storylines aided in small-screen verisimilitude, they still functioned as role modeling regarding wearing masks for safety.

Offscreen, celebrities used their status to mobilize their respective fanbases, tugging at our heartstrings along the way. On June 29, 2020, Hollywood heartthrob Patrick Dempsey took to his Instagram to encourage his followers to wear masks. Dempsey played successful neurosurgeon Derek Shepherd on 11 seasons of the hit ABC show *Grey's Anatomy*, and on the show, Dr. Shepherd's catchphrase is, "It's a beautiful day to save lives." Dempsey used that famous quote as the caption to an artful Instagram post showing him wearing a mask. The mask fits snugly on his cheeks, covers his nose, and disappears under his chin. With a picture, a signature quote, and a few hashtags, the megastar delivered a master class in sending all of the right messages to an audience primed to receive them – all while looking appropriately "McDreamy" (Dr. Shepherd's nickname in the show). Notably, one of the hashtags included in the post states #YourActionsSaveLives. This wording capitalized on the larger messaging in 2020 that centered on everyone doing their part, that we could end the pandemic through our own actions (for related work, see also Chapters 13 and 15, this volume).

Public Level

Whereas the individual level of influence emphasizes altering personal behavior as the way to resolve health threats, the public level recognizes that people make decisions about health within a political system. This level emphasizes that social determinants of health, such as living conditions and the unequal distribution of resources, as well as social norms and conditions, make it difficult if not impossible for people to *choose* healthier lifestyles. Thus, policymakers must pursue population-level actions, such as enacting laws and regulations, to alter the social environment in which people make choices about their health (Brown & Walsh-Childers, 1994; Rowbotham et al., 2019; Walsh-Childers & Brown, 2009).

Many of these policies strive to facilitate lifestyle choices by mandating behaviors (e.g., "no shots, no school"), restricting behaviors (e.g., bans on smoking in certain places), or (dis)incentivizing behaviors (e.g., taxes on tobacco products or sugary beverages; expanding food stamp programs so the stamps can be used at farmers' markets). However, not all health-related policies encourage individual lifestyle changes. Instead, policies help individuals improve health outcomes by requiring insurance companies to cover pre-existing conditions, eliminating sales tax on menstrual hygiene products, and providing lower-cost hearing aids. In the same way, policies can harm individuals, which we're seeing currently in the aftermath of the repeal of *Roe v. Wade* (Klibanoff, 2023; NPR Staff, 2023).

As the COVID-19 pandemic peaked at the end of 2020 and vaccines were still being developed, public health officials relied on testing for the virus to contain outbreaks (Mercer & Salit, 2021). Prior to the availability of at-home tests, coordinated efforts nationwide implored people to go to testing centers to find out if they had the virus. Unfortunately, testing centers were not equitably distributed. In our home state of Texas, most testing centers were on the wealthier, whiter side of town, leaving Black and Hispanic residents with few options for obtaining the test (McMinn et al., 2020). Federal legislators – many of whom live on these wealthier sides of town – wrangled with a bill that would have helped fund testing centers in these minority communities, but bipartisan dissension thwarted that effort (Martinez & Sparber, 2021). In 2021, history repeated itself when it was time for widespread vaccine distribution; minority communities struggled to access vaccines (Abba-Aji et al., 2022; Goodnough & Hoffmman, 2021).

Popular media plays an important role in setting the agenda and affecting public understanding, opinion, and acceptance of policy initiatives. Very briefly, agenda-setting refers to the ways in which media repeatedly cover certain topics, focusing audience attention on some issues and deflecting from others, effectively determining the matters that need more immediate action. While agenda-setting typically applies to news media (Rowbotham et al., 2019), it can encompass other forms of media (Turow & Coe, 1985).

Policymakers are not immune to popular media influences, both in their positions as members of society and as officials who need to attend carefully to the shared national agenda being represented – after all, they need the support of their constituents to maintain their status. Agenda-setting also holds implications for how those aforementioned constituents understand and accept policy initiatives. Indeed, Walsh-Childers and Braddock (2022) asserted that "the public's need to understand how government or corporate decisions affect them and their communities arguably is at least as important as their understanding of diet, exercise, drugs and other typical health topics" (p. 1779).

Conversations around HIV/AIDS exemplify popular media's effect on policy agendas. From 1981 onward, the media largely ignored or demonized a decade of death as (mostly) gay men died of AIDS (Otten, 1992; see also U.S. Department of Health and Human Services, 1991, for death statistics; Wallack, 1990). All the while, the gay community fought for research funding. In 1988, AIDS activist and gay, white artist David Wojnarowicz wore a customized jacket that read, "If I die of AIDS – forget burial – just drop my body on the steps of the F.D.A" (Laing, 2016). Three years later, it would be straight, Black athlete Magic Johnson who would move the needle on news coverage of HIV/AIDS (Brown & Basil, 1995; Flora et al., 1996; see also Chapter 15, this volume). When he announced that he was HIV-positive in 1991, Johnson garnered global news coverage that became dinner-table conversation. News media increased the volume of this conversation, allowing entertainers to tell their stories, and people listened. The 1993 film *Philadelphia* won multiple awards (IMDB, n.d.), and, in 1996, the musical *Rent* filled theater seats on Broadway (Jefferson, 1996). As the art scenes in L.A. and New York featured stories about HIV/AIDS, the political scene in D.C. also started to shift as President Bill Clinton's administration put its weight behind helping those with HIV/AIDS and eradicating its spread (Clinton Digital Library, n.d.). We saw the wheel continually turning as news coverage, entertainment media, and policies all advanced the public's understanding of HIV/AIDS.

Sociocultural Level

The public level and sociocultural level both focus on the context within which people negotiate health experiences and expectations. However, scholars considering the public level anticipate that public policy decisions will ultimately impinge on the individual's *ability to engage in recommended health behaviors* (e.g., Walsh-Childers, 2017); whereas those who interrogate the implications of media at the sociocultural level focus more on the manner in which discourse is constitutive of knowledge and values and the repercussions of social, political, and economic influences for people's *lived experiences and health outcomes* (e.g. Baglia & Foster, 2015; Lupton, 1994a; Seale, 2002; Thaker et al., 2019).

Research at the sociocultural level calls into question the ideological commitments mirrored in, constituted by, and rendered meaningful through social discourses, including the ubiquitous popular media. For example, one ideological commitment referred to in much of the health-related media research (regardless of level) entails the issue of responsibility for health, the focus on the individual, and the disregard of social and systemic causes of health disparities. Walsh-Childers (2017) noted this concern, even as her book predominantly concentrated on individual behaviors at the personal level. In the chapter where she briefly discussed public-level research and the need to acknowledge social/structural determinants of health, she observed that individual-level research dominates the field, adding, "this is probably not surprising in the United States given the centrality of individualism in our culture" (p. 425). Dutta-Bergman (2005), to whom she attributed this observation, actually critiqued the unquestioned reliance of dominant theoretical approaches on their ideological commitment to individualism.

Much of the work at the sociocultural level takes a critical-cultural stance, challenging existing beliefs about the particular practices and institutions that normalize and reinforce structures of power. Sociologist Lupton (1994b) exemplified this critical stance in her pivotal article "Toward the development of critical health communication praxis," notably published in the Health Communication discipline's flagship journal. Troubled by the reliance of Health Communication scholars on theories "too often limited to individualistic models of knowledge and behavior," Lupton maintained the need to attend to "the political, economic, and historical factors that shape a culture's response to and concepts of health, disease, and treatment issues" and recognize:

> health and ill-health states as being products of social systems and ideological processes; the identification of sickness as a form of social control; and biomedical treatment as an artifact of late capitalism in its view of the body as a mechanized commodity, which is the responsibility of the individual to maintain.
>
> *(p. 58)*

Critical scholars ultimately focus on structures of power in society; they call attention to who is advantaged and who is disadvantaged as well as whose voices are amplified and whose are silenced (Kline, 2014, 2022; Zoller & Kline, 2008). For example, a common critique of mainstream ideologies that contribute to health disparities involves the primacy of Western conceptualizations of medicine (Germov & Freij, 2019; Lantz et al., 2023; Turow & Coe, 1985). This assumption holds that all health threats can and should be treated using (Western) medicine, thereby expanding the purview of medical establishment control (medicalization), which relies on privileged medical authorities (professionalization), technological interventions (technologizing), and pharmaceutical cures (pharmaceuticalization) (Kline, 2003, 2011). Here again, we see reference to the individual vs. social responsibility issue as "medicalization takes a fundamentally individualizing stance. It is designed to fix or change one body at a time. As such, it eschews a focus on community supports and interventions" (Clarke, 2022, p. 10). Indeed, in their detailed analysis of the implications of medicalization for public and population health as well as health policy, Lantz et al. (2023) maintained that "medicalization and its focus on health at the micro or individual level presents one of the greatest challenges to improving population health in the United States" (p. 63). These ideological commitments remain so deeply entrenched that we tend to lose sight of the social, political, and economic structures that buttress them.

Despite millennia of medical systems that didn't hand out health care in amber-colored bottles, medicalization now constitutes "conventional" medicine, completely ignoring 3,000 to 5,000 years of traditions like acupuncture, moxibustion, herbal treatments, homeopathy, and holistic medicine (Ng et al., 2023). As art imitates life, mainstream medical shows have almost completely ignored thousands of years of healing systems. Since 1951, 137 medical-based television shows have aired in the United States alone (see Wikipedia, n.d. for an extensive list of worldwide medical dramas). Popular U.S. shows like *Trapper John, MD*, *St. Elsewhere*, *Scrubs* (Turow, 2010), *Chicago Hope*, *ER*, *Grey's Anatomy*, and *House, M.D.* (Foss, 2014) follow gaggles of doctors in white coats shuffling from room to room to see a patient who is admitted, diagnosed, treated, and discharged (or killed off) in a single episode. Though medical errors accounted for between 44,000 and 98,000 deaths each year in the 1990s, medical dramas from that era supported the preeminence of medical solutions to health threats with "mortality rates … so low that doctors rarely lose patients and [e]ven when patients are given low chances of survival, they usually pull through, without complications" (Foss, 2014, p. 232). At the same time, providing numerous examples from these shows, Foss contended that:

> *as long as fictional patients follow their physicians' advice*, they are encouraged to take responsibility for their health, especially in terms of illness prevention. TV doctors praise fictional "responsible" patients—those who live healthy lifestyles and criticize patients who do not
>
> *(p. 234, our emphasis)*

However, if they tried to treat themselves, they "were portrayed as foolish and often needed treatment for their choices" (p. 235). Thus, perhaps ironically, medical shows can reinforce ideological commitments to both the physician's unquestioned authority and individual responsibility. (For additional discussion of popular culture and medical errors, please see Chapter 12, this volume.)

In other genres, characters who dare to deviate from the medicalized model of treatment often become the punchline or a pale attempt at lip service. For example, despite evidence that home births cost less (Anderson & Gilkison, 2021) and constitute a safe birth plan for low-risk pregnancies (Hutton et al., 2019), few scripted TV shows portray giving birth at home as a reasonable alternative to the medicalized hospital birth. When *Gilmore Girls*, *Dharma & Greg*, and *Girlfriends* each had an episode where a central character planned a home-birth, the choice to give birth at home was depicted as irrational, midwives were "self-involved, disengaged, unhelpful, and generally mean," and two of the women ultimately choose a medicalized hospital birth in order to get pain medication (Kline, 2007, p. 24; see also Cummins, 2020).

Scholars from a number of disciplines also call attention to the stigmatization of certain individuals or groups, which "does not refer to inherent moral flaws of particular individuals or groups but rather to *the sociocultural process* by which members of marginalized groups are labeled by others as abnormal, shameful, or otherwise undesirable" (Jones & Corrigan, 2014, p. 9, our emphasis). While it's easy to conceptualize stigma as a psychological process that functions as a barrier to seeking health care, psychologist Hatzenbuehler (2016) discussed how structural stigma – the "societal level conditions, cultural norms, and institutional policies that constrain the opportunities, resources, and well-being of the stigmatized" (p. 742) – impacts the ability of marginalized groups to receive health care.

Though popular media is often a conduit for sustaining any number of often intersecting stigmatized identities (e.g., deafness, mental health, disability, weight, sexuality, drug addiction) (Else-Quest et al., 2023), we note more evidence of characters and the celebrities behind them role modeling positive representations while shifting away from negative stereotypes. Actors like Peter Dinklage (an actor who has dwarfism), Marlee Matlin (an actor who is deaf), and Easton Rocket Sweda (an actor who has autism) prove on- and off-screen that these differences aren't limitations to happy, healthy lives. In the sibling-centered TV show *This Is Us*, Sterling K. Brown's character Randall has a panic attack on-screen. Praised for its accurate portrayal of what 40 million Americans experience in one way or another, Brown wasn't content to let audiences think that brotherly love or an exercise routine is enough to solve anxiety (Holmes, 2017). Brown spoke openly in an interview with *People Magazine* about his own experiences in therapy, how he has no shame about seeing a therapist, and how he wished his character – and anyone suffering – would do the same (Mizoguchi, 2020; for related information on popular culture and mental health, please see Chapter 3, this volume).

Conclusion

In 1982, Gerbner et al. (1982) claimed that "[u]nlike other media, television is used relatively nonselectively. Most viewers watch by the clock rather than by the program. Television is like a ritual. It involves the average American household for 6 ½ hours a day in a *stable* and *repetitive* world of shows, news, and commercials" (p. 291, our emphasis). We're pretty sure that Gerbner and other media-effects scholars of his time (Bryant & Zillmann, 1994) didn't envision a world where viewers had access to 817,000 different TV shows (Nielsen, 2022) at any time of day, no matter where they were geographically, or a time when 142 million households all over the world could tune into a 2021 Korean dystopian thriller called *Squid Game* on Netflix (Rushe, 2021), just two years after the Korean black comedy thriller *Parasite* took home the 2019 Best Picture Academy Award. Add to that, people now watch reruns on a host of streaming services (Harris, 2023). Who would have thought that the medical show *ER*, which aired from 1994 to 2009, would be in the top 4 shows on Hulu in 2018, nearly 20 years since its premiere (Harnick, 2018)? In 2024, what we watch isn't limited by what producers decide to put on television; it isn't even constrained by time or location. We witness resurgences of popular media from years past that were produced and distributed for the first time under different contexts and with different social priorities and knowledge. Kim remembers showing Sut Jhally's (1995) *Dreamworlds* in one of the first classes that she taught as a newly minted assistant professor circa 1996 and being enticed by his notion that it's not about getting rid of problematic representations per se, but the need for more and different representations. Well, here we are.

Now, Health Communication scholars face the challenge of figuring out what these developments mean for popular media research. How are Health Communication scholars supposed to evaluate the implications of, say, international shows or reruns for health understanding and behaviors? How will researchers evaluate the implications for people living in one country consuming shows from another country? Should scholars include old television shows that have regained popularity in their studies? Given the deluge of entertainment options, how can scholars isolate "dominant" narratives that presumably influence audience attitudes, beliefs, and behaviors as they relate to health?

We have also seen the rise of news media outlets through mediums like podcasts and blogs. In fact, while podcasts can and do focus on a wide variety of themes, there's no denying that podcasts can serve as a source of news. Almost half of adult Americans listened to a podcast within the last year, and around one-third of podcast listeners say that they tune into podcasts as their source of news (Shearer et al., 2023). These news media also use social media to ostensibly disseminate information. In the midst of true journalism shared via social media, it is also easy to drown in misinformation (Suarez-Lledo & Alvarez-Galvez, 2021; Wang et al., 2019). For instance, in June 2023, when the submersible OceanGate went missing on its trek to the Titanic, social media was filled with commentators laughing about how Celine Dion's famous song "My Heart Will Go On*"* went on a Spotify-streaming tear. Those rumors were actually untrue, debunked by the reputable news source *USA Today* (Hudnall, 2023). It's important to add the adjective "reputable" because "over 3,000 outlets … call themselves newsrooms in America. That's before we add bloggers, podcasts, talk radio and the deluge of user-generated content" (Legg, 2021), which at any time can be rife with misinformation (see also Chapter 11, this volume).

Commercial advertisements are omnipresent. As of 2024, cable television still includes paid-for and scheduled commercial breaks, but websites feature pop-up ads, paid "suggested" posts, algorithms that decide what to show viewers based on their habits and the habits of people like them, and, of course, influencer marketing. Under the guise of "making content," people on the internet peddle products with discount codes and affiliate links. Influencers sell products that promise those scrolling will look or love or live like they do … if they buy this product first. So-called wellness influencers sell their lifestyle, although the receipt details the purchase of psoriasis drugs or nasal-based tanning products or colloidal silver to kill COVID-19 (see also Chapter 16, this volume).

These popular media messages become even more powerful because they are duplicated, replicated, and seemingly infinite. Media convergence has irrevocably altered the ways in which people partake in the media ecosystem. Not only do multiple platforms repeatedly push out a myriad of media content, but many of us can access all of it with just a swipe of our thumb on a smartphone screen. Podcasts, which were originally developed for the iPod, have outlived their intended distribution device and exist instead on platforms like Spotify, Apple Podcasts, Google Music, Audible, and more. Even the well-respected National Public Radio (NPR) produces podcast content that is never once pushed out via radio waves. NPR developed its very own app so all of their podcasts can be found in one place!

What used to be a show broadcast once a week on a specific cable TV channel is now a binge-able complete series we can watch over and over again. We have to wonder, though, do viewers come to different understandings of the messages in *Grey's Anatomy* if they watch one episode each week or ten episodes in one sitting? Should media scholars add binge-watching as a confounding variable when crafting studies to understand audience responses (e.g. Walter et al., 2018)? Ultimately, pieces of media are produced, fractured, repackaged, and consumed over and over again, all while still retaining the taste of the "subtle messages proposing a particular perspective about what is 'appropriate' and 'inappropriate,' 'desirable' and 'undesirable,' 'good' and 'bad,' and so on" (Sellnow, 2018, p. 3). In the Netflix series *Orange Is the New Black*, a character commented that she was tired of hearing people talk about "how they're turning their Twitter feeds into blogs, their blogs into books, and their books into Twitter feeds. It's exhausting!" Ironically, the protagonist of the show turned her prison sentence into a book and her book into a television show and her television show into a hashtag – #OITNB.

Remember Barbie? We love the fact that, in the *Barbie* movie, the eponymous character develops her own agency and is empowered by her autonomy. Margot Robbie's Barbie would definitely scream-sing "F*** the patriarchy!" along to Taylor Swift's "All Too Well (10 Minute Version) (Taylor's Version)." That should be celebrated. However, just as the voice of our internal feminist begins shouting that Barbie remains the quintessential icon of unobtainable beauty, the narrator of *Barbie* beats us to the punch. When Barbie spoke about not feeling pretty enough, Dame Helen Mirren broke in, "Note to filmmakers: Margot Robbie is not the right person to cast to make this point." Though she's older than the Barbie doll, Mirren is still hailed as one of the most beautiful women in Hollywood. She was even on the cover of the 2022 "Beautiful" issue of *People Magazine* at the age of 76, so perhaps it's a bit cheeky of Mirren to call out the filmmakers. After all, Mirren has managed what so many stars wish they could – decades of critical success that went hand-in-hand with positive press around her physical appearance. Regardless, Mirren wasn't wrong to point out that Robbie might rub some viewers the wrong way when talking about not feeling pretty enough. In fact, the *Barbie* movie doesn't shy away from the controversy wrapped around her waistline. In the movie, a "real-world" teenager named Sasha called out Barbie to her face, remarking on the doll's complicity in perpetuating the thin ideal: "You've been making women feel bad about themselves since you were invented."

There's another story going around, though, that shifts the narrative to focus on Barbie's aspirational side. That narrative points out that Barbie "has had over 250 inspirational careers, including astronaut, pilot, firefighter, journalist, and entrepreneur," as well as surgeon, CEO, "computer engineer, video game developer, Mars explorer, robotics engineer, and presidential candidate" (Mattel, n.d.). (Brianna actually bought that one when she was campaigning for a female candidate in Texas.) Kim still tears up watching the new advertisement that capitalized on this new image of Barbie and told us, "When a girl plays with Barbie, she imagines everything she can become" (imagine the possibilities, n.d.). Two things can be true at the same time – Barbie epitomizes a thin ideal to young girls that should be critiqued, *and* she can serve as a way for those same young girls to envision themselves in a wide range of professions, many of which are male-dominated. Yet, it does feel like PANTONE 219 C-colored, Barbie-pink commodity feminism where "feminist ideas and icons are appropriated for commercial purposes, emptied of their political significance and offered back to the public in a commodified form – usually in advertising" (Gill, 2008). Notably, Mattel made a lot of money, experiencing a 25% increase in toy sales after the movie's summer 2023 release (Verdon, 2023). It's motivational, but it's also calculated to sell dolls to a new generation. Commodity feminism is good for commerce.

Suggestions for Future Research

The popular media ecosystem is increasingly elaborate and tangled, having changed radically since the initial studies of media representations and effects (see Danesi, 2012, for a detailed media technology timeline). We realize this chapter raises more questions than answers, but we'd like to offer some broad suggestions for future research. First, scholars concerned with the implications of popular media for attitudes, beliefs, and behaviors must attend carefully to new developments in media effects theory as it is evolving in response to the contemporary popular media ecosystem. For example, talking about journalism and politics in the authoritative text *Media Effects: Advances in Theory and Research* (Oliver et al., 2020), Tsfati and Walter (2020) detailed how "changes in communication technologies, in media ecology, and in the political environment have shaken the assumptions that were at the core of political communication for decades in ways that have shaped effects research" (p. 36). Thus, they concluded that media effects scholars need to:

- reconceptualize the news with a focus on a larger universe of content and media that includes political comedy, user-generated comments, reactions, and memes;
- better conceptualize and operationalize the notion of audience exposure in the online environment;
- (take into consideration) a much broader array of dependent variables…as the outcome of news exposure, and the associations between these outcomes and immediate reactions such as likes or retweets should be further explored;
- pause to think about whether existing theories can shed light on new challenges and opportunities … before substituting old questions and theories for a new set of frameworks.

(p. 45)

Thus far, much of the popular media research related to Health Communication has relied on Cultivation Theory (Gerbner & Gross, 1976), Social Cognitive Theory (Bandura, 1977), Agenda-Setting Theory (McCombs & Shaw, 1972), and Framing Theory (Goffman, 1974; see Kline, 2017).

Yet, many other media theories can help researchers tease out the implications of today's chaotic media ecosystem for how people understand and react to popular media. To wit, Oliver et al.'s (2020) book "[contained] both new and updated content that reflects our media-saturated environments" including chapters on "social media, video games, mobile communication, and virtual technologies … narratives, positive media, the self and identity, media selection, and cross-cultural media effects" (p. 1).

Second, Health Communication scholars who want to broaden the scope of popular media research to take a more ecological approach in understanding the implications of popular media for health, illness, and wellness need to more actively and consistently embrace the contributions of interdisciplinary critical-cultural scholars in order to better integrate considerations of sociocultural context. This quest will likely be troublesome at times, as critical-cultural scholars often call into question taken-for-granted notions of what constitutes "best practices" when it comes to health promotion.

For instance, Lupton (2018) challenged the assumption that bodyweight is equivalent to health, detailing at length the ways in which social constructions of "obesity," "overweight," and the "obesity epidemic" (many of which play out in popular media) contribute to the pathologizing and medicalization of weight in ways that negatively affect fat embodiment and identity by contributing to stigmatization and victim-blaming. Indeed, Lupton purposely used the term "fat" as a means "to describe corpulent people in a positive, accepting manner" (in much the same way LGBTQ individuals appropriated the term "queer" as a "positive self-identifying and political term") and rejected the term "obesity," which "immediately places that person within the purview of medicine as someone who has the disease of 'obesity' and is therefore considered abnormal, inevitably unhealthy or at high risk of disease, requiring medical intervention to reduce his or her weight" (p. 3). One can see how Health Communication scholars might find it difficult to accommodate this perspective when one of the mainstays of health promotion is the need to entice people to lose weight through exercise and diet under the assumption that health problems like Type 2 diabetes, heart disease, and stroke are exacerbated when a person's body mass index (BMI) is greater than 30 (Office of Disease Prevention and Health Promotion, n.d.). We would point out that the ways in which "obesity" has been pathologized and medicalized in Western society participate in the discourses of the "thin ideal" we noted as a health threat at the outset of this chapter. An ecological approach necessitates panning out from media effects micro-level analyses to explore complex systemic influences constituted, maintained, and perpetuated in popular media.

In closing, popular media forms of entertainment, news, advertising, and social media obviously comprise a powerful force in our society at personal, public, and sociocultural levels. As the other chapters in this volume illuminate, understanding the popular media ecosystem and its implications for health, illness, and wellness knowledges and experiences constitutes an essential step for Health Communication scholars and practitioners.

References

Abba-Aji, M., Stuckler, D., Galea, S., & McKee, M. (2022). Ethnic/racial minorities' and migrants' access to COVID-19 vaccines: A systematic review of barriers and facilitators. *Journal of Migration and Health*, *5*, 100086–100086. https://doi.org/10.1016/j.jmh.2022.100086

Anderson, D. A., & Gilkison, G. M. (2021). The cost of home birth in the United States. *International Journal of Environmental Research and Public Health*, *18*(19), 10361. https://doi.org/10.3390/ijerph181910361

Baglia, J., & Foster, E. (2015). Mad men as health communication: Health-related themes in the hit AMC television series. *Health Communication*, *30*(1), 50–60. https://doi.org/10.1080/10410236.2013.835782

Bandura, A. (1977). *Social learning theory*. Prentice Hall.

Betz, D. E., & Ramsey, L. R. (2017). Should women be "all about that bass?": Diverse body-ideal messages and women's body image. *Body Image*, *22*, 18–31. https://doi.org/10.1016/j.bodyim.2017.04.004

Brown, J. D., & Walsh-Childers, K. (1994). Effects of media on personal and public health. In J. Bryant & D. Zillman (Eds.), *Media effects: Advances in theory and research* (pp. 389–415). Erlbaum. https://doi.org/10.4324/9781410602428

Brown, J. D., & Walsh-Childers, K. (2002). Effects of media on personal and public health. In J. Bryant & D. Zillmann (Eds.), *Media effects: Advances in theory and research* (2nd ed., pp. 453–488). Erlbaum.

Brown, W. J., & Basil, M. D. (1995). Media celebrities and public health: Responses to "Magic" Johnson's HIV disclosure and its impact on AIDS risk and high-risk behaviors. *Health Communication*, *7*(4), 345–370. https://doi.org/10.1207/s15327027hc0704_4

Bryant, J., & Zillmann, D. (1994). *Media effects: Advances in theory and research*. Erlbaum.

Cambra-Badii, I., Guardiola, E., & Baños, J.-E. (2022). The COVID-19 pandemic in serial medical dramas. *JAMA: The Journal of the American Medical Association*, *327*(1), 20–22. https://doi.org/10.1001/jama.2021.19779

Clarke, J. N. (2022). *When medicine goes awry: Case studies in medically caused suffering and death*. University of Toronto Press. https://doi.org/10.3138/9781487538064

Clinton Digital Library. (n.d.). An unprecedented problem: The Clinton administration and HIV/AIDS in the United States. https://clinton.presidentiallibraries.us/an-unprecedented-problem-the-clinton-administration-and-hiv/aids-in-the-united-states

Conkline, J. (2023). Beyonce vs. Taylor: How these superstars stack up against one another. *Forbes*. https://www.forbes.com/sites/justinconklin/2023/06/11/taylor-swift-vs-beyonce-how-these-super-stars-stack-up-against-one-another/?sh=7069b566718a

Cummins, M. W. (2020). Miracles and home births: The importance of media representations of birth. *Critical Studies in Media Communication*, *37*(1), 85–96. https://doi.org/10.1080/15295036.2019.1704037

Danesi, M. (2012). *Popular culture: Introductory perspectives* (3rd ed.). Rowman & Littlefield.

Dutta-Bergman, M. J. (2005). Theory and practice in health communication campaigns: A critical interrogation. *Health Communication*, *18*, 103–122. https://doi.org/10.1207/s15327027hc1802_1

Easton, A. (2020). The 'Law & Order: SVU' squad deals with Covid, community unrest, and personal stress in 22nd season, says EP. *Forbes*. https://www.forbes.com/sites/anneeaston/2020/11/11/the-law--order-svu-squad-deals-with-covid-community-unrest-and-personal-stress-in-22nd-season-says-ep/?sh=3acf793f3f36

Else-Quest, N. M., French, A. M., & Telfer, N. A. (2023). The intersectionality imperative: Calling in stigma and health research. *Stigma and Health*, *8*(3), 269–278. https://doi.org/10.1037/sah0000397

Flora, J. A., Schooler, C., Mays, V. M., & Cochran, S. D. (1996). Exploring a model of symbolic social communication: The case of 'Magic' Johnson. *Journal of Health Psychology*, *1*(3), 353–366. https://doi.org/10.1177/135910539600100308

Foss, K. A. (2014). From Welby to McDreamy: What TV teaches us about doctors, patients, and the health care system. In D. A. Macey, K. M. Ryan, & N. J. Springer (Eds.), *How television shapes our worldview: Media representations of social trends and change* (pp. 227–244). Lexington Books.

Gerbner, G., & Gross, L. (1976). Living with television: The violence profile. *Journal of Communication*, *26*(2), 172–199. https://doi.org/10.1111/j.1460-2466.1976.tb01397.x

Gerbner, G., Morgan, M., & Signorielli, N. (1982). Programing health portrayals: What viewers see, say, and do. In D. Pearl, L. Bouthilet, & J. Lazar (Eds.), *Television and behavior. Ten years of scientific progress and implications for the eighties – Volume II: Technical reviews* (pp. 291–307). National Institute of Mental Health.

Germov, J., & Freij, M. (2019). Media and health: Moral panics, miracles and medicalisation. In J. Germov (Ed.), *Second opinion: An introduction to health sociology* (6th ed., pp. 422–445). Oxford University Press.

Gill, R. (2008). Commodity feminism. In W. Donsbach (Ed.), *The International Encyclopedia of Communication* (1st ed., pp. 583–585). John Wiley & Sons. https://doi.org/10.1002/9781405186407.wbiecc055

Goffman, E. (1974). *Frame analysis: An essay on the organization of experience*. Northeastern University.

Goodnough, A., & Hoffmman, J. (2021). The wealthy are getting more vaccinations, even in poorer neighborhoods. *The New York Times*. https://www.nytimes.com/2021/02/02/health/white-people-covid-vaccines-minorities.html

Grabe, S., Hyde, J. S., & Ward, L. M. (2008). The role of the media in body image concerns among women: A meta-analysis of experimental and correlational studies. *Psychological Bulletin*, *134*(3), 460–476. https://doi.org/10.1037/0033-2909.134.3.460

Harnick, C. (2018). The second coming of ER: Why the medical drama's arrival on Hulu is the surprise TV success story of 2018. https://www.eonline.com/news/922453/the-second-coming-of-er-why-the-medical-drama-s-arrival-on-hulu-is-the-surprise-tv-success-story-of-2018

Harris, D. (2023). The complete list of streaming services in 2024 – 200+ services. https://agoodmovietowatch.com/how-to/complete-list-streaming-services/

Hatzenbuehler, M. L. (2016). Structural stigma and health inequalities: Research evidence and implications for psychological science. *The American Psychologist, 71*(8), 742–751. https://doi.org/10.1037/amp0000068
Holmes, L. (2017). 'This Is Us' totally captured the hard truth of panic attacks. *Huff Post*. https://www.huffpost.com/entry/this-is-us-panic-attack_n_58a74471e4b07602ad54617e
Huang, Q., Peng, W., & Ahn, S. (2021). When media become the mirror: A meta-analysis on media and body image. *Media Psychology, 24*(4), 437–489. https://doi.org/10.1080/15213269.2020.1737545
Hudnall, H. (2023). No, 'My Heart Will Go On' isn't on recent Billboard charts | Fact check. *USA Today*. https://www.usatoday.com/story/news/factcheck/2023/06/29/oceangate-submersible-hasnt-made-celine-dion-song-viral-fact-check/70366004007/
Hutton, E. K., Reitsma, A., Simioni, J., Brunton, G., & Kaufman, K. (2019). Perinatal or neonatal mortality among women who intend at the onset of labour to give birth at home compared to women of low obstetrical risk who intend to give birth in hospital: A systematic review and meta-analyses. *EClinicalMedicine, 14*, 59–70. https://doi.org/10.1016/j.eclinm.2019.07.005
Imagine the possibilities. (n.d.) https://www.youtube.com/watch?v=l1vnsqbnAkk
IMDB. (n.d.). Philadelphia Awards. https://www.imdb.com/title/tt0107818/awards/
James, E. S. (2021). 17 seasons in, Grey's Anatomy reimagined itself for the pandemic. But only a little bit. *Vox*. https://www.vox.com/culture/22465064/greys-anatomy-finale-season-17-recap-review-covid-19-beach
Jefferson, M. (1996). SUNDAY VIEW; 'Rent' Is brilliant and messy all at once. *The New York Times*. https://www.nytimes.com/1996/02/25/theater/sunday-view-rent-is-brilliant-and-messy-all-at-once.html
Jhally, S. (1995). Dreamworlds III: Desire, sex & power in music video. https://shop.mediaed.org/dreamworlds-3-p86.aspx
Jones, N., & Corrigan, P. W. (2014). Understanding stigma. In P. W. Corrigan (Ed.), *The stigma of disease and disability: Understanding causes and overcoming injustices* (pp. 9–34). American Psychological Association. https://doi.org/10.1037/14297-002
Klibanoff, E. (2023). A year after Dobbs decision, Texas has settled in to a post-abortion reality. *Texas Tribune*. https://www.texastribune.org/2023/06/23/texas-abortion-dobbs-roe-overturn/
Kline, K. N. (2003). Popular media and health: Images, effects, and institutions. In T. L. Thompson, A. M. Dorsey, K. I. Miller, & R. Parrott (Eds.), *Handbook of health communication* (pp. 557–581). Erlbaum.
Kline, K. N. (2006). A decade of research on health content in the media: The focus on health challenges and sociocultural context and attendant informational and ideological problems. *Journal of Health Communication, 11*(1), 43–59. https://doi.org/10.1080/10810730500461067
Kline, K. N. (2007). Midwife attended births in prime-time television: Craziness, controlling bitches, and ultimate capitulation. *Women & Language, 30*, 20–29.
Kline, K. N. (2011). Popular media and health: Images and effects. In T. L. Thompson, R. Parrott, & J. F. Nussbaum (Eds.), *Handbook of health communication* (2nd ed., pp. 252–267). Erlbaum.
Kline, K. N. (2014). Media and health, critical analysis of. In T. L. Thompson (Ed.), *Encyclopedia of health communication* (pp. 805–809). SAGE.
Kline, K. N. (2017). Popular media and exposure to health and risk messages. *Oxford research encyclopedia of communication*. http://communication.oxfordre.com/view/10.1093/acrefore/9780190228613.001.0001/acrefore-9780190228613-e-330
Kline, K. N. (2022). Critical rhetorical and strategic communication approaches to health research: Bridging the gap with PEN-3. In C. O. Airhihenbuwa & J. Iwelunmor (Eds.), *Health, culture, and place: From the tree to the forest* (pp. 55–68). U-Rise, LLC.
Kreps, G. L., Bonaguro, E. W., & Query, J. L. (1998). The history and development of the field of health communication. In L. D. Jackson & B. K. Duffy (Eds.), *Health communication research: A guide to developments and directions* (pp. 1–15). Greenwood.
Kreps, G. L., & Thornton, B. C. (1984). *Health communication* (1st ed.). Longman.
Laing, O. (2016). David Wojnarowicz: Still fighting prejudice 24 years after his death. *The Guardian*. https://www.theguardian.com/books/2016/may/13/david-wojnarowicz-close-to-the-knives-a-memoir-of-disintegration-artist-aids-activist
Lantz, P. M., Goldberg, D. S., & Gollust, S. E. (2023). The perils of medicalization for population health and health equity. *The Milbank Quarterly, 101*(S1), 61–82. https://doi.org/10.1111/1468-0009.12619
Leaper, C., & Bigler, R. S. (2018). Societal causes and consequences of gender typing of children's toys. In E. S. Weisgram & L. M. Dinella (Eds.), *Gender typing of children's toys: How early play experiences impact development* (pp. 287–308). American Psychological Association. https://doi.org/10.1037/0000077-013
Legg, H. (2021). Have you heard the news? But who owns what you're hearing and reading? We need to know. *USA Today*. https://www.usatoday.com/story/opinion/2021/05/14/mainstream-media-owner-ship-america-needs-news-transparency/5077719001/

Lemish, D. (2015). *Children and media: A global perspective*. John Wiley & Sons, Inc.
Lewis, B., & Lewis, J. (2015). *Health communication: A media and cultural studies approach*. Palgrave.
Lupton, D. (1994a). *Medicine as culture: Illness, disease, and the body in Western societies*. SAGE.
Lupton, D. (1994b). Toward the development of critical health communication praxis. *Health Communication*, *6*, 55–67. https://doi.org/10.1207/s15327027hc0601_4
Lupton, D. (2018). *Fat* (2nd ed.). Routledge. https://doi.org/10.4324/9781351029025
Martinez, M., & Sparber, S. (2021). As Texas expands COVID-19 vaccination eligibility, racial disparities persist among Black, Hispanic residents. *Texas Tribune*. https://www.texastribune.org/2021/03/19/texas-vaccine-race-disparities/
Mattel. (n.d.). Barbie fast facts. http://www.barbiemedia.com/about-barbie/fast-facts.html
McCombs, M. E., & Shaw, D. L. (1972). The agenda-setting function of mass media. *Public Opinion Quarterly*, *36*(2), 176–187. https://doi.org/ 10.1086/267990
McMinn, S., Carlsen, A., Jaspers, B., Talbot, R., & Adeline, S. (2020). In large Texas cities, access to coronavirus testing may depend on where you live. *NPR*. https://www.npr.org/sections/health-shots/2020/05/27/862215848/across-texas-black-and-hispanic-neighborhoods-have-fewer-coronavirus-testing-sit
Mercer, T. R., & Salit, M. (2021). Testing at scale during the COVID-19 pandemic. *Nature Reviews Genetics*, *22*(7), 415–426. https://doi.org/10.1038/s41576-021-00360-w
Mizoguchi, K. (2020). 'This Is Us' ' Sterling K. Brown breaks down Randall's meltdown, reflects on his own mental self-care. *People*. https://people.com/tv/this-is-us-sterling-k-brown-randall-meltdown-mental-self-care/
Neuendorf, K. A. (1990). Health images in the mass media. In E. B. Ray & L. Donohew (Eds.), *Communication and health: Systems and applications* (pp. 111–135). Erlbaum. https://doi.org/10.4324/9780203812280-15
Ng, J. Y., Dhawan, T., Fajardo, R.-G., Masood, H. A., Sunderji, S., Wieland, L. S., & Moher, D. (2023). The brief history of complementary, alternative, and integrative medicine terminology and the development and creation of an operational definition. *Integrative Medicine Research*, *12*(4), 100978–100978. https://doi.org/10.1016/j.imr.2023.100978
Nielsen. (2022). The video streaming industry has reached a tipping point. https://www.nielsen.com/insights/2022/state-of-play/
NPR Staff. (2023). New abortion laws changed their lives. 8 very personal stories. *NPR*. https://www.npr.org/sections/health-shots/2023/06/23/1183878942/abortion-bans-personal-stories-dobbs-anniversary
Office of Disease Prevention and Health Promotion. (n.d.). Healthy People 2030. U.S. Department of Health and Human Services. https://health.gov/healthypeople.
Oliver, M. B., Raney, A. A., & Bryant, J. (2020). *Media effects: Advances in theory and research* (4th ed.). Routledge.
Otten, A. L. (1992). The influence of the mass media on health policy. *Health Affairs*, *11*(4), 111–118. https://doi.org/10.1377/hlthaff.11.4.111
Rodriguez, G. (2018). The power of media literacy. https://www.nationaleatingdisorders.org/power-media-literacy/
Rowbotham, S., McKinnon, M., Marks, L., & Hawe, P. (2019). Research on media framing of public policies to prevent chronic disease: A narrative synthesis. *Social Science & Medicine*, *237*, 112428. https://doi.org/https://doi.org/10.1016/j.socscimed.2019.112428
Rushe, D. (2021). 142m households watched Squid Game, Netflix says as it adds 4.4m subscribers. *The Guardian*. https://www.theguardian.com/media/2021/oct/19/netflix-quarterly-results-subscribers-squid-game
Seale, C. (2002). *Media & health*. SAGE.
Sellnow, D. D. (2018). *The rhetorical power of popular culture: Considering media texts* (3rd ed.). SAGE. https://doi.org/10.4135/9781071800638
Shearer, E., Liedke, J., Matsa, K. E., Lipka, M., & Jurkowitz, M. (2023). Podcasts as a source of news and information. https://www.pewresearch.org/journalism/2023/04/18/podcasts-as-a-source-of-news-and-information/
Signorielli, N. (1993). *Mass media images and impact on health: A sourcebook*. Greenwood.
Spettigue, W., & Henderson, K. A. (2004). Eating disorders and the role of the media. *The Canadian Child and Adolescent Psychiatry Review*, *13*(1), 16–19.
Suarez-Lledo, V., & Alvarez-Galvez, J. (2021). Prevalence of health misinformation on social media: Systematic review. *Journal of Medical Internet Research*, *23*(1), e17187–e17187. https://doi.org/10.2196/17187
Thaker, J., Dutta, M. J., Nair, V., & Rao, V. P. (2019). Media portrayal stigma among gender and sexual minorities: Meaning, power, and resistance. In M. J. Dutta & D. B. Zapata (Eds.), *Communicating for social change: Meaning, power, and resistance* (pp. 383–407). Palgrave Macmillan. https://doi.org/10.1007/978-981-13-2005-7_18
Tsfati, Y., & Walter, N. (2020). The world of news and politics. In M. B. Oliver, A. A. Raney, & J. Bryant (Eds.), *Media effects: Advances in theory and research* (4th ed., pp. 36–50). Routledge. https://doi.org/10.4324/9780429491146-3

Turow, J. (2010). *Playing doctor: Television, storytelling, and medical power* (New and expanded ed.). University of Michigan Press.

Turow, J., & Coe, L. (1985). Curing television's ills: The portrayal of health care. *Journal of Communication, 35*, 36–51.

U.S. Department of Health and Human Services. (1991). Mortality attributable to HIV Infection/AIDS – United States, 1981–1990. *MMWR. Morbidity and Mortality Weekly Report, 40*(3), 41–44.

Verdon, J. (2023). Barbie movie boosted Mattel's sales, but investors held their applause. *Forbes*. https://www.forbes.com/sites/joanverdon/2023/10/25/barbie-movie-boosted-mattels-sales-but-investors-held-their-applause/?sh=69dcc1281bd4

Vorderer, P., Park, D. W., & Lutz, S. (2020). A history of media effects research traditions. In M. B. Oliver, A. A. Raney, & B. Jennings (Eds.), *Media effects: Advances in theory and research* (4th ed., pp. 1–15). Routledge. https://doi.org/10.4324/9780429491146-1

Wallack, L. (1990). Mass media and health promotion: Promise, problem, and challenge. In C. K. Atkin & L. Wallack (Eds.), *Mass communication and public health: Complexities and conflicts* (pp. 41–59). SAGE.

Walsh-Childers, K. (2017). *Mass media and health: Examining media impact on individuals and the health environment*. Routledge.

Walsh-Childers, K., & Braddock, J. (2022). Costs, evidence, context and values: Journalists' and policy experts' recommendations for U.S. health policy coverage. *Health Communication, 37*(14), 1778–1787. https://doi.org/10.1080/10410236.2021.1920711

Walsh-Childers, K., & Brown, J. D. (2009). Effects of media on personal and public health. In J. Bryant & M. B. Oliver (Eds.), *Media effects: Advances in theory and research* (pp. 469–489). Routledge.

Walter, N., Murphy, S. T., & Rosenthal, E. L. (2018). Narrative persuasion in a new media environment: The impact of binge-watching and second-screening. *Communication Research Reports, 35*(5), 402–412. https://doi.org/10.1080/08824096.2018.1525348

Wang, Y., McKee, M., Torbica, A., & Stuckler, D. (2019). Systematic literature review on the spread of health-related misinformation on social media. *Social Science & Medicine, 240*, 112552–112552. https://doi.org/10.1016/j.socscimed.2019.112552

Weisgram, E. S., & Dinella, L. M. (2018). *Gender typing of children's toys: How early play experiences impact development*. American Psychological Association.

Wikipedia. (n.d.). List of medical drama television programs. https://en.wikipedia.org/wiki/List_of_medical_drama_television_programs

Zoller, H. M., & Kline, K. N. (2008). Interpretive and critical research in health communication. In C. S. Beck (Ed.), *Communication yearbook* (Vol. 32, pp. 88–135). Routledge. https://doi.org/10.1080/23808985.2008.11679076

3

MENTAL ILLNESS AND POPULAR CULTURE

Heather Stuart

Introduction and Definitions

The first and possibly greatest challenge in considering the role of mental illness in popular culture lies in defining what constitutes popular culture (Hall, 2018). In his seminal work, Marshall McLuhan drew attention not only to the message but to the medium – the way in which the message was transmitted. Further, he suggested that modern communications form a cultural mosaic that gains meaning through individual interpretations (see Nye, 1971). From this perspective, individuals co-create popular notions of mental illness (including substance use disorders) as they interact with various information sources. Therefore, one view of "popular culture," and the one used in this chapter, is based on the active co-production of social meanings which reflect underlying attitudes and values (Fluck, 1987). Given that individuals interact with popular culture messaging to co-create meaning, it is useful to consider popular culture as one aspect of a broader socialization process that may include additional elements such as family values, religious beliefs, educational curricula, and peer cultures, all of which have helped form and be formed by popular cultural content in a reciprocal process.

Ohiagu and Okorie (2014, p. 96) defined popular culture as "all socially acquired traditions and lifestyles learned and made popular through the media." In this chapter, I will consider key channels of communication that transmit the content and values of popular culture pertaining to people living with mental illness, treatments, and health care providers. I do so by examining dominant portrayals of mental illness-related content in mass media, specifically news, entertainment, social media, music, and language.

Critical Issues and Topics

Communication comprises the foundation of culture, and mass media serves as a key conduits through which communication flows (Ohiagu & Okorie, 2014). Indeed, Ohiagu and Okorie indicated that the role of mass media in the transmission of culture is "nonnegotiable." With the addition of social media, they noted that people can share content, opinions, insights, and perspectives directly among themselves, turning communication into an interactive dialogue. Mass media not only mirrors societal norms and values, but it also reflect and maintains them. Indeed, according to Ohiagu and Okorie, media constitutes such a powerful socializing agent that politicians in some countries fear that unbalanced content will diminish national sovereignty, cultural autonomy, and cultural identity.

DOI: 10.4324/9781003436409-4

Notably, the media have created a vast store of negative imagery with some of the most horrifying and malignant images of madness. The media have also been responsible for some of the most gripping, sensitive, and award-winning depictions of people living with mental illness and the barriers they encounter. The fact that the former greatly outweighs the latter, and is more memorable, is of considerable concern to people living with mental illness, their family members, mental health professionals, and human rights advocates (Stuart & Sartorius, 2022).

Stuart (2006) noted that denigrating fictional images of people with mental illnesses frequent all forms of media. As well as being frequent, they are potent, highlighting violence, criminality, and unpredictability. These messages do little to convince the viewing public (including people with a mental illness) that they can recover and become productive members of society. The negative social stigma sparked by these images creates major barriers to treatment-seeking, recovery, and quality of life for people living with mental illness, their families, and all those who support them. Stigmatizing images of mental illness cultivate misinformation about crime and misconceptions about those who commit them. They also engender fear and rejection of people with mental illnesses and negatively influence the way in which the public evaluates mental health issues and mental health policy. Indeed, as Stuart claimed, some have used the presumption of dangerousness to justify forced legal action, coercive treatment, bullying, and other forms of victimization.

In addition to social stigma, media presentations of violence (suicide, homicide, and mass murders) can result in copy-cat behaviors (Domaradzki, 2021). According to Domaradzki, the idea that suicide reporting could create a contagion dates back to the late 18th century when a novel by Goethe, *The Sorrows of Young Werther*, was followed by numerous suicides across Europe. However, it wasn't until the early 1970s that researchers subjected suicide contagion to scientific scrutiny and dubbed it the *Werther effect*. In his review of studies focusing on news (n=65) and fictional stories (n=20), Domaradzki found that the vast majority (n=69) showed an association between media coverage and suicidality (both suicide attempts and suicides). Studies involving non-fictional people, particularly entertainers and politicians, were particularly triggering. For example, suicides increased by 10% in the United States following the suicide of actor Robin Williams, especially among males, many of whom used the same method (for related work on celebrity health narratives, please see Chapter 15, this volume). Non-celebrity suicides can also create contagion, especially if people of similar background or social status can identify with the individuals who died. As such, according to Domaradzki, responsible reporting avoids valorizing individuals who have taken their own lives or providing specific details about these incidents.

Schildkraut (2023) raised a similar red flag with respect to reporting of mass shootings, where reporters produced newspaper and television news stories at a rapid pace, and coverage often lasted for weeks. She argued that detailed information on the perpetrators (names, faces, pre-recorded manifestos, live feeds, etc.) as well as phone camera footage from people on the scene turn mass shooters into media celebrities. This notoriety rewards killers for their actions and can inspire copycat attacks. For one example, Schildkraut referenced the mass shooting at Marjory Stoneman Douglas High School in Florida, where threats and incidents of school violence increased by 300% in the first month after the attack, when media coverage was at its highest (see Klinger & Klinger, 2018), and 74 copycat threats occurred in the first 15 years following the Columbine shooting (see Follman, 2015).

As I have described in this section, two of the most critical issues to consider when examining the framing of mental illnesses in popular culture include the stigmatizing effects for people who are living with a mental illness and the harms that can flow from copycat violence.

Current Contributions and Research

The visualization of mental illnesses has a long history existing in most 'popular cultures' of the day (Stuart & Sartorius, 2022). Some of the most vivid depictions occurred in historical art and medical images dating back to at least the 16th century. Visual culture has been "saturated" with negative and frightening imagery of mental illness, treatments, and asylums (Eisenhauer, 2008). Contemporary popular culture can be distinguished from these historical moments in that mass media provides a key platform for negative imagery that can traverse the globe in an instant.

News Media

Stuart (2006) noted that a good story, particularly one that can be sensationalized, catches public attention. As a result, a reporter's job often entails ***selling*** the news rather than ***telling*** the news. News stories use cultural stereotypes to provide the context for the materials presented. In the case of news involving mental illnesses, stories often require the reader to draw on dominant cultural stereotypes and common-sense understandings of what it means to be mentally ill. Narratives feature sketchy or generic depictions, and audiences can easily identify the cultural frames being referenced and fill in the gaps. In the case of broadcast news, real-time visual images caught by news cameras that "don't lie" give overwhelming authentication to negative stereotypes, such as those linking mental illness to violence.

Aragonès et al. (2014) argued that journalists around the world have used psychiatric terminology pejoratively as a synonym for something untrustworthy, scary, unpredictable, and violent. For example, in their 2010 study of leading Spanish newspapers, 48% of the total texts reviewed (333 of 695) used clinical or psychiatric terms in this way to refer to irrational fears (81% of stories), incoherence (71%), or eccentricity (64%). Only 4% of the stories depicted people with a mental illness as victims. Bilić and Georgaca (2007) provided a second example. In the wake of Serbia's tumultuous sociopolitical situation, newspaper stories frequently likened the spread of post-traumatic stress disorder to an uncontrollable and malignant viral epidemic that was sweeping the nation. Journalistic accounts of people with PTSD committing violence used phrases, such as "bloodstained streets" or "personal and family tragedies," to highlight the association with violence and emphasize the impact of PTSD on broader family and community networks. Portrayals of perpetrators as quiet, normal-seeming people made the violence seem even more unpredictable and scary.

A content analysis of over 11,000 newspaper articles in major Canadian newspapers conducted by Whitley and Berry (2013) showed that 40% of the articles directly linked crime, violence, and dangerousness to mental illnesses. The voices of mental health professionals and people with lived experience of a mental illness were virtually nonexistent, and few articles spoke about treatment or recovery. However, importantly, we should not simply give voice to people with a mental illness. As Gwarjanski and Parrott (2018) determined, one in five newspaper articles about people with schizophrenia appearing in major US newspapers quoted an individual with schizophrenia (n=121); whereas, 435 did not. Almost half of the articles quoting someone with schizophrenia (45%) were framed in a stigmatizing way, illustrating the need for reporters to make a deliberate effort to provide a positive (or at least neutral) context for these quotes.

Entertainment Media

Entertainment media (movies and television) comprise a vast reservoir of negative and violent imagery depicting characters with a mental illness that both reflect and create cultural norms, attitudes, stereotypes, and beliefs that show us what to expect from a person with a mental illness and how to behave toward them. They can also portray deviant or criminal activities that are not normally publicly viewed, such as drug use, drug treatment, or sexual activity (Cape, 2003; Hersey, 2005). Similar to news, movies and television misinform the viewing public about the nature of mental illnesses by emphasizing the bizarre and violent (Owen, 2012). Thus, they serve as a catalog of stereotypic imagery that the public can draw upon when thinking about mental illness or interacting with other forms of media, such as when interpreting a news story.

Crime dramas have been particularly potent in linking mental illnesses to violence and criminality (Borecky, 2019; Parrott & Parrott, 2015). Borecky traced the evolution of the serial killer in U.S. crime dramas to the 1950s when the serial killer first emerged. Subsequently, the serial killer has become an archetype in crime dramas such as Alfred Hitchcock's *Psycho* (1960), Jonathan Demme's *Silence of the Lambs* (1991) and, more recently, television dramas such as *Criminal Minds*. Much of this material extends from the premise that people who commit grotesquely violent acts have a mental illness and need to be institutionalized (jailed) or killed. Unquestioned repetition of negative imagery – throughout history and across popular cultures – creates and maintains prejudice and discrimination, carrying it forward from one epoch to the next. When reporters describe a mass shooting or other incident as unimaginable or horrific, the public uses these negative archetypes to provide the interpretive frame. No mention of mental illness needs to be made (Stuart, 2006).

Socialization through popular culture begins early. Negative stereotypical content is evident in films and cartoons that target young children. Lawson and Fouts (2004) examined mental illness imagery in 40 full-length Disney animated films created between 1937 and 2001. They found that 85% contained references to characters with a mental illness, and 21% depicted the principal characters as mentally ill. In the *Beauty and the Beast*, for example, the townspeople referred to Belle and her father as mentally ill. The frequency of mental illness words increased as the film progressed, climaxing in a scene where the townspeople chained the father and took him away in a *lunacy wagon*. The *Lion King* presented the three hyenas as mentally ill with rolling eyes and high-pitched hysterical laughter. Ed, the *craziest* of them all, mistakenly gnawed on his own leg. The generic nature of the illnesses portrayed in children's television invites negative generalizations to all people with a mental illness (Stuart, 2006).

Negative imagery has also hounded psychiatrists and psychiatric treatments. Media has portrayed psychiatrists as malevolent, incompetent, or prone to sexual boundary violations, with treatments characterized as punitive or of no therapeutic value. For example, Gharaibeh (2005) reviewed 106 movies featuring 120 psychiatrists or therapists. Over half of the fictional therapists (44.9%) violated sexual (30.5%) or ethical boundaries (23.7%), and over half (47.5%) were depicted as clinically incompetent. Movies in this sample portrayed therapists as eccentric, bizarre, weird, and lethal. The classic and award-winning movie *One Flew Over the Cuckoo's Nest* not only gave us a chilling glimpse into the life inside a psychiatric institution, but it also vividly portrayed the punitive nature of psychiatric treatments (electroshocks and lobotomies) and the lack of morality of psychiatric staff who applied them. Is it any wonder that many people who have a mental illness avoid seeking treatment?

Social Media

Social media platforms have become an important source of health information, but also a frequent source of misinformation and stigmatizing content which cannot be easily deleted or corrected (see also Chapter 11, this volume). Analysis of social media content can provide meaningful clues as to the nature and content of stigmatizing and misinformed public attitudes and opinions. Li et al. (2018a) examined linguistic patterns of stigma expressions pertaining to suicidality in 6,632 posts on a popular Chinese microblogging service. Twelve percent of the posts contained misinformation about suicide, and up to a third reflected stigmatizing content. In a similar study of depression stigma involving 15,879 posts, Li et al. (2018b) classified 6% as reflecting depression-related stigma. Of these, the most frequent stigmatizing views depicted people with depression as unpredictable (39.3%), with depression presented as a sign of personal weakness (15.8%). Using a random sample of Twitter feeds, Robinson et al. (2019) assessed stigmatizing attitudes across five mental and five physical health conditions over 10, 72-hour windows in a 50-day period (1,300 tweets per condition). More posts in the sample stigmatized mental health conditions (12.9%) and trivialized mental health (14.3%) compared to physical health conditions (8.1 and 6.8%, respectively). Schizophrenia and HIV were the most stigmatized conditions in this study. These three studies provided examples of how social media blogs can transmit stigma and misinformation.

Youth have increasingly used social media platforms to post messages about their personal distress and suicidal ideation. Intahchomphoo (2018) reviewed the literature linking social media use to youth suicide between 2008 and 2016 (n=65 studies). Intahchomphoo found that social media posts have been used to encourage and pressure youth toward suicide through pro-suicide messages, cyberbullying, sexting (particularly sextortion), and by providing detailed information on self-harming techniques. Intahchomphoo's review demonstrated that we can easily find pro-suicide videos, some containing explicit and visually graphic content. Not only can such messaging hasten the planning process; it can also provide a forum for the development of suicide pacts.

At the same time, social media affords the opportunity to run prevention awareness campaigns targeting at-risk groups such as youth. Through group chats, social media can also facilitate support for youth facing mental health crises and provide information on the availability of crisis hotlines. Latha et al. (2020) evaluated the effectiveness of social media platforms in hosting three health promotion campaigns. One of the campaigns – *Buddies for Suicide Prevention* – was designed to create awareness for suicide prevention through script writing, slogan writing, poster making, and short film making organized for the public who wanted to participate. The campaign engaged Facebook and Instagram for five months. The posts received 32 likes and reached 2,058 people, showing that social media can be a powerful tool for spreading awareness. However, Pourmand et al. (2019) reported that, between 2007 and 2014, the number of websites including information on suicide methods tripled; whereas those designed to provide support to those thinking about suicide decreased by half.

Music

Music and song can also create and reinforce narratives about the nature of mental illnesses, and different musical genres have been linked to different representations. For example, both popular music and opera have been prolific in their presentations linking madness and suicide; whereas country music has more often linked alcohol use to suicide (Pavez et al., 2017).

In addition to the music, the musicians themselves have also represented various degrees of mental illness and substance use, and many have died as a result. Pavlova (2017, p. 13) argued that the music business has commercialized "the mad musician gimmick" for their own profit. One lucrative genre presented in music has been the mad musician genius, where the industry characterizes inspiration as an uncontrollable product of genius. The model of divine madness portrays the artist as gifted, lonely, separated from society, and cursed by inspiration and talent. This image occurs most prominently in rock and heavy metal, where it may be taken to the extreme.

Real-life examples of artists that struggle with mental illnesses or who have succumbed to them provide vivid support for the mad musician model and, in the case of overdose deaths or suicide, may touch off a contagion. Countervailing forces from popular music artists who have spoken out about their mental ill-health and used their music to portray their experiences may be signaling a new wave of mental health awareness activism (see also Chapter 15, this volume). Chan (2023) noted that musicians are increasingly speaking out to destigmatize mental health issues. For example, Adele and Alanis Morissette have spoken about their experiences with postpartum depression, and Guns N' Roses' Duff McKagan has described his experience of panic attacks. Bruce Springsteen has opened up about his father's schizophrenia and his own battles with mental illness. They believe that sharing their experiences will encourage the millions of fans that follow their work. Despite these attempts to destigmatize mental illnesses, Partridge (2020) argued that the master cultural narrative expressed through popular music and song is not predominantly altruistic but dark and introspective, exploring self-hatred, mental illness, and suicidality.

Musical theater has featured two dominant representations: the "personification model" and the "fragmentation model" (Perry, 2023, pp. 5–6). In the personification model, the mental illness becomes a character unto itself, separate from the person with the mental illness. This new character appears only to the audience and the person – not the other characters on the stage. The interactions between the person and the illness (often presented by a separate performer) position the mental illness as an antagonist that constantly works against the character, driving the person to make poor, irrational, and harmful decisions. This model reduces the representation of mental illness to the interactions between the illness and the person, effectively villainizing it. The fragmentation model depicts a character split into multiple performers who undergo a fractured state stemming from the mental illness. In some cases, the fragmented characters can remain on stage and work as one, providing a more holistic representation of how people with a mental illness are able to manage their symptoms and live successful lives in conjunction with their illness characters.

Both models use musical content and staging to create their effects. For example, Perry (2023) described the use of music in Dave Malloy's 2015 *Preludes*, where the main character confided symptoms of depression to his hypnotherapist. The fragmented music echoed the emotional distress of the character. At times, the piano chord progression created a sense of tonal motionlessness, illustrating the character's depression. When the character faced his trauma, the music became overwhelming and abrasive. Near the end of the show, the musical fragmentation lifted, and the music became melodical, signifying relief as the character worked through his trauma and depression.

According to Borecky (2019), serial crime dramas use music and sound to enhance the audience's emotions of disgust and intensify violent scenes, reinforcing the repeated demonization of mental illnesses that occur throughout the dramas. Far from illustrating the possibility and nature of recovery, as in some musical theater, in the serial killer crime drama, music plays a colluding role in linking mental illness to violence and heightens audience fear and disgust. For example, according to Borecky, *Criminal Minds* often juxtaposed romantic or soft music (such as Chicago's 1984 "You're the Inspiration") with scenes of horrific violence to create "semantic disturbance" resulting from the conflicting meanings that are generated between seeing and hearing (p. 8).

Language

According to Jacobs and Quinn (2022), language lies at the heart of popular culture. Words hold the power to transmit a negative or positive value judgment, either explicitly or implicitly. Our cognitive schemas about mental illnesses and the mentally ill facilitate the spread and reinforcement of stigmas. Individual cognitive biases shape the way that individuals remember information and share it through discourse and narratives present in newspapers, entertainment, and social media.

When ordinary language contains sensationalist words, misconceptions, or negative biases, it creates and maintains stigma (Bertolín & Porcel, 2021). The words that we use to describe mental illnesses and people who have experienced a mental illness can impact the likelihood that they will seek care, diminish their quality of life, promote self-stigma, and reduce chances for recovery. In the substance use field, for example, the use of pejorative words such as *substance abuser* as opposed to someone with a *substance use disorder* can sway professionals away from providing treatment in favor of punishment (Volkow et al., 2021).

In discussing the language of mental illness, Bolinger (2021) noted that pejorative terms employed to characterize an individual (e.g., he's *crazy*) not only diminish the targeted person but also reinforce a cultural stereotype that people who get dubbed as "crazy" should be dismissed or marginalized. In this way, pejorative uses of mental illness terms inflict two wrongs: one directed at the person and the other at the group.

Over the past 15–20 years, advocates have been calling for the use of *person-first* language as a means of reducing stigma. For example, the Mental Health Commission of Canada (2023) and the National Institute of Health in the United States (2023) indicated that person-first language should be used to combat stigma related to mental illnesses and suicide. Person-first language places the person before the impairment or disability (e.g., person with a mental illness). Person-first language sets the tone for inclusion rather than isolation, and various stakeholders have increasingly called for it in legislation, policy, health practice, the media, and day-to-day personal exchanges (Jensen et al., 2013). Stuart and Sartorius (2022, p. 94) summarized the content of media guidelines from anti-stigma initiatives in Australia, Canada, New Zealand, and the United Kingdom that were developed to assist news reporters in being more reflective about the words they use to describe people with a mental health problem or situations involving suicide. (I discuss the content of these guidelines more in the next section.)

Evidence exists that such practices may be effective. For example, Whitley and Wang (2017a) analyzed newspaper articles from print and online media in 20 best-selling newspapers in Canada between 2005 and 2015 (n=24,570). Researchers rated 21% of the articles as having a positive tone and 28% as having stigmatizing content. Over the study period, positive articles doubled, and articles with stigmatizing content decreased by a third. Whitley and Wang speculated that this change could have been related to the intensive activities of the Mental Health Commission of Canada in targeting journalists and supporting them to develop and disseminate media guidelines. Whitley and Wang (2017b) reported similar improvements in television news coverage between 2013 and 2015.

Recommendations for Practice

The largely negative portrayals of mental illnesses and the mentally ill in popular media both reflect and promote societal stigma. Consequently, it is important to consider how the mental health community can work more closely with popular media to promote more accurate and positive images of people with mental illnesses and support the importance of help-seeking. This section examines recommendations for practices that have the potential to provide alternate and positive views of mental illnesses and people who experience them.

Media Reporting

As previously mentioned, out of concern for the effects of sensationalized news reporting on stigma and copycat behaviors, many countries have developed media guidelines. Stuart and Sartorius (2022) overviewed these guidelines, which show considerable consistency in messaging from one country to the next, including the use of person-first language, avoiding derogatory terms, not linking criminality or dangerousness to mental illness, relying on credible sources rather than speculating about diagnoses or causes of events, and not using negative story frames, stereotypic imagery, and sensationalized headlines. As Stuart and Sartorius pointed out, countries have differed in the way in which media guidelines have been developed and the extent to which journalists have been invited or allowed to take a leadership role. Many advocacy groups also have developed guidelines without collaboration from journalists and assumed that journalists would accept and widely use them. A best-practice model would allow journalists to take the lead with support from relevant advocacy groups and subject matter experts.

In Canada, for example, Mindset is a journalist-to-journalist guide that was researched and written on behalf of the Canadian Journalism Forum on Violence and Trauma with support from the Mental Health Commission of Canada and the Canadian Broadcasting Corporation. It is now in its third edition and is widely used (Canadian Journalism Forum on Violence and Trauma, 2020).

With respect to entertainment media, Pirkis et al. (2006) recommended that the mental health sector make a concerted effort to collaborate with producers, directors, scriptwriters, and actors to minimize negative portrayals and maximize positive portrayals of people with mental illness. Fruitful relationships between these sectors would give entrance for mental health advocates to comment on inappropriate portrayals and help correct muddled or misleading information. Juncture points, such as the Mental Health Media Partnership in the U.S., could facilitate easy access to expertise, grassroots experiences, and knowledge transfer.

Stuart and Sartorius (2022) described one example that occurred in Australia where producers and scriptwriters of a popular teenage soap opera, *Home and Away*, worked with members of the advocacy community (*SANE Australia*) and clinicians to create a storyline in which one of the main characters experienced schizophrenia. The story developed over three months, and an estimated 1.5 million people viewed the shows. *Home and Away* presented and reinforced non-stigmatizing messages and recovery behaviors. Partnering with mental health experts facilitated a realistic and positive storyline, and the show provided a helpline number and a chatline. The actor who played the character experiencing schizophrenia participated in the publicity for the campaign. In the three months following the storyline, the show garnered extensive national media coverage and a 100% increase in helpline and online contacts. The show illustrated how someone could recover from schizophrenia, transmitting the important message that schizophrenia was treatable. It also demonstrated how a likable and previously "normal" individual could subsequently experience a mental illness and how the negative effects of stigma could impact the person and the family.

Respectful Language

Widespread support exists for language change from the mental health community, particularly from people who have a mental illness, their family members, and peer advocates (Stuart & Sartorius, 2022). Several authors (e.g., Lasalvia et al., 2015; Sartorius et al., 2014) have noted that some countries have made deliberate attempts to change diagnostic terms to avoid their negative and stigmatizing effects. One example discussed by these authors is the diagnostic term for schizophrenia being changed in Japan in a deliberate attempt to reduce stigma at the request of the Japanese Federation of Families of the Mentally Ill. The original term meant something akin to *mind-split disease*, which evoked negative stereotypes of dangerousness, unpredictability, and untreatability. In 2002, the Japanese Society of Psychiatry and Neurology changed the name of schizophrenia to reflect an *integration disorder*, considered to give a better impression about the treatability of the condition. As Sartorius et al. have noted, the name change was accompanied by a complete reformulation of the disorder by the Japanese Society of Psychiatry and Neurology, raising the question of whether language change alone suffices to erase negative imagery. In any case, Lasalvia et al. reported that the new terminology and reformulation made it easier for psychiatrists to inform patients and families of their diagnosis and facilitated education about the illness and use of psychosocial interventions. The increase in the percentage of people who were told about their diagnosis changed from 7% in 2002 to 70% in 2004.

Cheung (2018) suggested that, amid the ongoing debate about whether people with a mental illness who are receiving treatment constitute "patients," "consumers," "clients," "survivors," "service users," or "self-advocates," we are beginning to realize the power of letting people self-identify. Empowering people to use the terms that they prefer, rather than the terms that mental health providers have conferred, provides an opportunity to redress historical power imbalances (as those who confer a label have power) and begin the journey toward self-determination. It also recognizes that one size doesn't fit all. No term will work for everyone, so critical examination of our word choices when we speak about mental illnesses and speak to people living with mental illness is an important and potentially powerful stigma reduction strategy.

Inclusivity and Social Media

With the notable exception of *Home and Away*, people who live with mental illnesses and who, therefore, have expertise in managing their illness on a day-to-day basis seldom get included in the development of journalistic or fictional portrayals. In many cases, popular culture also excludes them from activities, such as mental health literacy or anti-stigma activities, that are explicitly designed to reduce social distance and improve inclusivity. Such exclusion implicitly places them in the position of receiving the good intentions and beneficence of others or as token participants, rather than actively engaged in, or leading these activities.

Social media can sidestep this problem by providing an opportunity for people with lived experience to tell their stories and provide a more realistic and sympathetic narrative of living with a mental illness. Betton et al. (2015) provided a striking example of how social media can be used by people with a mental illness to challenge negative and hurtful stereotypes. In 2023, thousands of people voiced their displeasure and offense about a Halloween costume that stereotyped a 'mental patient' (complete with meat cleavers, blood, and masks) advertised by a national supermarket chain in the UK (see BBC, 2013). Tweets rapidly went viral and criss-crossed various networks. The next day, the story comprised the lead item on the national news, indicating that mainstream media sourced their stories from Twitter. The supermarket in question and other retailers removed the costumes from sale. The supermarket apologized and made donations to England's *Time to Change* anti-stigma program. During the protest, people with lived experience of a mental illness posted selfies alongside text such as "this is what a real mental patient looks like." Posters used the hashtag almost 7,000 times in the span of 24 hours.

The media storm illustrated the democratizing and catalyzing effects of social media. In this case, Twitter users shared personal stories, ultimately influencing mainstream reporting and organizational behavior. This situation demonstrates that social media can be used to include and amplify individual voices to change the social narrative.

Future Directions

The *sledgehammer sensationalism* that has typically characterized depictions of mental illnesses in TV and the movies is starting to give way to more nuanced representations with occasionally sensitive movies such as *Silver Linings Playbook* or *A Beautiful Mind* (Lunn, 2020). The development of coalitions between mental health experts and media sources could encourage this trend with more accurate portrayals of people living with mental illnesses, the efficacy of supports, services, and treatments, as well as the possibilities for recovery. Both news and entertainment media could highlight some of the more structural factors that result in vast inequities in timely access to care for people with mental illness, as well as geographic inequities within and across countries. Changing the way in which people with mental illnesses are portrayed could have important impacts on public perceptions, which, in turn, could impact the perceptions people with mental illness have of themselves, as well as the social supports needed to support them.

As part of this effort, it is important to create a bank of credible information and expert contacts that can be quickly accessed by individuals creating media content. This resource bank may be particularly useful for reporters who have limited time to create stories when news events occur. While media guidelines have been created by a number of groups across the world, we need additional data on their effectiveness. Efforts to understand their key ingredients for success and barriers to their effective use could provide important information sufficient to reframe stories and minimize contagion.

Social media can reach a vast number of people quickly. In the future, more consideration could be given to the potential of social media to direct people experiencing a mental health crisis and who may be planning suicide to appropriate supports. Research in this area is just beginning to emerge.

For example, in their literature review, Robinson et al. (2016) identified only two studies that specifically targeted individuals who were suicidal to provide information on treatment and support resources. Another study included in their review (see Silenzio et al., 2009) found that a peer-driven preventative intervention was able to reach more than 18,000 individuals – a significantly larger number than could be reached through conventional means.

Anti-stigma programs increasingly use social media platforms to share their work and improve the public narrative. For example, New Zealand's *Like Minds Like Mine* Facebook page has featured a stigma watch component where members post and discuss media postings of concern that contain stigmatizing content. Australia's *Beyond Blue* has provided space for people to tell their personal stories of illness and recovery. The most promising aspect of advocacy proponents' use of social media entails how one story can go viral and be picked up by conventional media and backed by anti-stigma and other organizations in the mental health space. Social media allows individual experiences to be amplified such that spontaneous bursts of protest can bring about significant change in organizational behaviors (Stuart & Sartorius, 2022).

In addition to protest, social media platforms could also could be used to provide corrective information and to root out and eliminate misinformation. Smith and Seitz (2019) demonstrated the possibility of correcting misinformation using a fake Facebook feed in a survey-based experiment of 744 MTurk participants in the United States. Smith and Seitz provided participants with positive correcting information that changed their attitudes, while those provided with confirmatory misinformation retained their negative views. Their findings supported the immediate use of corrective messaging via social media. With the increasing use of artificial intelligence and the growing sophistication of natural language processing, both misinformation and people at risk of acting on misinformation could be identified for preventive intervention and corrective messaging (see also Chapter 11, this volume). After identifying susceptible sub-groups (such as youth on platforms sharing mental distress), public health gatekeeper interventions could be used to direct individuals to correct information and appropriate support services. Posts could also be monitored for concerning content (such as instructions on how to commit suicide) and removed or blocked.

We need to improve adherence to suicide reporting guidelines for news content presented online. Sumner et al. (2020) examined the content of over 600 news stories shared on a social networking platform. Sumner et al. determined that 60% of the articles named the individual, 59% used the word "suicide" in the title, 55% gave specific details about the place of the suicide, and 50% gave specific details about the method. They also unexpectedly found that outlets that paid closer adherence to the suicide guidelines had higher reader re-shares and positive engagement. Therefore, more robust efforts to improve safe reporting would not only have a beneficial effect for the public, but also for the publisher, who would have greater reach. In the future, the importance of safe reporting also could be widely disseminated by social media platforms. Perhaps, then, we could look forward to slow and incremental progress in the ways in which popular culture shapes the narrative of mental illness.

While the trend in the use of person-first language will likely continue, we lack clarity on the extent to which this trend can shift the current stereotypic narrative of mental illness. Scholars possess mixed opinions about whether good connotations can drive out bad, or whether innocent words eventually accumulate the negative baggage that was attached to the words they oust. Termed the *euphemistic treadmill*, the lifespan of a euphemism can be short-lived, and, in many cases, the euphemistic value of the term can be quickly diluted such that negative connotations reattach (Burridge, 2012). If, as suggested, people with a mental illness experience person-first language as more respectful and inclusive, at the very least, it may stave off their own personal stigmas and support their self-esteem. Future research will be needed to determine whether language change constitutes an efficacious tool for shifting the cultural narrative. Such incremental changes in other forms of mass media also will be needed to provide more sensitive and nuanced presentations of mental illnesses and the mentally ill in popular culture.

Final Thoughts

Popular culture comprises a powerful socializing force. Through various forms of mass media, popular culture shapes ideas about mental illnesses, people with mental illnesses, and appropriate behaviors toward them. Negative and horrifying imagery, made more vivid in movies and television, promotes social stigma, marginalization, and inequity. As well as shaping societal values, popular culture, through various communication channels, also reflects them. Content analysis of social media posts allows us a glimpse into these views and a way to monitor progress. As harmful as social media can be, it can also encompass a positive and democratizing force. It provides a place where people who have mental illnesses can share their experiences and give voice to their objections, sometimes bringing about important structural changes in the way organizations behave. The challenge for the future will be to break the cycle of misinformation and stigma that is promoted through mass media channels and supplant these with a store of more realistic and positive images that foster a respect for diversity and social inclusion.

Further Reading

Domaradzki, J. (2021). The Werther effect, the Papageno effect or no effect? A literature review. *International Journal of Environmental Research and Public Health, 18*, 1–21. https://doi.org/10.3390/ijerph18052396

Robinson, J., Cox, G., Bailey, E., Hetrick, S., Rodrigues, M., Fisher, S., & Herrman, H. (2016). Social media and suicide prevention: A systematic review. *Early Intervention Psychiatry, 10*, 103–121. https://doi.org/10.1111/eip.12229

Schildkraut, J. (2023). A call to the media to change reporting practices for the coverage of mass shootings. *Journal of Law & Policy, 60*, 273–272.

Stuart, H. (2006). Media portrayal of mental illness and its treatments: What effect does it have on people with mental illness? *CNS Drugs, 20*, 99–106. https://doi.org/10.2165/00023210-200620020-00002

Stuart, H., & Sartorius, N. (2022). *Paradigms lost, paradigms found. Lessons learned in the fight against the stigma of mental illness* (2nd ed.). Oxford University Press.

References

Aragonès, E., López-Muntaner, J., Ceruelo, S., & Basora, J. (2014). Reinforcing stigmatization: Coverage of mental illness in Spanish newspapers. *Journal of Health Communication, 19*(11), 1248–1258. https://doi.org/10.1080/10810730.2013.872726

BBC. (2013). Asda and Tesco withdraw Halloween patient outfits. https://www.bbc.com/news/uk-24278768

Bertolín, G. J., & Porcel, T. A. (2021). Mental health: Stigma, language and nosology. *OSP Journal of Health Care and Medicine*, 2(2), 1–6.

Betton, V., Borschmann, R., Docherty, M., Coleman, S., Brown, M., & Henderson, C. (2015). The role of social media in reducing stigma and discrimination. *British Journal of Psychiatry, 206*(6), 443–444. https://doi.org/10.1192/bjp.bp.114.152835

Bilić, B., & Georgaca, E. (2007). Representations of "mental illness" in Serbian newspapers: A critical discourse analysis. *Qualitative Research in Psychology, 4*(1–2), 167–186. https://doi.org/10.1080/14780880701473573

Bolinger, R. J. (2021). The language of mental illness. In J. Khoo & R. K. Sterken (Eds.), *The Routledge handbook of social and political philosophy of language* (pp. 389–404). Routledge. https://doi.org/10.4324/9781410606686-12

Borecky, A. J. (2019). *Music and the monster: Sounding fear and mental illness in Criminal Minds* [Master's Thesis, University of Tennessee]. https://trace.tennessee.edu/utk_gradthes

Burridge, K. (2012). Euphemism and language change: The sixth and seventh ages. *Lexis, 7*, 65–92. https://doi.org/10.4000/lexis.355

Canadian Journalism Forum on Violence and Trauma. (2020). MINDSET Reporting on mental health.

Cape, G. S. (2003). Addiction, stigma and movies. *Acta Psychiatrica Scandinavica, 107*(3), 163–169. https://doi.org/10.1034/j.1600-0447.2003.00075.x

Chan, A. (2023, October 9). Musicians who have opened up about their mental health struggles. *Bilboard.* https://news.yahoo.com/musicians-opened-mental-health-struggles-180031260.html

Cheung, I. (2018). Minding our language. *Philosophical Forum, 49*(4), 5–7.

Demme, J. (1991). *Silence of the lambs*. Orion Pictures.

Domaradzki, J. (2021). The Werther effect, the Papageno effect or no effect? A literature review. *International Journal of Environmental Research and Public Health*, *18*(5), 1–21. https://doi.org/10.3390/ijerph18052396

Eisenhauer, J. (2008). A visual culture of stigma: Critically examining representations of mental illness. *Art Education*, *61*(5), 13–18. https://doi.org/10.1080/00043125.2008.11518991

Fluck, W. (1987). Popular culture as a mode of socialization. A theory about the social functions of popular cultural forms. *The Journal of Popular Culture*, *21*(3), 31–46. https://doi.org/10.1111/j.0022-3840.1987.2103_31.x

Follman, M. (2015, November/December). Inside the race to stop the next mass shooter. *Mother Jones*, 15. https://www.motherjones.com/politics/2015/10/mass-shootings-threat-assessment-shooter-fbi-columbine/

Gharaibeh, N. M. (2005). The psychiatrist's image in commercially available American movies. *Acta Psychiatrica Scandinavica*, *111*(4), 316–319. https://doi.org/10.1111/j.1600-0447.2004.00489.x

Gwarjanski, A. R., & Parrott, S. (2018). Schizophrenia in the news: The role of news frames in shaping online reader dialogue about mental illness. *Health Communication*, *33*(8), 954–961. https://doi.org/10.1080/10410236.2017.1323320

Hall, S. (2018). Popular culture, politics and history. *Cultural Studies*, *32*(6), 929–952. https://doi.org/10.1080/09502386.2018.1521623

Hersey, C. (2005). Script(ing) treatment: Representations of recovery from addiction in Hollywood film. *Contemporary Drug Problems*, *32*(3), 467–493. https://doi.org/10.1177/009145090503200308

Hitchcock, Alfred. (1960). *Psycho*. Paramount Pictures.

Intahchomphoo, C. (2018). Social media and youth suicide: A systematic review. *Research Papers*, *13*, 1–18. https://aisel.aisnet.org/ecis2018_rp/13

Jacobs, S., & Quinn, J. (2022). Cultural reproduction of mental illness stigma and stereotypes. *Social Science and Medicine*, *292*, 1–9. https://doi.org/10.1016/j.socscimed.2021.114552

Jensen, M. E., Pease, E. A., Lambert, K., Hickman, D. R., Robinson, O., McCoy, K. T., Barut, J. K., Musker, K. M., Olive, D., Noll, C., Ramirez, J., Cogliser, D., & King, J. K. (2013). Championing person-first language: A call to psychiatric mental health nurses. *Journal of the American Psychiatric Nurses Association*, *19*(3), 146–151. https://doi.org/10.1177/1078390313489729

Klinger, A., & Klinger, A. (2018). *30 days since Parkland : School-based violent incidents and threats from School-based threats of violence : 30 days after Parkland*. The Educator's School Safety Network. www.eSchoolSafety.org

Lasalvia, A., Penta, E., Sartorius, N., & Henderson, S. (2015). Should the label "schizophrenia" be abandoned? *Schizophrenia Research*, *162*(1–3), 276–284. https://doi.org/10.1016/j.schres.2015.01.031

Latha, K., Meena, K. S., Pravitha, M. R., Dasgupta, M., & Chaturvedi, S. K. (2020). Effective use of social media platforms for promotion of mental health awareness. *Journal of Education and Health Promotion*, *9*(124), 1–6. https://doi.org/10.4103/jehp.jehp_90_20

Lawson, A., & Fouts, G. (2004). Mental illness in Disney animated films. *Canadian Journal of Psychiatry*, *49*(5), 310–314. https://doi.org/10.1177/070674370404900506

Li, A., Huang, X., Jiao, D., O'Dea, B., Zhu, T., & Christensen, H. (2018a). An analysis of stigma and suicide literacy in responses to suicides broadcast on social media. *Asia-Pacific Psychiatry*, *10*(1), 1–8. https://doi.org/10.1111/appy.12314

Li, A., Jiao, D., & Zhu, T. (2018b). Detecting depression stigma on social media: A linguistic analysis. *Journal of Affective Disorders*, *232*(16), 358–362. https://doi.org/10.1016/j.jad.2018.02.087

Lunn, O. (2020). From "Bunny Boiler" stigmas to brave storytelling, a time of mental health narratives in popular culture. *British Vogue*. https://www.vogue.co.uk/arts-and-lifestyle/article/mental-health-narrative#:~:text=From%20%27Bunny%20Boiler%27%20Stigmas%20To,t%20always%20been%20the%20case

Mental Health Commission of Canada. (2023, November 15). Language matters. https://mentalhealthcommission.ca/resource/language-matters/

National Institutes of Health. (2023, November 15). Person-first and destigmatizing language. https://www.nih.gov/nih-style-guide/person-first-destigmatizing-language

Nye, R. B. (1971). Notes for an introduction to a discussion of popular culture. *Journal of Popular Culture*, *4*(4), 1031–1038.

Ohiagu, O. P., & Okorie, V. O. (2014). Social media: Shaping and transmitting popular culture. *Covenant Journal of Communication*, *2*(1), 93–108. http://journals.covenantuniversity.edu.ng/index.php/cjoc/article/view/57

Owen, P. R. (2012). Portrayals of schizophrenia by entertainment media: A content analysis of contemporary movies. *Psychiatric Services*, *63*(7), 655–659. https://doi.org/10.1176/appi.ps.201100371

Parrott, S., & Parrott, C. T. (2015). Law & disorder: The portrayal of mental illness in U.S. crime dramas. *Journal of Broadcasting and Electronic Media*, *59*(4), 640–657. https://doi.org/10.1080/08838151.2015.1093486

Partridge, C. (2020). Suicide, angst, and popular music. In M. Coward-Gibbs (Ed.), *Death, culture and leisure: Playing dead* (pp. 189–208). Emerald Group Publishing Ltd. https://doi.org/10.1108/978-1-83909-037-020201020

Pavez, F., Saura, E., Perez, G., & Marset P. (2017). Social representation of psychiatry and mental disorders examined through the analysis of music as a cultural product. *Music and Medicine*, *9*(4), 247–253.

Pavlova, E. (2017). Selling madness: How mental illness has been commercialised in the music business. *Billboard*, 13–15. http://www.billboard.com/articles/news/56996/evanescence-

Perry, M. (2023). *"Voices in my head:" Representations of mental illness in contemporary American musical theatre* [Master of Music, University of Massachusetts Amherst]. https://doi.org/10.7275/35040821

Pirkis, J., Blood, R. W., Francis, C., & McCallum, K. (2006). On-screen portrayals of mental illness: Extent, nature, and impacts. *Journal of Health Communication*, *11*(5), 523–541. https://doi.org/10.1080/10810730600755889

Pourmand, A., Roberson, J., Caggiula, A., Monsalve, N., Rahimi, M., & Torres-Llenza, V. (2019). Social media and suicide: A review of technology-based epidemiology and risk assessment. *Telemedicine and e-Health*, 25, *10*, 880–888. https://doi.org/10.1089/tmj.2018.0203

Robinson, J., Cox, G., Bailey, E., Hetrick, S., Rodrigues, M., Fisher, S., & Herrman, H. (2016). Social media and suicide prevention: A systematic review. *Early Intervention in Psychiatry*, *10*(2), 103–121. https://doi.org/10.1111/eip.12229

Robinson, P., Turk, D., Jilka, S., & Cella, M. (2019). Measuring attitudes towards mental health using social media: Investigating stigma and trivialisation. *Social Psychiatry and Psychiatric Epidemiology*, *54*(1), 51–58. https://doi.org/10.1007/s00127-018-1571-5

Sartorius, N., Chiu, H., Heok, K. E., Lee, M. S., Ouyang, W. C., Sato, M., Yang, Y. K., & Yu, X. (2014). Name change for schizophrenia. *Schizophrenia Bulletin*, *40*(2), 255–258. https://doi.org/10.1093/schbul/sbt231

Schildkraut, J. (2023). A call to the media to change reporting practices for the coverage of mass shootings. *Journal of Law & Policy*, *60*, 273–272. https://heinonline.org/HOL/License

Silenzio, V. M. B., Duberstein, P. R., Tang, W., Lu, N., Tu, X., & Homan, C. M. (2009). Connecting the invisible dots: Reaching lesbian, gay, and bisexual adolescents and young adults at risk for suicide through online social networks. *Social Science and Medicine*, *69*(3), 469–474. https://doi.org/10.1016/j.socscimed.2009.05.029

Smith, C. N., & Seitz, H. H. (2019). Correcting misinformation about neuroscience via social media. *Science Communication*, *41*(6), 790–819. https://doi.org/10.1177/1075547019890073

Stuart, H. (2006). Media portrayal of mental illness and its treatments: What effect does it have on people with mental illness? *CNS Drugs*, *20*(2), 99–106. https://doi.org/10.2165/00023210-200620020-00002

Stuart, H., & Sartorius, N. (2022). *Paradigms lost, paradigms found. Lessons learned in the fight against the stigma of mental illness* (2nd ed.). Oxford University Press.

Sumner, S. A., Burke, M., & Kooti, F. (2020). Adherence to suicide reporting guidelines by news shared on a social networking platform. *Proceedings of the National Academy of Sciences of the United States of America*, *117*(28), 16267–16272. https://doi.org/10.1073/pnas.2001230117

Volkow, N. D., Gordon, J. A., & Koob, G. F. (2021). Choosing appropriate language to reduce the stigma around mental illness and substance use disorders. *Neuropsychopharmacology*, *46*(13), 2230–2232. https://doi.org/10.1038/s41386-021-01069-4

Whitley, R., & Berry, S. (2013). Trends in newspaper coverage of mental illness in Canada: 2005-2010. *Canadian Journal of Psychiatry*, *58*(2), 107–112. https://doi.org/10.1177/070674371305800208

Whitley, R., & Wang, J. W. (2017a). Good news? A longitudinal analysis of newspaper portrayals of mental illness in Canada 2005 to 2015. *Canadian Journal of Psychiatry*, *62*(4), 278–285. https://doi.org/10.1177/0706743716675856

Whitley, R., & Wang, J. W. (2017b). Television coverage of mental illness in Canada: 2013–2015. *Social Psychiatry and Psychiatric Epidemiology*, *52*(2), 241–244. https://doi.org/10.1007/s00127-016-1330-4

4
FOOD IN POPULAR CULTURE

Alane Presswood

It is summer 2023, and I'm rewatching HBO's *Game of Thrones.* I'm not teaching this summer, so my days are largely unscheduled, and one of the best parts about working in communication and media studies has always been the ability to claim that time spent immersed in popular culture artifacts counts as work. I am struck by how young the Stark siblings look, far more so than when I watched the HBO fantasy epic as it aired live in 2011. This awareness makes me more attuned to how Sansa Stark's fondness for lemon cakes throughout the show's first season symbolizes her character's youth, sweetness, and naivete – and her slow loss of interest in the treat accompanies the loss of that innocence.

To reach the show on Max (the streaming service formerly known as HBO Max), I have to click past a long list of cooking and food competition titles: *Diners, Drive-Ins, and Dives; BBQ USA; Beat Bobby Flay; Worst Cooks in America* … HBO's parent company Warner Media merged with Discovery, Inc. in 2022, and now legacy HBO shows like *The Wire* live nestled next to unscripted Food Network content. When initial Covid-19 shutdowns in 2020 brought about unprecedented logistical challenges for the entertainment industry, David Zaslav (then the CEO of Discovery) praised the ingenuity of home-produced, unscripted lifestyle programming on the Food Network and the Cooking Channel, saying that shows produced by hosts in their own homes "[felt] significantly more authentic" and "the audience is going with it" (Hayes, 2020).

Despite the whiplash that I feel at seeing multiple Emmy-award winning dramatic series slotted next to Guy Fieri, Zaslav's actions reflect the truth that food television is now the fastest-growing subgenre of unscripted television (O'Connell, 2019). The Food Network alone boasts more than 560 shows on its official roster of programming. Combined with their competitor The Cooking Channel and original programming like Netflix's *Nailed It* or Bravo's *Top Chef,* the thrall of food and cooking programming is undeniable. Offerings include vehicles for aging actresses and performers like Valerie Bertinelli, Patricia Heaton, and Trisha Yearwood; increasingly ludicrous competition shows for professional chefs and amateurs alike; snappy educational shows on food science hosted by trained chefs like David Chang or Samin Nosrat, who seamlessly cross the divide between the culinary and media industries; and high production value documentaries like *Chef's Table.*

Elsewhere, in the summer 2023, news outlets were briefly enamored with the concept of "girl dinner," sparked by TikTok user Olivia Maher. Maher posted a video of a simple bread and cheese spread in May 2023, labeled it "girl dinner" and joked about its similarity to "medieval peasant" food as often depicted in fiction. The concept immediately struck a chord; the hashtag #girldinner

DOI: 10.4324/9781003436409-5

now has 1.4 billion views on TikTok, and the discourse about what exactly counts as girl dinner has grown equally fast. Roy (2023) explained that "girl dinner represents a conscious choice to opt out of the tyranny of cooking and doing the dishes ... [it's] made by one person, for the consumption and enjoyment of one person" (para. 14). Yet, what exactly counts as girl dinner? Some posters explained that the crux of the idea lies in its low-effort nature and asserted that girl dinner comprises whatever can be grabbed out of the fridge without thought or laborious preparation: leftover pasta, pickles, applesauce, hardboiled eggs, cold cuts ... Others looked askance at some of the more artfully curated, charcuterie-esque "girl dinner" plates, worried that the style of dining was barely masked disordered eating and that its celebratory moment in pop culture would promote calorie restriction and other harmful behaviors.

For me, seeing what other women put on their plates scratches the itch that I always feel to understand how other people act, behave, and consume when they are home alone. However, what do these examples collectively say about the intersection of food and popular culture (other than that this author maybe spends too much time watching television)? Popular culture can be a difficult subject to nail down. Parasecoli (2014) defined popular culture as:

> the totality of ideas, values, embodied experiences, representations, material items, practices, social relations, organizations, and institutions that are conceived, produced, experienced, and reciprocally connected within environments influenced by markets and consumption, with or without the specific economic goal of reaping a profit.
>
> *(p. 323)*

When it comes to the intersections of food and health, popular culture offers a seemingly unlimited number of examples to draw from: film, television, literature, social media, advertising, and more all provide ample fodder for the exploration of how popular culture depictions of food and eating impact the choices we make regarding our own physical and mental health.

However, when exploring *food* and popular culture – as opposed to, say, religion, sport, or romance – we cannot avoid the fact that food is necessary for continued existence. So, how do we come to understand the role of a subject with significant material implications on our physical health that also constitutes a frequent metaphorical stand-in for culture, connection, for family, and power? This chapter examines both the emotional and physical dimensions of food's relationship to health and wellbeing as depicted in popular culture.

Emotional and Social Well-Being

In the 2007 romantic comedy *Waitress* (and its 2016 Broadway adaptation of the same name), Jenna, a reluctantly pregnant waitress scheming to escape her abusive husband, used her talent for baking pies to cope with and express her feelings. Immediately after taking the pregnancy test, Jenna closed her eyes and described "bad baby pie" to her friends: "a quiche of egg and brie cheese with a smoked ham center." Later, in bed after a fight with her husband, she thought about "Pregnant, miserable, self-pitying loser pie: lumpy oatmeal with fruitcake mashed in. Flambé, of course."

Jenna's tactic illustrates Lawson's (2009) assertion that people use food "to perform the self and employ autobiographical strategies to reveal aspects of their personal domestic lives to their audience" ("Confessing the Self" section, para. 2). Food – the ingredients we use, the recipes we share, the restaurants we patronize, the conversations we participate in – entails a crucial part of how we express individuality and assert our identity. Sometimes those messages express who we are or believe ourselves to be; other times they communicate how we want to act or the positions that we endorse. Because "food represents a discursive constellation of power and knowledge," food choices reveal what group we consider ourselves to belong to, who our allies are, and who we sit in opposition to (Mikulak, 2013, p. 85). To return to *Game of Thrones* for another example, friends repeatedly gave the youngest Stark daughter Arya a wolf-shaped pastry to quietly signal their loyalty to her family as she embarked on a dangerous journey. Food discourse in popular culture, ranging broadly from film and television to marketing and advertising campaigns, reveals how we connect the purchase, preparation, and consumption of food to matters of personal identity, gender, cultural history and belonging, and family dynamics – a constantly renegotiated array of understandings about who we are and how we fit in with the people around us.

Food and Consumption as Indicators of Personal Identity

In real life, consumers purchase and consume goods and services in ways that serve to consolidate and validate their personal identity (Pierce et al., 2003; Sirgy, 1985). According to Zhu et al. (2019), consumers can achieve self-congruity by consuming a brand with an image/personality that aligns with either their actual or ideal self. Actual self-congruency may occur when a functional brand's "utilitarian" qualities fit with the consumer's perception of their actual self, and ideal self-congruity may occur when a symbolic brand's "value-expressive" qualities fit with the consumer's perception of their ideal self. Simply put, when the foods we purchase, eat, and share reaffirm what we already know about ourselves, we feel good; however, when our choices contradict existing parts of our self-image, it leads to conflict (Reed et al., 2012).

For example, in April 2023, trans influencer Dylan Mulvaney (who grew a popular following on TikTok through her "Days of Being a Girl" series, wherein she chronicled her process of coming out as a trans woman and her day-to-day life) posted a sponsored video promoting Bud Light that included a can with a photo of her on it. Bud Light immediately received vitriolic protest from swaths of conservative beer drinkers, who protested the brand's decision to go "woke" and felt abandoned by their champion beverage. Bud Light sales dropped precipitously, with the brand actually losing its long-standing status as the top-selling beer in the nation (Brooks, 2023). Musician Kid Rock filmed himself shooting cases of Bud Light in protest, and countless copycat videos of outraged men committing violence against cans of beer followed (Holpuch, 2023).

Other brands have found their alignment with patrons' political identities similarly fraught. When Goya Foods CEO Robert Unanue made a public statement in spring 2020 stating that the U.S. was "truly blessed … to have a leader like President Trump, who is a builder" (Taylor, 2020, para. 4), Unanue's remarks brought swift criticism from a variety of public figures. Actor, activist, and playwright Lin-Manuel Miranda tweeted, "We learned to bake bread in this pandemic, we can learn to make our own adobo con pimienta. Bye" (Lin-Manuel Miranda [@Lin_Manuel], 2020). Similarly, Representative Alexandria Ocasio-Cortez retweeted news of the press conference with the caption, "Oh look, it's the sound of me Googling 'how to make your own Adobo'" (Alexandria Ocasio-Cortez [@AOC], 2020).

Opponents were upset that a brand like Goya, which holds particular importance for immigrants from Latin America, would praise Trump when the former president was personally and politically outspoken against immigrants. Ironically, the boycott endorsed by liberal politicians like Ocasio-Cortez sparked a corresponding counter-protest "buycott" from Trump supporters that actually resulted in a 22% short-term increase in the company's sales (Holpuch, 2023).

Food can also represent struggles for power and control in smaller cultural units, like family systems. In HBO's *Succession*, the wealthy Roy family (fictional media moguls analogous to the real-life Murdochs, who own Fox News) hold top-tier access to the best food and restaurants imaginable. Rao (2023) noted that, "for those [characters] with meaningful status in 'Succession,' food doesn't exist for pleasure or nourishment—it barely exists at all" (para. 5). Rejecting food demonstrates the tightly exercised control that correlates with success in this cutthroat world, and learning the cues of the moneyed elite surrounding when (not) to eat marks one of the easiest ways for characters who come late to the party of wealth and status to demonstrate hard-earned lessons of belonging (McCarthy, 2021; Pérez, 2023). Those on the periphery of belonging are among the fastest to weaponize knowledge about consumption; Tom Wambsgans, the husband of the only Roy daughter and a man well-acquainted with being shunned by people with more power, quickly observed when a younger family member's clueless date is "wolfing all the canapés like a famished warthog" (Rao, para. 6). Kintner et al. (1981) found a significant relationship between dysfunctional families and disordered or dysfunctional systems of eating; when family is a place of trauma, rather than a place of safety, food loses its ability to nurture and becomes just one more battleground to navigate dangerous dynamics.

As a point of contrast, dinner played a pivotal role in helping one family come together and make peace with the reality of their situation in Netflix's *Don't Look Up.* After spending the majority of the film trying and failing to raise awareness and find a solution for the impending impact of a large comet that could throw the planet off its orbit, the protagonists of the film – several astronomers and their family – gathered around a dinner table. Their conversation remained conspicuously mundane as the scene cut between the cozy domesticity of their dinner table and reaction shots around the world of the beginnings of the comet's impact. "The apple pie is actually storebought, but you really can't tell," one diner noted. "If I'm to be completely honest, which at this point, why not, I actually like the junky taste of storebought better than homemade," another responded. Amid some lighthearted protestations, another friend joined in: "I know what he means, it's like a childhood memory thing." The thing of it is … we really did have everything, didn't we? I mean, if you think about it." Everything boiled down to a quiet hour or two together, around a table, coming together over nostalgic foods and precious memories.

Food and the Performance of Gender

Food provides strong connections to political identity and group affiliation in part because it aligns with strong cultural messages about gender roles and expected behavior (Belasco, 2008; Swenson, 2009). Inness (2001) explained that gender coding in food and kitchen culture extends far beyond cookbooks, televised cooking shows, and women's magazines – indeed, candy bars, TV dinners, and even cultural texts that might at the outset seem to have little to do with food all reveal deeply embedded details of our own social kitchen culture.

Whether depicted in film, television, literature, marketing, or education, gendered categories, portrayals, or understandings of food are far from arbitrary; indeed, "the control of food production and consumption is inextricably tied up with issues of power and position" (Julier & Lindenfeld, 2005, p. 4). According to Swenson (2009), "cooking culture has made gender a natural and normal part of discourse about the kitchen" (p. 39). Gendered depictions of kitchen culture often reveal deep insecurities that permeate through multiple levels of society:

> Assumptions about male and female food predilections are so ingrained that they are hardly noticed. Hiding in plain sight are expectations that women are more preoccupied with dieting, more likely to be vegetarian, more worried about health altogether. Men are widely assumed to like meat in general, steak in particular, and such things as hot sauce or milk, while women are supposed to prefer light and insubstantial food, but also desserts, chocolate, and candy.
>
> *(Freedman, 2021, p. 106)*

More often than not, published food discourse and cooking advice promote quite conservative, traditional views on gender and sexuality (Vester, 2015). Accordingly, the associations made between women and various food items in popular culture reflect conflicting and difficult-to-achieve ideals of femininity. Popular culture codes light fare like salads and vegetables as feminine to promote adherence to popular beauty standards of a lean, trim, disciplined body and associates confections like cake and candy with the expectations that women are demure and sweet – just recall the nursery rhyme proclaiming that little girls are made of "sugar and spice and everything nice" (Cairns et al., 2010; Nathanson, 2015; Presswood, 2019). Decades after Carrie and Miranda ate them in a season 3 episode of *Sex and the City* in July 2000, Magnolia Bakery's pink cupcakes still represent a specific aspirational brand of single-urban-womanhood (Levy, 2018).

If sweet and light fare are culturally associated with femininity, men and masculinity are connected with meat – particularly substantial, unmanipulated cuts of red meat like steaks and ribs – to emphasize their culturally assigned role as predators and providers (Contois, 2020). This connection between men, masculinity, and meat spans decades and cultures and reflects beliefs that the male body is naturally larger and stronger than the female body, as well as beliefs that red meat comprises a status symbol reflecting financial success and comfort (Contois, 2020; Harbottle, 2004; Rozin et al., 2012).

Of course, the prevalence and predominance of gendered food scripts do not mean that these associations are natural or inevitable; they are still culturally constructed and subject to the limiting influence of our heteronormative and patriarchal culture. Lettuce is not inherently for women any more than a ribeye steak is innately better suited for men. However, the food itself is real; timeless, material, natural. While some consumers might find gendered associations with food constraining, others find them a useful shortcut for impression management. Neuhaus (2003) found that performing gender through food choices and kitchen culture allows individuals to adhere to social norms, reducing cognitive load and smoothing social cohesion. According to Contois, these contradictions between choice and obligation, the material and the symbolic, are precisely what renders food a "uniquely meaningful and anxious arena within consumer culture" (p. 130).

Food as Demonstration of Cultural Identity and Social Power

In addition to revelations about gender, social behaviors, and political power, food provides a way to navigate cultural identity and belonging, especially for members of minoritized populations.

The pilot episode of ABC's *Fresh Off the Boat*, a family sitcom based on the life of chef Eddie Huang as his family adjusted to a new life after moving to Orlando from Washington, D.C. in the 1990s, prominently featured what is often referred to in immigrant culinary circles as the "lunchbox moment."

> The lunchbox moment has become such a touchstone both because it's recognizable for many and because it's an editor's dream. It cleanly illustrates, in personal essays, children's books, or standup routines, how food that's delicious in the context of the home becomes disgusting in public, the moment a brown child recognizes this divide, and the heartbreak of the child (usually) choosing to perform whiteness rather than get bullied again."
>
> *(Saxena, 2021, para. 3)*

Eddie became upset on his first day at his new middle school when, just as he thought that he had started to bond with his new classmates, they recoiled in disgust when he pulled out his packed lunch: "What is that? It's gross … Ying Ding's eating worms! Dude, that smells nasty!" Eddie's white classmates jeered over his meek protestations of, "It's Chinese food … my mom made it." Eddie ended up eating lunch "outside, with the janitor." At home, Eddie implored his mother to buy him Lunchables: "I need white-people lunch," he explained. "That gets me a seat at the table. And then you get to change the rules … I'm not trying to eat with the janitor for the rest of my life" (Shelton, 2018). Eddie learned the next day that not even bringing a Lunchable enabled him to gain access to the whiteness he sought – another student threw a racial slur at him at lunch and reminded him that, as a student of color and the new kid, he sat the lowest in the power hierarchy of the middle school cafeteria.

In a nonfictional example, popular cookbook author and YouTube host Priya Krishna explained that, after a classmate said her lunchbox smelled like "rotten curry," she asked her mom for peanut butter and jelly sandwiches for lunch (Naik, 2020). It might be hard for some readers to conceptualize children facing a backlash for bringing Asian noodle dishes to a school cafeteria, given the current ubiquity of Asian American cuisine in the U.S. More than 45,000 Chinese takeout restaurants operate in the U.S.; more restaurants than all the McDonald's, KFCs, Pizza Huts, Taco Bells, and Wendy's in the country combined (Feng, 2021).

However, just like our gendered associations with food grow and change, the cultural experiences of food and dining are dynamic and can evolve quickly, even for characters in the examples cited above. On *Fresh Off the Boat,* Eddie's younger brother had no trouble with his Chinese bagged lunch at school. Veit (2013) explained that in the early 20th century, some considered the concept of foods like stews – anything with many ingredients and sauces mixed in one dish – to be dangerously foreign and likely to "imperil digestion" (p. 123). Today, those classifications include undeniably American staples like chili, lasagna, and broccoli casserole. Other immigrant cuisines face similar arcs from the unimaginably foreign to the everyday as they grow in popularity in a new context or location.

Film and television can ease the transition of these cultures and cuisines from foreign to familiar. Studio Ghibli movies constitute one such source of exposure to a cuisine that differs from what many white American children experience at home. The studio has produced 22 animated feature-length films since 1985, including favorites like *My Neighbor Totoro*, *Ponyo*, *Howl's Moving Castle*, *Princess Mononoke*, and the 2003 winner of the Academy Award for Best Animated Feature, *Spirited Away*. Retired director and studio co-founder Hayao Miyazaki's final film, *The Boy and The Heron*, earned $12.8 million in its opening weekend in December 2023, making it the first original anime title in history to top the North American box-office chart (McClintock, 2023). Hui (2020) explained that "Studio Ghibli's food portrayal tends to be associated with a whole range of positive emotional appeals from palatability (the bacon and eggs in *Howl's Moving Castle*), to healing power (Chihiro and the rice balls), to warmth and transformation (Ponyo and the ham)" (p. 118).

Ghibli movies feature loving, artfully crafted portrayals of Japanese dishes like onigiri, ramen, and bento, all things Japanese children might be likely to bring to school in a lunchbox. Animations of a single plate or dish often contain the level of artistic skill or detail one might expect to see dedicated to an entire background illustration (Cavallaro, 2015, p. 146). Entwining these beautiful images tightly within characters' narrative arcs and journeys toward conflict resolution reduces the "foreignness" of such dishes and helps young Americans approach new cuisines with empathy and curiosity. Wright-Ruiz (2023) asserted:

> The narratives [in Ghibli movies] slow down to accommodate the cooking, eating, and sharing of food … From the tiniest details of a cooking sequence, like an eight-year-old chopping vegetables in a way that suggests she's had to do it for years because of an absent parent… the focus on preparing and enjoying food seems to make these animated worlds come to life.
> *(para. 6)*

Because the United States, and Hollywood particularly, comprise such prolific and influential producers of cultural content, American children often do not encounter media and traditions from other cultures until young adulthood, at which point forms like film and literature can take on a lingering academic/intellectualized status (Darling-Wolf, 2015). Food, with its multi-sensory tangibility and its connections to everyday living, can be an accessible entry point into understanding and accepting other cultures.

The lunchbox moment experienced a playful inversion in summer 2023 as workers in China embraced the hashtag #whitepeoplefood, uploading pictures of lunches containing raw vegetables, deli meats, and dry crackers as a humorous jab at white Western culture – described as an "insult to gastronomy" by some young Chinese professionals (Cao & Feng, 2023). The mostly good-natured trend arose to poke fun at the casual, on-the-go way many Westerners eat, particularly when at school or work; "compared with the warm, flavorful and elaborately prepared food people from China are used to, meals made with a handful of cold and unseasoned ingredients can seem underwhelming or just plain inedible" (Liu et al., 2023, para. 4). One Japanese student explained that "I was kinda surprised that I saw people just bringing veggies in ziplock for lunch when I was an exchange student in the States," as many Asian cultures historically placed a higher value on eating warm, home-cooked food for all meals (as opposed to the cold sandwiches commonly found in the U.S.) (Wong, 2023, para. 19).

Other captions seen on photos shared to the #whitepeoplefood hashtag included "Food of suffering" and "What death must feel like" (Liu et al., 2023, para. 5). These pointed critiques can call to mind decades of bias against traditional Chinese foods as part of the U.S.'s long history of anti-immigrant bias, but participants in the trend also genuinely acknowledged the convenience of these low-effort lunches, alleviating guilt when workers didn't have time to dedicate to savoring a well-made meal in the middle of the day (Li, 2023). The trend showcases the humor and curiosity to be found in members of one culture adapting to both the benefits and the drawbacks of increased exposure to another culture.

Food can also serve as a way for fans of various popular culture artifacts to materially connect with the world of their fandom. Tie-in cookbooks are available for *Harry Potter*, *Star Wars*, *Game of Thrones*, *Gilmore Girls*, *Outlander*, *The Walking Dead* (questionable, in my opinion), *Orange is the New Black*, *Star Trek*, *Doctor Who*, *Firefly*, *Supernatural*, a variety of DC and Marvel properties, and more. While fans of *The Lord of the Rings* cannot experience a flight to Mordor on the back of a great eagle, they certainly can cook up "The Prancing Pony's Potato Garlic Soup" from Robert Tuesley Anderson's 2020 cookbook, *Recipes from the World of Tolkien*. As Reinhard et al. (2021) wrote,

> eating the food represented in the text allows the fan to experience a different type of emotional attachment—a more sensual attachment that allows them to increase their identification with the text [and] blur the line between their physical, everyday lives and the mediated, even fantastical, situations of the text.
>
> *(p. 10)*

Ultimately, the tangible, comfortable, shared nature of food provides fertile grounds for exploring areas that feel unfamiliar or frightening (tense family interactions, the interplay between different cultures) and creating a shareable bond or experience related to the parts of life we wish could be more prominent or longer-lasting (fantasy and fandom).

Physical Well-Being

The intersections between food and well-being are not limited to the realm of metaphor; food has literal implications on physical wellness and bodily composition as well. Popular culture plays a key role in mediating which foods are perceived as healthy or unhealthy, how much food we should consume, the impact of food on our bodies, and how food can treat or interact with other forms of physical illness.

Consumption and Cultural Understandings of Body Size

Mass communication scholars have understood for more than 50 years that television shapes the attitudes and behaviors of audiences (Alper & Leidy, 1969). Much of the foundational research into these effects, such as the report published by the Surgeon General's Scientific Advisory Committee on Television and Social Behavior (1972), was focused on the connections between violent television programming and aggressive behavior in children. However, by the early 1980s, scholars widely agreed that television could be used to model and influence prosocial behaviors as well – positive or socially desirable attitudes like altruism, friendliness, and the ability to self-regulate fear and apprehension (Lowery & Defleur, 1995). Extrapolating to a 21st century context, we also know that television viewing, social media use, and other media exposure impact the internal beliefs of audiences. For teenagers and young adults, television and digital media content have a significant impact on body image and impressions of their own sexuality and agency (Rousseau & Eggermont, 2018; Vandenbosch & Eggermont, 2012). Media influences on consumption can be explored through two seemingly opposite issues of body image: obesity and eating disorders like anorexia nervosa. As explained by Hefner et al. (2014),

> Factors such as media use and body image dissatisfaction are shared by both obesity and anorexia as potential activators, depending on the individual. These body-related concerns are not two ends of the spectrum, but rather two sides of the same coin.
>
> *(p. 190)*

In the second season of Netflix's *Heartstopper*, teenage Charlie repeatedly turned down invitations to ice cream or listlessly pushed meals around his plate. After facing bullying, an abusive partner, and a forced outing in season one, Charlie now had a family who supports him, a loving boyfriend, caring friends … and yet, as he told his concerned boyfriend Nick when he asked why Charlie wasn't eating much: "Some days I'm fine and other days I control it. I used to do it a lot last year when everything at school was really bad. Sometimes it feels like the only thing I can control in my life." (For further information on body image and popular culture, please see Chapter 5, this volume.)

Waldman (2015) wrote that "the act of starving yourself is one of the most alienating experiences you can possibly have … Starving doesn't transform your life into one glorious act of self-expression. Starving silences who you really are" (para. 55). In contrast to the ways in which food serves as a bonding agent – between lovers, between generations of family, between a diaspora and their motherland – refusing food renders a body a stranger to everything that should seem familiar, natural, good. In *Heartstopper*, when Charlie rejected Nick's proffered ice cream cone or ham sandwich, a shadow passed over the larger boy's face; the act never just involved a refusal of food itself, but a rejection of a bid for connection and caretaking.

Eating disorders occupy a contentious place in popular culture. Newman (2014) suggested that shows which attempt to leverage humor out of eating disorders often fall flat because "eating disorders and disordered eating are commonly misunderstood, whereby the sufferer is perceived as making poor choices and the depth of the disorder is not fully comprehended" (p. 241). While it is possible to effectively wring humor out of serious illness – as *Crazy Ex-Girlfriend* did with borderline personality disorder or *United States of Tara* did with dissociative identity disorders, or medical shows like *Scrubs* have done with any manner of ailments (all shows which were critically acclaimed) – the use of slapstick humor to poke fun at people with eating disorders tends to create repulsion or shame rather than commiseration and a sense of being gently seen and understood.

If not eating enough food entails a fraught minefield, then so too does eating too much food. American sitcoms often employ a "fat past" as a comedic punchline (e.g., the characters of Monica in *Friends* or Schmidt in *New Girl*). Scripts routinely reference characters' pasts as fat people to explain their current-day dating decisions, display exaggerated character traits, or simply provide comic relief (Gullage, 2014; Himes & Thompson, 2007).

Schmitz (2000) provided an alternative to fatness-as-punchline with his discussion of Jackie Gleason's iconic 1955 portrayal of Ralph Kramden in the sitcom *The Honeymooners.* Gleason created and starred in *The Honeymooners* as Ralph Kramden, a New York City bus driver. The show followed the daily exploits of Ralph, his (thin) wife Alice, and Ralph's best friend. While Ralph was regularly the subject of remarks and jokes surrounding his weight, he actively responded to and moved through those remarks, rather than being passively relegated to the butt of the joke:

> Fatness was not his essential being, not his determining reality. [Gleason] exhibited his size as the source of his energy, as the sign of his genius ... He was fat, no doubt about that, but the impression he gave was more of boundless energy, of a great deal going on beneath his smooth surface.
>
> *(Schmitz, 2000, p. 100)*

Reality television has been fertile ground for portrayals of obesity. *The Biggest Loser* ran for 17 seasons on NBC, beginning in 2004. Obese contestants competed to win a cash prize by losing the highest percentage of body weight compared to their starting weight. Over the past two decades, the show has often been criticized for its punitive tactics, and most contestants gained back the majority of the weight they lost (or ended up heavier than their starting weight). Science generally agrees that dieting, particularly if it involves severe calorie restriction, doesn't work, and weight cycling (gaining and losing large amounts of body weight repeatedly) threatens physical health more than simply maintaining a higher overall weight (see, e.g., Lowe et al., 2013). Reality television "isolates the travails of drinkers, smokers, junk food addicts, the overweight, the sedentary: those who can be seen as victims of their own lifestyle choices" (Silk et al., 2011, p. 374). Obesity and weight loss are complicated and poorly understood by the general public and many medical professionals, but reality television clings to obesity and weight loss as a moral battleground, perpetuating problems of self-acceptance and social integration for the forty-plus percent of Americans who live with obesity (Fryar et al., 2021).

Food as Medicine

Folk wisdom from cultures across the world advocates that the best cure for common ailments like a cold or flu is a steaming hot bowl of chicken soup (Alpert, 2023). It's such a well-known trope that Campbell's leans on it in their television advertising, positioning chicken soup as a loving way for mothers to treat their children's ailments (Parkin, 2006). We've already discussed the emotional healing dimensions of food. Can food heal the body as well as the soul? The medical community does support dietary intervention as a specialized treatment in specific circumstances; for example, the ketogenic diet can help control seizures in patients with medication-resistant epilepsy, and prediabetic patients are advised to reduce their risk for type two diabetes through dietary management (Sami et al., 2017; Sourbron et al., 2020). However, Freedman (2021) explained:

> Our society frames the relationship between food and health in terms of a science of nutrition, so that in theory, there should be agreed-upon evidence for beneficial versus harmful diets... [but] even when dietary advice is clear and consistent, it doesn't align with what people like to eat, or with what is being advertised or what is cheap and readily available.
>
> *(p. 89)*

While the idea of eating a balanced diet in pursuit of health *feels* logical, many consumers lack either the appropriate information about what a healthy diet is or the logistical means to access and afford one. Furthermore, substituting food for medication can set a dangerous precedent, especially when the constraints of socioeconomic status are brought into the conversation. As one notable example, Steve Jobs (former Apple CEO) briefly tried a "fruitarian" diet (a strict vegetarian regime that prioritized fruit) in early attempts to mitigate the effects of his pancreatic cancer (Isaacson, 2021). Jobs' diet didn't *cause* his cancer, but other research has linked a fruitarian diet to temporary dementia associated with vitamin B12 deficiency (Storti et al., 2021). When actor Ashton Kutcher was cast to portray the tech founder in a 2013 biopic, his attempts to mimic the diet landed him in the hospital days before filming began (Stieg, 2019).

The participation of celebrities like Jobs and Kutcher in extreme food trends contributes to a "health halo" around those choices, or "biased inference about a product's broader healthfulness based on incomplete information" (Gonzales et al., 2023, p. 244). Seeing celebrities recommend specific diets or supplements can encourage the lay public to adopt those behaviors regardless of whether they are a sensible choice within someone's individual lifestyle, and the dangers of those choices can swiftly outweigh the benefits for individuals who lack consistent access to a personal physician (for related work on celebrity health narratives, see Chapter 15, this volume).

Conclusion

In summary, representations of food in popular culture strongly impact consumers' socioemotional well-being, including our individual understandings of personal identity, gender, cultural history and belonging, and family dynamics. Food discourse in popular culture also impacts physical dimensions of individual health and well-being; film/television, advertising, social media, and celebrity culture all communicate messages about what type of body is desirable, what foods can be consumed to maintain an ideal body, and which food choices are healthy or unhealthy.

Belasco (2008) asserted that the question of "what's for dinner" can be answered by exploring three interdependent points of consideration: identity, or considerations of pleasure, preference, and creativity; responsibility, or the economic and systemic consequences of our choices; and convenience, the variables of price, availability, and ease. To that equation, this chapter has added the dimension of popular culture as the avenue through which we come to learn about these influential variables. We can't taste the food that we see on television or in internet advertisements, but it nonetheless influences how we behave and interact:

> the inclusion of culinary imagery in film creates a tension within the viewer, exciting the appetite but refusing fulfillment, drawing out desire and attaching it to objects unconnected to the slaking of one's thirst or the glutting of one's appetite.
>
> *(Keller, 2014, p. 5)*

For Health Communication scholars, these intersections between food and popular culture can be leveraged to uncover how patients are learning about healthy practices and who or what influences their choices; to understand trending popular concerns about conditions or medications; and even to explore how to situate best-practice recommendations in appropriate cultural contexts. Whether we decide to buy an extra box of Eggo frozen waffles after watching Netflix's *Stranger Things* or hit the gym a little harder after seeing those super-hero physiques in the latest Marvel movie, our choices surrounding which foods we buy, eat, and celebrate intertwine with the popular culture messaging that we consume.

References

Alexandria Ocasio-Cortez [@AOC]. (2020, July 10). Oh look, it's the sound of me Googling "how to make your own Adobo" [Tweet]. *Twitter*. https://twitter.com/AOC/status/1281383352315125762

Alper, S. W., & Leidy, T. R. (1969). The impact of information transmission through television. *Public Opinion Quarterly*, *33*(4), 556–562. https://doi-org.rlib.pace.edu/10.1086/267744

Alpert, J. S. (2023). The universal panacea: Chicken soup. *The American Journal of Medicine*, *136*(12), 1131–1132. https://doi.org/10.1016/j.amjmed.2023.02.003

Belasco, W. (2008). *Food*. Bloomsbury.
Brooks, K. J. (2023, June 15). Modelo Especial is the new top-selling beer brand in the U.S. *CBS News*. https://www.cbsnews.com/news/bud-light-no-longer-best-selling-beer-boycott-sales/
Cairns, K., Johnston, J., & Baumann, S. (2010). Caring about food: Doing gender in the foodie kitchen. *Gender & Society*, *24*(5), 591–615. https://doi.org/10.1177/0891243210383419
Cao, A., & Feng, E. (2023, July 10). This is not a joke: Chinese people are eating — and poking fun at — #whitepeoplefood. *NPR*. https://www.npr.org/sections/goatsandsoda/2023/07/10/1185780577/this-is-not-a-joke-chinese-people-are-eating-and-poking-fun-at-whitepeoplefood
Cavallaro, D. (2015). *The anime art of Hayao Miyazaki*. McFarland.
Contois, E. J. H. (2020). *Diners, dudes, and diets: How gender and power collide in food media and culture*. University of North Carolina Press Books.
Darling-Wolf, F. (2015). *Imagining the global: Transnational media and global audiences*. University of Michigan Press. https://doi.org/10.2307/j.ctv65sw7r.10
Feng, Z. (2021, November 24). What I learned eating at 8,000 Chinese restaurants. *BBC*. https://www.bbc.com/news/world-us-canada-59356176
Freedman, P. (2021). *Why food matters*. Yale University Press.
Fryar, C., Carroll, M., & Afful, J. (2021, February 5). Prevalence of overweight, obesity, and severe obesity among adults aged 20 and over: United States, 1960–1962 through 2017–2018. *CDC*. https://www.cdc.gov/nchs/data/hestat/obesity-adult-17-18/obesity-adult.htm
Gonzales, G. E., Berry, C., Meng, M. D., & Leary, R. B. (2023). Identifying and addressing the "health halo" surrounding plant-based meat alternatives in limited-information environments. *Journal of Public Policy & Marketing*, *42*(3), 242–261. https://doi.org/10.1177/07439156221150919
Gullage, A. (2014). Fat Monica, fat suits, and Friends. *Feminist Media Studies*, *14*(2), 178–189. https://doi.org/10.1080/14680777.2012.724026
Harbottle, L. (2004). *Food for health, food for wealth: Ethnic and gender identities in British Iranian communities* (1st ed.). Berghahn Books.
Hayes, D. (2020, May 11). Food Network, cooking shoots get cheaper, more timely in trend to last beyond COVID-19, Discovery CEO David Zaslav says. *Deadline*. https://deadline.com/2020/05/food-network-cooking-channel-shoots-get-cheaper-more-timely-in-a-trend-to-last-beyond-covid-19-discovery-ceo-david-zaslav-says-1202931522/
Hefner, V., Woodward, K., Figge, L., Bevan, J. L., Santora, N., & Baloch, S. (2014). The influence of television and film viewing on midlife women's body image, disordered eating, and food choice. *Media Psychology*, *17*(2), 185–207. https://doi.org/10.1080/15213269.2013.838903
Himes, S. M., & Thompson, J. K. (2007). Fat stigmatization in television shows and movies: A content analysis. *Obesity*, *15*(3), 712–718. https://doi.org/10.1038/oby.2007.635
Holpuch, A. (2023, August 16). Behind the backlash against Bud Light. *The New York Times*. https://www.nytimes.com/article/bud-light-boycott.html
Hui, G. S. (2020). Stimulating thought rather than appetite: On Takahata Isao's animation aesthetics. *The Japanese Journal of Animation Studies*, *21*(1), 111–125.
Inness, S. A. (Ed.). (2001). *Kitchen culture in America: Popular representations of food, gender, and race*. University of Pennsylvania Press.
Isaacson, W. (2021). *Steve Jobs*. Simon and Schuster.
Julier, A., & Lindenfeld, L. (2005). Mapping men onto the menu: Masculinities and food. *Food and Foodways*, *13*(1–2), 1–16. https://doi.org/10.1080/07409710590915346
Keller, J. R. (2014). *Food, film and culture: A genre study*. McFarland.
Kintner, M., Boss, P. G., & Johnson, N. (1981). The relationship between dysfunctional family environments and family member food intake. *Journal of Marriage and Family*, *43*(3), 633–641. https://doi.org/10.2307/351764
Lawson, J. (2009). Food confessions: Disclosing the self through the performance of food. *M/C Journal, 12*(5). https://doi.org/10.5204/mcj.199
Levy, N. (2018, June 6). How a 'Sex and the City' cameo for the West Village's Magnolia Bakery launched a cupcake empire. *amNewYork*. https://www.amny.com/lifestyle/eat-and-drink/sex-and-the-city-magnolia-bakery-1-19003312/
Li, L. (2023, June 21). Why 'White people food' is going viral on Chinese social media. *The Washington Post*. https://webcache.googleusercontent.com/search?q=cache:wIUKTRqDeVAJ:https://www.washingtonpost.com/world/2023/06/21/china-white-people-food-viral-social-media/&hl=en&gl=us
Lin-Manuel Miranda [@Lin_Manuel]. (2020, July 10). We learned to bake bread in this pandemic, we can learn to make our own adobo con pimienta. Bye. [Tweet]. *Twitter*. https://twitter.com/Lin_Manuel/status/1281585507743543297

Liu, D., Huang, L., & Zhao, M. (2023, July 3). Chinese social media users are not impressed with your ham sandwich. *NBC News*. https://www.nbcnews.com/news/world/china-white-people-food-rcna91547
Lowe, M. R., Doshi, S. D., Katterman, S. N., & Feig, E. H. (2013). Dieting and restrained eating as prospective predictors of weight gain. *Frontiers in Psychology*, *4*, 577. https://doi.org/10.3389/fpsyg.2013.00577
Lowery, S., & Defleur, M. (1995). *Milestones in mass communication research* (3rd ed.). Pearson.
McCarthy, A. (2021, November 22). In 'Succession,' food exists only to create more misery. *Eater*. https://www.eater.com/2021/11/22/22796396/hbo-succession-food-is-misery
McClintock, P. (2023, December 10). Box office: Hayao Miyazaki's 'The Boy and the Heron' soars to record $12.8m U.S. opening. *The Hollywood Reporter*. https://www.hollywoodreporter.com/movies/movie-news/boy-and-the-heron-box-office-opening-1235732076/
Mikulak, M. (2013). *The politics of the pantry: Stories, food, and social change*. McGill-Queen's University Press.
Naik, P. (2020, December). Priya Krishna: Cheering on Indian-ish food. *National Geographic Traveller India*, *9*(6), 24–37.
Nathanson, E. (2015). Sweet sisterhood: Cupcakes as sites of feminized consumption and production. In E. Levine (Ed.), *Cupcakes, pinterest, and ladyporn: Feminized popular culture in the early twenty-first century* (pp. 249–268). University of Illinois Press.
Neuhaus, J. (2003). *Manly meals and mom's home cooking: Cookbooks and gender in modern America*. Johns Hopkins University Press.
Newman, E. L. (2014). "It's Not okay": FX's *Starved* and eating disorders as entertainment. *The Communication Review*, *17*(3), 233–244. https://doi.org/10.1080/10714421.2014.930275
O'Connell, M. (2019, July 19). Welcome to peak food TV: Inside Hollywood's growing hunger for culinary shows. *The Hollywood Reporter*. https://www.hollywoodreporter.com/movies/movie-features/gordon-ramsay-more-hollywoods-growing-hunger-food-tv-shows-1225214/
Parasecoli, F. (2014). Food and popular culture. In P. Freedman, J. E. Chaplin, & K. Albala (Eds.), *Food in time and place: The American Historical Association companion to food history* (pp. 322–339). University of California Press.
Parkin, K. J. (2006). *Food is love: Food advertising and gender roles in modern America*. University of Pennsylvania Press.
Pérez, L. (2023, May 31). The powerful hidden message behind the food in "Succession." *Tapas*. http://www.tapasmagazine.es/en/the-powerful-occult-message-behind-the-succession-eating/
Pierce, J. L., Kostova, T., & Dirks, K. T. (2003). The state of psychological ownership: Integrating and extending a century of research. *Review of General Psychology*, *7*(1), 84–107. https://doi.org/10.1037/1089-2680.7.1.84
Presswood, A. (2019). *Food blogs, postfeminism, and the communication of expertise: Digital domestics*. Lexington Books.
Rao, T. (2023, May 16). On 'Succession,' if you're eating, you're losing. *The New York Times*. https://www.nytimes.com/2023/05/16/dining/hbo-succession-food.html
Reed, A., Forehand, M. R., Puntoni, S., & Warlop, L. (2012). Identity-based consumer behavior. *International Journal of Research in Marketing*, *29*(4), 310–321. https://doi.org/10.1016/j.ijresmar.2012.08.002
Reinhard, C. D., Largent, J. E., & Chin, B. (2021). Introduction: Food culture and fandom. In Reinhard, C. D., Largent, J. E., & Chin, B. (Eds.), *Eating fandom: Intersections between fans and food cultures* (pp. 1–14). Routledge.
Rousseau, A., & Eggermont, S. (2018). Tween television and peers: Reinforcing social agents in early adolescents' body surveillance and self-objectification. *Journal of Research on Adolescence*, *28*(4), 807–823. https://doi.org/10.1111/jora.12367
Roy, J. (2023, July 8). Is it a meal? A snack? No, it's 'girl dinner.' *The New York Times*. https://www.nytimes.com/2023/07/08/style/girl-dinner.html
Rozin, P., Hormes, J. M., Faith, M. S., & Wansink, B. (2012). Is meat male? A quantitative multimethod framework to establish metaphoric relationships. *Journal of Consumer Research*, *39*(3), 629–643. https://doi.org/10.1086/664970
Sami, W., Ansari, T., Butt, N. S., & Hamid, M. R. A. (2017). Effect of diet on type 2 diabetes mellitus: A review. *International Journal of Health Sciences*, *11*(2), 65–71.
Saxena, J. (2021, February 8). Children of immigrants all know the lunchbox moment. That doesn't mean they relate. *Eater*. https://www.eater.com/22239499/lunchbox-moment-pop-culture-tropes
Schmitz, N. (2000). Humor's body: Jackie Gleason, Roseanne, and some others. *Arizona Quarterly: A Journal of American Literature, Culture, and Theory*, *56*(2), 97–109. https://doi.org/10.1353/arq.2000.0021
Shelton, L. (Director). (2018, February 4). Pilot (1). In *Fresh Off the Boat*. ABC.

Silk, M., Francombe, J., & Bachelor, F. (2011). The biggest loser: The discursive constitution of fatness. *Intellect, 1*(3), 369–389. https://doi.org/10.1386/iscc.1.3.369_1

Sirgy, M. J. (1985). Using self-congruity and ideal congruity to predict purchase motivation. *Journal of Business Research, 13*(3), 195–206. https://doi.org/10.1016/0148-2963(85)90026-8

Sourbron, J., Klinkenberg, S., van Kuijk, S. M. J., Lagae, L., Lambrechts, D., Braakman, H. M. H., & Majoie, M. (2020). Ketogenic diet for the treatment of pediatric epilepsy: Review and meta-analysis. *Child's Nervous System: ChNS: Official Journal of the International Society for Pediatric Neurosurgery, 36*(6), 1099–1109. https://doi.org/10.1007/s00381-020-04578-7

Stieg, C. (2019, October 3). Ashton Kutcher tried Steve Jobs' all-fruit diet—And it didn't go well. *CNBC*. https://www.cnbc.com/2019/10/03/ashton-kutcher-steve-jobs-fruit-diet-health-effects.html

Storti, B., Nastasi, G., Acampora, R., Ferri, F., Isella, V., Ferrarese, C., Appollonio, I., & Tremolizzo, L. (2021). A case of reversible dementia due to a strictly fruitarian diet. *Neurology: Clinical Practice, 11*(5), e784–e786. https://doi.org/10.1212/CPJ.0000000000001005

Surgeon General's Scientific Advisory Committee on Television and Social Behavior. (1972). *Television and growing up: The impact of televised violence.* https://profiles.nlm.nih.gov/101584932X543

Swenson, R. (2009). Domestic divo? Televised treatments of masculinity, femininity and food. *Critical Studies in Media Communication, 26*(1), 36–53. https://doi.org/10.1080/15295030802684034

Taylor, D. B. (2020, July 10). Goya foods boycott takes off after CEO Bob Unanue praises Trump. *The New York Times*. https://www.nytimes.com/2020/07/10/business/goya-boycott.html

Vandenbosch, L., & Eggermont, S. (2012). Understanding sexual objectification: A comprehensive approach toward media exposure and girls' internalization of beauty ideals, self-objectification, and body surveillance: Media, adolescent girls, and self-objectification. *Journal of Communication, 62*(5), 869–887. https://doi.org/10.1111/j.1460-2466.2012.01667.x

Veit, H. Z. (2013). *Modern food, moral food: Self-control, science, and the rise of modern American eating in the early twentieth century*. University of North Carolina Press.

Vester, K. (2015). *A taste of power: Food and American identities*. University of California Press.

Waldman, K. (2015, December 7). We need to reject the false narratives around anorexia. I can start by telling my story. *Slate Magazine*. http://www.slate.com/articles/double_x/cover_story/2015/12/we_need_to_reject_the_false_narratives_around_anorexia.html

Wong, M. H. (2023, July 2). #Whitepeoplemeals: The story behind China's 'coldest' food trend. *CNN*. https://www.cnn.com/travel/article/white-people-meals-chinas-food-trend-intl-hnk/index.html

Wright-Ruiz, K. (2023, June 24). Miyazaki's magical food: An ode to anime's best cooking scenes. *Serious Eats*. https://www.seriouseats.com/studio-ghibli-anime-best-food-scenes

Zhu, X., Teng, L., Foti, L., & Yuan, Y. (2019). Using self-congruence theory to explain the interaction effects of brand type and celebrity type on consumer attitude formation. *Journal of Business Research, 103*, 301–309. https://doi.org/10.1016/j.jbusres.2019.01.055

5

POPULAR CULTURE AND THE OPPOSITIONAL GAZES OF BLACK WOMEN'S BODIES

Mister v. Celie

Rokeshia Renné Ashley

The Color Purple is a film based on Alice Walker's epistolary novel published in 1982, a winner of the 1983 Pulitzer Prize for Fiction and the American Book Award (Harris, 1984). American media has tended to only focus on a particular Black writer at a time, and, during that period, Harris hailed Walker as the spokesperson for Black women. Indeed, scholars have referred to the historical novel as the quintessential statement of Black women's experience (Bobo, 2004; Talebian Sedehi, 2014; Udoette, 2014).

Director Blitz Bazawule reimagined the novel-turned-film, stage, and Broadway play as a musical again in 2023. The cinematic presentation provided a vivid depiction of a story weaving the lives of women under the patriarchy of men: Celie (Phylicia Pearl Mpasi and Fantasia Barrino), Nettie (Halle Bailey and Ciara), Shug Avery (Taraji P. Henson), Sophia (Danielle Brooks), and Squeak or Mary Agnes (H.E.R.). Although some may not have read the novel, the 2023 film included many household-name celebrities that underscored a powerful representation of sisterhood, trauma, resilience, and grief.

This story encompassed a tale of a time, centering on race, gender, and domesticity in the actions, or lack thereof, by the protagonist Celie as she responded to the controlling grip and abusive powers of, first, her father, then her dominant husband (Ross, 1988). In the book and film's most formidable quote, Celie finally asserted her freedom, self-agency, and autonomy by exclaiming, "I'm poor, I'm Black, and I may be ugly, but I'm here." This resounding statement foregrounded the emphasis on Celie's class, self-perception, and body image. Given critiques of the book and previous film in terms of their interactions with race, feminism, abuse, and many other concepts (Bobo, 1989; Harris, 1984; Henderson, 1985), the 2023 film affords a more contemporary conversation about women's body image in general, as well as a critical lens on how Black women may be viewed.

In this chapter, I discuss the male/popular culture third-party gaze and its disdain for Black women, its impact on self-esteem, and decision-making in body modification for Black women. After situating this chapter in salient literature on body image representations, I use the characters of *The Color Purple* to illustrate the importance of body image for mental and physical well-being.

 DOI: 10.4324/9781003436409-6

Introducing *The Color Purple*

Set in the early 1900s in rural Georgia, *The Color Purple* is a fictional tale of a woman facing consistent hardships from her youth through adulthood; however, she demonstrated resilience through the reclamation of her autonomy, self-esteem, and body. The movie first showed Celie as an adolescent who was pregnant with her second child. Viewers come to know that she was bearing the children of her father. Her father, Pa, purportedly sent her children "to be with God," but he actually sold them to a couple who eventually relocated to West Africa. As an adolescent, Celie's father groomed her to consider her appearance as "grotesque." Her father described her as worthless and inadequate. Her father constructed her body image, impacted by dominant depictions of beauty. Celie was the direct deviant from mainstream, white beauty standards. She was dark-skinned, with West African facial features, and coarse, coily hair. Celie toiled in her father's store and fields like a beast of burden and was the unwilling receptacle for his semen.

During Celie's childbearing years, she received support from her sister, Nettie. Nettie was fair-skinned, with more Eurocentric adjacent facial features. Nettie attended school, and she displayed an imagination beyond the circumstances in which the girls live. Nettie envisioned herself and her sister as royalty from Africa. Nettie's imagination provided the foundation of her self-esteem, and her view of herself stemmed from how others upheld her. Pa eventually sold Celie off to marry Mister, a farmer who continued the verbal, emotional, and physical abuse against her. Mister forced Celie to work in his home and tend to his children and his land. Nettie tried to join her sister at Mister's home once their father attempted to rape Nettie. Instead of a safe haven, Mister put Nettie out in the middle of the night after she refused his advances to sleep with her.

At Mister's home, Celie encountered many women – Shug Avery, Sophia, and Mary Agnes, who became an extension of support that helped her develop her self-esteem and gave her the courage to reclaim her life and body as her own. Shug Avery held particular importance. Shug Avery was a celebrity songstress who popped into town to visit her father, the town minister, and Mister (Albert), who was her previous lover. As Shug waltzed into Mister's home, she became intrigued by Celie's docile and submissive character and almost hellbent on encouraging her to stand up to her abusive husband. Shug urged Celie to explore her body and come to the realization that her body was not just for the gaze and purposes of men, but also for herself.

For the purposes of this chapter, I focus on Celie. Markedly, Celie's body image constituted the subject of consistent commentary throughout the story, being characterized as "ugly as sin" by her Pa, through to the very end where she finally gained bodily autonomy and identity. As I will discuss further, much of Celie's existence was steeped in her body image, given the lack of worthiness projected onto her by dominant, patriarchal figures in her life, her own self-concept, and her subsequent enactment of agency near the end of the film. In opposition to such gaze, I situate the sisterhood's, including Shug Avery and Nettie's treatments of Celie and Celie's conception of them as a reflection of hooks' (2012) oppositional gaze and the women as active spectators. In doing so, I demonstrate how such depictions reflect or rejects contemporary popular culture's idealistic yet unfavorable representation of the Black woman's body and further discuss major debates and critical issues facing Black women in relationship to their body image.

Because of space constraints, I do not critique or discuss the differences between the book, screenplay, or film, nor do I discuss the sexuality or sexual encounters of the characters or domestic violence. Instead, I employ the 2023 movie as an exemplar of contemporary popular culture's idealistic yet unfavorable representation of the Black woman's body.

Stereotypical Black Women's Body Image

Our lived experiences are inherently impacted by the body we live in (Cash, 2004). The bodies in which we live – whether fat, skinny, tall, or short – and the bodies that exist on and around the spectrums of what others dominantly treat as beautiful or handsome are also impacted by the popular images of the body that we see in popular culture. The differences between those bodies also vary in the capacity of abilities. As we exist in our bodies, we perceptively measure and judge our bodies and, arguably, maybe others as well (Slade, 1994). In its formal conception, Schilder (1950, p. 11) defined body image as "the picture of our own body which we form in our mind, that is to say the way in which the body appears to ourselves." Body image, as a concept, continuously morphs in its operationalization but encompasses the multidimensional self-attitude of an individual's own body which has a relationship with self-esteem and psychosocial modification (Cash & Henry, 1995). Self-perception, affect, cognitions, and behaviors in response to one's physical attributes comprise body image. General body image concerns typically pertain to size, weight, and shape (Polivy et al., 2013). We hold a mental representation and picture of our bodies in our thoughts that construct the form, size, and shape in estimation, and feelings about body parts, whether one is satisfied or dissatisfied (Slade, 1988). This "inside view" (the self-perspective of body image) includes the psychological experience of the individual that entails a composition of body images and not just a singular body image (Cash & Pruzinsky, 1990).

This composition of body image is comprised of the "outside view," i.e., the stereotyping of third-parties' bodies (Cash & Pruzinsky, 1990). Kwate and Threadcraft (2015) argued that mainstream dominant popular culture presents Black women in stereotypical imaging (see also Hughes, 2021). For Black women, such stereotypical treatment includes body types and representations of heavy-set nurturing women like the Mammy or Madea. Kwate and Threadcraft asserted that such presentations feature "Black women as overweight, asexual, and [un]threatening servants, hypermaternal if not ultrafeminine" (pp. 213–214). Alternatively, they could be presented with an athletic, masculine body, like professional tennis player Serena Williams. Body shape, size, complexion, hair texture, and facial features impact the differential treatment of Black women (Ashley & Jung, 2017). These stereotypical images rarely depict Black women as beautiful or attractive; they may be hypersexualized or objectified, but never just pretty. Notably, research has supported that being beautiful constitutes an occasion for self-agency and for a woman to distinguish her value (Ashley, 2021; Ashley & Jung, 2017). Such stereotypical images, and a list of others, have a damaging impact on Black women, which includes me.

Ironically, the majority of body image research has examined the disturbances related to white, college-aged women or comparative studies with other racial and/or ethnic groups. For example, Cash and Green (1986) examined the relationships between body weight and body image, finding that the perceptual, cognitive, and emotive aspects of body image change when body weight changes. Also, Black female college students have more flexible criteria for perceiving fatness than their white counterparts (Rucker & Cash, 1992). According to Lovejoy (2001, p. 239), major ethnic differences in body image exist between Black and white women, so much so that:

> Black women may develop a strong positive self-valuation and an alternative beauty aesthetic to resist societal stigmatization … and positive body image among Black women may sometimes reflect a defensive need to deny health problems such as compulsive overeating and obesity.

Furthermore, identification with each racial group contributes to the body satisfaction and beauty ideals adopted by Black female college students (Awad et al., 2015; Hesse-Biber et al., 2010). The aforementioned, highly cited research almost encompasses the type of studies that summarize the field. These studies support insight into Black women's body image. However, a void exists in scholarship about the limitations and misunderstandings of the Black woman's body, and work to date lacks cultural clarity and astute accountability for the nuances that emphasize the underpinnings of body image related to the *Others* (see related arguments by Stanton et al., 2022). Considering such a gap, and as a Black woman, mother, and researcher, I argue that we should address this important issue related to women whose general lived experience and race are congruent. As Cash and Henry (1995, p. 20) affirmed, "As body-image experiences often mirror the cultural context, intercultural and racial/ethnic diversity has been observed in body satisfaction."

This examination of Celie in *The Color Purple* equips us not only with a powerful popular culture text for exploring representations of body image treatments; it also illustrates the centrality of body issue concerns for both physical and mental health. Through the various mediums of *The Color Purple*, Celie's self-esteem entails an underlying thread that weaves a cloth of how patriarchy, the dominance of beauty standards, and gazes impact self-perception and self-worthiness. According to Szabó (2015, p. 1354), "Body image is one of the significant components of the individual's self-concept that provides the opportunity to reach a more healthy physical and mental state."

Celie

According to Muhammad and McArthur (2015, p. 134), "popular culture serves as a central influence on the racialized and gendered identity construction of Black girls." This influence creates a complex dual relationship where Black women have to negotiate Black culture and dominant culture, what bell hooks called "double jeopardy" (2015), where representations of Black women are often based in a negative or derogatory manner.

As the film began, Celie was pregnant. Of course, during and after pregnancy, a birthing person's body undergoes significant changes that may include weight gain (Carter-Edwards et al., 2010). As a girl in her mid-teen years, Celie worked in her Pa's store and carried his children. As an adult, she could bear no more children. (The novel alludes to a forced hysterectomy.) She envisioned herself as poor, unattractive, talentless, insignificant, and uneducated (Harris, 1984). Celie believed that she was ugly, with 4C hair, dark skin, full lips, a wide nose, and breathy nostrils. Black women's identities are shaped by the representations of Black girlhood, which includes them being judged by their hair (Muhammad & McArthur, 2015). Under her housedress is a full figure, voluptuous breasts, wide hips, and round buttocks – all directly deviant from dominant beauty standards, even differing from Black beauty ideals (see related work by Hughes, 2021).

Dark skin tone is often a characteristic that causes Black women to be excluded (Blackman-Richards et al., 2023). In the color hierarchy, or colorism, acceptable complexions rely on skin tone gradations, with extremes of white, Black, or light dark. Even hair texture, if it is more coarse and coily, leads to Black women experiencing texturism, where some experience preferential treatment based on the texture of one's curls (Shephard, 2018).

The othering that Celie experienced exemplifies how Black bodies have had an extensive history of being divergent from white, dominant, and popular beauty standards. One of the primary images of the Black woman's body was Saartjie Baartman, a Khoisan woman from the Cape of South Africa who was paraded throughout Europe because of her "deviant" body type. In my previous work (Ashley, 2021, p. 668), I discussed how her "body was characterized as strange, primitive, grotesque, lascivious, unfeminine, and obscene." Artists depicted her body in caricatures that over-exaggerated her buttocks, breasts, and other body parts, and welcomed the "male gaze onto Black women's bodies in popular culture" (LaVoulle & Lewis Ellison, 2017, p. 70). Baartman's body served as the underpinning for the objectification of the Black woman's body. Dating back to the 1800s, when some regarded Saartjie Baartman as the quintessential body type for Black women's bodies (Ashley, 2021), she was popularly exploited throughout Europe where white audiences gazed and groped her large buttocks and genitals (Ashley, 2021). Popular culture impacts how we produce and reproduce images of Black women's bodies (see related argument by Awad et al., 2015; Hughes, 2021). Although Baartman's and Celie's storylines were incongruent, the Black female body remains constant as others gazed and gawked upon Celie's facial features and complexion.

The Gazes

hooks (2012) described the outside view or *gaze*, or power of looking, on Black women by patriarchal figures and its impact on Black spectatorship. The racialized power relations entrenched in the gaze for so much time only allowed the right of the gaze to slave owners (their children and counterparts). However, in this chapter, I connect this gaze to the patriarchal dominance of Mister and how Mister's gaze aligns with the popular cultural gaze of the Others, and the Others' (Sisterhood) inside view of Celie as the oppositional gaze.

Mister's physical, verbal, emotional, and sexual abuse all work in tandem to oppress Celie, exemplifying popular culture's oppressive, dominant, and abusive relationship to Black women and their bodies (for related work, please see Stanton et al., 2022). *The Color Purple*'s continuous conversations about Celie's ugliness, as described by her father, her husband, and then herself at the end, work to reinforce the power of the popular culture gaze and reproduce themselves.

The oppositional gaze constitutes the women's support and outside view of Celie: Nettie and Shug showing Celie herself in the mirror. Nettie allowed Celie to see herself in a full-body mirror when describing their assumed African royal ancestry. Nettie wrapped Celie in cloth with African-style prints and enabled Celie to envision herself through the eyes of her doting and loving sister. Mirror scenes aid in the development of the ego (Ross, 1988).

hooks (2012, p. 308) noted that "[e]ven in the worst circumstances of domination, the ability to manipulate one's gaze in the face of structures of domination that would contain it, opens up the possibility of agency." In Celie's relationship with Mister, she seemingly had no power, autonomy, or authority; however, based on Foucault (1984), a possibility of resistance remains. Resistance came through her interactions with her sister Nettie and Shug, both offering her an oppositional outside view or gaze of herself, other than what had been started by her father and reinforced by her husband, Mister. In her resistance, Celie transformed and modified her look, equipping her to resist by changing the adornments and attachments that she used. hooks (2012, p. 116) told us that "[s]paces of agency exist for Black people, wherein we can both interrogate the gaze of the Other but also look back, and at one another, naming what we see."

Young Nettie

Nettie is Celie's younger sister (portrayed in the 2023 film by Hailee Bailey, a fair-skinned, petite 20-something-year-old). Celie and Nettie have distinctively different features. Celie is dark-skinned, and Nettie is light-skinned. In the film, Nettie attends school, and other characters treat her as possessing more power than Celie. Nettie – fairer complexioned and much prettier – lives a softer existence, educated, and affirming the confidence and power to turn away her Pa's and Mister's sexual advances. Trying to escape the advances of her father, Nettie goes to Celie's new home only to find that Mister would try to have sex with her too.

First, Nettie was petitioned by Mister, after failing at singing, "You got some real pretty teeth, Nettie…and your skin dazzle my eyes like the moon lights the night, that's a real pretty dress and your shoes look just right on them pretty little feet." To which she retorted, "Now you lying. I'm a tomboy and I live to climb trees. I got corns, bunions, and blisters. Ain't nothing pretty about my feet."

Their complexions proved central to the behaviors that they encountered – i.e., colorism, the prejudicial and discriminatory treatment toward people with darker skin (Ashley, 2020). Skin complexion has an impact on attitudes toward Black people (Mucherah & Frazier, 2013). Along with

Nettie's lighter skin tone, she had facial features that more closely resembled white, European features, such as high cheekbones and a slender nose with small nostrils (Zhang et al., 2009). Faal (2021) and Taylor (1993) called the preference for white features "featurism." Faal (2021) also suggested that the world tries to "fix" Black women's bodies to assimilate to white bodies. Notably, exposure to dominant beauty standards may impact Black women's body satisfaction (Awad et al., 2015; Stanton et al., 2022; Walker Gautier, 2021).

Popular culture tends to treat a small nose, thin lips, fair skin, tall stature, light hair, and a slim as idealistic features of a woman. Women's attractiveness is related to individuals having features that are closely associated with fairer skin and Caucasoid features (Bond & Cash, 1992; Mucherah & Frazier, 2013). With attractiveness and proximity to white features and fair complexion comes the estimation of a women's value. For example, Bond and Cash found that Black women idealize light skin and that Black men preferred light-skinned women and exalted them. On the other hand, darker skin has disadvantages and brings emotional pain.

Mister petitioned Alfonso, the girls' Pa, for Nettie's hand as his wife. Pa responded by saying that Nettie was too smart. Instead, he sold Celie for a cow and a couple of eggs, describing her as "ugly as homemade sin, but will work hard like a man." Mister responded with, "Celie? That's what you call that thing walking round in your store? I don't want that." According to Thompson and Keith (2001), complexion is so important that it could determine one's self-worth, attitude, and identity. Thompson and Keith asserted that complexion can correspond to socioeconomic status; a woman who is poor is likely to be darker and have low self-esteem, while those with a light hue tend to be better economically and socially positioned with positive self-esteem.

Shug Avery

Black women who possess body and facial features that are popular in the dominant mainstream are more likely to be successful, socially and economically (Ashley, 2020: Hamermesh, 2011). Black popular culture describes Black women's bodies in various ways: slim thick, voluptuous, and athletic builds among others. Mister had a loose woman on the side, Shug Avery, "a woman who won't let no one man tie her down." Celie wanted to be a loose woman. Celie discovered a picture of Shug Avery on her nightstand. Shug's photo exuded glamour, layered with a powder blue, wide-brimmed, feathered hat, large costume jewelry, lace fan, and a background with jacquard velvet drapes and fringe. Shug presented an idealized appearance and stardom, much comparable to Josephine Baker, Dorothy Dandridge, or Beyoncé. In her presence, Shug embodied a sexualized performance, one mirroring Beyoncé's feminism and the Black feminist body (Weidhase (2015). In that moment, Shug's body comprised a site of asserting her feminism, using her body as a contestation to the oppressive dwelling of Mister. In Shug, we see a self-actualized pop star and a feminist agent for change.

Celie is entrenched with Shug Avery. As Shug lounged in the tub with the morning light shining through the drapes, Celie washed her back and body, saying that she felt like "I'm praying." Shug reintroduced Celie to her body. This time, Celie's view of herself comes in a mirror big enough to only capture the reflection of her head and shoulders. Celie gleefully giggled at the surprise of her appearance, augmented by red lipstick. In all of her glamour, Shug also engaged in the Bad Bitch Barbie trope (LaVoulle & Lewis Ellison, 2017). As such, she actively objectified herself, used her body for profitability, actively negotiated her image, and imparted such representation onto Celie. She celebrated her body while also commodifying it. As LaVoulle and Lewis Ellison noted, the Bad Bitch Barbie "should not be viewed as negative or vulgar, but as an alternative characterization that embodies past and present research about the historical representations and perceptions of Black women, their bodies, and their voices" (p. 67).

The *Bad Bitch Barbie* comprises a contradiction in terms because it represents both a Western/European beauty ideal of long straight hair and keen features as well as Black standards of beauty: voluptuous hips, a small waist, and a large derriere. In the same way, the *Bad Bitch Barbie* directly objectified the Black female body while simultaneously representing a performance in feminism. A *Bad Bitch Barbie* entails an image of a woman who rises against opposition and stands her ground. She comprises both a Black feminist and someone who acknowledges that intersectionality and racism exist. The *Bad Bitch Barbie* holds a specific role in supporting Black women who are not oversexualized commodities, but who understand the histories of racialized and sexualized representations of Black women (LaVoulle & Lewis Ellison, 2017).

The perception of one's body image may be internalized by idealized appearances (Erickson, 2020; see also related work by Awad et al., 2015; Jiotsa et al., 2021; Papageorgiou et al., 2022; Stanton et al., 2022). Like Beyoncé, Shug offered an ideal body image that is unattainable (LaVoulle & Lewis Ellison, 2017). Invariably defined, Erickson noted that the most recent usages of body dysmorphia have been to describe feelings of insecurity related to one's appearance and may assume flaws in themselves that may be very minor or not there at all and perhaps may change or hide the perceived deficits. Body dysmorphic disorder is considered an obsessive-compulsive disorder, in which individuals proceed to modify their appearance using harmful exercises, diets, cosmetic or plastic surgeries, and Black-market methods (Ashley & Jung, 2017; Erickson, 2020). References to physical appearances may elicit symptoms of the disorder, having negative behaviors or thoughts.

Mainstream Gaze: Mister's Gaze and its Congruency to Mainstream Popular Culture

"Until you do right by me everything you touch gone crumble," said Celie. Celie's statement to Mister reinforced her new agency and marked the dismissal of his gaze upon her. Celie, finally gaining her self-autonomy, rejected Mister's negative assertions of her class, complexion, and body image. Shortly after Celie's dismissal, Mister's land became infested with bugs, and he had to torch the entire plot. During that same period, Celie's Pa passed, marking the death of another gaze. These outside views, or gazes, typically have a negative impact on Black women's inside view, contributing to, but not limited to, body dysmorphia, eating disorders, and body modification.

I liken mainstream popular culture's gaze on Black women's bodies to the male gazes in the film Celie. Black women who are dark and have non-Eurocentric facial features are more likely experience trauma related to their self-esteem and tend to experience less success in attracting worthy spouses or attaining social and economic success because of dominant beauty standards (Haddad, 2022; Perloff, 2014; Shephard, 2018; Thompson & Keith, 2001). To be clear, I do not agree with nor support the aforementioned perspective; however, the literature and the examination of this film certainly suggest it.

Yet, this film also affirms a way for Black women to establish their own self-esteem, autonomy, and agency. Celie overwhelmingly longed to look at herself, and she shifted her reality, whether imagining herself in African garb as royalty with her sister or as a songstress alongside Shug. As Celie loosed herself, she reimagined her reality and adopted the oppositional gaze of herself; that new envisioning of self gives way for her to engage in agency and autonomy.

In my work, I strive to restore autonomy for women's bodies, which have been a consistent and historical target for male dominance that actualizes as exploitation, whether it be sexual, commodifying, or physical aggression. Given the pervasiveness of this treatment, especially in popular culture, women can develop a complex and sometimes painful relationship with their own bodies, making it difficult to assess, look in the mirror, adjust, modify, or just be (Ross, 1988; Stanton et al., 2022). According to Ross,

> To confront the body is to confront not only an individual's abuse but also the abuse of women's bodies throughout history; as the external symbol of women's enslavement, this abuse represents for a woman a reminder of her degradation and her consignment to an inferior status.
> *(p. 70)*

In the case of *The Color Purple*, Mister's (popular culture) gaze is oppressive, and the Sisterhood oppositional gaze of Nettie and Shug is uplifting and transformative.

Discussion

Overall, this chapter strived to foreground the male/popular culture third-party gaze and its disdain for Black women, its impact on self-esteem, and decision-making in body modification for Black women. After situating this chapter in salient literature on body image representations, I used the characters of *The Color Purple* to illustrate the importance of body image for mental and physical well-being. Being satisfied with one's body image is related to one's overall health outcomes (see, e.g., Go et al., 2024; Gustat et al., 2017; Rodgers et al., 2023).

Research has clearly documented connections between eating disorders and body dissatisfaction (see, e.g., Castellano et al., 2021; Feingold & Mazzella, 1998; Lovejoy, 2001; Mallerum et al., 2023). More specifically to Black women's body image, disturbances to body image more closely relate to racially related markers that determine the treatment of Black women, including complexion, facial features, and hair texture (see, e.g., Awad et al., 2015; Mucherah & Frazier, 2013). Studies related to complexion document how Black women may decide to alter their complexion based on offshoots from racism, which can have harmful effects (see, e.g., Ashley & Jung, 2017). For example, skin whitening is a multibillion-dollar industry that grows from the imposition of colorist and racist structures, while also exposing users to skin irritation issues and body dysmorphia (Ashley, 2020; Williams, 2022). With popular culture serving as one of the factors that contribute to self-perception and body image, significant growth has occurred in Black women choosing to augment their facial features (Rohrich & Bolden, 2010; Williams, 2022). For example, in this chapter, I compared Shug to Beyoncé. What does it take to look like Beyoncé? What lengths should women go to obtain the *Bad Bitch Barbie* look? Thus, establishing a dangerous undertaking of trying to attain a particularly commodifiable appearance.

Furthermore, longstanding debates and conversations continue considering "good" hair, determining the favorability of textures among Black women (Shepherd, 2018). As popular culture examines and modifies Black women's bodies, their bodies continue to function as commodities. As mentioned previously, we see how Mister buys Celie from her father. Although not considered attractive, her body still had value. According to Thompson and Keith (2001), women who experience lower self-esteem may have fewer opportunities related to economic and social status. Thus, Celie had fewer opportunities. Also, Shug Avery demonstrated how a woman can harness her own power and create economically beneficial means through her body, but it came with a contemporary cost.

Even though *The Color Purple* occurred at a different historical time, popular culture still objectifies the bodies of Black women. According to Young (1997), "The treatment of Black women's bodies in nineteenth-century Europe and the United States is considered the foundation upon which Black women's commodification and objectification is based" (p. 706). As such, Black women's bodies are often only depicted as useful for sexual performance and accepting of the gazes of third parties (Ashley, 2021). Whether objectification is useful for Black women (i.e., to self-commodify like Shug Avery) or it is harmful (i.e., to be raped like Celie), we require further exploration of issues pertaining to Black women's bodies and further understanding of their various functionalities as they relate to the well-being of Black women.

Although more studies have focused on Black women's body image (see, e.g., Chacón & Langlais, 2024; López-Guimerà et al., 2010; Rodgers et al., 2023), we need more inclusive research related to beauty that does not attempt to discuss the beauty standards of white women or the dominant culture. Studies should more frequently address issues of hair, lips, nose, hips, and buttocks in relation to attractiveness while also accounting for complexion (Taylor, 1993). Also, consider how featurism may impact intragroup and inter-group bias in patient-provider communication. Black women should critically examine images in media to question the representations that they consume (LaVoulle & Lewis Ellison, 2017).

In this chapter, I have explored the representation of Black women's bodies in popular culture through a prevalent example – *The Color Purple*. I close by emphasizing that the ways in which popular culture chooses to depict and discuss body image matters. Other chapters in this collection underscore the powerful and persuasive voices of celebrities (see Chapter 15) and social influencers (see Chapter 16), as well as how various genres include compelling examples about health, wellness, and well-being. The bodies that we see on screen and the ways in which those bodies get presented and treated permeate our culture and hold significance for those who watch, follow, and then reflect on their own bodies. This area remains one ripe for both investigation and work on how to shift popular culture narratives for more inclusive, balanced representations of "acceptable" and "desirable" bodies.

References

Ashley, R. R. (2020). #DemABleach: Sources' roles and functions in health information seeking behavior in a cultural health practice, *Howard Journal of Communications, 32*, 352–365. https://doi.org/10.1080/10646175.2020.1818648

Ashley, R. R. (2021). # ModernBaartmans: Black women's reimagining of Saartjie Baartman. *Journal of Black Studies, 52*(7), 667–687.

Ashley, R. R., & Jung, J. (2017). # BlackBodiesMatter: Cross-Cultural examination of Black women's motivation to engage in body modification. *Journal of Black Studies, 48*(3), 235–255.

Awad, G. H., Norwood, C., Taylor, D. S., Martinez, M., McClain, S., Jones, B., Holman, A., & Chapman-Hilliard, C. (2015). Beauty and body image concerns among African American college women. *Journal of Black Psychology, 41*(6), 540–564.

Blackman-Richards, N., Jiménez, J. V., & Pusey-Reid, E. (2023). Deconstructing standards of whiteness to establish the power of Black women. In T. B. Johnson (Ed.), *The experiences of Black women diversity practitioners in historically white institutions* (pp. 167–191). IGI Global.

Bobo, J. (1989). Sifting through the controversy: Reading *The Color Purple*. *Callaloo, 39*, 332–342.

Bobo, J. (2004). *The Color Purple*: Black women as cultural readers. In J. Bobo, C. Hudley & C. Mitchel (Eds.), *The Black studies reader* (pp. 189–204). Routledge.

Bond, S., & Cash, T. F. (1992). Black beauty: Skin color and body images among African-American college women. *Journal of Applied Social Psychology, 22*, 874–888.

Carter-Edwards, L., Bastian, L. A., Revels, J., Durham, H., Lokhnygina, Y., Amamoo, M. A., & Ostbye, T. (2010). Body image and body satisfaction differ by race in overweight postpartum mothers. *Journal of Women's Health, 19*(2), 305–311.

Cash, T. F. (2004). Body image: Past, present, and future. *Body image, 1*(1), 1–5.

Cash, T. F., & Green, G. K. (1986). Body weight and body image among college women: Perception, cognition, and affect. *Journal of Personality Assessment, 50*(2), 290–301.

Cash, T. F., & Henry, P. E. (1995). Women's body images: The results of a national survey in the USA. *Sex Roles, 33*, 19–28.

Cash, T. F., & Pruzinsky, T. (Eds.) (1990). *Body images: Development, deviance, and change*. Guilford Press.

Castellano, S., Rizzoto, A., Neri, S., Currenti, W., Guerrera, C. S., Pirrone, C., Coco, M., & Di Corrado, D. (2021). The relationship between body dissatisfaction and eating disorder symptoms in young women aspiring fashion models: The mediating role of stress. *European Journal of Investigation in Health, Psychology, and Education, 11*(2), 607–615.

Chacón, V., & Langlais, M. R. (2024). Unmasking the impact: Instagram use, body image satisfaction, and the mediating role of body ideals for Black American emerging adult women. *Sexuality & Culture*, 28, 1757–1774.

Erickson, M. (2020). Body dysmorphia in the age of the Internet. Unpublished thesis. University of California, Stanislaus.

Faal, S. (2021). "Oh no she didn't!"—No literally, she didn't: Meghan Markle, Kate Middleton, and the politics of tears. https://edspace.american.edu/atrium/portfolio-item/faal-sirra-oh-no-she-didnt-no-literally-she-didnt/

Feingold, A., & Mazzella, R. (1998). Gender differences in body image are increasing. *Psychological Science*, *9*(3), 190–195.

Foucault, M. (1984). *The foucault reader*. Vintage.

Go, P. H., Loh, H. Y., Chung, K. R., & Ramadas, A. (2024). Body (dis)satisfaction and health screening behaviors: A systematic review of observational studies. *Journal of Health Psychology*, *29*(2), 137–155. https://doi.org/10.1177/13591053231189413

Gustat, J., Carton, T. W., Shahien, A. A., & Andersen, L. (2017). Body image satisfaction among Blacks. *Health Education & Behavior*, *44*(1), 131–140.

Haddad, G. (2022). *The impact of social media on body dissatisfaction and dysmorphia in adolescents in the U.S.* [Unpublished master's essay]. Graduate School of Public Health, University of Pittsburgh.

Hamermesh, D. S. (2011). *Beauty pays: Why attractive people are more successful*. Princeton University Press.

Harris, T. (1984, December). On *The Color Purple*, stereotypes, and silence. *Black American Literature Forum*, *18*(4), 155–161. https://doi.org/10.2307/2904291

Henderson, M. G. (1985). *The Color Purple*: Revisions and redefinitions. *SAGE: A Scholarly Journal on Black Women, 2*(1), 14–18.

Hesse-Biber, S., Livingstone, S., Ramirez, D., Barko, E. B., & Johnson, A. L. (2010). Racial identity and body image among Black female college students attending predominately White colleges. *Sex Roles*, *63*, 697–711.

hooks, b. (2012). The oppositional gaze: Black female spectators. In M. Diawara (Ed.), *Black American Cinema* (pp. 288–302). Routledge.

hooks, b. (2015). *Ain't I a woman : Black women and feminism* (2nd ed.). Routledge.

Hughes, E. (2021). "I'm supposed to be thick:" Managing body image anxieties among African American women. *Journal of Black Studies*, *52*(3), 310–330. https://doi.org/10.1177/0021934720972440

Jiotsa, B., Naccache, B., Duval, M., Rocher, B., & Grall-Bronnec, M. (2021). Social media use and body image disorders: Association between frequency of comparing one's own physical appearance to that of people being followed on social media and body image and drive for thinness. *International Journal of Environmental Research and Public Health*, *18*(6), 2880.

Kwate, N. O. A., & Threadcraft, S. (2015). Perceiving the Black female body: Race and gender in police constructions of body weight. *Race and Social Problems*, *7*, 213–226.

LaVoulle, C., & Lewis Ellison, T. (2017). The bad bitch Barbie craze and Beyoncé African American women's bodies as commodities in Hip-Hop culture, images, and media. *Taboo: The Journal of Culture and Education*, *16*(2), 65–84.

López-Guimerà, G., Levine, M. P., Sánchez-Carracedo, D., & Fauquet, J. (2010). Influence of mass media on body image and eating disordered attitudes and behaviors in females: A review of effects and processes. *Media Psychology*, *13*(4), 387–416.

Lovejoy, M. (2001). Disturbances in the social body: Differences in body image and eating problems among African American and white women. *Gender & Society*, *15*(2), 239–261.

Mallerum, G. K., Sharma, P., Kattula, D., Singh, S., & Pavuluru, P. (2023). Body image perception, eating disorder behavior, self-esteem and quality of life: a cross-sectional study among female medical students. *Journal of Eating Disorders*, *11*, 225.

Mucherah, W., & Frazier, A. D. (2013). How deep is skin-deep? The relationship between skin color satisfaction, estimation of body image, and self-esteem among women of African descent. *Journal of Applied Social Psychology*, *43*(6), 1177–1184.

Muhammad, G. E., & McArthur, S. A. (2015). "Styled by their perceptions": Black adolescent girls interpret representations of Black females in popular culture. *Multicultural Perspectives*, *17*(3), 133–140.

Papageorgiou, A., Fisher, C., & Cross, D. (2022). "Why don't I look like her?" How adolescent girls view social media and its connection to body image. *BMC Women's Health*, *22*, 261.

Perloff, R. M. (2014). Social media effects on young women's body image concerns: Theoretical perspectives and an agenda for research. *Sex Roles*, *71*(11), 363–377. https://doi.org/10.1007/s11199-014-0384-6

Polivy, J., Herman, C. P., & Pliner, P. (2013). Perception and evaluation of body image: The meaning of body shape and size. In J. M. Olson & M. P. Zanna (Eds.), *Self-Inference Processes* (pp. 87–114). Psychology Press.

Rodgers, R. F., Laveway, K., Campos, P., & de Carvelho, P. H. (2023). Body image as a global mental health concern. *Global Mental Health, 10*, e9.

Rohrich, R. J., & Bolden, K. (2010). Ethnic rhinoplasty. *Clinics in Plastic Surgery, 37*(2), 353–370.

Ross, D. W. (1988). Celie in the looking glass: The desire for selfhood in "The Color Purple." *Modern Fiction Studies, 34*(1), 69–84.

Rucker III, C. E., & Cash, T. F. (1992). Body images, body-size perceptions, and eating behaviors among African-American and white college women. *International Journal of Eating Disorders, 12*(3), 291–299.

Schilder, P. (1950). *The image and appearance of the human body: Studies in the constructive energies of the psyche*. Routledge.

Shepherd, J. M. (2018). Don't touch my crown: Texturism as an extension of colorism in the natural hair community (Unpublished thesis). Texas State University, San Marcos.

Slade, P. D. (1988). Body image in anorexia nervosa. *The British Journal of Psychiatry, 153*(S2), 20–22.

Slade, P. D. (1994). What is body image? *Behaviour Research and Therapy, 32*(5), 497–502. https://doi.org/10.1016/0005-7967(94)90136-8

Stanton, A. G., Avery, L. A., Matsuzaka, S., & Epinel, S. (2022). Black women's experiences of gendered, racial, sexual objectification, body image, and depressive symptoms. *Body Image, 41*, 443–452.

Szabó, M. K. (2015). The relationship between body image and self-esteem. *European Psychiatry, 30*, 1354.

Talebian Sedehi, K. (2014). *The Color Purple* and women's time. *Journal of Language Teaching and Research*, 5(6), 1328–1333.

Taylor, J. (1993). Reaction to Penn et al.'s "On the Desirability of Own-Group Preference." *Journal of Black Psychology, 19*(3), 333–335. https://doi.org/10.1177/00957984930193009

Thompson, M. S., & Keith, V. M. (2001). The Blacker the berry: Gender, skin tone, 35 self-esteem, and self-efficacy. *Gender and Society, 15*, 336–357.

Udoette, M. (2014). Female consciousness in Alice Walker's *The Color Purple*. *IJSELL: International Journal on Studies in English Language and Literature, 2*(5), 74–80.

Walker Gautier, S. (2021). Black beauty: Womanist consciousness as a protective factor in Black women's body image satisfaction. *Journal of Black Psychology, 47*(8), 631–656.

Weidhase, N. (2015). 'Beyoncé feminism' and the contestation of the Black feminist body. *Celebrity Studies, 6*(1), 128–131. https://doi.org/10.1080/19392397.2015.1005389

Williams, B. (2022, May 5). 5 plastic surgery trends for Black Women. *Yahoo! News*. https://news.yahoo.com/5-plastic-surgery-trends-Black-160832600.html

Young, J. (1997). The re-objectification and re-commodification of Saartjie Baartman in Suzan-Lori Park's Venus. *African American Review, 31*(4), 699–708.

Zhang, Y., Dixon, T. L., & Conrad, K. (2009). Rap music videos and African American women's body image: The moderating role of ethnic identity. *Journal of Communication, 59*(2), 262–278.

6

SEXUAL HEALTH AND POPULAR CULTURE

Jay Baglia

Introduction

In the 2011 film, *Hysteria*, the young Dr. Joseph Mortimer Granville (Hugh Dancy) convinced London's "leading specialist in women's medicine," the older Dr. Dalrymple (Jonathan Pryce), to make use of an invention in their work treating women suffering from hysteria in the late 19th century: an electric vibrator. Each of these physicians had been employing their practiced hands to their female patients' "most gentle areas" with "good, steady pressure" in order to treat hysteria. With so many patients, however, they succumbed to hand cramping. The application of the vibrator was a marked success, and the pair promoted "Dr. Dalrymple's Electro-Vibratory Massage Theatre" with advertisements, encouraging patients to "Get in the Pink of Health Today!" Dalrymple called hysteria "the plague of our time," characterized by melancholia, weeping, anxiety, and frigidity, all "stemming from a woman's overactive uterus." The film, set in 1880, featured a series of women of varying ages and dispositions describing their symptoms. One said it's "just a feeling." Another labeled it as "a hungering." An opera diva complained that she "cannot sing." The Electro-Vibratory Massage Theatre resulted in a parade of satisfied patients; a montage reveals them exiting the confines of the treatment room elated.

In addition to hysteria, diagnoses of the 19th century contributed mightily to the social construction inherent in much medical discourse. In addition to diagnoses of nymphomania and spermatorrhea, the late 19th century marked the first time when public health officials labeled and distinguished homosexuality and heterosexuality (Hart & Wellings, 2002; Wheeler, 2017). According to Wheeler, because of the science of public health and the professionalization of medicine, definitions and surveillance of sexual conduct moved inevitably from theological frameworks to those of medical science and the human sciences and from acts ("crimes against nature") to identities.

Differences in how sexual desire is experienced, studied, and reported are, of course, central to the study of sexual health. Alfred Kinsey's work in the late 1940s and early 1950s, the debut of *Playboy* magazine and its imitators, and Masters and Johnson in the 1960s (Robinson, 1976) transformed mediated coverage and public communication of sex and sexuality. Meanwhile, the birth control pill became widely available in the early 1960s, followed by distinct changes in the upsurge of nudity in mainstream films (Wolf, 2020) and the sexual revolution (Allyn, 2016) including the Stonewall riots (Halkitis, 2019). Shere Hite's (1976) *Hite Report: A Nationwide Study of Female Sexuality* emerged at the pinnacle of second-wave feminism. In the 1980s, the AIDS crisis raised new concerns about

DOI: 10.4324/9781003436409-7

sexual health as well as the extent to which the press covered it (Treichler, 1999). The continued fight for civil rights, LGBTQ+ rights, and women's rights have persisted along with astonishing advances and monumental changes in the transmission and consumption of media.

In this chapter, I offer examples of how sexual health topics are broached in popular culture, including film and television, advertising, social media, and news. Before transitioning into examples, however, I provide definitions and an historical context for how we, today, view sexual health in and through popular culture.

With regard to the popular culture of the late-19th century, Sigmund Freud compared the details of his cases with popular short stories (e.g., Perkins Gilman's "The Yellow Wallpaper") and novels of the late 19th and early 20th centuries (Showalter, 1993). However, whether patients mimicked fiction or the popular hysteria literature of his time inspired Freud's case narratives, there remains today a slipperiness regarding how popular culture informs our understanding of gendered bodies, sexual health, and health in general.

In this chapter, I draw on various forms of popular culture in order to demonstrate different ways in which the media have framed sexual health. Other chapters in this volume influenced my decisions about which sexual health topics to include and what not to include. For example, the editor made a conscious choice to create chapters for representations of women's health and LGBTQIA+ health – both of which can and do intersect with sexual health (see Chapters 7 and 8, this volume). For the purposes of this chapter, I have endeavored to limit the literature search for sexual health topics to avoid overlap with those chapters found elsewhere in this collection. At the same time, I also chose not to select examples of sexual health topics that could be interpreted – whether by what I included or failed to include – as strictly heteronormative. Specifically, I remain mindful that gender roles, the expansion of what we consider in terms of sexual identity, and the trans movement definitely belong in conversations about sexual health.

On the other hand, sexual health is not necessarily implicated when performing a search on gender roles and health in popular culture. For example, in a content analysis, Hether and Murphy (2009) listed the 10 most common health issues in a comprehensive study of almost 1,300 storylines from the 10 most popular American television programs between 2004 and 2006. Defining health issues as "something dealing with disease, injury, or disability" (p. 813), the authors identified the ten top issues for male and female characters, but not one explicitly focuses on sexual health. In a follow-up study, Pariera et al. (2014) looked explicitly for sexual and reproductive health content in a similarly sized set of popular prime time shows from the years 2009 to 2011. In their rationale, they remarked that "[w]hile sexual content is pervasive and growing, little is understood about how health issues resulting from sexual activity are portrayed" (p. 700).

This chapter's review of sexual health in popular culture, then, does *not* include scholarship related to sexual behavior, orientation, and/or identity if such research does not also directly encompass discussions of health and well-being, including mental health. Finally, digital sources sometimes do and often do not satisfy the definition of "popular culture." Digital sources, including social media, have pages and posts which vary significantly in terms of views. Therefore, when I considered examples from digital platforms – such as Instagram and TikTok – my decision to integrate those references to sexual health as popular culture depended a great deal on whether or not a specific post went "viral" or otherwise reached tens of thousands of views, thus satisfying the criterion of "popular."

Finally, sexual health and popular culture encompass a necessarily multidisciplinary area of inquiry. In addition to being of interest to Health Communication researchers, scholars in fields as methodologically and theoretically diverse as anthropology, education, health promotion, journalism, literary criticism, media studies, philosophy, primary care, psychology, sexology, sociology, and women's and gender studies have generated an extensive reservoir of knowledge, with new questions constantly being posed. Therefore, I treated my search as correspondingly ecumenical in nature and reference multiple disciplines.

With these parameters in mind, in this chapter, I chose to address 1) sex education and advice, 2) performance and desire, and 3) sexually transmitted infections (STIs). Particularly in light of social media, advertising, and television, these categories provide abundant examples of how multiple informal channels broach sexual health. First, however, it is practical to *define* sexual health. Following this brief section, I will take up the topics identified above.

Defining Sexual Health

The World Health Organization's (WHO) definition of "health" as "a state of complete physical, mental, and social well-being and not merely the absence of disease or infirmity" (1948, p. 100) originated in 1946 and has remained unchanged (despite calls to change or adapt it). In 1975, WHO defined "sexual health" as:

> the integration of the somatic, emotional, intellectual, and social aspects of sexual being, in ways that are positively enriching and that enhance personality, communication, and love. Thus the notion of sexual health implies a positive approach to human sexuality, and the purpose of sexual health care should be the enhancement of life and personal relationships and not merely counseling and care related to procreation or sexuality transmitted diseases.
>
> *(p. 41)*

This definition contrasted with the historical genesis of the study of sex and sexuality that had emerged in the mid-19th century. Although the WHO's definition of "health" hasn't changed, the 1975 definition has evolved considerably to include pleasure, well-being, safety, and emerging identities in 2006.

> Sexual health is a state of physical, emotional, mental and social well-being in relation to sexuality; it is not merely the absence of disease, dysfunction, or infirmity. Sexual health requires a positive and respectful approach to sexuality and sexual relationships, as well as the possibility of having pleasurable and safe sexual experiences, free of coercion, discrimination and violence. For sexual health to be attained and maintained, the sexual rights of all persons must be protected and fulfilled
>
> *(2006, p. 3)*

This updated definition eliminated *personal* relationships (in favor of *sexual* relationships) and any mention of procreation. Indeed, the WHO's (2010) sexual health program acknowledged the need to distinguish reproductive from sexual health. The question of how to define sexual health remains unsettled; in fact, Starrs and Anderson (2016) discussed and critiqued definitions used by a range of stakeholders. For the purpose of providing a starting point for this discussion of sexual health and popular culture, the WHO statement comprises the most recognized and employed definitive source.

Media shapes norms for health generally (Seale, 2002) and sexual health in particular (Collins et al., 2017; Pariera et al., 2014; Ward et al., 2006). Typically cast as "informal" channels for information about sex, popular media serves as a source across the lifespan (Graf & Patrick, 2015; see also Chapter 24, this volume). Kunkel et al. (2005) identified television as a normalizing force regarding expectations and attitudes for teenagers. Meanwhile, Brown et al. (2005) refer to media generally as a "sexual super peer" (p. 420). While sexual *content* in popular media is pervasive, the media has displayed sexually healthy behavior or communication about healthy sexual behavior far less frequently (Collins et al., 2017; Hust et al., 2008; White et al., 2023). By and large, mediated scripts tend to be both gendered and heteronormative (Hust et al., 2008; Seabrook et al., 2017). The messages that popular media sources *do* send about sex are often intertextual and include how to talk about sex as well as how to behave sexually (Dillman Carpentier et al., 2017).

The popular Netflix series *Never Have I Ever* provided a compelling example of intertextuality. Devi Vishwakumar (Maitreyi Ramakrishnan), Fabiola Torres (Lee Rodriguez), and Eleanor Wong (Ramona Young) are best friends at Sherman Oaks High School in Los Angeles. In Season One, antagonist and academic rival Ben Gross (Jaren Lewison) derisively nicknamed the racially diverse trio of freshmen as "The U.N." (unfuckable nerds). As seniors in Season Four, each had reached a sexual awakening, acknowledging their respective sexual identities and preferences, and experimenting with partners. In Season Four's first episode, Fabiola, Eleanor, and Devi met in Devi's bedroom, talking about how the latter recently lost her virginity – a stated goal of Devi's since Season One. Surprisingly, her first experience of sexual intercourse occurred with the aforementioned Ben. In chorus, Eleanor and Fabiola were incredulous, "You had sex with Ben Gross?" Devi, sitting on her bed, answered in the affirmative. Fabiola quickly followed up, "How was it?" Devi replied, "Ok. I think." Eleanor asked, "Did you have an orgasm?" Devi admitted, "No," disappointment evident in her facial expression. Fabiola asked if Ben did. Devi guessed, "I think so." Eleanor inquired as to how many positions they tried. Devi responded quickly (but with some insecurity), "One," and then, "How many were we supposed to do?" Eleanor answered confidently, "I think like four to five." Wincing, Fabiola confirmed this perspective, "They definitely do four to five on [HBO television series] *Euphoria*." Devi demanded immediately, "Do you think Ben wanted to have *Euphoria* sex?" Fabiola responded unhesitatingly, "Who doesn't?"

Whether through television, film, music, stand-up comedy, comics, advertising, news, or social media – consciously or unconsciously – adolescents and adults alike can find validation of their bodies and sexual experiences through popular culture.

Sex Education and Advice

Lameiras-Fernández et al. (2021) defined sex education "as any combination of learning experiences aimed at facilitating voluntary behavior conducive to sexual health" (p. 2555). Between abstinence education, the COVID-19 pandemic, and the proliferation of online content not only including social media sites but also magazines and streaming video, more and more people are turning to their phones, tablets, and laptops to find answers to their questions about sexual health.

I begin with the sex education dispensed not in the middle school classroom by an indefatigable science teacher to a mix of curious and cringing 13-year-olds, but by largely amorphous columnists and/or authoritative medical experts found in popular magazines for teens and adults alike. Döring (2021) maintained that not only does traditional, formal sex education tend to be targeted to specific audiences, but also that it tends to focus on risk, the "danger" in Vance's (1992) *Pleasure and Danger*. While not always less targeted, informal sex education includes ever-expanding media options, but also the capability of more user-generated content, in addition to the ability to comment and interact with other users. I start this section with advice columns in magazines (encompassing both print and digital formats) before moving to social media.

Sexual Advice in Magazines

Cosmopolitan magazine has remained relatively unchanged over the last few decades, but the publication now offers a digital version to accompany its traditional, slick print version. The print version greets me at the supermarket checkout line, an unwavering presence over the course of my adulthood. Helen Gurley Brown introduced *Cosmopolitan* to "modern" women in the 1960s specifically to offer women reading material that was not about the domestic sphere (Mackin & Thornborrow, 2003). Its website (2023) bills *Cosmopolitan* as "the biggest young women's media brand in the world" (para. 3), and it dispenses sex advice in most issues through columns such as "Love," "Sex &

Relationships," and "Ask Him Anything," each of which is regularly featured both in the print version and on the website.

Cosmo, as well as a dozen or so other well-known magazines, caters to women by offering a balance of fashion, entertainment, current events, and – to a greater or lesser degree – advice about love, sex, and relationships. Appealing to a younger demographic of 14- to 17-year-olds, its publisher structures *Seventeen* similarly. Since the 1980s, these kinds of magazines have sought – again, to varying degrees – to improve sexual health and destigmatize sex (Boynton & Callaghan, 2006). For example, a February 4, 2021 issue of *Cosmopolitan* featured an article titled, "At-Home STI Kits for When You *Need* to Get Tested." Written at the height of the COVID pandemic, it advised readers matter-of-factly that "just because people are home now doesn't mean STIs are going away" (Andrews & Hsieh, 2021, para. 2). The authors acknowledged the difficulty in getting in-person appointments and reviewed about a half dozen testing options available through vendors with home delivery and mail-away results. As I scrolled through the article, I noted both a survey about the practice of halting non-emergency medical appointments as well as an invitation to join "Cosmo Unlocked" if I wanted to be "the best at sex," gaining access to "the real juicy stuff." A September 12, 2022 issue chronicled the experience of former *Big Bang Theory* co-star and current *Jeopardy!* host Mayim Bialik's visit to her gynecologist for her pap smear (Berry, 2022). The article included playful photos of Bialik in her clinic-issued paper gown, a screenshot of her Instagram post about the visit, and gentle urging for "individuals with vaginas" to schedule a visit to maintain sexual health.

Women's magazines have been frequent sites for analysis of sexual health content. Clarke (2010) examined *Cosmopolitan* and *Glamour* from 2000 to 2007 and discovered a paradox. In those years, these magazines simultaneously promoted sex as "ubiquitous, pleasurable, and casual" and STIs as "fearsome, rampant, gruesome, and repulsive" (p. 564). Wegmann (2013) retraced the breadcrumbs which accounted, in part, for the turn made in the 1990s by magazines catering to girls from a "risk" frame to a "desire" frame. McCabe (2005) identified virginity, contraception, and masturbation as topics addressed 25% of the time in question and answer advice columns in girls' magazines during the late 1990s. However, while acknowledging desire, curiosity, and agency, this format also tended to reinforce heteronormativity and medicalization through reliance on medical expert testimony.

Wegmann (2013) pointed out that, despite the preponderance of studies focusing on the sexual discourse of girls' magazines between 1998 and 2007, including *Seventeen*, none examined sexual health specifically. As Wegmann asserted, this finding holds significance because those years spanned both the Bill Clinton and George W. Bush administrations, when the "U.S. Federal Government instituted an abstinence-only curriculum policy for public schools" (p. 495). Wegmann's analysis confirmed the editorial commitment to valuing and respecting young readers of *Seventeen* and acknowledging their interest in sex. However, despite the regular inclusion and encouragement of contraceptive use, articles rarely incorporated instructions on how to use condoms and other contraceptive methods. Furthermore, the messages about contraception use implied zero responsibility on the part of male partners to participate.

Studies of men's magazines have revealed similar failures or resistance to addressing contraception use and instead focus on sex as a set of skills to improve heteronormative pleasure (Porter et al., 2017) or hegemonic performances of sexuality with the erect penis as central and indicative of masculinity (Owen & Campbell 2018). Unfortunately, Anstiss and Lyons (2014) reported that, while men do pen anonymous queries to popular men's health magazines for general health questions, they reinforced hegemonic performances with topics organized around pain and injuries, wrapped in an aura of stoicism and self-reliance, and an explicit distancing from the feminine. For example, according to Anstiss and Lyons, one help-seeker framed his query in a way that encompasses all three themes: "The skin on the back of my hands is dry and painful. Do I need to take a trip to a girly nail parlour, or are there some home remedies?" (p. 1365).

While not focused on advice columns per se, D'Enbeau (2011) provided a feminist textual analysis of the advertising in *Bust* – a pro-sex, third-wave feminist magazine with a target audience of 18- to 34-year-old women – and concluded that sex enhancement commodity advertising (including dildos and vibrators) can exist in conjunction with the magazine's stated commitment to feminism (including protest feminism), embrace sexual minority identities, and provide informal sexual health advice. Furthermore, companies marketed the use of these products without any endorsement or expectation of heteronormative relationships (or any relationships), instead often promoting them as an enhancement for self-pleasure.

Sexual Health on Social Media

Magazine advice columns notwithstanding, clear evidence demonstrates that informal, mediated sexual health content holds the potential to enhance traditional, formal mechanisms of delivering comprehensive sexual health education. Both the pop culture material – through characters, scenes, and plotlines – and the willingness to introduce more topics have reduced the pervasive neoliberal heteronormativity. This finding holds incredible importance, especially in those ultraconservative bastions which only endorse abstinence. While unplanned pregnancies and STIs represent two dangers of sexual activity, Allen (2021) advanced the idea of "breathing life" into sex education by embracing pleasure, sex positivity, and sexual well-being as complementary topics. Two social media spaces providing education about sexual health include TikTok and Instagram, both visually-based sites. The content generators on these sites seem to have answered Boynton and Callaghan's (2006) call for collaborative work that corrects many of the challenges required to eliminate media's inconsistent, outdated, and incorrect messages regarding sexual health.

Teens and young adults (15- to 24-year-olds), in particular, seek information about sexual health online (Fowler et al., 2021). In a content analysis of TikTok, employing the hashtag #sexeducation, Fowler et al. found sexual pleasure to be the most pervasive theme after female anatomy. While sex education also comprised a prevalent theme, the majority of these short videos about sex education were critical, singling out the curriculum as limited, with an overemphasis on STIs dominating the critique. While expanding the scope of sexual education content to topics beyond the dangers of STIs and unplanned pregnancies is absolutely necessary, Fowler et al. reported two concerns. First, the very nature of researching online – which allows for the perception of privacy – perpetuates the passive consumption of video and limits communication in terms of asking questions and perception-checking. Second, the overwhelming majority of TikTok videos are user-generated, and misinformation abounds, with little chance of oversight and corrections (see also Chapter 11, this volume). Without aspiring to restore the "old, linear 'expert message sender to receiver' approach" (Kreps & Neuhauser, 2010, p. 330), social media platforms – like TikTok – offer motivated health professionals a chance to engage with their young audiences. Through the hashtag #TikTokDoc, Stein et al. (2022) found that OB/Gyn physicians employed explanatory, documentary, comedic, communal, and interactive forms, resulting in both credibility and relatability to their audiences, generating sexual health information that could be accessible, entertaining, and interactive.

With over 23 million views, #TikTokDoc "yoxlyhealth" presents Sex Myths (#seggsfacts) from a clinical exam room with pulsing electronic music in the background. Her facial expressions and hand gestures accompanied the voiceover "Nope" as she debunked the myths "masturbation is harmful," "no smell = healthy vagina," "pubic hair is unhygienic," "you can't get pregnant on your period," and "frequent sex will loosen your vagina." The plentiful comments (close to 3000) engaged with several of the myths, generating animated clashes among viewers. In other TikTok videos, yoxlyhealth drew viewers' questions out of coffee cup and answered them with a clear, nonjudgmental tone. She read the questions verbatim – including slang – and translated the slang into clinical terms ("cum" to "ejaculate," for example) as she answered. A more general overview of #TikTokDoc revealed a wide variety of sexual topics including pleasure, hygiene, and a seemingly infinite number of questions about normalcy in terms of appearances, partners, and practices.

Without question, not all the docs on #TikTokDoc have the presence, production values, or followers of yoxlyhealth, but the popular hashtag's efforts are laudable. While discussing lay expertise and YouTube, Johnston (2016) emphasized presentation styles, trust, and viewer engagement of content producers in the area of sexual health curriculum to produce "the illusion of face-to-face interaction" (p. 76). Such attention effectively cultivates a parasocial relationship between "expert" and audience. This delivery method differs from the anonymous or disembodied expert discussed earlier in the magazine context.

Sciberras and Tanner (2023) explored infographics content – visually but not video-based – on Instagram in order to examine empowering representations of feminine sexuality. Following Carmody (2005), Sciberras and Tanner emphasized pleasure and ethical sexual intimacy by focusing their critical discourse analysis on posts of feminist and/or queer educators that feature colorful illustrations and text. As with yoxlyhealth on TikTok (among others), pleasure-based sex education also emphasizes unlearning misinformation (myths) while celebrating and normalizing consent, curiosity, and exploration. An illustration by @shrimpteeth, for example, featured two people sitting, facing each other, and kissing, with what appears to be a sex toy at hand. The caption read, "Sex is an experience not a performance," a perspective that emphasizes presence, play, improvisation, and possibility, rather than the less-than-sexy focus on sexual *function*. One respondent (@ruby_rare) posted an Instagram that depicted a pointed, embodied finger moving toward (but not reaching) an "OK" hand gesture's chasm with the message, "It's not all about penetration." This post served to decenter penile-vaginal penetration as the (heterosexual) sex act of choice. As with TikTok and YouTube, Instagram offers interactivity between the Instagram poster and her followers as well as among followers.

In this brave not-so-new-anymore world of social media, most sites allow users to provide feedback and comments to producers of content, including both pushing back against and embracing the capital "D" discourse of big pharma. In the next section of this chapter, I turn to advertising and marketing efforts of pharmaceutical companies who have profited considerably in the arena of sexual health. "Condition branding" constitutes, perhaps, a somewhat nicer way of saying "disease mongering," with the same implications: companies develop conditions for the drugs in the pipeline, repurpose existing drugs for new conditions, and solicit physician buy-in through a variety of incentives (Meixel et al. 2015; Syed et al. 2021).

Performance and Desire

Approximately 20 minutes into Amy Schumer's 2023 Netflix special *Emergency Contact*, she turned to the topic of post-partum sex. Dressed cheerfully in pink with white slip-on tennis shoes, she shared her doctor's admonition following the caesarean delivery of her newborn baby boy: "You cannot have sex for six weeks." After joking that she could easily wait six *years* after her C-section, she changed the topic to the conditions of her pregnancy. Well into her first pregnancy, she felt relief to receive a diagnosis for her chronic nausea and vomiting. Cloaked in the medicalese *hyperemesis gravidarum*, this perpetual queasiness with a name prompted her to ask, "So what do 'we' do?" Her care team explained, "We haven't been able to study it because it only happens to women." After pausing for the knowing audience applause inspired by her trademark cynicism, Schumer continued. She confided how her providers followed up this disappointing news with an offer of a new medical breakthrough: "If your husband wants, we now have chewable Viagra." Ms. Schumer goaded the crowd by making a pouty face, channeling a would-be erectile dysfunction sufferer who whined: "I want to get hard, but I don't want to take a *pill*."

As I demonstrated in my 2005 book, *The Viagra Ad Venture: Masculinity, Media, and the Performance of Sexual Health*, Pfizer Pharmaceuticals joined others at the table when they recast "impotence" as erectile dysfunction (ED) in the early 1990s. Such a rhetorical shift arguably decreased the social stigma of a condition that implicates the man as much as the physiological workings of male arousal. I examined the construction and use of the Sexual Health Inventory for Men (SHIM) to show how Pfizer Pharmaceuticals created a Likert-scale questionnaire, the results of which would declare any man in need of their little blue pill. Meanwhile, Pfizer also wooed physicians both by offering continuing medical education (CME) credits (often in exotic locales) and by encouraging pharmaceutical reps to provide monetary and other rewards to elite prescribers.

Based on the non-fiction "*Hard Sell: The Evolution of a Viagra Salesman*" by former drug rep Jamie Reidy (2005), the 2010 romantic comedy "*Love and Other Drugs*" dramatized the tactics employed by Pfizer. Without question, Viagra became enormously successful. With sales in excess of a billion dollars a year, two competitors – Levitra and Cialis – quickly followed in the years after its debut in 1998. In my analysis (Baglia, 2005), I focused on how news media and Pfizer's marketing promote very narrow definitions of masculinity and negate other possibilities for sexual play. As an example of their commitment to a heteronormative platform, Pfizer failed to market the product to gay men until more than 15 years after its launch (Williams, 2015), even though no good reason existed for why pharmaceutical firms producing erectile dysfunction drugs ignored the gay male market for so long. With Viagra's commercial success, other pharmaceutical companies sought a similarly profitable product. Tiefer (2006) provided a timeline for the promotion of Female Sexual Dysfunction (FSD), identifying the FDA approval of Viagra (sildenafil citrate) in 1998 as the "blast-off point" in the pharmaceutical pursuit for a pink pill that would solve the newly created and ambiguous problem of Female Sexual Arousal Disorder (FSAD).

Advertising and Women's Desire

Known as the long-awaited versions of a female Viagra, Addyi and Vyleesi were approved by the FDA in 2015 and 2019, respectively, to treat hypoactive sexual desire disorder (HSDD). Unlike Viagra, which is taken as needed, Addyi is taken daily. Vyleesi (bremelanotide) is a self-administered injection. Much earlier, in 2001, the FDA approved a product called the Eros clitoral therapy device (CTD) to treat female sexual dysfunction (FSD), also known as sexual arousal disorder (SAD), precursors to HSDD.

Flore (2019) pointed to the lead-up in the approval of Addyi by calling attention to the deployment of "social and digital media platforms including Facebook and Twitter, which mobilized discourses of post-feminism to reconfigure narratives of intimacy to lobby the FDA" (p. 3). Looking at 29 studies (including Flore's), Dan and Pauer (2023) focused on the social construction of low libido in women in public communication research. By examining strategic communication of key stakeholders (drug/device manufacturers), news stories (including advice columns), and examples in popular entertainment (such as *Sex and the City* and *Oprah!*), Dan and Pauer identified three frames from these studies: 1) the empowered frame, 2) the handmaid frame, and 3) the rejector frame. The empowered frame positions women as rightful beneficiaries in the use of treatment. The handmaid frame, on the other hand, identifies male partners as the beneficiaries, and the rejector frame envisions pharmacological- or device-responses to low libido as meddling and ignorant of the complexity inherent in human sexuality. Not surprisingly, among these frames, Dan and Pauer claimed that the empowered frame was overdetermined by strategic communication from pharmaceutical campaign messages; the discourse posited access to pharmaceutical treatment for increased desire as a 21st century women's rightful claim. The empowered frame also appeared most frequently. This embrace of biomedical solutions for a questionable diagnosis becomes operational through what Fishman and Mamo (2001) called "ideologies-in-progress" (p. 183). Unsurprisingly, pharmaceutical companies (along with news media and entertainment industries) have influenced attitudes about sexual health; performance and desire is but one entrée – prevention is another. While the development and improvement of contraceptive pills have long been in the domain of the pharmaceutical industry's marketing arm, promoting a product that sought to control sexual health targeted a much younger demographic.

Before turning to future directions for sexual health in popular culture research, I focus on sexually transmitted infections (STIs) and, especially, the launch of Merck Pharmaceutical's Gardasil vaccine and how it has been represented in popular culture.

Sexually Transmitted Infections (STIs)

HBO's *Girls*, written by Lena Dunham, premiered in 2012 and followed four friends navigating life in New York City following college. Dunham played Hannah Horvath, a writer, and the series revolved around the pursuit of meaningful employment and navigating the often-vexing terrain of sexual possibility. In Season One's third episode, Hannah tested positive for HPV. In discussing this unpleasant diagnosis with her friend Shoshanna (Zosia Mamet), she learned that her other friend, Jessa, also had HPV. According to Jessa, "all adventurous women do." Rogers (2016) employed this line from the script, observing the show's acknowledgment of HPV's commonality. However, Rogers also noted the stigma of the virus as well as – from the perspective of different characters in varying contexts – the fickle meaning of HPV. For example, Hannah reproduced Jessa's characterization when she posted "All adventurous women do" on her Twitter feed, but, earlier in the episode, in a brief skirmish with her roommate, Marnie (Allison Williams), she deflected Marnie's reminder that the rent was due when she pleaded, "But, I have pre-cancer!" For Rogers, the show both did and did not offer helpful representations of sexual health in that it did suggest an intervention and focused on the *source* of the infection (e.g., How does Hannah contract HPV?). Hannah spent a considerable amount of time trying to figure out how she contracted HPV, whereas the episode did not pursue how she – and others (including the viewing audience) – might avoid HPV in the future.

Conversely, in his analysis, Rogers (2016) appreciated the candid, somewhat stigma-free discussion of HPV that Hannah had, both with her friends and with her sexual partners. Returning to Amy Schumer's 2023 Netflix special, *Emergency Contact*, the 41-year-old comic briefly engaged with a younger (under 30) member of the audience when she looked at her and said, "You are definitely vaccinated for HPV. And I feel bad for you. You're missing out on an important character-building experience. We all had it." Here, Schumer both named the condition, its (controversial) solution and then contextualized it as a remarkably common problem.

In a reading of *Girls* as a postfeminist text, Kissling (2017) described the show (along with other postfeminist television shows) as emphasizing "individualism and choice" for 21st-century urban women, presenting both their successes and shortfalls as resulting from personal agency "rather than collective action or structural impediments" (p. 211). Notably, such shows impose the assumption of responsibility on young women regarding any of the dangers of sexual activity. Kissling detailed how Hannah confronted her current sex partner, Adam (Adam Driver), suggesting she picked up HPV from him. He claimed "angrily" that it wasn't possible "because he's been tested" (p. 214). Taking Adam's word for it, Kissling narrated how Hannah then contacted her old college boyfriend, Elijah. Hannah told Elijah that she and Adam have been having protected sex – which may have been true (but probably wasn't) – and Adam's been tested. Elijah responded, "Well, that's absurd." Hannah wanted to know why, and Elijah replied knowingly, "Because there is no test for men" (p. 215). Kissling concluded that shows like *Girls* – while delivering accurate sexual health information through realistic dialogue – reify the neoliberal sensibilities where sexual freedom "means also being responsible for not-so-independent (heterosexual) men who can't be relied upon to carry and use condoms or to know they may be carriers of HPV even if they can't be tested" (p. 220).

The FDA approved Merck's Gardasil in 2006 (McLemore, 2006). Beginning in 2007, it became recommended as a routine vaccination for girls aged 11 and 12. Thompson (2010) reported in her analysis of the public discourse around Gardasil's FDA approval that the director of the clinical trials suggested that girls *and* boys, aged 9 to 15, and 16- to 26-year-old girls and young women gain the most benefit from the vaccine. As the above examples from *Girls* imply and Thompson's epidemiological data underscored:

> [w]hile countless women learn about the important of regular gynecological exams, men have no established protocol, no annual exam, or comprehensive health education directing their lives. In matters of sexual and reproductive health, it continues to be far more common for men to attend to matters of sexual health only if or when visible symptoms of infection are evident.
> *(p. 123)*

Furthermore, HPV is spread *skin-to-skin*, so while condoms are useful and, in fact, most likely do inhibit some of the spread of HPV, they are not foolproof. In the *Girls* episode described above, Hannah revealed her own blind spot to this fact when, wrapped in a towel and sitting on her bed, she performed a half-hearted pelvic exam and then Googled "stuff that gets up around the sides of the condom."

Polzer and Knabe (2012) argued that, for girls, the Merck marketing suggested even the risk of *pending* sexual activity must be controlled through a biotechnical intervention in the form of the Gardasil vaccine. Furthermore, the subtext implied an emergent adolescence *without* the vaccine serves to pathologize sexual behavior itself. In other words, the prospect of human papillomavirus and the danger of cervical cancer makes sexual activity too risky; only Gardasil protects those (with vaginas) who want to engage in sex.

Malkowski (2014) investigated Merck's direct-to-consumer advertisements and concluded that they invoke complacency among female consumers. Following Thompson (2010), Malkowski advocated for Health Communication researchers to continue the work of deconstructing dominant medical discourses.

By the time that many of these types of pharmaceutical products get to market, the news media readily and willingly embraced them (Fishman & Casarett, 2006). Science legitimates much of the newsworthiness of news, whether newspaper or magazine, radio or television (Nelkin, 1996). Furthermore, science wants the public to learn of its inventions, developmental advancements, and breakthroughs (Glasser, 2008). Despite the misinterpretations of complex scientific information by journalists (Dentzer, 2009), the scientific community benefits when the news shares its work (Briggs & Hallin, 2016). More to the point, however, the media rarely raises questions about the science. Dubriwny's (2013) analysis of the Gardasil debate observed how Texas Governor Rick Perry initially signed a mandate that all Texas girls would get the vaccine before beginning sixth grade. Many (postfeminist) women considered the sexual agency that came from the vaccine as a positive choice. Texas conservatives raised a stink over Perry's executive order, as Dubriwny detailed it, because a vaccine that protects against HPV endorses promiscuity. In this skilled analysis of public communication, Dubriwny noted how agency constitutes – at once – something young women want but also something that conservatives don't want them to have. Perry reversed course. Meanwhile, the debate about whether boys should be vaccinated disappeared entirely. To close the loop on *Girls* (which, again, premiered in 2012, five years after the launch of Gardasil), the show did not recognize at all that either Hannah or Adam might have been vaccinated.

Whether we're talking about sexual advice, desire, or protection, Foucault's (1978) biopower – "the diverse techniques for achieving the subjugation of bodies" (p. 140) – becomes a useful theoretical concept, particularly (but not exclusively) when we consider the landscape of biomedicalization (Clark et al., 2003). In other areas, we can applaud the significant advances that have been made in bringing to the fore those subjugated bodies that have been made invisible by the dominant texts and images in popular culture. In their analysis of sexuality and disability in the Netflix series, *Special,*

Davies et al. (2022) summoned Foucault when they referenced his insistence on accepting scientific authority as "truth" – particularly in the realm of medicine – as early as the 17th century. As "authentic" knowledge production, medical discourse is "unquestionably true" (p. 53). They presented both disability studies and queer theories as examples of practices that destabilize binaries and orient us all to discourses of normalcy. I would add that feminist theory, indeed any critical theory, does this as well.

Future Directions

The COVID-19 pandemic had an interesting effect on marketing. With significant decreases in commuting and increases in commercial-free streaming services, more advertising dollars found their way to social media sites (Carey et al., 2022; Szalai, 2021). TikTok, Instagram, YouTube, X (formerly Twitter), and even Meta/Facebook (along with anything "new" coming down the pike) remain rich areas for the analysis of sexual health in popular culture. Although television isn't delivered in the same way today as in its first 40 years of existence – with limited channels and the sense that we were all watching the same thing – the fact remains that audiences of television programs are (or can be) enormous and their chatter about what happens in a scene, an episode, a season, or over an entire series finds its way into the news, and onto fan sites and other social media sites.

In this chapter, I have endeavored to capture topics to maximize range across different channels that deliver popular culture, and yet I would have liked to include so much more. Before moving to a summary of dominant theories and methodologies, along with some un(der)tapped topics, I will provide an example of the mediated breadth of a single show.

The series *"Sex Education*" remains one of the most popular on Netflix (Tauty et al., 2021). Key characters include Otis Milburn (Asa Butterfield), a high school student at Moordale Secondary School in England, and his mother Jean (Gillian Anderson), who works as a sex therapist. Despite his limited (or maybe nonexistent) experiences with sex in Season One, Otis expressed considerable knowledge about anatomy and many of the features of its charms, chaff, and challenges. Classmate Maeve Wiley (Emma Mackey) self-identified as a school "pariah," owing to the reputation gained through having multiple sex partners. In one episode, Otis was speaking with Maeve after class when they heard a concerning cry of pain coming from an old abandoned building on the school grounds. They found Adam (Adam Groff), who had become concerned about his above-average erect penis. Adam experienced priapism after ingesting three Viagra tablets. Otis, who had already exhibited his considerable acumen about sex and sexual health to Maeve, advised Adam that time is the most likely remedy. While not explicitly discussed, Adam had taken what amounted to an overdose of Viagra because he thought that the medicine would help him to ejaculate, which he had trouble accomplishing with his girlfriend. Importantly, Otis encouraged Adam to become comfortable with himself, to "own his narrative." But, Otis did not correct Adam's misconception, not for Adam, and not for the audience. Independent of this fact, Maeve recognized an opportunity and, the next day, suggested that she and Otis go into business. She would find the clients and handle the financials; Otis would dispense the advice.

As with plenty of contemporary television, sexual content is explicit, expansive, and frequently educational. Most importantly, the promise of incorporating contemporary, audience-centered examples into formal sexual health curricula encourages productive dialogue and debate. News articles have been written about *Sex Education*, along with YouTube clips, and page after page of TikTok clips (Larson, 2020; Poniewozik, 2019). The patterns of media rearticulation of this show have been impressive, and, clearly, the uses of media are fulfilling for its legions of fans, who want to piece together their favorite characters and controversies for contemplation and communication.

With so many more newspapers and magazines in digital form now than 20 years ago, I think that a huge opportunity exists not only for the visual analysis of accompanying illustrations and advertising but also for examinations of comments and co-opting, which abound in Web 2.0. The lived experiences of sexually diverse readers come through the comments for consideration, especially in fan sites and general news commentary for and about television shows such as *Orange Is the New Black, Special, Never Have I Ever, Heartstopper, Sex Education,* and *Never, Rarely, Sometimes, Always*. These shows engage with themes and storylines attractive to sexual minorities and/or tackle provocative subject matter.

Finally, I'd like to list some subjects which space did not permit me to explore but that I found extremely enticing as sexual health topics. These topics include the mediated representations of sexual assault investigations (which frequently include a biomedical component), cosmetic genital surgery (i.e., labiaplasty and phalloplasty), premature ejaculation – also referred to (somewhat conflictingly) as ejaculatory control, vasectomies (especially in light of the *Roe v. Wade* reversal decision), vulvodynia (pain in and around the vagina), and sex addiction. For now, many of these topics remain in the news and, in some cases, through marketing and advertising.

The summer blockbuster movie of 2023 was, without question, *Barbie*. In a memorable scene, Stereotypical Barbie (Margot Robbie) and Ken (Ryan Gosling) have emerged in the real world, and Barbie found herself explaining that she doesn't have a vagina, and Ken doesn't have a penis. "We don't have genitals," she summarized. With this scene in mind, I'm troubled, in the realm of cosmetic genital surgery, by the "option" of labiaplasty – which, again occupies this disconcerting liminal space between postfeminist agency and biopower's normalcy – being advertised on more than one plastic surgery website as the "Barbie Procedure."

Consider how businesses pitch this procedure: "Many women suffer from enlarged labia minora (the inner genital lips). Some may not like the appearance of their large, uneven or thick labia" (De La Cruz Plastic Surgery, n.d., para. 1). The website lists the advantages of genital beautification (or vaginal rejuvenation), but it doesn't clarify the name: the "Barbie Procedure." *Jezebel* columnist Katie Baker (2013) voiced concern in her article, "Unhappy with your gross vagina? Why not try 'the Barbie'?" Baker asked, "Why the fuck do women want their vulvas to look like they're made out of plastic?" (para. 5). We know the film *Barbie* ended with Stereotypical Barbie going to see her gynecologist, presumably with her new, real genitals. We might all hope to have this kind of transformative awakening through popular culture. Until then, we have a lot of work to do.

Further Reading

Aggleton, P., Parker, R., & Thomas, F. (Eds.) (2015). *Culture, health, and sexuality.* Routledge. A multidisciplinary look in nineteen chapters at the socio-cultural factors which intersect with sexuality and sexual health.

Allen, L., & Rasmussen, M. L. (2017). **Palgrave Handbook of sexuality education.* Palgrave. 34 chapters exploring how and where sex education is taught (and could be taught).

Kuhn, A. (2016). *The power of the image: Cultural representations of sex and sexuality.* Routledge. How visual art creates expectations for sexual normalcy as well as novel reimaginings.

McRuer, R., & Mollow, A. (Eds.). (2012). *Sex and disability.* Duke University Press. Seventeen chapters explore how sex and disability are closely related topics across multiple disciplines.

Spurgas, A. (2021). *Diagnosing desire: Biopolitics and femininity into the twenty-first century.* Ohio University Press. How cultural studies interprets neoliberalism, sex, gender, and whiteness and their role in feminine sexuality.

References

Allen, L. (2021). *Breathing life into sexuality education.* Palgrave.

Allyn, D. (2016). *Make love, not war: The sexual revolution: An unfettered history.* Routledge.

Andrews, T., & Hsieh, C. (2021, February 4). Here are your STI testing options if you can't get an appointment with your doctor because of the coronavirus. *Cosmopolitan.* https://www.cosmopolitan.com/sex-love/a27533540/at-home-sti-std-test-kits/

Anstiss, D., & Lyons, A. (2014). From men to the media and back again: Help-seeking in popular men's magazines. *Journal of Health Psychology, 19,* 1358–1370.

Baglia, J. (2005). *The Viagra ad venture: Masculinity, media, and the performance of sexual health.* Peter Lang.

Baker, K. (2013, January 18). Unhappy with your gross vagina? Why not try "The Barbie"? *Jezebel.* https://jezebel.com/unhappy-with-your-gross-vagina-why-not-try-the-barbie-5977025

Berry, E. (2022, September 12). Fans rally around Mayim Bialik after her pap smear post on Instagram. *Cosmopolitan.* https://www.cosmopolitan.com/entertainment/celebs/a41169739/mayim-bialik-health-pap-smear-mammogram-instagram-news/

Boynton, P., & Callaghan, W. (2006). Understanding media coverage of sex: A practical discussion paper for sexologists and journalists. *Sexual and Relationship Therapy, 21,* 333–346.

Briggs, C. L., & Hallin, D. C. (2016). *Making health public: How news coverage is remaking media, medicine, and contemporary life.* Routledge.

Brown, J., Halpern, C. T., & L'Engle, K. L. (2005). Mass media as a sexual super peer for early maturing girls. *Journal of Adolescent Health, 36,* 420–427.

Carey, J., Gallent, J. S., & Stipp, H. (2022). The COVID-19 pandemic and consumer media behavior. In G. Einav (Ed.), *Transitioning media in a post COVID world: Digital transformation, immersive technologies, and consumer behavior* (pp. 1–17). Springer International Publishing.

Carmody, M. (2005) Ethical erotics: Reconceptualizing anti-rape education. *Sexualities, 8,* 465–480.

Clarke, A., Shim, J., Mamo, L., Fosket, J., & Fishman, J. (2003). Biomedicalization: technoscientific transformations of health, illness, and U.S. biomedicine." *American Sociological Review, 68,* 161–194

Clarke, J. (2010). The paradoxical portrayal of the risk of sexually transmitted infections and sexuality in U.S. magazines *Glamour* and *Cosmopolitan,* 2000-2007. *Health, Risk, and Society, 12,* 560–574.

Collins, R., Strasburger, V., Brown, J., Donnerstein E., Lenhart, A., & Ward, L. M. (2017). Sexual media and childhood well-being and health. *Pediatrics, 140* (Supplement 2), S162–166.

Cosmopolitan (2023, December). "About us." *Cosmopolitan Magazine.* https://www.cosmopolitan.com/about/a26950060/about-us-contact-information-masthead/

Dan, V., & Pauer, C. (2023). Empowered, handmaid, or rejector? The framing of low libido in women according to scholarly investigations of public communication. *Health Communication, 38,* 705–713. https://doi.org/10.1080/10410236.2021.1971356

Davies, A., Maich, K., Belcher, C., Cagulada, E., DeWelles, M., & van Rhijn, T. (2022). A critical examination of the intersection of sexuality and disability in *Special,* a Netflix series. In M. Jeffries (Ed.) *In disability representation in film, TV, and print media* (pp. 44–64). Routledge.

De La Cruz Plastic Surgery (n.d.). Barbie procedure for genital beautification. https://www.delacruzplasticsurgery.com/barbie-procedure-labiaplasty

D'Enbeau, S. (2011). Sex, feminism, and advertising: The politics of advertising feminism in a competitive marketplace. *Journal of Communication Inquiry, 35,* 53–69.

Dentzer, S. (2009). Communicating medical news: The pitfalls of health care journalism. *New England Journal of Medicine, 360,* 1–3. https://doi.org/10.1056/NEJMp0805753

Dillman Carpentier, F., Stevens, E., Wu, L., & Seely, N. (2017). Sex, love, and risk-n-responsibility: A content analysis of entertainment television. *Mass Communication, and Society, 20,* 686–709.

Döring, N. (2021). Sex education on social media. In A. D. Lykins (Ed.) *Encyclopedia of sexuality and gender* (pp. 1–12). Springer Nature Switzerland. https://doi.org/10.1007/978-3-319-59531-3_64-1

Dubriwny, T. (2013). *The vulnerable empowered woman: Feminism, postfeminism, and women's health.* Rutgers University Press.

Fishman, J., & Casarett, D. (2006). Mass media and medicine: When the most trusted media mislead. *Mayo Clinic Proceedings, 81,* 291–293.

Fishman, J., & Mamo, L. (2001). What's in a disorder?: A cultural analysis of medical and pharmaceutical constructions of male and female sexual dysfunctions. *Women & Therapy, 24,* 179–193.

Flore, J. (2019). Intimate tablets: Digital advocacy and post-feminist pharmaceuticals. *Feminist Media Studies, 19,* 3–18. https://doi.org/ 10.1080/14680777.2017.1393834

Foucault, M. (1978), *History of sexuality, Volume 1.* Random House.

Fowler, L., Schoen, L., & Morain, S. (2021). Sex education on TikTok: A content analysis of themes. *Health Promotion Practice, 23,* 739–742.

Glasser, S. (2008). The media and clinical research. In S. Glasser (Ed.) *Essentials of clinical research* (pp. 329–333). Springer.

Graf, A. S., & Patrick, J. H. (2015). Foundations of life-long sexual health literacy. *Health Education, 115,* 56–70

Halkitis, P. (2019). The Stonewall riots, the AIDS epidemic, and the public's health. *American Journal of Public Health, 109,* 851–852.

Hart, G., & Wellings, K. (2002). Sexual behavior and its medicalization: In sickness and in health. *BMJ [British Medical Journal], 324,* 896–900.

Hether, H., & Murphy, S. (2009). Sex roles in health storylines on prime time television: A content analysis. *Sex Roles, 62,* 810–821. https://doi.org/10.1007/s11199-009-9654-0.

Hite, S. (1976). *The Hite report: A nationwide study of female sexuality.* Seven Stories Press.

Hust, S., Brown, J., & L'Engle, K. (2008). Boys will be boys and girls better be prepared: An analysis of the rare sexual health messages in young adolecents' media. *Mass Communication & Society, 11,* 3–23.

Johnston, J. (2016). Subscribing to sex edutainment: Sex education, online video, and the YouTube star. *Television & New Media, 18,* 76–92.

Kissling, E. (2017). All postfeminist women do: Women's sexual and reproductive health in television comedy. In M. Nash & I. Whelehan (Eds.) *Reading Lena Dunham's* Girls: *Feminism, postfeminism, authenticity and gendered performance in contemporary television* (pp. 209–223). Palgrave MacMillan.

Kreps, G., & Neuhauser, L. (2010). New directions in eHealth communication: Opportunities and challenges. *Patient Education and Counseling, 78,* 329–336.

Kunkel, D., Eyal, K., Finnerty, K., Biely, E., & Donnerstein, E. (2005). Sex on TV 4: A Kaiser Family Foundation Report (Report No. 4). Kaiser Family Foundation.

Lameiras-Fernández, M., Martínez-Román, R., Carrera-Fernández, M. V., & Rodríguez-Castro, Y. (2021). Sex education in the spotlight: What is working? Systematic review. *International Journal of Environmental Research and Public Health, 18,* 2555–2586.

Larson, S. (2020, January 18). *Sex Education,* season 2: The doctor is in. *The New Yorker.* https://www.newyorker.com/culture/on-television/sex-education-season-2-the-doctor-is-in.

Mackin, D., & Thornborrow, J. (2003). Branding and discourse: The case of *Cosmopolitan. Discourse & Society, 144,* 453–471.

Malkowski, J. (2014). Confessions of a pharmaceutical company: Voice, narrative, and the case of Gardasil. *Health Communication, 29,* 81–92.

McCabe, J. (2005) Who are the experts? Medicalization in teen magazine advice columns. In L. Bass (Ed.) *Sociological studies of children and youth* (pp. 153–191). Elsevier.

McLemore, M, (2006). Gardasil: Introducing the new human papillomavirus vaccine, *Clinical Journal of Oncology Nursing, 10,* 559–560.

Meixel, A., Yanchar, E., & Fugh-Berman, A. (2015). Hypoactive sexual desire disorder: Inventing a disease to sell low libido. *Journal of Medical Ethics, 41,* 859–862.

Nelkin, D. (1996). An uneasy relationship: The tensions between medicine and the media. *Lancet, 347,* 1600–1603.

Owen, C., & Campbell, C. (2018). How do men's magazines talk about penises? *Journal of Health Psychology, 23,* 332–344.

Pariera, K., Hether, H., Murphy, S., de Castro Buffington, S., & Baezconde-Garbanati, L. (2014). Portrayals of reproductive and sexual health on primetime television, *Health Communication, 29,* 698–706.

Polzer, J., & Knabe, S. (2012). From desire to disease: Human papillomavirus (HPV) and the medicalization of nascent female sexuality. *The Journal of Sex Research, 49,* 344–352. https://doi.org/10.1080/00224499.2011.644598

Poniewozik, J. (2019, January 9). Review: *Sex Education*, a sweet teen comedy of modern lust. *The New York Times*. https://www.nytimes.com/2019/01/09/arts/television/sex-education-review-netflix.html

Porter, C., Douglas, N., & Collumbien, M. (2017). Enhance her pleasure—and your grip strength: *Men's Health* magazine and pseudo-reciprocal pleasure. *Culture, Health, & Sexuality, 19,* 738–751.

Reidy, J. (2005). *The hard sell: Evolution of a Viagra salesman.* Andrews McMeel Publishing.

Robinson, P. (1976). *The modernization of sex.* Harper & Row.

Rogers, B. (2016). "All adventurous women do": HPV, narrative, and HBO's *Girls. Health Communication, 31,* 83–96.

Sciberras, R., & Tanner, C. (2023). "Sex is so much more than penis in vagina": Sex education, pleasure and ethical erotics on Instagram. *Sex Education,* 1–14. https://doi.org/10.1080/14681811.2023.2199976

Seabrook, R., Ward, L. M., Cortina, L., Giaccardi, S., & Lippman, J. (2017). Girl power or powerless girl? Television, sexual scripts, and sexual agency in sexually active young women. *Psychology of Women Quarterly, 41,* 240–253. https://doi.org/10.1177/0361684316677028

Seale, C. (2002). *Media & health.* SAGE.

Showalter, E. (1993). On hysterical narrative. *Narrative, 1,* 24–35.

Starrs, A., & Anderson, R. (2016). Definitions and debates: Sexual health and sexual rights. *The Brown Journal of World Affairs, 22,* 7–23.

Stein, K., Yao, Y., & Aitamurto, T. (2022). Examining communicative forms in #TikTokDocs' sexual health videos, *International Journal of Communication, 16,* 1309–1331.

Syed, S., Dixson, B., Constantino, E., & Regan, J. (2021). The law and practice of off-label prescribing and physician promotion. *Journal of the American Academy of Psychiatry and the Law, 49,* 1–7.

Szalai, G. (2021, December 5). Social media ad market to overtake TV in 2022, Zenith forecasts. *Hollywood Reporter*. https://www.hollywoodreporter.com/business/business-news/advertising-market-recovery-covid-social-media-overtake-tv-1235055453/

Tauty, S., Martin, P., Bourmaud, A., Chapoton, B., La Rochebrochard, E., & Alberti, C. (2021). Sexual health promotion messages for young people in Netflix most-watched series content (2015-2020): A mixed-methods analysis study. *BMJ Open [British Medical Journal], 11:* e052626.

Tiefer, L. (2006). Female sexual dysfunction: A case study of disease mongering and activist resistance. *PLoS Medicine, 3*(4), e178. https://doi.org/10.1371/journal.pmed.0030178

Thompson, M. (2010). Who's guarding what? A poststructural feminist analysis of Gardasil discourses, *Health Communication, 25,* 119–130.

Treicher, P. (1999). *How to have a theory in an epidemic: Cultural chronicles of AIDS.* Duke University Press.

Vance, C. (Ed.) (1992). *Pleasure and danger. Exploring female sexuality.* Pandora.

Ward, L. M., Day, K., & Epstein, M. (2006). Uncommonly good: Exploring how mass media may be a positive influence on young women's sexual health and development. *New Directions for Child and Adolescent Development, 112,* 57–70.

Wegmann, J. (2013). It must be true – I read it in "Seventeen" Magazine: US popular culture and sexual messages in an era of abstinence-only education. *Sex Education: Sexuality, Society, and Learning, 13*(5), 494–508. https://doi.org/10.1080/14681811.2013.765358

Wheeler, L. A. (2017). Inventing sexuality: Ideologies, identities, and practices in the Gilded Age and Progressive Era. In C. Nichols & N. Unger (Eds) *A companion to the gilded age and progressive era* (pp. 102–115). Wiley & Sons.

White, A., Boehm, M., Glackin, E., & Bleakley, A. (2023). How sexual information sources are related to emerging adults' sex-positive scripts and sexual communication, *Sexuality & Culture, 27,* 1224–1245.

Williams, M. E. (2015, October 22). Gay men buy Viagra, too: We demand our gay ED ad! *Salon*. https://www.salon.com/2015/10/22/wheres_our_gay_ed_ad/

WHO. (1948). *Preamble to the Constitution of the World Health Organization*. Official records of the World Health Organization, no. 2, p. 100. https://www.who.int/about/accountability/governance/constitution

WHO. (1975). Education and treatment in human sexuality: The training of health professionals (Technical Report Series, No. 572). https://iris.who.int/handle/10665/38247

WHO. (2006). Defining sexual health: Report of a technical consultation on sexual health, 28–31 January 2002. https://www.cesas.lu/perch/resources/whodefiningsexualhealth.pdf

WHO. (2010). Developing sexual health programmes: A framework for action. Defining sexual health (Report No. WHO/RHR/HRP/10.22). http://whqlibdoc.who.int/hq/2010/WHO_RHR_HRP_10.22_eng.pdf

Wolf, D. (Director). (2020). *Skin: A history of nudity in the movies*. Plausible Films.

7

THEY DON'T LOOK SICK

Popular Culture and Women's Health

Sarah LeBlanc

Golden Girls (1985–1992; NBC) did not shy away from health issues, leading conversations about older adults using contraception to keep themselves safe from STDs, how heart attack symptoms for women look different than those of men, and how AIDS is not a bad person disease (Sheknows, 2017). In 1989, *Golden Girls* featured a two-part episode where Dorothy (Bea Arthur) complained about not being able to shake a cold that came on a few weeks prior (S5.E1; S5.E2). She visited two or three doctors, only to be told her symptoms were "psychosomatic" or maybe she was depressed. Only after she spoke with her neighbor, Dr. Harry Weston (Richard Mulligan), a pediatric doctor with professional contacts, who introduced to another doctor did she receive a diagnosis of chronic fatigue syndrome.

Nearly 25 years after the airing of those 2 episodes, many women still experience the brushed-off "because they don't look sick" response or aren't believed. This 25-year-old plot line is reflected today (Thompson et al., 2023). Entertainment health narratives provide either a positive distraction or can be harmful if diseases are portrayed inaccurately (Collins et al., 2024). For better or worse, television can set expectations for what to expect; what we watch influences our behaviors, beliefs, values, and attitudes (Bessett & Murawsky, 2017). For example, early research on mediated depictions of postpartum depression (PPD) focused on PPD being a result of traumatic events (Fenton Stitt, 2012; Tropp, 2012). Tropp also asserted that some media representations attributed weak attachment between the mother and the baby to an external event, such as a coma, an affair, or the baby being cut out of the mother's womb and taken from the mother. When looking at more contemporary shows, LeBlanc (2021) determined that they presented attachment to be based on something internal going on with the mother. In that piece, I argued that the gender makeup of the writer's room changed, with the postpartum storyline in *Black-ish* based on the real-life experiences of the head writer (Ellenbogen, 2017) and the one in *Workin' Moms* based on the leading lady, Catherine Reitman's, real-life experience (Reitman, 2019).

This chapter provides an overview of how women's health is communicated and portrayed in popular culture. Given the vast definition of women's health, I use my background as a maternal health and menstrual communication scholar and a Generation Xer to determine which health issues I cover in this chapter. Specifically, I focus on menstruation, cancer, and dementia, given that other topics will be addressed elsewhere in this collection or have been explored in prior research. For example, Johnson (2018) overviewed how HIV/AIDS had been portrayed on television and my earlier research

 DOI: 10.4324/9781003436409-8

(LeBlanc, 2021) discussed postpartum depression. For issues such as mental health, sexual health, and neurological health, please see other chapters in this volume.

This chapter features select examples from television, movies, and books. I refrained from focusing exclusively on popular medical dramas such as *Grey's Anatomy, ER, Chicago Hope, House,* etc., but I do mention *Grey's Anatomy* in the dementia section. I made this choice mainly because avid viewers of medical dramas have been found to have more fatalistic attitudes toward health, do not take their health concerns as seriously as they need to, or even have a negative influence on health-related matters (Chung, 2014; Hoffman et al., 2017; Ye & Ward, 2010). Furthermore, only 6% of diagnoses may be affiliated with common diseases (Meyer & Yermal, 2021). I want to give this chapter a more contemporary look at women's health, relying on examples from my lifetime as a Generation Xer.

"A Woman's Cycle Is Shameful"

As a menstruation communication researcher, I pay attention to different forms of popular culture for mentions of menstruation. More often than not, I finish a book or a series without any mention. When I do find a mention, I get excited in an "*OMG! They mentioned menstruation*" kind of moment. For example, a series of books about seven siblings, known in literary circles as the Bergman Brothers series by Chloe Leise, integrated menstruation or a period act in nearly every book of the series. Each brother noted how they grew up knowing about menstruation because their father was a doctor, and they had two sisters. I looked forward to each book in the series because I wanted to know how the next sibling would tackle menstruation or how menstruation would show up while I was lost in their world.

Menstruation constitutes an intimate but integral part of women's health, but limited scholarship exists on how popular culture addresses menstruation. Exemplars include Rosewarne's (2012) overview of menstruation in television before 2012, Kissling's (2002) examination of menstruation storylines, and an undergraduate honors thesis (Tropp, 2012). Popular culture is starting to embrace menstruation as Yuko (2017a) dubbed 2017 as the year of menstrual cameos.

Keeping menstruation out of popular culture works to perpetuate cultural preferences for treating it as invisible and unspoken (Chaney, 2017). This treatment is evident in American and British literature and films as menstruation is rarely found to be a theme or a plot device (Kasenko, 2019). Menstruation became a more frequent topic in popular culture around 2016, after Jennifer Weisser-Wolf (2017) dubbed 2015 the year of menstruation,[1] which could have led to more movies and television mentioning menstruation (Todd, 2016). For a future book chapter, some colleagues and I are investigating fiction books written by female authors since 2017 to determine how books may frame or talk about menstruation; we are finding more and more books mention menstruation, even going as far as to make menstrual products a murder weapon (LeBlanc et al., under development).

This section addresses how menstruation has been represented and what these representations communicate about women's health. Specifically, this section highlights three sub-themes that weave society's menstrual narrative by characters using language that supports or refutes the narrative.

Menstruation is shameful or secret. The lessons that we learn about periods stay with us, and we pass these on to future generations (Aragòn & Cooke-Jackson, 2021). Popular culture depicts menstruation as shameful and secretive, supporting the master societal narrative (Delaney et al., 1988). We see this scenario play out in *Anne with an E* (2017–2019), a Netflix adaptation of *Anne of Green Gables*. After watching the episode (S1.E5), I discovered this adaptation was the first to discuss menstruation since the book's release in 1908 (Yuko, 2017b); the original book did not talk about menstruation. When Anne shared with her female classmates that she was menstruating, one told her, "No one is supposed to know. A woman's cycle is shameful."

Another show that tackled menstruation and puberty was *The Babysitter's Club* (2020–2021; Netflix). Notably, published four decades earlier, the book on which this episode is based, also titled *Kristy's Big Day* (1987), did not address menstruation. In *Kristy's Big Day,* Kristy experienced menarche at the reception following the wedding of her mom (Alicia Silverstone) to Watson (Mark Feuerstein). Kristy ran to the bathroom with her friends trailing after her. The girls figured out the problem; Marianne, Kristy's best friend, handed Kristy a pad through the door and explained how to put it on. Kristy's club friends assisted Kristy in her moment of need, but Kristy still shared her menarche with her mom. Kristy's mom asked Kristy if she had any questions, but Kristy explained that her friends helped her out. This storyline could potentially spark conversations about menstruation between real-life mothers and daughters as Kristy and her mom made it look easy. This example demonstrates how not all menarche experiences end with "we don't talk about menses."

While plotlines or themes may keep menstruation silent or treat it as shameful, menstrual products are a different story. Menstruation as a storyline started in 1970 with the publication of *Are You There God? It's Me, Margaret* (1970) by Judy Blume, but the book was not made into a feature film until 2023. In it, the characters verbally communicated about menstruation, and the film featured unused pads. However, most of the signs of menstruation remained hidden. This presentation affirmed that the act of menstruating should be hidden, but products may be visible.

Some films, such as *She's the Man (2006)*, framed tampons as a device to help with bloody noses. More recently, the Netflix show *XO Kitty* (2023) showcased one girl in detention having the male detention supervisor ask the other students if anyone had a tampon or pad. This scene was used as a distraction so that two other students could sneak back into detention (S1.E7). In the scene, two fellow female classmates held up a pad and a tampon, which the menstruating girl grabbed as she headed to the ladies' room.

In *The Queen's Gambit* (S1. E2), a fellow female chess competitor handed Beth Harmon a sanitary napkin and asked Beth if she knew how to use it. In *Anne with an E*, Marilla Cuthbert instructed Anne Shirley on how she must wear cotton cloth, rinse the cloth in cold water, and then wash it in hot water during her monthly cycle (S1, E5). This scene between Anne and Marilla is how *Anne with an E* stayed true to what products were like in the early 19th century, but it defied the notion that the act is hidden, as the water turned red when Anne attempted to wash her sheets. This scene marked one of the first times that red water, instead of blue water, became visible on television.

Women are treated differently. When women talk about our periods, we are told "[t]hat's normal," as evident in a scene from the Amazon Prime show "*Harlem*" Tye, one of the four prominent females featured in the show, passed out on the subway, and her friend Quinn rushed her to the hospital (S1.E6). After waiting for four hours, the doctor informed Tye that her back pain and fainting were due to her cycle and that everything was normal. "Is having it for 11 days, normal?" she asked. The doctor reminded Tye and her friend Quinn that each body is different. Tye sought help from the doctor, only to be shut down and assured that her menstruation was "normal."

Tye's experience underscores the message to viewers that, even when women speak up about a medical problem, they are told that what they are experiencing is not out of the ordinary. As such, they don't require treatment or medication, and protests to the contrary could be considered "hysterical" or "drug seeking." In the prior example, Tye wanted something stronger than aspirin and became assertive when her concerns and requests were dismissed, at one point even being labeled a drug seeker. The tendency to keep medical concerns quiet begins with menstruation but carries with women as they mature. For example, LeBlanc et al. (2023) determined that new mothers keep quiet about PPD symptoms for many of the same reasons, such as the perception that they are seeking drugs or that what they are feeling is normal. The 2020 documentary, *Ms. Diagnosis* (Regan, 2020), showcased how women with heart problems are labeled as being depressed or anxious.

Don't Tell Dad. Popular culture representations of menstruation routinely depict it as a family problem, something parents must solve. Kissling's (2002) examined shows such as *Rosanne*, *7th*

Heaven, King of the Hill, and *Something So Right.* Kissling's takeaways include: menstruation and/or menarche signify differences between girls and boys, comprise awkward situations for fathers, and position mothers as the ones to assist with their child's menarche. In the last 20 years, these themes continue to be played out in films and television.

Fathers, or males in general, in popular culture continue to treat menstruation as an awkward experience. *Modern Family's "Red Alert"* episode (S10.E16) featured teenage daughter Lilly locked in the bathroom while her male parents, Cam and Mitchell, fretted over what to do outside the bathroom door. Mitchell announced that he would leave and "tackle his fear of the feminine hygiene aisle," which mirrored Hank Hill's situation in *King of the Hill* (Kissling, 2002). Mitchell returned with a plethora of products, framing menstrual product buying as an overwhelming experience for men. David, in *Schitt's Creek,* watched his boss's stepdaughter as a favor to his boss, and, incidentally, the stepdaughter started her period during their time that they were together (S2.E10). David yelled through the bathroom door that Alexis, his sister, had products under the sink. The word menstruation or period was not mentioned, but viewers could see David nonverbally communicate the awkwardness of having to be the one handling menarche.

In the 2017 Angel Soft commercial, *Just Dad,* when a dad followed his daughter to the bathroom where she closed the door on him. The dad leaned against the door frame with crossed arms and commented, "What? You're becoming a woman?" When his daughter communicated discomfort by saying, "Dad-ad," he left, saying, "I'm leaving." This scene in the commercial signifies how menstruation can be an awkward time for fathers (Kissling, 2002) but also how daughters don't necessarily want to communicate with their dad about menstruation.

Fathers in popular culture indicate assumptions that behavioral issues are correlated to menstruation. In *To All the Boys I've Loved Before,* Dr. Covey and Kitty, his youngest daughter, discussed Lara Jean, the main character and middle daughter.

Dr. Covey:	What's her problem?
Kitty:	Moon day?
Dr. Covey:	"Moon day"? Menstruation is science. It has nothing to do with the moon.
Kitty:	Says you, Doctor Man. But the goddess within says it's a sacred rhythm that represents the deepest cycle of womanhood.

This exchange connected Lara Jean's problem with menstruation, which viewers don't know to be true or not.

In *Modern Family's Red Alert,* Cam sent a group message to the females in the family, seeking help for Lily. All the female characters – minus Claire, Mitchell's sister – appeared at some point during the episode to assist Lily. First, Gloria, her step-grandmother who was originally from Colombia in South America, arrived to assist Lily. Gloria's Colombian heritage played a role in how she approached Lily's menarche. In Colombia, a "Godmother" applies the powdered caravurú, a vegetable-based rub, on the young girl's skin. The young girl also inhales a hot spice mix (Zuluaga & Andersson, 2013). Zuluaga and Andersson found that young Colombian girls who participated in rites were less likely to have dysmenorrhea than those who did not.

In addition to Gloria, Lily's female cousins arrived to provide help, each arriving with a different perspective on how to approach menstruation. Alex, who tended to be scholastic, represented the educational importance of menstruation, bringing in and later reading brochures on biology and menstruation. Haley, Alex's older sister who often was the comic relief, offered the humor aspect of menstruation by sharing with Lily how periods provided her a "get out of jail free card." In the end, though, Lily opened the bathroom door for Mitchell and Cam, and they discussed her menarche as a family (off-screen), providing a conclusion that dads can talk about menstruation.

"Did the 'red peony' bloom?[2]" If dads can find comfort in talking about menstruation, then surely moms can do the same. This section examines popular culture representations of how mothers and daughters deal with menstruation. More recently, television shows and movies have provided a trend of mothers assisting their daughters with menstruation, including *Black-ish, The Queen's Gambit, The Middle, Turning Red* (2022), and *Are You There, God? It's Me, Margaret* (2023). When Mei-Mei turned into a red panda in *Turning Red,* her mom, Ming, ran into the bathroom listing off the menstrual products and medicine in the house. When Margaret (of *Are You There God),* finally got her period, she yelled for her mom (Barbara). They cried happy tears in the bathroom, and Barbara (Rachel McAdams) asked if she needed help learning how to put pads on. Margaret declined, saying that she had been practicing for months (Blume, 1970; Craig & Blume, 2023).

Not only are moms helpful, but they often communicate excitement when their daughter experiences menarche. "*The Middle*" (2009–2018; ABC), which centered on the Heck family in Indiana, captured this moment when Sue (only daughter; Eden Sher) awoke Frankie (her mom; Patricia Heaton) in the middle of the night during a family camping trip to let her know her period started. Suddenly, a bear appeared, and Brick, the youngest child (Atticus Shaffer), explained that bears are attracted to the menstruation scent. Before the bear appeared, though, Frankie expressed excitement for Sue, but Sue asked Frankie to keep it quiet, supporting the notion that menstruation experiences should be kept secret. The request represented how menstruation can be a bonding moment between mother and daughter.

In the series *Black-ish (*2014–2022; ABC), Diane (Marsai Martin) experienced menarche but did not seek out support from her mom in the episode, "*First and Last*" (S4.E6). Her twin brother Jack (Miles Brown) called on big sister Zoey (Yara Shahidi) to assist Diane. Diane's teacher told Bow (mom; Tracee Ellis Ross) that Diane's period had started, as she met Bow in the carline to explain the sweatpants that Diane wore. Word got out among other family members. When Bow's mother, Alicia Johnson (Anna Devere Smith), arrived, she wanted to highlight the spirituality and "mark the sacred right of Diane's first cycle" (S4.E6). Dre's (dad; Anthony Anderson) mom, Ruby (Jennifer Lewis), entered the conversation, but Diane interrupted, explaining how she learned about menstruation in health class and had the Flow app. Eventually, the grandmothers, mom, sister, and Diane bonded over shared memories of menarche and what menstruation means to reproductive health, ending the episode with the unspoken message of how menarche is different for everyone but we shouldn't avoid talking about it.

Messy and Gross. *Black-ish's* ending scene took menstruation away from the shame and secretiveness and instead brought the conversation into the open. My favorite line from *Blackish*'s *First and Last* occurred when Diane described the period as gross and messy. Anne Shirley felt the same way. Rosewarne (2012) characterized on-screen versions of menstruation as pretty awful experiences for nearly everyone. Amazon Prime's *The Wilds* (2020-2021) constituted a good example of menstruation being messy, even for those not involved. *The Wilds* featured eight teenage girls trapped on an island. As they waited for rescue, each recalled how and why they got there. On day 16 (S1.E8), the girls each took an edible gummy bear and began playing in the water. As four of the girls had a chicken fight in the water, Rachel (Reign Edwards) removed herself from Dot's (Shannon Berry) shoulders. Leah (Sarah Pidgeon) approached Dot and found blood on her right shoulder. As they looked for an injury, Rachel announced "It is me," became embarrassed, and ran off, while another castaway said, "Shark week for Rachel." Later, Rachel's twin sister, Nora (Helena Howard), humored Rachel by telling her that, in some cultures, one's menstruation is the height of spiritual power. However, Rachel confessed that this marked her first period in years, as having a regular period would mean being sidelined during the climax of her swimming career. She admitted that her coach had her on NuvaRing, and her body became more machine-like. Rachel's bout with her cycle exemplified how female athletes' bodies often get treated like machines rather than a womanly, female body (George, 2005) and how society turns to euphemisms to describe their monthly visitor (Urban & Holtzman, 2023). For many Generation Xers, the 1995 movie *Clueless* introduced us to the euphemism "Crimson Wave," when Cher (Alicia Silverstone) used it as an excuse for being tardy to class. A search on the internet estimates that over 5,000 different euphemisms around the world exist for menstruation.

As the examples mentioned thus far indicate, the messiness of a period marks the beginning of a woman's reproductive health. *Game of Thrones* not only addressed the messiness of menstruation but captured a mother-in-law/daughter's communication about the act. Sansa (Sophie Turner; *Game of Thrones*, 2011–2019; S2.E7) awoke from a nightmare, pulled down her covers, parted her legs, and discovered her sheets stained with red. She immediately started to cry and panic. She began to cut the stain out with a knife as her lady maid, Shae (Sibel Kekilli), entered her chamber and attempted to help Sansa hide the evidence. Later, though, Queen Cersei, Sansa's future mother-in-law (Lena Headey), spoke with Sansa, who explained that she thought the period would be less messy. Sansa also admitted that, with her first period, she understood her physical readiness to carry a baby – a thought that no longer excited her.

In the past decade, popular culture has begun to embrace menstruation storylines. Like a period, the trend is starting slowly but appears to be picking up with more storylines coming forward. Popular culture provides valuable lessons about the importance of menstruation and teaches viewers to break the code of silence regarding menstruation. However, it has rarely been treated as an important issue to women's health. In the next section, we will see how that is not so true when it comes to cancer.

"I can't have a glass of wine before I put poison in my body from chemo."

Cleo Shearer entered my orbit during the Season 1 of *Get Organized with The Home Edit* on Netflix. I became a fan and instantly started following her on Instagram. In 2021, she felt a lump in her breast, but she ignored it. She felt the lump again in February 2022. One month later, she received the diagnosis of *mammary carcinoma*, an aggressive form of breast cancer. As I watched Season 2 of *Get Organized,* I watched Cleo's breast cancer journey play out on Instagram.

Cleo Shearer's story is just the latest breast cancer storyline that caught my attention. I remember the episode of *Beverly Hills 90210* when Brenda, Kelly, and Donna performed self-breast exams instead of studying for the SATs (S1.E18). While all three girls said, "All clear," Brenda's reaction suggested otherwise. Brenda's discovery turns out to be a benign lump. The airing and watching of this episode introduced viewers to breast cancer, self-breast exams, and a family history of breast cancer. Art mimics real life, or in this case, real life mimics art. In 2015, actress Shannen Doherty was diagnosed with breast cancer but went into remission in 2017. In 2020, she announced that cancer had returned. In June 2023, Shannen publicly shared that she underwent surgery in January to remove and biopsy a tumor in her brain. In late November 2023, Shannen announced the cancer had moved to her bones (e.g., Bacher, 2023; for related work, please see Chapter 15, this volume).

The original *Beverly Hills 90210* introduced me to breast cancer on television; however, the controversial situational comedy *All in the Family* first aired a breast cancer storyline (S4.E15) in the 1970s. Not wanting to worry her husband, Edith only told her daughter-in-law, Gloria, and her neighbor that she felt something. Notably, during this groundbreaking episode, no character uttered the words "lump" or "breast cancer," as both were deemed too controversial at that time. Brenda and Edith kept their initial discoveries a secret from their friends and family but later disclosed their diagnosis. They managed their privacy boundaries and chose whom to disclose to (Petronio, 2002). Women find that they do disclose to family, mainly so they won't think they are going through the illness alone (Chang & Garcia Saavedra, 2021). Second, both shows demonstrated that the storyline of finding a lump can be wrapped up quickly. In the years to follow, many television shows featured the cancer storyline throughout the season.

Breast Cancer. Much of the communication and popular culture scholarship on breast cancer focuses on *Sex in the City*'s Samantha and *Desperate Housewives*' Lynette (Fernández-Morales, 2009; Gray, 2007). Unlike the examples mentioned above, Samantha's and Lynette's storylines played out throughout a season instead of just one episode. Samantha's storyline extended over the final eight episodes of *Sex in the City*. Blackwelder (2020) quoted Kim Cattrall (Samantha; SITC) sharing that the greatest compliment to her portrayal of a woman with breast cancer was when others approached her to thank her for helping them get through their cancer battles. Popular culture, or specifically in this case *Sex in the City*, brought to light how women could take control of their health, fight the disease, and assist in increasing acceptance and understanding of cancer.

During Season 4 of *Parenthood* (NBC; 2010–2015), Kristina Braverman received a breast cancer diagnosis. She fought cancer and the chemo side effects throughout Season 4 of the show, and the show captured her hair loss, extreme sickness from therapy, and chemotherapy treatment. Gabrielson (2018) noted how some television characters described chemotherapy as putting poison in their bodies, and Kristina was no exception. She said, "Funny thing is I can't have a glass of wine before I put poison in my body from chemo." Maggie Bloom (*A Million Little Things*; ABC, 2018-2023) received notification that her breast cancer had returned in Season 1, and, initially, she didn't want to fight it. However, her new set of friends encouraged her as they communicated hope and strength. She later changed her mind and began chemotherapy. In the Season 2 premiere (S2.E1), Maggie learned that she was cancer-free, but the episode closed with a confession to her boyfriend, himself a breast cancer survivor, that she feared the first shower after the "all clear" because she found a lump when she took her first shower at the end of her first breast cancer battle.

As with Kristina, Maggie, Samantha, and Lynette, viewers could watch the different stages of addressing breast cancer. We saw the diagnosis. We viewed the disclosure of cancer to friends and family. We witnessed the struggle of losing hair and appetite. We witnessed the aftereffects. We understood the love and support each character had. However, viewers don't typically get to witness the latent long-term cancer effects (Ellingson & Borofka, 2018).

Presence of Other Cancers. Breast cancer is not the only cancer to find its way into the plotlines of television shows or movies. The 1998 blockbuster film, *Stepmom,* introduced us to Jackie (Susan Sarandon), who spent most of the film silently fighting lymphoma. After chemotherapy and seeking out a specialist on the opposite coast, we learned that Jackie's latest scans revealed that her lymphoma was terminal. Only after Isabel (Julia Roberts), Jackie's ex-husband's fiancée, loses the address to a birthday party does Jackie's secret come out. The audience heard Jackie flushing the toilet after vomiting, watched her spending time in a hospital bed and smoking a joint, and observed her wearing a portable chemo dispenser. Unlike in the breast cancer storylines, viewers didn't witness Jackie losing her hair or suffering the side effects of chemotherapy.

Garam (2022) wrote that she was excited to see another movie, not mentioned in her piece, where the main character had ovarian cancer, but pointed out that, unless we read the plot line, we would have no idea what type of cancer the character had. Viewers did see the character wearing head wraps, looking wan, and writhing in pain to conclude that they had cancer. Fernández-Morales (2009) argued that cancer storylines are best left for soap operas because they have time to develop the storyline to include denial and the impacts of the disease on family, femininity, and body.

Some may suggest that Fernández-Morales' (2009) argument is antiquated after some cancer storylines in primetime television dramas. Kastor (1990) wrote about fans who ran to their telephones to talk to friends when Patricia Wettig's character, Nancy (*30-something*) was diagnosed with ovarian cancer. In the 90s, ovarian cancer was one of the hardest cancers to diagnose, often leaving doctors diagnosing it in later stages (Monroe, 1990). Nancy's ovarian cancer was found in stage 1, a diagnosis that went against the norm (Monroe, 1990). For the rest of the season, nearly 25 million flocked to the television to watch Nancy's battle with the cancer, describing Nancy as a character of hope (Napoli, 2018).

While Nancy's character survived her battle with ovarian cancer, not all characters are as lucky. *Tiny Beautiful Things* never really showed a character being sick with cancer, repeating the trend where viewers were told that she was sick but did not witness signs of her illness until the character was near death. The mini-series followed a woman, Claire Pierce (Kathryn Hahn), who reluctantly became an advice columnist. The show switched between Claire's present day and her past, especially diving into her relationship with her mother, who viewers learned died from cervical cancer at 43. Again, the film revealed that Claire's mom Frankie Weaver (Merritt Wever) had cervical cancer, but it did not include the progression of the disease. In the last episode, a flashback took the audience to the hospital where Frankie was confined to a bed and struggling to breathe. When Frankie learned of her diagnosis, young Claire (Sarah Pidgeon) wanted her to fight the disease, but Frankie wanted to maintain "normality" and thought in terms of quality of life instead of quantity of life.

Frankie's approach differed from Judy (Linda Cardellini), a character in *Dead to Me.* Judy learned in the first episode of Season 3 that she had stage 4 ovarian cancer. Garam (2022) described how Judy received a port and left with a gauze bandage visible (an indication of the port). She used a cold cap, which is worn to reduce or prevent hair loss, accurately portraying the infusion center. This portrayal highlighted how cancer patients feel when cancer entertainment narratives allow them to channel their cancer-related emotions (Collins et al., 2024). Garam wrote, "It's clear that someone who had gone through a cancer diagnosis and treatment contributed to this storyline" (para. 21).

Cancer and race. *Midnight Club* (Netflix 2022) was set in a hospice and followed eight terminally ill teens. In the pilot episode (S1.E1), we met Ilonka (Iman Benson), an overachieving 17-year-old Black female who started coughing up blood just days before graduation. A few minutes later, the episode made clear that Ilonka had thyroid cancer; by 10 minutes and 45 seconds into the show, the storyline jumped forward to her 18th birthday and revealed that the cancer had metastasized to her lungs. She was now considered terminal. She then chose to attend Brightcliff House, a hospice for teens outside of Seattle. *Midnight Club* captured Ilonka's story pre-diagnosis, diagnosis, post-2 rounds of chemo, entering hospice, and admitting, near the end of the pilot episode, that she didn't want to die from the disease. The show provided one of the rare opportunities in popular culture to witness non-Caucasian women living with cancer.

During the writing of this section, I kept thinking, "But what about non-white cancer patients? Ilonka can't be the only one." I studied actresses' biographies and roles to find examples of non-Caucasian characters with cancer. My long days of coming up empty are not surprising as Kim (2022) found that most cancer storylines focus on white patients and white doctors. I did, however, find some examples. In the pilot of *L.A. Law* (S1.E1; NBC 1986-87), Alfre Woodard played a woman dying of leukemia, a role for which she later won the Emmy Award for Outstanding Guest Actress in a Drama Series. Queen Latifah, in the film *Last Holiday,* decided to go on her dream trip and spend every cent she had after receiving a cancer diagnosis from a faulty X-ray machine. Viewers later learned that she didn't have cancer. Diahann Carroll, known for her roles in *Dynasty* and *A Different World,* survived breast cancer and later went on to share her story in *1 a Minute*, a 2010 documentary that chronicled the diagnosis and treatment of breast cancer survivors, including famous international celebrities. More recently, Reese Witherspoon's May 2023 book club selection, *Did You Hear About Kitty Karr* by Crystal Smith, mentioned cancer deaths. Kitty Karr, a woman who could pass as white, discovered that her Black mother, Hazel, died of breast cancer, and Kitty died from lung cancer from years of smoking, the catalyst for the novel as her death uncovered many family secrets.

Popular culture frames women's fights with cancer in different ways, depending on the time of diagnosis, race, and type of cancer (Kim, 2022). First, popular culture depicts breast cancer as treatable. Hence, the lesson from 90210 is just as important today as it was in 1991. Second, women battle breast cancer. As evident in each of the above-mentioned shows, these storylines often continue throughout one regular season. Third, it seems that some women characters are less likely to fight against their cancer diagnosis when they are told that they are in stage 4 or they are terminal. Ilonka, a younger female character, is the exception. Finally, the portrayal of cancer has been more accurate when one of the writers has experience with cancer and cancer diagnoses (Garam, 2022), and shows rarely feature diverse characters living with cancer (Kim, 2022).

"She's Forgetting You"

As a child of the 80s, I remember several episodes revolving around women and losing their memories. The first one I always think of is *Family Ties*, which ran on NBC for seven seasons (1982–1989). The show centered on the life of the Keatons: Steven, Elyse, Alex, Mallory, Jennifer, and later Andy. In a 1987 episode, the Keatons were surprised by a visit from Elyse's (Meredith Baxter) Aunt Rosemary (S6, E9). The family, especially eldest daughter Mallory (Justine Bateman), noted Rosemary's actions and forgetfulness, and, before the final credits, a doctor diagnosed Rosemary (Barbara Barrie) with early-onset Alzheimer's. Witherspoon (2012) wrote, "Barrie plays with dignity her role of the effervescent and fiercely independent woman struggling to understand her forgetfulness" (para. 2). Witherspoon's observation captures the opposite of how portrayals of dementia in popular culture are usually portrayed negatively and cause social distance between those with and without dementia (Gerritsen et al., 2014).

Nearly 15 years later, I encountered the Alzheimer's, or dementia, storyline again as I read Nicholas Sparks' *The Notebook.* Sparks (1996) wrote in detail about Allie Hamilton and the diagnosis that led to her entering an assisted living facility in the chapter, *Winter for Two*. The description of the disease started with simple acts such as forgetfulness and confusion, moved into more serious events, and finally climaxed when Allie got lost while driving home. Later, actress Gena Rowlands, as late-in-life Allie Hamilton, portrayed dementia on screen when the featured book was made into a movie (2004). Her portrayal was often through dialogue, such as when a nurse encouraged her to play the piano and Allie questioned if she knew how (Cassavetes, 2004). Thain (2018) argued that the film took a less realistic approach to dementia as "Allie" experienced "moments of full lucidity" (p. 25), but to be fair, she had these moments within the book as well.

A few years later, *Grey's Anatomy* became a widespread phenomenon (2007-present; ABC). While I tried to stay away from medical dramas in this chapter, I must refer to *Grey's* in this section. At the end of the series premiere, viewers met Ellis Gray (Kate Burton), Meredith's mom, as a resident of Roseridge Home for Extended Care. Just like Allie Hamilton mentioned above, Ellis had a moment of lucidity, but Ellis was often portrayed on screen with gaps in memory, agitation, and aggressiveness. Ellis Gray was not the only resident from Seattle General to wind up in Roseridge Home, as Adele Webber (Loretta Devine), wife of the head of surgery Richard Webber (Jack Pickens, Jr.), moved into the home. Adele's storyline provided unique insight in that viewers encountered Adele before Alzheimer's and then played witness to her decline and subsequent death (DiZazzo-Miller & Pociask 2015).

Barrie, Rowlands, Burton, and Devine portrayed aging characters with dementia, a common theme among cultural depictions and frames regarding dementia and Alzheimer's (Low & Purwaningrum, 2020). According to Low and Purwaningrum, these portrayals often include the character losing their memory, mind, or identity, and then acting unpredictably. Yet, this pattern contrasted with Mama Coco in the 2017 film *Coco* (Pixar). The movie depicted Mama Coco as confined to a wheelchair. The film hinted at Mama Coco's memory disorder, as when Coco referred to Miguel as her deceased husband, Julio, but never overtly revealed that Mama Coco has dementia. Miguel told the audience that "[s]he has some trouble remembering things, but it's good to talk to her anyways" (Unkrich & Molina, 2017).

Like Allie Hamilton in *The Notebook,* Mama Coco had a moment of full lucidity when Miguel returned from the Land of the Dead and began singing "Remember Me." This moment prompted Coco to open a drawer containing all the letters that her father had sent her, a catalyst to ending the "no music" rule in the family.

Finally, the health issue of dementia/Alzheimer's played an instrumental role in the fourth season of *This is Us,* continuing until the end of the NBC series (2016-2022). Unlike *Family Ties, The Notebook,* and *Coco*, I didn't watch *This is Us* as it aired, but I do recall hearing about Rebecca's

(Mandy Moore) memory decline. Hoffman et al. (2022) described the storyline as following Rebecca's memory decline and subsequent diagnosis of Alzheimer's disease, the plot line mirroring Allie Hamilton's and Adele Webber's. However, their research focused on the conflict between Randall and Kevin regarding Rebecca's care, not the toll that dementia had on the individual. Randall and Kevin's struggles are important to note since Rebecca didn't die until the second-to-last episode of the series, enabling the show to capture the toll the disease had on the individual and the family. In portraying Rebecca's slow mental decline, Mandy Moore told *Variety*:

> This poor woman who lost a child, who lost a spouse, then finds herself at this juncture of her life in cognitive decline, with a degenerative brain disease. It's just very, very sad. But I also feel buoyed by the fact that we're able to represent this situation that millions of people find themselves and their families in and for people to feel a sense of community and not feel like an anomaly and hopefully feel a little less alone.
>
> *(Maas & Longeretta, 2022, para. 10)*

The *This Is Us* storyline prompted a reduction in stigma regarding dementia and Alzheimer's (Urban, 2022). The storyline also sparked communication about dementia among viewing families, from not only the right course of action (Hoffman et al., 2022) to how family systems impact the identity changes of the afflicted individual (Stuart et al., 2021). *This Is Us* narrated a story that millions of families around the country encounter, but instead of just focusing on the grief and sadness (Strause, 2022), the storyline concentrated on the nuances, such as the best course of action for treatment and quality of life (Stuart et al., 2021). Some critics hailed that the storyline focused on the family's grief but also capitalized on Rebecca and her wishes for her life while showcasing that Rebecca was much more than her diagnosis (Weatherhead, 2022). Before reading the popular culture press and never watching the show past the first season, I could not imagine what life would be like living with an aging parent fighting dementia; however, the popular press wrote about how families cope (Strause, 2022; Urban, 2022; Weatherhead, 2022), or how the disease impacts the parent. What I can empathize with is the grief of watching a loved one deteriorate slowly.

Conclusion

One outcome of examining how popular culture communicates about menstruation, cancer, and dementia is how popular culture brings awareness to how differently women and their caregivers and family members communicate (and/or fail to communicate) about women's health issues. In this chapter, I discussed mediated representations of three women's health concerns – menstruation, cancer, and dementia.

Although Haley in *Modern Family* referenced menstruation as a "get out of jail free card," I also presented other examples that reveal a range of mediated responses by characters to menstruation. As such, contemporary mediated communication contradicts some of the master society narratives, opening the door for education about menstruation as well as instruction to families about how to communicate about menstruation.

I shared that the mediated representations of cancer typically include finding lumps, seeing a doctor, undergoing a biopsy, and receiving a diagnosis. Although Lange (2023) provided an overview of how humor has been used to talk about cancer in popular culture, this chapter provides examples of the drama, the risks, and the grief associated with cancer. Yet, popular culture also showcases characters who are ready to tackle cancer.

Finally, dementia storylines showcased how families in films and television talk about and deal with the illness as they slowly watch their loved ones deteriorate. *Coco* explained to young children how it is okay to still communicate with their elders, even if their elders don't remember them. Critics praised *This is Us* because of the focus on Kevin and Randall and how they each presented competing but complementary approaches to handling dementia. Because of this approach, Kevin, Randall, and Rebecca opened up lines of communication, moving together as a unit in their approach. How popular culture showcases a health issue helps us talk about illnesses by discussing the popular culture we consume (Lange, 2023).

Using popular culture to talk about issues does provide educational components (see Dutta et al., 2019; also Chapter 17, this volume), but not in a comprehensive or coherent manner. For example, recent plotlines involving menstruation demonstrate either friends or parents attempting to educate their daughters/friends about the issue. We are taught disease prevention, such as how to do self-checks on our breasts for demarcations or look for lumps, but we aren't taught what makes a cramp normal or not normal. We are taught the early symptoms of dementia but not necessarily how the disease progresses. As the chapter underscores, today's popular culture provides useful but incomplete information about critical women's health issues.

The field of communication experiences a gap in research that examines women's health issues outside the area of breast cancer. I hope that this chapter can be a catalyst for a younger group of scholars to pick up the torch and address this gap. Maybe, when pop culture and academic research stop silencing women's health, we can stop silencing ourselves as well.

In Fall 2022, I got the idea to write about television shows and menstruation. I put the idea down on my list and then became more mindful of what I was watching. It was also during the fall semester that my colleagues and I proposed our menstrual literature framing chapter. I then became more aware of what I was reading. During Spring 2023, the focus of my health communication course centered on women's health. It was then that I noticed a big gap in television storylines and in research regarding women's health. We are entering a new era where it is not just one sex or gender in the writer's room, and I hope that an increase in women writers will mean women's health will be less invisible in our popular culture.

Notes

1 In 2015, following the Fox News-sponsored Republican Debate, then-candidate Donald Trump described Megyn Kelly as having blood coming out of her eyes, "blood coming out of her…whatever" (Crawford & Waldman, 2023).
2 Quotation is from Turning Red (Shi, 2022).

References

Aragón, A., & Cooke-Jackson, A. (2021). The sex talk was taboo…so was wearing a tampon: Sexual and menstrual health conversations among young Latina and Latinx women and gender minorities. In A. Cooke-Jackson & V. Rubinsky (Eds.), *Communicating intimate health,* (pp. 33–50). Lexington.

Bacher, D. (2023, November). Shannon Doherty wants to 'embrace life' as cancer has spread toher bones: 'My greatest memory is yet to come' (exclusive). *People*. https://people.com/shannendoherty-embrace-life-cancer-spread-to-bones-cover-exclusive-8407406

Bessett, D., & Murawsky, S. (2017). "I guess I do have to take back what I said before, about television": Pregnant women's understandings and use of televisual representations of childbearing. *Sociology of Health & Illness, 40,* 478–493. https://doi.o.rg/10.1111/1467-9566.12658

Blackwelder, C. (2020, October 23). Breast cancer on TV: A history of the disease's depiction throughout the years. https://abcnews.go.com/GMA/Culture/breast-cancer-tv-history-diseases-depiction-years/story?id=73764613

Blume, J. (1970). *Are you there, God? It's me, Margaret.* Bradbury Press.

Cassavetes, N. (2004). *The notebook.* New Line Cinema.

Chaney, J. (2017). On TV, a girl's first period as a mark of female power. *Vulture*. https://www.vulture.com/2017/11/blackish-alias-grace-big-mouth-period-episodes.html

Chang, W. L., & Garcia Saavedra, D. E. (2021). To tell or not to tell: A quantitative analysis identifying the individual, relational, and cultural factors that affect the maternal disclosure of their breast cancer diagnosis and treatment to their daughters. *Kentucky Journal of Communication, 40,* 50–67.

Chung, J. E. (2014). Medical dramas and viewer perception of health: Testing cultivation effects. *Human Communication Research, 40,* 333–349. https://doi.org/10.1111/here.12026

Collins, M. K. R., Lazard, A. J., McKenzie, A. M. H., & Varma, T. (2024). "It's nothing like cancer": Young adults with cancer reflect on memorable entertainment narratives. *Health Communication, 39*(3), 552–562. https://doi.org/10.1080/10410236.2023.2174403

Craig, K. F., & Blume, J. (2023)—*Are you there God? It's me, Margaret.* Lionsgate.

Crawford, B. J., & Waldman, E. G. (2023). *Menstruation matters: Challenging the law's silence on periods.* NYU Press.

Delaney, J., Lupton, M. J., & Toth, E. (Eds.). (1988). *The curse: A cultural history of menstruation.* University of Illinois Press.

DiZazzo-Miller, R., & Pociask, F. D. (2015). Dementia in the context of disability. *Physical & Occupational Therapy in Geriatrics, 33,* 139–151. https://doi.org/10.3109/02703181.2015.1014126

Dutta, M. J., Jaur-Gill, S., & Tan, N. (2019). Cultivation in health and risk messaging. In *Oxford Research of Encyclopedia of Communication, online.* Oxford University Press. https://doi.org/10.1093/acrefore/9780190228613.013.289

Ellenbogen, R. (2017, October 17). 'Black-ish' star Tracee Ellis Ross: Postpartum depression episode 'made me cry.' *International Business Times.* https://www.ibtimes.com/black-ish-star-tracee-ellis-ross-postpartum-depression-episode-made-me-cry-2599397

Ellingson, L., & Borofkat, K. G. E. (2018)—Long-term cancer survivors' everyday embodiment. *Health Communication, 35,* 180–191. https://doi.org/10.1080/10410236.2018.1550470

Fenton Stitt, J. (2012). Tom vs. Brooke: Or postpartum as bad mothering postpartum. In E. Podnieks (Ed.). *Mediating moms: Mothers in popular culture* (pp. 339–357). McGill-Queen's University.

Fernández-Morales, M. (2009). Illness, genre, and gender in contemporary television fiction: Representations of female cancer in *Sex in the City* and *Desperate Housewives. Women's Studies, 36,* 670–691. https://doi.org/10.1080/00497870909302I752

Gabrielson, T. (2018). Life at all costs: The biopolitics of chemotherapy in contemporary television and film. In J. Lawrence & S. M. Wiebe (Eds.), *Biopolitical disaster* (pp. 188–200). Routledge.

Garam, J. (2022, December 23). What Netflix's "Dead to Me" got right about cancer: It's all in the details. *Medium.* https://medium.com/@jennifergaram/what-netflixs-dead-to-me-got-right-about-cancer-b7257cfa7e79

Gerritsen, D. L., Kuin, Y., & Nijboer, J. (2014). Dementia in the movies: The clinical picture. *Aging & Mental Health, 18,* 276–280. https://doi.org/10.1080/13607863.2013.837150

George, M. (2005). Making sense of muscle: The body experiences of collegiate women athletes. *Sociological Inquiry, 75,* 317–345. https://doi.org/10.1111/j.1475-682X.2005.00125.x

Gray, J. B. (2007). Interpersonal communication and the illness experience in the *Sex in the City* breast cancer narrative. *Communication Quarterly, 55,* 397–414. https://doi.org10.1080/01463370701657889

Hoffman, B. L., Shensa, A., Wessel, C., Hoffman, R., & Primack, B. A. (2017). Exposure to fictional medical television and health: A systematic review. *Health Education Research, 32,* 107–123. https://doi.org/10.1093/her/cyx034

Hoffman, B. L., Sidani, J. E., Wang, Y., Chang, J., & Burke, J. G. (2022). "It encourages family discussion": A mixed-methods examination of the *This is Us* Alzheimer's disease and caregiving storyline. *Journal of Health Communication, 27,* 382–393. https://doi.org/10.1080/10810739.2022.2111620

Johnson, M. A. (2018). *HIV on TV: Popular culture's epidemic.* Lexington.

Kasenko, J. (2019). Tracing menstruation in British and American culture. Strategies of invisibilization, stigmatization, and the question of im-purity in historical and cultural context. *New Horizons in English Studies, 4,* 144–157. https://doi.org/10.17951/nh.2019.144-157

Kastor, E. (1990, January 23). The shock of 'thirtysomething.' *Washington Post.* https://www.washingtonpost.com/archive/lifestyle/1990/01/23/the-shock-of-thirtysomething/eb4bdf0e-4850-469f-a4dd-84cf7d27a3c8/

Kim, G. (2022). Examining diversity: A content analysis of cancer depictions on primetime scripted television. *Journal of Cancer Education, 37,* 1842–1848. https://doi.org/10.1007/s13187-021-02050-x

Kissling, E. A. (2002). On the rag on screen: Menarche in film and television. *Sex Roles, 46,* 5–12. https://doi.org/10.1023/A:1016029416750

Lange, L. (2023). Cancertainment: How entertainment may help people with (and without) cancer? In M. Szabat & J. Piaksecki (Eds.), *Approaches to death and dying: Bioethical and cultural perspectives* (pp. 151–164). Jagiellonian University Press.

LeBlanc, S. S. (2021). It isn't all happy tears: The changing nature of how PPD is portrayed in situational comedies. In M. A. Johnson & C. J. Olson (Eds.), *Quieting the madness: Entertainment media's shift into more accurate depictions of mental illness* (pp. 134–148). Routledge.

LeBlanc, S. S., Mitchell, R. P., Butcher, L., Russell, J., & Navarro, J. (2023). "No one ever talked about…": New mothers, anxiety, and the postpartum discourse. *Southern Communication Journal, 88(3),* 195–210. https://doi.org/10.1080/1041794X.2023.2182905

LeBlanc, S. S., Wagner, S., & White, K. K. (in development). Tears, joy, and blood: Depictions of menstruation in literature. In B. J. Epstein & R. Neve (Eds.), *Heroines with periods: Finding menstruation in contemporary literature*. *Peitho.*

Low, L., & Purwaningrum, F. (2020). Negative stereotypes, fear and social distance: A systematic review of depictions of dementia in popular culture in the context of stigma. *BMC Geriatrics, 20,* 477–493. https://doi.org/10.1186/s12877-020-01754-x

Maas, J., & Longeretta, E. (2022, May 17). 'This is Us' creator Dan Fogelman and star Mandy Moore on saying goodbye to Rebecca ahead of the finale. *Variety*. https://variety.com/2022/tv/news/this-is-us-rebecca-dead-mandy-moore-1235264308/

Meyer, M. D. E., & Yermal, A. L. (2021). Representing illness in medical melodramas on television: A qualitative content analysis of medical diagnoses in *Grey's Anatomy. Qualitative Research Reports in Communication, 22,* 22–29. https://doi.org/10.1080/17459435.2020.1819139

Monroe, L. R. (1990, February 27). When TV and life part company: Health: 'thirtysomething's Nancy Weston may recover from her ovarian cancer. Many other women won't be so lucky. *Los Angeles Times.* https://www.latimes.com/archives/la-xpm-1990-02-27-vw-1462-story.html

Napoli, J. (2018, June 11). 'thirtysomething' cast on Nancy's cancer, Gary's death & LGBTQ representation. *TVInsider*. https://www.tvinsider.com/695338/thirtysomething-reunion-atx-festival-2018/

Petronio, S. (2002). *Boundaries of privacy: Dialectics of disclosure.* SUNY Press.

Regan, T. (2020). *Ms.Diagnosed.* American Medical Women's Association.

Reitman, C. (2019). Catherine Reitman is on a mission to depict complex, imperfect moms on TV. *Evoke*. https://www.evoke.org/articles/october-2019/fresh-takes/catherine-reitman-mission-to-depict-imperfect-workin-moms-on-tv

Rosewarne, L. (2012). *Periods in pop culture: Menstruation in film and television.* Lexington.

SheKnows (2017, February 10). 6 times the Golden Girls were women's health pioneers. *Sheknows*. https://www.sheknows.com/health-and-wellness/articles/1131837/golden-girls-were-womens-health-pioneers/

Shi, D. (Director). (2022). *Turning red.* Pixar Animation.

Smith, C. (2023). *Did you hear about Kitty Karr?* Henry Holt and Co.

Sparks, N. (1996). *The notebook.* Grand Central Publishing.

Strause, J. (2022, June 3). *'This is Us'* team on destigmatizing aging and illness: "We were telling the story of millions of families." *The Hollywood Reporter.* https://www.hollywoodreporter.com/tv/tv-features/this-is-us-alzeihmers-aging-illness-tv-1235158599/

Stuart, L. B., Jones, C. H., & Windle, G. (2021). A qualitative systematic review of the role of families in supporting communication in people with dementia. *International Journal of Language and Communication Disorders, 57,* 1130–1153. https://doi.org/10.1111/1460-6984.12738

Thain, A. (2018). *Film and television as a psychotherapeutic tool.* Unpublished dissertation. Michigan School of Professional Psychology.

Thompson, C. M., Babu, S., & Makos, S. (2023). Women's experiences of health-related communicative disenfranchisement. *Health Communication, 38,* 3135–3146. https://doi.org/10.1080/10410236.2022.2137772

Todd, C. A. (2016, July 7). 7 important menstruation moments from movies & TV. *Refinery29.* https://www.refinery29.com/en-us/2016/07/115887/menstruation-movie-scenes-tv-shows

Tropp, L. (2012). Off their rockers: Representations of postpartum depression. In L. C. Rubin's (Ed.). *Mental illness in the media* (pp. 77–91). McFarland.

Unkrich, L., & Molina, A. (2017). *Coco.* Pixar Animation Studios.

Urban, (2022, September 16). "This Us" reduced dementia stigma; Researchers find NBC hit show encouraged family discussion on aging. *AARP.* https://www.aarp.org/health/conditions-treatments/info-2022/this-is-us-dementia-story.html#:~:text=As%20the%20millions%20of%20faithful,of%20care%20she%20should%20receive

Urban, A., & Holtzman, M. (2023). Menstrual stigma and Twitter. *Sociological Focus, 56,* 483–496. https://doi.org/10.1080/00380237.2023.2243588

Weatherhead, S. (2022, May 20). How 'This is Us' handled Alzheimer's with dignity and grace. *Collider.* https://collider.com/this-is-us-alzheimers-why-its-good/

Weisser-Wolf, J. (2017). *Periods gone public: Taking a stand for menstrual equity.* Skyhorse.

Witherspoon, C. (2012, December 23). Forget me not. *IMBD.* https://www.imdb.com/title/tt0577409/?ref_=ttep_ep9

Ye, Y., & Ward, K. E. (2010). The depiction of illness and related matters in two top-ranked primetime network medical dramas in the United States: A content analysis. *Journal of Health Communication, 15,* 555–570. https://doi.org/10.1080/10810730.2010.492564

Yuko, E. (2017a). 2017 was a big year for periods on TV. *SheKnows.* https://www.sheknows.com/health-and-wellness/articles/1137604/periods-on-tv-2017/

Yuko, E. (2017b). Why it matters that "Anne with an E" has a period episode. *Pacific Standard.* https://psmag.com/social-justice/half-the-population-suffers-through-it

Zuluaga, G., & Andersson, N. (2013). Initiation rites at menarche and self-reported dysmenorrhea among indigenous women of the Colombian Amazon: A cross-sectional study. *BMJ [British Medical Journal] Open*, 3. http://doi.org/10.1136/bmjopen-2012-002012

8

THE INTERSECTION OF LGBTQ+ IDENTITIES AND POPULAR CULTURE

Examining the Stigmas, Stories, and Social Realities of Mediated Health Discourses

Raffi Sarkissian and Michaela D. E. Meyer

Mass media for much of the 20th century has depicted non-heteronormative gender or sexuality as a contemporary and ongoing social health problem – framing LGBTQ[1] identities as a disorder, an illness, a perversion, or a crime. Indeed, from its inception in the 1950s up to 1973, the American Psychiatric Association categorized homosexuality as a personality disorder (Burgess, 2023; Kunzel, 2018). The law, up through 2003, considered private consenting sex between same-sex adults to be illegal. Media and popular culture played an integral role in these cultural and ideological constructions. In one of the first collections of queer research in the Communication discipline, Larry Gross penned a "state of the union" style chapter regarding the representation of gay and lesbian characters on television, noting, "the manner of that representation will itself reflect the biases and interests of those elites who define the public agenda" (1994, p. 143). Gross proceeded to explain that, by 1983, "nearly all mass media attention to gay men was in the context of AIDS-related stories, and because this coverage seems to have exhausted the news media's limited interest in gay people, lesbians became even less visible than before (if possible)" (p. 145).

Although Gross's analysis is now over 30 years old, it still rings true to contemporary social politics regarding LGBTQ health representations in media. In June 2023, the Human Rights Campaign declared a national state of emergency due to the increasing number of anti-LGBTQ bills introduced and passed across the country (HRC Staff, 2023). Many of these bills prohibit gender-affirming care for trans and gender non-conforming youth, while others target teaching LGBTQ history and drag performances, all of which have far-reaching effects on the health, safety, and rights of all citizens. At the same time, popular culture has never been more replete with LGBTQ images, narratives, and advocacy. In fact, according to GLAAD's (2022) 17th annual Where We Are on TV report, out of the 775 series-regular characters on the 2021-2022 prime-time slate, 92 (11.9%) of them are LGBTQ. That's not only a jump of 2.8% from the previous year's 9.1% but also a record-high percentage for broadcast television. These two phenomena – anti-LGBTQ health messaging and a record number of LGBTQ media images – are inextricably connected. In fact, the vector of health is integral to

 DOI: 10.4324/9781003436409-9

understanding how LGBTQ people and representations have operated and are currently operating in popular culture.

For the purposes of this chapter, we define "popular culture" primarily as film and television produced by dominant media industries in the 20th and 21st centuries in conjunction with the participatory practices of social media that, albeit more fragmented, make up large swaths of what's popular or trending. As LGBTQ-identified authors who live in the U.S. American social system and have experienced health concerns related to our identities through this lens, we approach media and popular culture from a critical-constructionist lens where the images on screen and the discourses distributed across all sorts of platforms do not simply reflect or unidirectionally affect reality, but rather are co-constitutive of our realities. Hollywood cinema, for instance, did not invent gay and lesbian stereotypes, but it played a powerful role in regulating and reinforcing them. Activists and everyday users on TikTok may not directly change oppressive laws, but they certainly contribute to steering popular sentiment and providing language to make sense of our cultural environment.

To organize our observations related to LGBTQ health representations in media, we divide this chapter into three sections. First, **Stigmas and Stereotypes** overviews media that laid the foundation for some of the deeply embedded connotations of LGBTQ people *as* health issues during the rise of visual mass media – as social problems, as threats to society. Second, **Intersectional Specificities** highlights how several more recent images of LGBTQ characters can serve as case studies for how LGBTQ people live with and navigate through a variety of health afflictions. Third, **The Rise of Participatory Culture and Social Media** considers the proliferation of LGBTQ images, stories, identities, politics, and advocacy through social media. Together, these sections provide varying perspectives on what the intersection of health and LGBTQ discourses looks like. Obviously, this chapter is necessarily incomplete – we cannot cover each and every possible LGBTQ image across the vast history of mass media – however, we offer it as a starting point to understand how the intersection of health and LGBTQ discourses in popular culture has been framed and may continue to be framed by media moving forward.

Stigmas and Stereotypes

For much of the 20th and early 21st century, LGBTQ representations in media and popular culture were rife with health stigmas – mental illness, criminality, sexual contagion, threats to society – due to rampant stereotypes and enduring tropes largely established during the Classical Hollywood Cinema era (1920s to 1960s). During most of this time, the Motion Picture Production Code (or Hays Code), a coordinated effort to self-sanitize their films to avoid outside regulation, governed all studios. The Production Code forbade various images, language, and representations, including "sex perversion," which was meant to censor any explicit acknowledgment of homosexuality on screen (Benshoff & Griffin, 2006; Russo, 1987). This regulation inevitably led to the proliferation of hidden codes, stereotypes, and connotations to insinuate gender and sexual variance.

One of the dominant stereotypes of this era encompassed coding gay men and lesbians as villains, predators, and murderers (Dhaenens, 2013). While these films never directly addressed their sexual orientation, the use of innuendo, thinly veiled metaphors, winking performances, and suggestive dialogue in films like *Dracula's Daughter* (1936), *The Maltese Falcon* (1941), *Rope* (1947), *Caged* (1950), and *Suddenly Last Summer* (1959) – notably cataloged in *The Celluloid Closet* (Epstein & Friedman, 1995) – firmly established queer characters as dangers to society. These depictions would be echoed decades later in sensationalized Hollywood releases like *Cruising* (1980), *Silence of the Lambs* (1991), and *Basic Instinct* (1992) while more nuanced depictions of queer villains in films like *The Talented Mr. Ripley* (1999), *Monster* (2003), and *Notes on a Scandal* (2006) would attempt to complicate such historic associations. This tradition even extended to children's media as animated villains like Ursula in *The Little Mermaid* (1989), Jafar in *Aladdin* (1992), and Scar in *The Lion King*

(1994), among others, were also queer-coded characters, entangling and flattening together traits like unattractive beauty standards, effeminacy, or villain-as-sissy with evil and treachery (Li-Vollmer & LaPointe, 2003).

Trauma and self-loathing also entail common frames for LGBTQ identities and experiences in popular culture, particularly as mainstream narratives attempt to sympathize with – or rather, pity – queer characters in the second half of the century. In Friedkin's (1970) *The Boys in the Band*, a group of gay friends gather for a private birthday celebration, drinking, dancing, and teasing each other in a refreshing representation of community and belonging. Yet, a party-game-gone-wrong eventually reveals deep traumatic wounds, turning the night into a pity party with the guest of honor eviscerating their host:

> You're a sad and pathetic man. You're a homosexual and you don't want to be. But there's nothing you can do to change it … You may very well one day know a heterosexual life if you want it desperately enough, if you pursue it with the fervor with which you annihilate. But you'll always be homosexual as well. Always, Michael. Always. Until the day you die.

In *The Children's Hour* (Wyler, 1961), an unruly child at an all-girls boarding school makes up a false rumor about what she "saw" between her two teachers, Martha and Karen. The lie spread and destroyed the school, but, in its wake, Martha (Shirley McClaine) broke down to Karen (Audrey Hepburn), revealing an ounce of truth to the rumor. Amid her hysterical cries, she confessed, "I'm guilty … It's all my fault. I've ruined your life and I've ruined my own. I swear I didn't know it. I didn't mean it. Oh, I feel so sick and dirty I can't stand it anymore." Significantly, while released at the tail end of the Production Code, *The Children's Hour* refrained from ever explicitly using terms like lesbian, homosexuality, or others, making such queerness still "unspeakable." At the end of the film, Karen dramatically charged into Martha's room and stared in horror as the camera panned to a shadow of Martha's dangling feet. Martha's demise marked a fate all too familiar not only for queer characters in media, but for numerous LGBTQ people in the U.S.

Just as LGBTQ movements gained traction in the 1970s and 1980s, including active challenges to homophobic stories in film, television, and news, the AIDS crisis further contributed to the media's construction of queer people as innately tied to disease and illness. Like the U.S. government's response, Hollywood studios largely remained silent on AIDS for much of the 1980s. Independent films like *Buddies* (1985) and *Parting Glances* (1986) and the made-for-TV movie genre, starting with 1985's *An Early Frost*, ushered in the first representations of AIDS in popular culture (Benshoff & Griffin, 2006). One of the biggest media events to raise public awareness about AIDS, though, occurred when closeted Hollywood star Rock Hudson announced that he had HIV in July 1985, prompting *Life* magazine to run a cover that read: "NOW NO ONE IS SAFE FROM AIDS" (Gross, 2001). Hudson died three months later, and the uptick in news hysteria only managed to strengthen the association between gay men, in particular, and the disease.

Death is thus the most enduring trope for queer characters on screen. What first served as an easy way to punish villains and unruly characters under the Production Code, fatal queer narratives have more recently turned into a reliable formula for straight actors in prestigious films. William Hurt in *The Kiss of the Spider Woman* (1985), Tom Hanks in *Philadelphia* (1993), Hilary Swank in *Boys Don't Cry* (1999), Charlize Theron in *Monster* (2003), Sean Penn in *Milk* (2008), Jared Leto and Matthew McConaughey in *Dallas Buyers Club* (2013), Rami Malek in *Bohemian Rhapsody* (2018), and Brendan Fraser in *The Whale* (2022) all won Oscars for playing LGBTQ or AIDS-afflicted characters who died or faced inevitable death in their respective films. This trope extended to television as well, where the death of a queer character on *The 100* in 2016 functioned as the catalyst for "Bury Your Gays," an Autostraddle list and critique of the frequent deaths of lesbian and bisexual female characters (Reise, 2023). The publication of this list sparked discourse across social media, trade publications, and media industries on the expendability of queer characters in popular media (for related work, see Chapter 9, this volume).

By the 1990s, despite commercial markets paying more attention to LGBTQ inclusion, LGBTQ narratives were still short-lived or mired in familiar traumas and self-loathing. Edgy television episodes included LGBTQ characters as guest stars or token supporting cast members, the subject of "very special" episodes about coming out, in ways that served the straight characters' story arcs and, by extension, the series' progressive politics (M. D. E. Meyer, 2003, 2009). Thus, shows during this period often defined queer characters "by their problem" or social issues in television narratives. The task of disassociating them from their "issues" so they could exist as their own fully realized characters proved too tall an order (Fuqua, 1994). With rare exceptions like *Will & Grace* or *Ellen* (which many scholars still found wildly problematic in their framing of LGBTQ characters – see Battles & Hilton Morrow, 2002; Dow, 2001), television's representational politics through the end of the 20th century was emblematic of a long history of queerness first as a health issue in and of itself, then as a social problem to be solved either through disposing of the characters or finding assimilationist, limited ways to incorporate their inclusion in society. Through a critical constructionist perspective, these industrial patterns shape the very meaning of being queer in/through popular culture.

Therefore, epistemologically, by the early 2000s, numerous patterns represented LGBTQ identities in media. Lynne Joyrich (2009) outlined five common patterns including *inferring sexuality* where filmmakers marked sexuality as an identity but entirely desexualized the character (such as Matt in *Melrose Place* or *Buffy The Vampire Slayer*'s Willow and Tara); *detecting sexuality* where a character's sexual identity gets revealed over the course of a narrative – either by oneself or by others (such as Anna on *One Tree Hill* or Dave on *Glee*); *conferring sexuality* where the queerness of a particular show or character becomes known to the audience but is not specifically designated in the text through dialogue or identity claims (such as *Smallville* or *Xena*); *enlightening sexuality* where a character identified as LGBTQ occupies a position of "knowing" or wisdom that other characters around them lack (such as Carter Haywood in *Spin City* or Javier in *Smiley*), and *disclosing sexuality* where the narrative centers on the process of disclosing one's sexual identity or desires as part of the media narrative (such as *Ellen*, or the more recent *Heartstopper*). These patterns influence how media narratively imagines LGBTQ characters, and in each instance, sexuality plays a central role in defining the character's story arc. Historically, it has been rare for media narratives to create layered images of LGBTQ identities with intersectional concerns such as health, disability, and neurodivergence.

Intersectional Specificities

In this section, we highlight some contemporary series that feature queer characters who suffer from and/or navigate various health issues. These examples explore how a character's queerness informs, contextualizes, and/or affects how they experience various health afflictions and vice versa. What makes this turn in the 21st century unique is that television and streaming services relied on memoirs and autobiographical experiences of LGBTQ individuals, making the fictionalized retelling semi-autobiographical in nature. As a result, the stories avoid characters who "happen to be" queer or "happen to have" X disease or affliction. Rather, the combination of health and queer intersections both inform and texture the characters' navigation of the health condition, of the healthcare system, and of queer relationships and community.

The Netflix Niche

Although certainly not the only streaming platform to address LGBTQ issues, Netflix is perhaps the most prolific and garners the most attention. Upon its announcement in 2007 that the company intended to transition from direct-to-home DVD rentals to streaming technology, the Netflix model rapidly disrupted traditional media industry approaches to content creation and distribution. After several years of success, Netflix began planning to launch its own original content line, with its first major offering, *House of Cards*, premiering in 2013. Although the series did not explicitly interrogate LGBTQ issues, the show revealed in Season 1 that protagonist Frank Underwood (played by actor Kevin Spacey) had a romance with one of his military colleagues prior to starting his political career. This narrative returned later in Season 5 of the series when the show disclosed that Underwood had another male lover, and his sexuality became a liability for his election campaign (Donnelly, 2017). The release of Season 5 occurred just months before Spacey faced allegations of numerous sexual assault violations, leading to Netflix canceling both the series and the actor (Kennedy, 2017) and distancing itself from long-standing stereotypes of gay men as pedophiles and sexual abusers (Gartner, 1999; E. J. Meyer, 2015).

Given the overlap between the fictionalized content in *House of Cards* and Spacey's real-life issues with sexuality, it is not surprising that Netflix then leaned into more positive semi-autobiographical scripted series to address LGBTQ issues. Poised to appeal to niche audiences and able to take more risks with content creation than broadcast networks, Netflix created and distributed numerous series that portrayed more complex images of LGBTQ populations, many of which have overlaps with health narratives. For example, *Heartstopper* (2022-present) entails a British coming-of-age story created by Alice Oseman, who began writing and illustrating *Heartstopper* as a webcomic when they were just 22 years old. The narrative of *Heartstopper* follows the queer love story of protagonists Nick and Charlie (who actually appeared as secondary characters in Oseman's previously published YA novel *Solitaire*). Wang (2022) described the series as representing "queer joy" and a diverse range of coming out and sexual identity stories.

Season two of *Heartstopper* revealed that protagonist Charlie suffered from disordered eating (see related discussion in Chapter 5, this volume). In Episode 5, "Heat," Charlie, Nick, and their classmates were on a school trip to Paris. Early in the episode, Charlie skipped eating breakfast, prompting Nick to put a croissant in his backpack. While touring a museum, the camera shot from Charlie's point of view as his vision blurred, his surroundings became fuzzy, and he ultimately passed out. Once he regained consciousness, Nick started a conversation:

> *Nick:* Charlie, I notice you don't really eat a lot generally. I feel like it's gotten worse recently, like you eat less than you used to …
>
> *Charlie:* I'm sorry, I'm really sorry. I know I don't eat like normal people. Some days I'm fine, but other days I feel like I need to control it. I used to do it a lot last year when everything at school was really bad – sometimes it feels like the only thing I can control in my life.
>
> *(Oseman & Lyn, 2023)*

Nick empathized with Charlie and reiterated that as his boyfriend, he wanted to know what was going on with Charlie, both good and bad. As the season progressed, the pattern continued. After Charlie attended and then left a dinner at Nick's house, Nick's mother observed, "Charlie didn't eat much," and the camera showed Nick googling eating disorders on his cell phone. This representation is rare in popular culture, despite the fact that epidemiological studies have noted a disproportionate number of gay men with eating disorders compared to their heterosexual counterparts (Arcelus et al., 2018). In fact, gay men are ten times more likely to experience disordered eating than heterosexual men (Strong et al., 2000). Addressing this issue in a narrative promoting "queer joy" provides a humanized version of navigating health concerns surrounding disordered eating.

Other semi-autobiographical series on Netflix skillfully interrogated intersections between LGBTQ identities and disability. *Special* (2019–2021) was an American comedy-drama based on the memoir "I'm Special: And Other Lies We Tell Ourselves." The series chronicled the protagonist's life as a gay man with cerebral palsy in Los Angeles, portrayed by writer and creator Ryan

O'Connell. The series attracted quite a bit of popular attention, culminating in four Emmy nominations: one for Outstanding Short Form Comedy or Drama Series and three for performances by O'Connell, Jessica Hecht (who plays Ryan's mother), and Punam Patel (who plays Ryan's best friend). Analyzing Season 1 of *Special*, Davies et al. (2021) argued that the series not only provided a complex and productive representation of a gay character but also "works within and against homonormative politics through a cripping of normative gay forms of representation in its emphasis on disability and CP" (p. 58).

One of the most unique features of the narrative in *Special* involved its representation of various types of disability. In Season 2, Episode 5, "Ryan Joins the Crips," Ryan navigated his life and questioned his internalized ableism. When pitching an article idea to his editor, he quipped, "I haven't spent much time with my disabled brethren – so really, do I have no disabled friends because of my internalized ableism, or have I just not found the right group of people?" (Kashyap & Johnson, 2021). This question occupied Ryan's mind after meeting Henry, a neurodivergent gay man who identified as on the autism spectrum, in the previous episode. In this scene, the editor clearly talked down to Ryan and insulted him numerous times. Taken together, the episode poignantly represented how society treats both queerness and disability; in one recent study of LGBTQ people living with disabilities, participants reported experiencing verbal abuse (42.5%), sexual assault (17.4%), and social exclusion based on their disability and/or gender identity (50.3%) in the past 12 months (Amos et al., 2023; see related work in Chapter 6, this volume).

Henry invited Ryan to a disabled support group of friends that he frequented, and Ryan finally decided to attend. As they walked toward the support group meeting place in a park, Henry visibly stimmed (a repetitive behavioral pattern associated with autism) and a stranger passing by stared. Henry noticed and immediately called the man out, saying,

> I'm stimming honey – self-stimulatory behavior is occasionally a symptom of people like me that were diagnosed with Aspbergers, but that term is now problematic because – whoops – it was coined by Nazis, so technically now we are all just somewhere on the autistic spectrum, neurodiverse if you're nasty. But I mostly identify as hot!
>
> *(Kashyap & Johnson, 2021)*

Once they arrived, they joined a broad group of characters with various types of disabilities. They took turns sharing their experiences navigating the world with their disabilities, and Ryan shared, "I thought I was done dealing with my CP but it still trolls me all the time. Uber drivers ask what's wrong with me. Strangers come up to me at the gym to congratulate me simply on exercising" (Kashyap & Johnson, 2021). One of the participants in the group responded with "Ewwww – inspiration porn!" – a term used by disability advocates to challenge the "paternalistic relationship between those with disabilities and those without" (Hoggatt, 2023, p. 210). After the group meeting, Henry eventually kissed Ryan and asked him out. Ryan agreed to go on a date which was featured later in the episode. Henry arrived for the date, and it began the following exchange:

> *Ryan:* "I am loving your mesh shirt/skirt combo!"
>
> *Henry:* "Me? Ryan, you shouldn't have! Yeah, I totally fuck with skirts. I think it's because growing up people would stare at me and I was like well if you're gonna do that, I might as well give em something to look at."
>
> *Ryan:* "For me it's always kind of been the opposite. You know, blend in, don't draw attention to your disability."
>
> *Henry:* "Ok, not to speak in bumper sticker here but you can fight who you are, but that's a fight you are never gonna win. So, you might as well embrace it."
>
> *Ryan:* "Yeah, I know – I'm getting there – it's just a journey, you know."
>
> *(Kashyap & Johnson, 2021)*

Ryan's journey continued throughout the season when he realized that he had to pause his relationship with Henry in order to deal with his feelings for Tanner, his neurotypical, able-bodied ex-boyfriend. Ryan resumed his relationship with Tanner only to realize over the course of the second season that his disability, and Tanner's inability to understand it, ultimately made it impossible for them to continue their relationship.

To date, many other series on Netflix have interrogated the overlap of LGBTQ identities and health issues including *Feel Good* (addiction and recovery), *Atypical* (excessive exercise), *Sex Education* (physical and emotional abuse), *Young Royals* (ADHD), *Heartbreak High* (Autism), *AJ and the Queen* (blindness), and *Merli Sapere Aude* (HIV diagnosis and PREP), just to name a few.

Reframing the AIDS Crisis in Pose

Pose (2018–2021) was a fictional series about New York City's underground ball culture set within the AIDS crisis of the late 1980s through the 1990s. Balls entail competitions where "houses" compete on the floor to see who best emulates various aesthetic categories like "royalty" and "butch queen realness." Airing on cable network FX, *Pose* offered significant interventions in representations of queer HIV-positive characters and the personal, political, and medical stakes of the AIDS crisis on queer communities during this time period. The series featured a large ensemble cast, made up largely of queer actors of color and/or trans actors, led by MJ Rodriguez and Billy Porter, who play Blanca and Pray Tell, respectively.

While fictional, the series borrowed from documentaries and passed-down oral histories of New York City's ball and house communities to ground the narrative. Both Blanca and Pray Tell were diagnosed as HIV positive in the first season, and AIDS became a persistent story attribute that more richly informed their character development and the direction of the series. Blanca's primary journey across *Pose*'s three seasons included taking on the role of a house mother, the term for a maternal figure who takes in and oversees an evolving group of ball participants who seek guidance, community, and care. Throughout the decade that the series spanned, she also became a business entrepreneur and, eventually, a nurse. Pray Tell served as the primary emcee of the weekly balls, providing much of the show's charismatic charm but also had ongoing story arcs including an intergenerational love affair, his alcoholism, and a fraught relationship with his family. By the end of the series, Pray Tell succumbed to AIDS complications after lending his trial medications to a younger character without access to such drugs.

The AIDS crisis did not simply provide historical context in *Pose*; it encompassed, part and parcel, the series' physical sets and story locations. Season 2's premiere episode opened with Blanca and Pray Tell in 1990 visiting Hart Island, a mass burial site for unclaimed bodies, many of whom were AIDS victims. Outside of the primary sets – the ball floor and various characters' apartments – HIV testing clinics, hospital rooms with dying AIDS patients, funeral services, and protest actions became a staple of the show's locations. Throughout seasons two and three, *Pose* also incorporated ACT UP meetings and protests, emulating – and in some instances recreating – documented public actions by the activist group protesting the CDC and government's inaction on AIDS (Morris, 2012). A running gag featured between Pray Tell and Nurse Judy (Sandra Bernhard) about which character will attend 1,000 funeral services first – dark humor emblematic of the times – exemplified the centrality, and intentionally repetitive nature, of set decisions.

Unlike popular media before it, especially on television, *Pose* centered queer characters and how HIV and the AIDS crisis not only informed their development, but the specific identity histories and legacies queer individuals inherit as part of the LGBTQ community. The show did not isolate these characters within an otherwise all-straight and cis ensemble, treat their story arcs as temporary, depict their health affliction as just an individual obstacle, or suggest a fatal demise as the only function for characters with AIDS. *Pose* situated HIV and AIDS as a core historical and generational feature contextualizing and enriching both character and story, not simply a narrative problem to resolve.

Work in Progress: Complicating LGBTQ Mental Health Concerns

Within the first minute of the pilot episode of *Work in Progress* (2019–2022), viewers witness protagonist Abby McEnany at her therapist's office, announcing:

> I'm going to kill myself in 180 days if things don't get better. I think it will hurt some people but in a way I'm doing them a huge service. I'm giving them a gift. I mean, I'm 45, I'm fat, I'm this queer dyke who hasn't done shit in her life and this is my identity?
>
> *(McEnany & Mason, 2019)*

She described how someone at work bought her almonds from Costco, presumably because of her fluctuating weight. "So I laid out 180 almonds," continued Abby, "and every day I'm just going to throw one away, and then at the end, when there's one last almond left and I don't feel any better, I'm done. I'm out. Because I'm sick of it. I'm sick of struggling" (McEnany & Mason, 2019). She kept talking until she noticed her therapist was unresponsive and realized, as her friends put it later at a game night, that she killed her therapist with her problems.

This type of dark humor pervaded the Showtime series in its deft representation of many layered mental health issues experienced by LGBTQ populations. Despite numerous scholars finding that LGBTQ populations experience mental health concerns more than their heterosexual counterparts (Grant et al., 2014), very few representations in media offer stories that extend beyond generic coming-out narratives or simply marking queerness as associated with mental illness. Notably, *Work in Progress* aired at the same time as queer women and non-binary individuals reported significant increases in utilizing mental health services during the pandemic (presumably linked to the broader online availability of such services providing a wider network of choice for patients) and reported higher rates of satisfaction with their mental health care providers (Simpson, 2023). In the second season, when Abby tried out new therapists, the camera focused on a list of 12 names and addresses in her notebook with lines already through many of them. In Season 2, Episode 2, several flashbacks showed a child and teen Abby at several different therapist offices due to her anxieties. This episode includes title cards before every new therapist – "Therapist #1 Dr. Mel" – including her makeshift therapists like "Therapist #4: Lunch Lady Dawn." This sustained emphasis throughout the series on Abby's therapy history and current struggles finding a new therapist normalized the trials and tribulations of seeking care for conditions like anxiety, depression, and obsessive-compulsive disorder that Abby experienced. The framing and narrative structure of the many different therapists, past and present, also highlighted the labor of seeking such care, not to mention the privilege and access to therapy afforded by Abby's middle-class upbringing and current office job.

Season 2 of *Work in Progress* also addressed the start of the COVID-19 pandemic when social distancing and the shutdown of many aspects of social life coincided with the racial reckoning after George Floyd's death. The series contended with how a relatively privileged person like Abby navigates isolation, loneliness, and networks of care as a queer person also battling depression, OCD, and past suicidal ideation. The show spotlighted the highs and lows of Abby's anxieties, news fatigue, and struggles with (unwittingly) drafting her employer's diversity statement while, at the same time, dropping off alcohol at friends' doorsteps, watering her neighbor's plants, and being with family after her father's hospitalization for a suicide attempt. Thus, *Work in Progress* critically and refreshingly represented the mundane existence of being queer *and* day-to-day living with mental health issues.

Finally, both seasons of *Work in Progress* offered a meta representation of *Saturday Night Live*'s 1990s skit character Pat, played by Julia Sweeney. Abby revealed on a date in Episode 1 that "the character, Pat … who nobody could tell was a man or a woman, ruined my life" (McEnany & Mason, 2019). In a subsequent flashback, a college-aged Abby arrived at a party as someone muttered, "Pat's here," in a nod to how the "joke" of Pat's gender ambiguity contributed to our culture's inhospitable treatment of trans and gender non-conforming people at a specific point of visibility in the 1990s. In the show, Sweeney played herself and, after a happenstance meeting with Abby, continuously attempted to rectify and "fix" the harm that Pat caused, which also revealed Sweeney's attachment to her own self-preservation. These scenes demonstrated the show's unique approach to addressing the trauma and anxieties that queer and gender-nonconforming people like Abby carry as a result of a long history of unchallenged representations of marginalized communities in media and popular culture.

The Long Life of "Reality" Television and LGBTQ Representation

Since the advent of reality television as a genre, communication scholars have challenged the terminology "reality" in reference to its representations. On the one hand, reality television offers an opportunity to represent *actual* LGBTQ people as competitors or contestants in their narratives. On the other hand, the politics of being out in these spaces have evolved over time. In early reality television programming from social shows like MTV's *The Real World* to competition shows like *Survivor*, having a queer character (overwhelmingly a white gay man) became part of normalized casting practices to tout the "diversity" of the "real world" (Choi, 2015; Kachgal, 2004). In these contexts, the degree to which the "character" is an out version of themselves varied. Other types of reality programming specifically mark queerness at the center of the program, such as *Queer Eye for the Straight Guy* (Meyer & Kelley, 2004; Sender, 2006) or *Boy Meets Boy* (Bennett, 2006). Thus, depending on the type of reality program (social vs. competition), the representation of LGBTQ people, framing and sharing their stories in "confessional" style diary room sessions, and/or interviews with producers outside of the watchful eyes of their castmates ultimately led to a wide variety of representations of LGBTQ identity (Rahman, 2008).

The television series *Big Brother* stands out as one of the longest-running reality shows on US television, broadcasting 26 seasons over the past 21 years. In each of those seasons, 16 houseguests have entered the *Big Brother* house, cut off from all information and communication from the outside world, to compete in a series of competitions, hoping to be one of the last two houseguests standing at the end. The previously evicted houseguests, who become members of the "jury," cast their vote for which of the remaining two players wins on finale night. *Big Brother* exists primarily as a social game – hinging on an individual's ability to cultivate meaningful relationships with housemates and carefully balance showing themselves as a competitor who will "get blood on their hands" while simultaneously not being too ruthless or unlikable so that a "bitter jury" votes against them at the end. Seasons to date have recorded the houseguests with 24-hour camera footage, some of which the production staff then edited and cut into episodes, and some of which is only available on the "live feeds" where viewers could watch inside the house in real-time. This structure promoted the Foucauldian notion of the panopticon, where participants expected and tolerated constant surveillance (Sears & Godderis, 2011). Thus, invested viewers could learn far more about each contestant than what has been presented in more scripted, pre-recorded reality series.

Big Brother US has often featured at least one LGBTQ-identified contestant (only two seasons have not) – although the degree to which they claimed this identity varied. Some contestants used their sexual and/or gender positionality as part of their initial pitch to be accepted onto the series; others disclosed this information in their introduction to other houseguests. In other cases, houseguests revealed their sexual and/or gender identity later on – either in the house as the series aired or outside the house after their series concluded. Depending on when and where the participants were in their sexual and/or gender identity journey, their days in the *Big Brother* house only represented a specific sliver of their life timeline. In fact, to date, casting directors have seemed to purposefully cast LGBTQ characters far more so than casting based on racial diversity. Dixon's (2019) work found that, although the LGBTQ community makes up about 4% of the total U.S. population, they account for 12% of *Big Brother US* contestants. As of the 26th finished season, this percentage had not changed: of the 431 total contestants to date, 51 were LGBTQ-identified: 31 gay men, 6 lesbian women, 12 bisexual, 1 transgender, and 1 non-binary.

Although LGBTQ individuals might be represented on *Big Brother*, the show has relied on larger social stereotypes and stigmas. R. Fox (2013), who competed in Season 12 of the series, identified after the fact that producers and other castmates framed his performance in the series through tropes of the "crying gay man" and the "gay villain." Andy Herron became the first gay winner of the series in Season 15; however, castmates and numerous fans described him as a "rat floater" and attributed his win to the controversy surrounding runner-up Gina Marie Zimmerman's participation in homophobic and racist commentary in the house (Gale, 2013). Herron's positionality in the house had him frequently serving as a purveyor of information across alliances. Thornborrow and Morris (2004) explained that success in *Big Brother* often relied on being able to "manage gossip talk strategically to establish social relationships within the house" (p. 246), adding another trope to representations of gay men as "gossiping queens" and social butterflies.

Throughout many seasons of the show, the LGBTQ houseguests have various overlapping health concerns – many of them shown as mental in orientation. In *Big Brother 25*, the gay male houseguest was evicted in the third week because he was "bossy" and domineering, and the lesbian houseguest was targeted shortly thereafter for being paranoid and overly emotional. In *Big Brother 17*, transgender houseguest Audrey Middleton was targeted for eviction, and the entire week's footage chronicled her "meltdown" where she socially isolated herself, hid under blankets and behind sunglasses, and generally disobeyed all house rules until her eviction. For good or ill, *Big Brother* is a staple of LGBTQ representation on television, particularly as it has been syndicated internationally in numerous countries and manages to be successful in various cultural contexts, awakening "a generation of young queers" (Peters & Smith, 2023).

The Rise of Participatory Culture and Social Media

Media industries created and produced the examples used in our last section for corporate profit. However, from a critical media and cultural studies perspective, popular culture extends beyond what industries produce for mass consumption – what sells most; it is also culture produced *by* and *for* the people (Hall, 2019). Long before the advent of the Internet, the field of fan studies explored the myriad ways in which media consumers were also often media producers (Gray et al., 2017; Jenkins, 2006; Meyer & Tucker, 2007). Fans circulated all kinds of original creations – fan fiction (Baughman & Meyer, 2007), fan art (Dennis, 2010), and fanzines (Triggs, 2006) through cultivated interpersonal and mass-mediated social networks. Others turned to the increasing accessibility of video starting in the 1980s to document and archive the lives and conditions of people with HIV and AIDS, for instance, when the mainstream media industries ignored the epidemic and its casualties (Juhasz, 1995). With Apple's introduction of the iPhone in 2007, along with other advancements in technology, a rapid turn to digital technologies and affordances vastly broadened access for everyday media consumers to produce and distribute original media creations. YouTube and social media have been a boon for content creators beyond simple access to technology – unbeholden to mass audience appeal and gatekept industry capital, these platforms allow multiple communities at any intersection imaginable to find each other, create their own media, and sometimes even break into mainstream visibility. In this section, we highlight just a few online communities, campaigns, and creators that have given voice to queer people navigating health and safety issues, as well as advocating for various forms of health and care.

YouTube's open and accessible video distribution platform and social functionality (commenting, linking, subscribing, etc.) have made it a popular space for queer people seeking help, care, and community. Wuest (2014) observed the reciprocal and communal function of coming out videos on YouTube for gay users in the late 2000s. Horak (2014) and Raun (2016) both published analyses of transitioning videos for trans audiences during those same early YouTube days. In September of 2010, sex columnist Dan Savage uploaded a YouTube video with his husband, urging gay youth that "it gets better" in response to a string of national reports of gay teen suicides. This video quickly turned into one of the earliest online viral campaigns, encouraging everyday users as well as celebrities, politicians, sports teams, and all types of businesses – from Lady Gaga and Barack Obama to compilations from Pixar, Apple, and Google employees – to upload their own "it gets better" videos directly addressed to vulnerable queer youth. Preceding social media tag campaigns like the ALS Challenge or hashtag activism like #BlackLivesMatter and #MeToo, the It Gets Better campaign largely spread via blogs, Facebook, news coverage, and fans of famous personalities who uploaded their own It Gets Better messages. While the most viewed videos typically featured the big-name accounts – and largely cis, white, male, and wealthy figures – digging deeper into the searches revealed tens of thousands of everyday users uploading their own messages, some of which challenged the viral refrain that life for queer youth necessarily encompasses a linear, positive trajectory – that a journey to healthy selfhood may have many ups and downs (Compton, 2020; Michaelsen, 2017). It Gets Better has since turned into a non-profit organization that creates projects for education and uplift related to LGBTQ youth, but its legacy will always be tied to its massive grassroots spread that started with one video uploaded to YouTube (Compton, 2020).

Social media has also become an indispensable tool and platform for visibility and activism, particularly for trans people in response to state and socio-cultural violence. Stern (2018) wrote about trans actress-activist Laverne Cox's popularization of the hashtag #TransIsBeautiful on her social media posts starting in 2015. Since then, the hashtag has amassed millions of posts by trans people across Tumblr, Twitter, Instagram, TikTok, and other social media platforms. Samer (2019) expanded our understanding of participatory culture by theorizing how "trans Instagram" is "a space where trans celebrities, artists, and activists craft their own visions for trans community and culture" (p. 544). In 2018, following the Trump administration's memo to prohibit the use of "transgender" as well as other terms like "vulnerable" and "diversity" from CDC reports and documents – the first of many efforts by the Trump White House to roll back state protections for trans citizens – users on social media made #WillNotBeErased trend with accompanying GIFs and images.

In a different, hybrid form of media representation, Gays Against Guns (GAG for short) – formed days after the Pulse nightclub shooting in 2016 which killed 49, mostly queer, people – is a direct-action group that engages in protests, boycotts, and public disruptions to call out and pressure companies and the government to change our gun laws. The organization's website stated, "Most gun deaths in the U.S. are suicides and LGBTQ people are overrepresented among suicide victims" and "LGBTQ people are also the most likely minority to be the victim of a hate crime" (Gays Against Guns, 2023, para 1). To date, GAG has used multimedia approaches by recording and posting their public actions on social media, running a podcast called RADIO GAG, and the organization was the subject of *Gays Against Guns: The Movie*. The synergy of LGBTQ activism and its direct relation to harm reduction illustrates how social media users can actively shape cultural discourse.

Given the rise of influencer and creator culture in the age of social media, we must analyze the ways these technologies and platforms both limit and afford visibility to queer, disabled, and otherwise marginalized and/or intersectional perspectives. In the short lifespan of social media, a long history of LGBTQ censorship already exists from YouTube to TikTok, including flagging queer content on these platforms as adult or shadow-banned (Bensinger & Albergotti, 2019; C. Fox, 2020). More recently, the same has been observed with TikTok videos from user accounts created by individuals with disabilities, again inhibiting content that intentionally promotes disability activism (Rauchberg, 2020). Imani Barbarin (also penning the account name Crutches & Spice on many platforms) has managed to break through both the censorship and the noise of social media platforms. A disability rights blogger, content creator, and activist, Barbarin "writes from the perspective of a black woman with Cerebral Palsy" (Crutches & Spice, n.d., para 1). Barbarin gained more cultural visibility and prominence by joining TikTok during the early days of the COVID-19 pandemic. As of Fall 2023, she has amassed more than half a million followers and nearly 50 million likes. Addressing the possibility of herself being shadow-banned, Barbarin (2020) remarked in one video, "I know that TikTok actively suppresses the videos of Black, disabled, fat, and queer people, and I am all those things." Many of Barbarin's videos responded to various ableist media content, positioning her voice as an intersectional critique of these discourses.

Along with an increasing number of other examples of participatory media culture and practices, the campaigns and accounts we have highlighted – whether strategically organized or organically viral and diffuse – demonstrate *people's* use of media, either individually or collectively, to make visible, popularize, educate, and advocate LGBTQ issues that intersect with health issues such as care, safety, and the general livelihood of queer people.

Conclusion

In this chapter, we have presented a broad vision of how LGBTQ images intersect with health and popular culture over time. From early representations focused largely on reifying stigmas and promoting stereotypes, to early 21st-century images attempting to position LGBTQ issues as part of cultural assimilation, to more contemporary intersectional representations and real-life storytelling/activism from LGBTQ populations, we have traced how these issues began and continue to beget popular culture discourses. While our analysis is admittedly not exhaustive, we feel that it paints a clear lineage of the ways in which health issues have been framed against and among LGBTQ images. With continued technological advances, extended competition in and among media industries that promote both fragmentation and media convergence simultaneously, we anticipate these patterns and tropes will continue to recycle, expand, and evolve in popular media culture.

Note

1 Throughout this essay, we use both "queer" and the acronym LGBTQ to include many forms of non-heteronormative identities and positionalities. We recognize that these terms are limiting in explaining and parsing the range of identifications associated with the broader LGBTQ+ community. We encourage readers to build on and further complicate the myriad ways in which health in media and popular culture intersect with a multitude of non-normative identities and experiences.

References

Amos, N., Hill, A. O., Lyons, A., Bigby, C., Carman, M., Parsons, M., & Bourne, A. (2023). Factors associated with experiences of abuse among lesbian, gay, bisexual, trans, queer, and asexual (LGBTQA+) adults with disability in Australia. *Disability and Health Journal, 16*(2), 101408.

Arcelus, J., Fernandez-Aranda, F., & Bouman, W. P. (2018). Eating disorders and disordered eating in the LGBTQ population. In L. K. Anderson & S. B. Murray (Eds.), *Clinical handbook of complex and atypical eating disorders* (p. 327–343). Oxford University Press.

Barbarin, I. [crutches_and_spice]. (2020, August 27). To the people that brought it to my attention I may be sh@dowb@nned #lgbt #thicc. [video]. *TikTok*. https://www.tiktok.com/@crutches_and_spice/video/6865836864935316742

Battles, K., & Hilton-Morrow, W. (2002). Gay characters in conventional spaces: *Will and Grace* and the situation comedy genre. *Critical Studies in Media Communication, 19*, 87–106.

Baughman, L., & Meyer, M. D. E. (2007). Slashing *Alias*: Viewer appropriation of Lauren Reed as commentary on female/female desire. In S. Abbott & S. Brown (Eds.), *Investigating alias: Secrets and spies* (pp. 174–185). I.B. Taurus & Co Ltd.

Bennett, J. A. (2006). In defense of gaydar: Reality television and the politics of the glace. *Critical Media Studies in Communication, 23*, 408–425.

Benshoff, H., & Griffin, S. (2006). *Queer images: A history of gay and lesbian film in America*. Rowman and Littlefield Publishers.

Bensinger, G., & Albergotti, R. (2019, August 14). YouTube discriminates against LGBT content by unfairly culling it, suit alleges. *The Washington Post*. https://www.washingtonpost.com/technology/2019/08/14/youtube-discriminates-against-lgbt-content-by-unfairly-culling-it-suit-alleges/

Burgess, S. (2023). *LGBT inclusion in American life: Pop culture, political imagination, and civil rights*. New York University Press.

Choi, H. (2015). White men still dominate reality television: Discriminatory casting and the need for regulation. *Hastings Communication & Entertainment Law Journal, 37*, 163–200.

Compton, J. (2020, September 21). 'It gets better': How a viral video fueled a movement for LGBTQ youth. *NBC News*. https://www.nbcnews.com/feature/nbc-out/it-gets-better-how-viral-video-fueled-movement-lgbtq-youth-n1240608

Crutches & Spice. (n.d.). About. https://crutchesandspice.com/about/

Davies, A., Maich, K., Belcher, C, Cagulada, E. DeWelles, M., & van Rhijn, T. (2021). A critical examination of the intersection of sexuality and disability in *Special,* a Netflix series. In M. S. Jeffress (Ed.), *Disability representation in film, TV, and print media* (pp. 44–64). Routledge.

Dennis, J. P. (2010). Drawing desire: Male youth and homoerotic fan art. *Journal of LGBT Youth, 7*(1), 6–28.

Dhaenens, F. (2013). The fantastic queer: Reading gay representations in *Torchwood* and *True Blood* as articulations of queer resistance. *Critical Studies in Media Communication, 30*(2), 102–116.

Dixon, V. (2019, August 26). *Big Brother*'s diversity problem by the numbers: A deep dive into casting data might explain why the reality show is constantly accused of bias. *Vince Dixon Portfolio*. https://vincedixon-portfolio.com/app/big-brother-diversity/

Donnelly, M. (2017, June). *House of Cards* revisits Frank Underwood's sexuality (and it's a huge liability). *The Wrap*. https://www.thewrap.com/house-of-cards-frank-underwood-sexuality-liability/

Dow, B. J. (2001). *Ellen*, television, and the politics of gay and lesbian visibility. *Critical Media Studies in Communication, 18*, 123–141.

Epstein, R., & Friedman, J. (Directors). (1995). *The celluloid closet.* Sony Pictures Classics.

Fox, C. (2020, September 10). TikTok admits restricting some LGBT hashtags. *BBC*. https://www.bbc.com/news/technology-54102575

Fox, R. (2013). "You are not allowed to talk about production": Narratization on (and off) the set of CBS' Big Brother. *Critical Studies in Media Communication, 30*, 189–208.

Friedkin, W. (Director). (1970). *The Boys in the Band.* Cinema Center Films.

Fuqua, J. (1994). There's a queer in my soap: The homophobia/AIDS storyline on *One Life to Live*. In R. C. Allen (Ed.). *To be continued…: Soap operas around the world* (pp. 199–212). Routledge.

Gale, D. (2013, September 17). *Big Brother* 15 Spoiler: Andy Herren wins to be first "out and proud" winner and salvage some good press for CBS. *Entertainment News*. https://www.celebdirtylaundry.com/2013/big-brother-15-spoiler-andy-herren-wins-winner/

Gartner, R. B. (1999). Sexual victimization of boys by men: Meanings and consequences. *Journal of Gay & Lesbian Psychology, 32*(2), 1–33.

Gays Against Guns (2023). About us. https://web.archive.org/web/20230927214348/ https://www.gaysagainst-guns.net/about

GLAAD Media Institute. (2022). Where we are on TV. https://glaad.org/whereweareontv21/

Grant, J. E., Odlaug, B. L., Derbyshire, K., Schreiber, L. R. N., Lust, K., & Christenson, G. (2014). Mental health and clinical correlates in lesbian, gay, bisexual and queer young adults. *Journal of American College Health, 62*, 75–78.

Gray, J., Sandvoss, C., & Harrington, C. L. (Eds.). (2017). *Fandom: Identities and communities in a mediated world.* New York University Press.

Gross, L. (1994). What is wrong with this picture? Lesbian women and gay men on television. In R. J. Ringer (Ed.), *Queer words, queer images: Communication and the construction of homosexuality* (pp. 143–158). New York University Press.

Gross, L. (2001). *Up from invisibility: Lesbians, gay men, and the media in America.* Columbia University Press.

Hall, S. (2019). Notes on deconstructing 'the popular.' In D. Morley (Ed.), *Essential essays, volume 1: Foundations of cultural studies* (pp. 347–361). Duke University Press.

HRC Staff. (2023). For the first time ever, Human Rights Campaign officially declares 'state of emergency' for LGBTQ+ Americans. *Human Rights Campaign,* https://www.hrc.org/press-releases/for-the-first-time-ever-human-rights-campaign-officially-declares-state-of-emergency-for-lgbtq-americans-issues-national-warning-and-guidebook-to-ensure-safety-for-lgbtq-residents-and-travelers

Hoggatt, M. J. (2023). Night to shine and inspiration porn: An examination of practices in disability ministry. *Journal of Disability & Religion, 27*, 210–222.

Horak, L. (2014). Trans on YouTube: Intimacy, visibility, temporality. *Transgender Studies Quarterly, 1*(4), 572–585.

Jenkins, H. (2006). *Fans, bloggers, and gamers: Exploring participatory culture*. New York University Press.

Joyrich, L. (2009). Epistemology of the console. In G. Davis & G. Needham (Eds.), *Queer TV: Theories, histories, politics* (pp. 15–47). Routledge.

Juhasz, A. (1995). *AIDS TV: Identity, community, and alternative video.* Duke University Press.

Kachgal, T. (2004). "Look at *The Real World.* There's always a gay teen on there": Sexual citizenship and youth-targeted reality television. *Feminist Media Studies, 4*, 361–364.

Kashyap, K. (Writer), & Johnson, C. (Director). (2021, May 20). Ryan joins the crips (Season 2, Episode 5) [TV series episode]. In R. O'Connell (Executive Producer), *Special.* Warner Bros. Television; That's Wonderful Productions; Campfire; Stage 13.

Kennedy, M. (2017, October). *House of Cards* canceled as fallout continues for Kevin Spacey. *The Wrap,* https://web.archive.org/web/20171102194521/http://www.twincities.com/2017/10/30/kevin-spacey-slammed-for-timing-of-coming-out-as-gay

Kunzel, R. (2018). The rise of gay rights and the disavowal of disability in the United States. In M. A. Rembis, C. J. Kudlick, & K. Nielson (Eds.), *The Oxford handbook of disability history* (pp. 459–476). Oxford University Press.

Li-Vollmer, M., & LaPointe, M. E. (2003). Gender transgression and villainy in animated film. *Popular Communication,* 1(2), 89–110.

McEnany, A., & Mason, T. (Writers), & Mason, T. (Director). (2019, December 8). 180 almonds (Season 1, Episode 1) [TV series episode]. In A. McEnany, T. Mason, & L. Wachowski (Executive Producers), *Work in Progress*. Tessa Films.

Meyer, E. J. (2015). The personal is political: LGBTQ education research and policy since 1993. *Educational Forum, 79*(4), 347–352.

Meyer, M. D. E. (2003). "It's me. I'm it.": Defining adolescent sexual identity through relational dialectics in *Dawson's Creek. Communication Quarterly, 51*(3), 262–276.

Meyer, M. D. E. (2009). "I'm just trying to find my way like most kids": Bisexuality, adolescence and the drama of *One Tree Hill. Sexuality & Culture, 13*(4), 237–251.

Meyer, M. D. E., & Kelley, J. (2004). Queering the eye?: The politics of gay white men and gender (in)visibility. *Feminist Media Studies, 4*(2), 214–217.

Meyer, M. D. E., & Tucker, M. (2007). Textual poaching and beyond: Fan communities and fandoms in the age of the Internet. *Review of Communication, 7*(1), 103–116.

Michaelsen, A. (2017). Feeling differently together: The *It Gets Better Project* as an unlikely intimate public of LGBT peers. *Emotion, Space and Society, 25*, 144–149.

Morris, C. E. III. (2012). ACT UP 25: HIV/AIDS, archival queers, and mnemonic world making. *Quarterly Journal of Speech, 98*, 49–53.

Oseman, A. (Writer) & Lyn, E. (Director). (2023, August 3). Heat (Season 2, Episode 5) [TV series episode]. In P. Walter (Executive Producer), *Heartstopper*. See-Saw Films.

Peters, A., & Smith S. (2023, March 28). How *Big Brother* blazed the trail for LGBTQ+ representation on TV. *Dazed.* https://www.dazeddigital.com/film-tv/article/58519/1/how-big-brother-blazed-the-trail-for-lgbtq-representation-on-tv

Rahman, M. (2008). Jade's confession: Racism and the dialectics of celebrity. *Social Semiotics, 18*(2), 133–148.

Rauchberg, J. S. (2020). TikTok's digital eugenics: Challenging ableism and algorithmic erasure through disability activism. *Flow.* https://www.flowjournal.org/2020/09/tiktok-digital-eugenics/

Raun, T. (2016). *Out online: Trans self-representation and community building on YouTube*. Routledge.

Reise. (2023, February 27). All 230 dead lesbians and bisexual characters on TV, and how they died. *Autostraddle.* https://www.autostraddle.com/all-65-dead-lesbian-and-bisexual-characters-on-tv-and-how-they-died-312315/

Russo, V. (1987). *The celluloid closet: Homosexuality in the movies*. Harper & Row.

Samer, R. (2019). Remixing transfeminist futures. *TSQ: Transgender Studies Quarterly, 6*(4), 539–555.
Sears, C. A., & Godderis, R. (2011). Roar like a tiger on TV? *Feminist Media Studies, 11*(2), 181–195.
Sender, K. (2006). Queens for a day: *Queer Eye for the Straight Guy* and the neoliberal project. *Critical Media Studies in Communication, 23*, 131–151.
Simpson, E. C. (2023). *Experiences of queer women and nonbinary individuals with mental health care services during the COVID-19 pandemic*. Dissertation Abstracts International: Section B: The Sciences and Engineering, 84(8-B), 2003. Antioch University.
Stern, D. (2018). #TransIsBeautiful: The polymediated, intersectional feminism of Laverne Cox. In K. V. Anderson (Ed.), *Women, feminism, and pop politics* (pp. 77–97). Peter Lang.
Strong, S. M., Williamson, D. A., Netemeyer, R. G., & Geer, J. H. (2000). Eating disorder symptoms and concerns about body differ as a function of gender and sexual orientation. *Journal of Social and Clinical Psychology, 19*(2), 240–255.
Thornborrow, J., & Morris, D. (2004). Gossip as strategy: The management of talk about others on reality TV show *Big Brother*. *Journal of Sociolinguistics, 8*(2), 246–271.
Triggs, T. (2006). Scissors and glue: Punk fanzines and the creation of a DIY aesthetic. *Journal of Design History, 19*(1), 69–83.
Wang, L. (2022, November). For writer Alice Oseman, *Heartstopper* fulfills a years-long crush: The mastermind behind the YA rom-com talks queer joy and watching their beloved comic come to life. https://www.netflix.com/tudum/articles/alice-oseman-heartstopper-queer-comfort
Wyler, W. (Director). (1961). *The children's hour*. The Mirisch Company.
Wuest, B. (2014). Stories like mine: Coming out videos and queer identities on YouTube. In C. Pullen (Ed.), *Queer youth and media cultures* (pp. 19–33). Palgrave Macmillan UK.

9

"DEATH LOVES TO BE REPRESENTED"

Death, Dying, and Palliative Care in Popular Culture

Michael Hviid Jacobsen and Adriana Teodorescu

Introduction

Death is undoubtedly a difficult phenomenon to understand and to deal with. Most people prefer to avoid death and live happily without ever having to confront it. However, whether we like it or not, death *is* part of life – it cannot be wished away or wiped out. Yet, despite all our fears about and discomfort with death, it also seems as if we are constantly curious about it, we want to get to know about and get acquainted with it (although mostly at a safe distance), and sometimes we even seem to wallow in it (see, e.g., Ariès, 1974; Choron, 1963). Death is, indeed, terrifying, but nevertheless still a thrill.

In his classic collection of iconographic images of death throughout history, French historian Philippe Ariès (1985, p. 1) stated that "[d]eath loves to be represented." Although humans love to represent death, death in and of itself – lacking the agency and emotions that we normally ascribe to humans – really loves nothing. However, *we*, humans, seem to nurture a continuous fascination with the topics of death and dying. For this reason, death and dying comprise recurring themes in culture and popular culture, classic and contemporary, and continuously constitute some of the favorite topics of representation.

Throughout human history – since cave drawings, wood carvings, and early pieces of poetry – people have tried to come to terms with and understand death in pictorial portrayal (Llewellyn, 1997; Townsend, 2008) and writing (see, e.g., Teodorescu, 2015). Death has thus entailed an important and recurring theme of realistic as well as purely fictional accounts and representations. In this chapter, we provide some insights into and illustrations of how death and dying can be understood by way of different popular cultural sources, such as movies and literature. These popular culture artifacts can function as critical commentaries on contemporary death culture by putting it into historical perspective as well as serving as important learning resources both for lay audiences and for scholars interested in death and dying. In this chapter, due to limitations of space, we only provide some selected examples. However, we offer an analysis of the purposes that popular cultural descriptions and depictions of death and dying may serve in an apparently paradoxical society which, on the one hand, finds death unpleasant and disgusting and, on the other, wallows in death-related images and stories.

DOI: 10.4324/9781003436409-10

Death's Great Disappearing Act

Death has always been a part and parcel of human life – for all practical intents and purposes, something inescapable and unavoidable. However, throughout human history, we have gradually become less accustomed to witnessing death as a first-hand and direct experience. Contrary to people living in prehistorical times, for whom death was something they could not avoid seeing, hearing, touching, or smelling, in contemporary society, we live sanitized and deodorized lives so that death does not typically contaminate or interfere with our lives. Researchers into our attitude toward death and dying agree that, with modern society, death has been increasingly sequestrated from our world of first-hand experience. Over the years, people have tabooed, denied, hidden, and forbidden references to death, and we, thus, have become alienated from the experience of death (see, e.g., Ariès, 1974; Bauman, 1992; Elias, 1985). Whereas our ancestors would be much more familiar with death and also how to deal with it – although they sometimes feared it just as much as we seem to do – today, death has moved behind the screens of society and into the darkness of function-designed institutions, professional expertise, and successful repression. Ariès described this evolution as the culmination of an extended historical development leading from the "tamed death" of the Middle Ages to the 'forbidden death' of modern times. For this reason, as Freud (1915/2001) observed in his reflections on the modern death mentality at the threshold of World War I, modern people have come to believe themselves to be non-mortal – a view supported by Ariès a few generations later. Since we seldom see or experience death, it seems unlikely that we will ever die.

Death, however, actually did not disappear during the 20th century. Rather, our experience with it increasingly became second-hand or vicarious – contact with real death moved into the hands of the medical profession and its representation into the realm of popular culture. In fact, death has, since the dawn of time, been depicted by people and particularly by artists and writers, but with the development of modern mass media technologies as vessels for the reproduction and distribution of images and text on a large scale, such material has now become publicly available in books, photographs, in the theater and on the silver screen. As Freud (1915/2001) suggested, in order to satisfy curiosity, individuals in contemporary society seek depictions out instead in "the world of fiction, in literature and in the theater compensation for what has been lost in life" (p. 291). Following this lead, Gorer (1955) famously insisted that death – rather than birth, procreation, and sexuality – during the 20th century gradually became the most unmentionable topic of modern society. According to Gorer, this development meant that death turned into an almost pornographic phenomenon that was surrounded by widespread public prudery, but, in privacy, writers used the obscenity of death for morbid entertainment through the mass consumption of "detective stories, thrillers, Westerns, war stories, spy stories, science fiction, and eventually horror comics" (p. 51).

The pornography of death mentioned by Gorer (1955) is not a thing of the past – we still wallow in images and stories of death and dying through various sources of popular culture and the media (see, e.g., Berridge, 2002; Foltyn, 2008; Tercier, 2013). Today, our encounter and experience with death – real and fictional – are, therefore, highly mediated as compared to previously in human history and much more so than only a century or two ago. The rise of electronic communication and information media has turned death into a spectacle, something we mostly observe from afar as part of entertainment or news stories. Whereas Ariès (1974) described our relationship in the Western world toward death during the 20th century as forbidden, we have now rather entered what Jacobsen (2016) characterized as the age of "spectacular death" in which a cornucopia of mediatized and commercialized images of death proliferate: real images of victims of war and terrorist acts, natural disasters, or violent crimes, but also images of fictional deaths from blood-dripping horror movies (e.g., *Final Destination*, 2000; *It*, 2017; *Hereditary*, 2018) and crime stories (e.g., *Gone Girl*, by Flynn, 2012; *Into the Water*, by Hawkins, 2017, both adapted into movies). Creative artists continue to make death a spectacle in their art installations and exhibitions (see Graeber, 2023); literature and movies spawn a multitude of very different representations of death from the autobiographical (see, e.g., *The Year of Magical Thinking* by Didion, 2005) to the purely fictional (e.g., Zusak, 2007), and the world of music (e.g., Dell & Hickey, 2017) and poetry (e.g., Young, 2010) provide myriad insights into the thoughts and feelings associated with death and grief. Our contemporary thanatographic imagination has been, therefore, shaped as much by real events of actual death as by artistic and creative inventions from the realm of popular culture and marketing.

Death has, thus, not disappeared but has been transformed into something to be observed, sold, and consumed – it is part of a growing commercialized industry advertising and selling products and experiences to a death-craving audience. Think, for example, of the revival of the use of the skull in a variety of different consumer contexts in contemporary popular culture and marketing (Kearl, 2015). Does this constant exposure to images of and stories about death then mean that we have embraced and accepted death? Probably not. As Durkin discussed, perhaps the saturation of entertainment-related death themes in American and more broadly Western mass media "is simply an extension of, or another configuration of, death denial. By rendering death into humor and entertainment, we effectively neutralize it" (2003, p. 47). Perhaps death in popular culture, as already Freud (1915/2001) suggested, comprises just another sophisticated way of repressing and distancing ourselves from "the real thing" while, at the same time, it might be, like the other face of the same coin, an attempt to explore possible meanings that could be assigned to this great unknown that lies at the heart of what we call death. In this sense, popular culture resembles a life buoy: it may help to advance in the water without guaranteeing, once removed, that it will keep drowning at bay.

Depicting and Representing Death

The sources of our creative and imaginative ways of dealing with and depicting death are many and seemingly inexhaustible and can be dated back to prehistoric times (e.g., The Royal Tombs of Ur, 2600 – 2000 BCE, a group of Sumerian tombs; see Porterfield, 2020). We find no shortage of attempts to write about or visually depict death and dying. Iconic images from medieval and Renaissance periods of "The Triumph of Death," "Danse Macabre," "Death and the Maiden," and the many "Vanitas" paintings – sometimes subsumed under the heading of *memento mori* – all encompass part of our rich historical cultural heritage from the Middle Ages to contemporary society. From simple cave drawings to contemporary sculptures, paintings, and computerized types of visual artwork, from ancient poetry to contemporary novels and autobiographies, from wood carvings, paintings, and still photography to contemporary television series and movies, changes in technology have profoundly transformed representations of death.

For example, with the invention of the printing press during the 15th century (replacing the woodblock printing practice), descriptions of death could suddenly appear in writings (the diverse *ars moriendi* typical of the late Middle Ages, but also pamphlets and newspapers) (Ariès, 1974; Vovelle, 1983/2001) now reaching a large reading audience; whereas, previously the scriptures and holy texts were reserved only for the initiated few. With the development of the camera in the 19th century, snapshots of moments of actual death and of those already dead (such as the many photographic images of dead children at that time) and the filming of dying processes became possible. Think of the photography of the French soldier taken at the moment of his death at the Battle of Verdun in 1916 (Capa, 1936), the harrowing images (photos and movies) of thousands of Jews killed in concentration camps during World War II (United States Holocaust Memorial Museum, 1945) or the award-winning image of the street execution of Nguyễn Văn Lém in Saigon in 1968 (Adams, 1968). With the invention of radio broadcasts and television during the 20th century, and not least with the explosively growing numbers of listeners and viewers, representations of death moved into the household. With the development of the internet during the 1990s, a multitude of images, news, and stories about death was just one click away. As technology changes, so does the representation of death and its outreach.

Together with sex, death constitutes perhaps one of the most lasting, largest, and most profitable industries of representation in popular culture. In contemporary popular culture, "death sells" and "death is in" as Berridge (2002, p. 26) concisely remarked. Death competes mainly with love or sex for attention in most types of popular culture. Love is undoubtedly the most favorite topic in literary fiction, music, and movies – and always has been. We know "erotic novels," "love songs," and "romantic movies," but we also crave horror, crime, disaster, and death, especially within our Western societies that tend to suppress violence (see, e.g., Bruckner, 2011). Although death lags far behind the interest in love, romance, and sex, it nevertheless remains one of those topics in constant supply and demand (particularly amongst so-called 'deathniks'), simply because we continue to be so curious about it. If we took death – or love for that matter – out of popular culture, it would turn out to be a much-diminished realm and result in a significant decrease in profit rates and an immediate public demand for more sex and more death.

Death – like love, romance, and sex – can be depicted and represented in a variety of widely different ways, depending on the type of death, the thematic framing of death (see, e.g., Dollimore, 1998; Tsagaris, 2023), the means of representation (see, e.g., Sullivan & Goldberg, 2013), and the specific perspective and agenda of the writer, artist, or producer (see, e.g., Teodorescu, 2015; Teodorescu & Jacobsen, 2020). Death can be represented for various purposes: entertainment, provocation, education, illumination, or other. Moreover, death can be approached from different genres of representation: humor, tragedy, drama, or horror. In addition, as with any other fictional material, the topics of death and dying can be either dramatized, distilled, or distorted by the techniques of representation (Hills & Hills, 1968). Importantly, we should remember potentially significant differences between "description" and "representation;" whereas the former is mostly mimetic and mirroring "reality as it is," the latter actively interprets, angles, and provides a perspective on that which is being represented (see Ankersmit, 1996).

Representations of death and dying, therefore, often comprise more than plain illustration and rather attempts at interpretation. Death and dying are indeed multi-dimensional and multi-faceted phenomena, with many different faces and framings depending on the actual circumstances depicted: who dies, how do people die, where do they die, when do they die, why do they die, etc. These variables obviously also impact what gets presented on screen or in other cultural artifacts. Moreover, what were the experiences and emotions involved in death and dying: was it a peaceful death, an extended period of agony and pain, was death swift, "natural," dramatic or other? Was it death due to accident, violence in the streets, during warfare, capital punishment or something else? Did it take place on the battlefield, in the hospital, at home, in hospice, nursing home or somewhere else? Answering such questions informs the concrete ways in which artists/writers/filmmakers capture topics of death and dying in specific pieces of popular culture.

Contrary to high-brow or so-called "fine" art or literature intended only for stimulating a small, exclusive, exquisite, or elite circle of viewers and readers, popular culture (sometimes used as a derogatory term) aims for some sort of mass consumption audience (hence the notion of "popular" culture; see Storey, 2003). Popular cultural products – such as books, films, television series, or music (on death in music, see Dell & Hickey, 2017; Kastenbaum, 2003) – target large-scale consumption and include representations of death for a variety of reasons. Whereas some are purely entertainment-based, playing commercially on the innate human curiosity for seeing or reading about death (e.g., video games as *Resident Evil*, 1996 or *I Am Dead*, 2020; comic books as *The Sandman,* by Gaiman, 1989 – present), others may be more ideological and directed toward dissolving the taboo and repression of death in contemporary society (e.g. Doughty, 2019).

Humans are (probably) the only species that contemplates death and not only knows that it must die but also knows that it knows it (Bauman, 1992). For this reason, death is and remains the ultimate and archetypal uncanny (Freud, 1919/2003) – at one and the same time something familiar (because we carry it within us from birth and cannot stop thinking about it) and strange (because most have never tried to die and only seldom meet people who are dying). Death is absent presence and present absence, and this duality is exactly what representations of death and dying seek to capture and combine. As once suggested by Epicurus trying to specify why we should not fear death: When we are here, death is not, and when death is, we are no longer here. The banality of this insight may perhaps risk overshadowing its deeper representative meaning (Jones, 1992).

Death is difficult to represent exactly because the representation is always nothing but "presentation" – we present the aspects of death that we somehow know about or can contemplate, but we expect or imagine that more exists to death than that. In his incisive analysis of death and mourning in Charlotte Brontë's novel *Villette*, Stewart rightly stated, "Death marks the impossible limit of representation, while at the same time death is an inevitability of representation" (1993, p. 51). This well-phrased paradox rests on the fact that death cannot be represented, simply because we do not know what it actually feels like being dead and thus cannot *re*-present it. However, at the same time, exactly since we cannot live and experience death while still being alive, we ultimately need to resort to representation. After all, such attempts constitute all that we can attain. Despite this challenge to representation, no shortage of attempts within popular culture at representing death exists, as we explore next.

Death and Dying in Literature

In this section, we will first discuss the representation of death and dying in literature. Death has been part and parcel of literary work as far back as the human capacity for expressing ideas in writing (Ariès, 2008). Going back thousands of years, death has remained an integral part of religious writings, philosophical treatises, and poetic pieces of work. As far back as the Gilgamesh Epic, dating back almost 5,000 years to Mesopotamian culture, the topics of death and the human quest for immortality loom large (e.g., *The Iliad* and *The Odyssey* (Homer, 8th century BCE/2011), *Beowulf*, circa 8th–11th century). In such writings, which were for a long time not intended for popular or public use (since the vast majority of people could not read or write until quite recently in human history), authors described death – our fear, trembling, and powerlessness when confronted with it (and hence as a justification of religious faith) – in great detail.

It is worth dwelling a little on the connection between literature and popular culture. We discussed above the distinction between fine art and popular culture, with literature included in the first part. However, we note more nuances in what literature means and how it functions within the postmodern world. For example, the same literary writings can be high and low in relation to culture, depending on their interpretation and use by the public, their space of dissemination, their format (e.g., e-book or printed book), etc. In this sense, Collins (2010) argued that literature suffered a process of democratization and that it influences popular culture, being, at the same time, impacted by cultural changes reflected in various proportions within its pages.

With the gradual development and expansion of writing and reading skills and the revolutions in publication and production capacities, the literary representation of death and dying has intensified immensely. According to American sociologist Michael C. Kearl, "[r]are is literature in which death does not function as a central motif or plot device" (1989, p. 381). Although this observation comprises perhaps a bit of an exaggeration, even if a specific piece of fiction deals with love, infidelity, treason, or tedious everyday travail (or some other seemingly non-death-related topics), death is almost destined somehow to be part of the plot. Someone will often be taken ill and die during the story (or the already dead will …) and, in this way, death and dying enter the storyline. Sometimes, death and dying merely comprise a side-story or simply narrative devices that help propel the action; other times it constitutes the main plot, often but not always, involving, besides a functional centrality (frequent, for instance, within crime fiction) a fundamental position within the possible interpretative networks of the fiction. *The Death of Ivan Ilyich* by Tolstoy (1886) entails perhaps one of the most famous writings in which death played both a central and significant role, transcending the basic instrumental function of a story trigger, and coagulating the entire field of possible interpretations, so that all paths lead to death. The short novel explored how the awareness of mortality becomes irrefutable and how death is a singular and extremely personal event that cannot be truly shared with others.

Indeed, literary productions, such as the Tolstoian short novel, succeed not only in representing death in the most basic understanding – that of re-presenting, of bringing death in literature as a subject – but also in making its representations meaningful for both personal epiphanies in relation to mortality and finitude, observable at the level of fictional characters and conveyable to the level of readers, and for building knowledge concerning various social and cultural aspects of death and dying. As Teodorescu observed (2015), epistemologically speaking, representing death in literature encompasses both a mimetic and semiotic dimension, meaning that literary representations have the power to generate knowledge regarding "real," extra-fictional death by mirroring reality and, at the same time, by divorcing reality in terms of language and images of death. Still, this power is not intrinsic to every literary production and, to complicate things, not always in strict correlation with their aesthetic achievements (although this is often the case) and must be seen rather as a potential that is activated depending on different variables.

Amid the diversity of literary works representing death and dying, with a careful thanatological eye, one can observe an entire (sub-)genre of literary fiction consisting in heterogeneous writing (many of them novels), in terms of style and aesthetic stakes and achievements, revolving around the idea that death is necessary for life. In fact, we assert that death represents the most stable axis that, once removed would generate chaos on multiple levels, from the most personal one to the macro level of human history (Saramago, 2005/2009; see also Teodorescu, 2019). These works share two key facts: all comprise Western productions, and all can be tracked down at least to the beginning of the 20th century. To name but a few: *All Men Are Mortal* (de Beauvoir, 1946/1955), *Larger than Life* (Buzzati, 1960/1967), *When I Was a Work of Art* (Schmitt, 2002), *Vincent, the Immortal One* (Suceavă, 2008), *The Postmortal* (Magary, 2011), *The Bible for the Ants* (Mitroi, 2013), and probably the most well-known work which illustrates the total necessity of death in the world, Saramago's *Death at Intervals*. Beyond their specific vision of both existence and literature, they elaborate narrative arguments in favor of death, which means not only that they advocate for the acceptance of death (which would come as a conclusion of understanding that death is not a negotiable or cancellable event), but that they advocate for death as such (the imperfect conclusion of acknowledging that death is the most fundamental and untransferable ontological experience). Thus, the fact that death is constitutive to human beings, but also, in extenso, to human societies and cultures – an aspect otherwise fully acknowledged and used as an epistemological argument by the sociology of death and dying (see Kastenbaum, 2007) – is converted into an argument in favor of maintaining death in our societies, which otherwise would fall apart. In fact, until death would truly become optional, it functions as a strong argument for keeping death in our social imaginaries.

In a narrative poem written in 1926, the modern Peruvian poet living in Paris, Cesar Vallejo described the necessity of death in terms that are emblematic for our arguments here. According to him, death encompasses the most imperative and the most irrevocable of all human necessities so that "our need to die outweighs our need to be born and live. We might simply not have been born, but we couldn't have died. Until today no one said: I need to be born. Instead, on the contrary, we often say that we must die" (1926/2022, p. 350, our translation). Indeed, these literary works primarily represent not death as such but the idea that death is necessary, with the great exception of the *Book Thief* (Zusak, 2007, p. 555), where the author presents death as an entity *haunted by humans* (see Teodorescu, 2019).

Built upon the "appealing to nature" logical fallacy (i.e., if something *is* natural, then something *ought to* be natural), such a thanato-literary approach limits imagination in relation to how a world without death would look and, implicitly, in relation to death itself. From this perspective, these literary productions – exercises of limited or self-censored imagination – are cathartic and propose an epistemic closure to the millennial obsession with death and the practical possibilities of transcending it physically.

For this (sub-)genre that tests immortality only to embrace mortality, death is, apparently paradoxical, at least as much centrifugal from the point of view of the content of representation – in the sense that the literary images and ideas related to death tend to be gradually diluted and become either non-specific or commonsensical (a sort of defeat of the creative powers of literature in the face of common thinking and stereotypes), fostering cohesion in terms of representation, so that the representation of death is consistent and observable within the literary narrative(s). To put it in other words, and alluding also to the title of our chapter, while death loves to be represented, those able to manage or in charge of its representations tame this enthusiasm and openness by choosing more rigid forms that can be suspected to be destined to offer relief in the face of death. Claiming that depicting death serves as "the great humaniser" (Jacobsen, 2017, p. 1) resonates with the broader contemporary approach of death (death studies included) that aims at shedding light on the need to reintegrate mortality in how we understand the world, talk about our lives, and make sense of them. Far from the tendency (also rooted in postmodernity) to deny them, it is also true that the risk might be to positivise it and disregard the magnitude of death in people's lives (if it were only to think of the death of significant others) and its un-human, un-domesticable side.

All these aspects regarding this literary sub-genre must be further questioned and elaborated, and perhaps a sociology of immortality, as envisaged by some contemporary death scholars (see Jacobsen, 2017), could provide the theoretical framework for such an endeavor, making sure that stereotypes and other shortcuts in interpreting the meanings of death will not pollute critical thinking and sociological imagination (see Mills, 1959/2000) applied to death and dying. Moreover, a sociology of immortality could be extremely suited for exploring literary fiction where immortality is no longer seen as a direct failure of not recognizing that death is necessary. For example, good candidates for a postmortal sociological analysis would be the short stories exploring possible afterlives gathered in the volume *Sum. Forty Tales from the Afterlife* (Eagleman, 2009); *How to Stop Time* (Haigg, 2017), a novel that deconstructs immortality in a postmodern vein, celebrating the eternity of the moment (see Bauman, 1992) because an indefinitely extended life could bring forgetfulness and relational emptiness, or *White Noise* (DeLillo, 1985), a novel in which, as shown by Jacobsen and Runge (2020), death played a central role, and the authors treated multiple topics relevant for a sociology of death, dying, and immortality (such as death anxiety, medicalization, commodification, and postmodern mediatization of death) with great finesse.

One of the strengths of a sociology of immortality applied to popular culture is that it could incorporate aspects relevant to Health Communication, especially in relation to mental health, communication about death and dying, and communication during end-of-life (for related works, please see Keeley, 2016; Keeley & Yingling, 2007). For example, it could provide theoretical frameworks for understanding and deepening the popular discourses on longevity and the pursuit of immortality (including a pathological fear of death, or on the contrary, an abnormal lack of it) as cultural products both reflecting and shaping specific beliefs and attitudes towards death and patterns of communicating about it in different settings, from the most intimate ones to healthcare facilities. At the same time, the intersection between sociology of immortality, popular culture, and Health Communication could illuminate how the thanatic layers of health-related narratives participate in constructing individual behaviors (e.g., diet, exercise, prevention) and public perceptions of what a good life and a good death mean, also considering the various communication channels of popular culture (media, literature, cinema) and the ethical implications in social policies centered on well-being (see, e.g., Nichels & Tenzek, 2022; Tenzek & Nichels, 2019).

The difficulties in assessing how representing death in literature functions as a tool for acknowledging, imagining, and thinking about death grow exponentially when literature means poetry because representation tends to be understood more as a narrative than simply a symbolic device (see Pavel, 1989), and poetry, on the other hand (although certainly not accurate for some modern and lots of postmodern poems), as anti-narrative. Moreover, some problematized poetry in terms of language and metaphor (see Picard, 1995), so that, from this perspective, sometimes death can be envisioned as unfitted for poetry, as '[t]he thing about death is: it isn't symbolic, but very real' (Young, 2010, p. xxii). Still, poetry can be understood as a continuous search for meaning and for conquering portions of reality where no one has ever reached with the help of (ordinary) words, while death has, according to Michel Picard (1995, p. 35), a cultural and linguistic nature that precedes any experience of it. Hence, due to the pervasive nature of death in terms of meanings (lacking an ultimate linguistic referent), poetry endeavors to chart the domain of the ineffable. Representation of death in poetry is a valid process both socially and aesthetically, but, in this case, the semiotic and creative part of representation is the prominent one. Young confessed that he edited the volume of poetry, *The Art of Losing. Poems of Grief and Healing*, calling it a "poetry of necessity" (p. xv) because ordinary words often fail to assist people during their grief process. This "necessity" is both personal and social and could be examined more from the perspective of the sociology of death, dying, and bereavement (with a focus on social articulations of what is personal in the way people experience and conceptualize death) and of Health Communication (paying attention to the capacity of language and culture in creating powerful tools to be used in conversation regarding, for example, end-of-life issues).

Death and Dying in Popular Films and Television Series

As several death scholars have shown, at first glance, popular culture (Kearl, 2015; Penfold-Mounce, 2018; Teodorescu & Jacobsen, 2020) – and here we refer mostly to its cinematographic and visual dimensions – appears as a territory where death flourishes, being astonishingly reinvigorated from what an entire interpretative direction within the field of death studies called, regarding Western modernity, *the denial of death* (see Robert & Tradii, 2019). In fact, in this equation, both variables – the social world as such and popular culture as a special microcosm grafted on the former one and endowed with visibility – were each suspected not to be quite what they seemed to be in relation to their approaches to death. Thus, while the idea of a death that tends to be denied by an era marked by decreasing mortality rates – that throws death to the peripheries of social visibility – remains mainstream especially (paradoxically!) within popular culture, some death scholars disagree with the denial thesis. Scholars have argued that death was never truly forbidden, but, on the contrary, freed from rigid expressions, death in our postmodern social worlds has been revived into new forms and personalized rituals (Poirier, 2001; Walter, 1994), as attested by popular culture.

Furthermore, despite its uneven composition (structurally, stylistically, and aesthetically), popular culture, and particularly its cinematic component, is widely recognized as a catalyst for the inherent human fascination with representing death and dying for the purpose of gaining knowledge and for vicarious experiences of death. By navigating the intersection between tangible reality and mediated reality, popular culture can enable learning in relation to finitude, one's own mortality and the death of others (see Penfold-Mounce, 2018; Teodorescu & Jacobsen, 2020). However, scholars also regard popular culture and its cinematographic productions with skepticism because of their supposed lack of authenticity, high degree of shallowness, and the avid entertainment market they create (Horkheimer & Adorno, 1947/2007). This critique becomes even more pertinent in the context of filmic depictions of death because of their capacity to generate, as previously addressed in the opening of this chapter, 'spectacular' effects (Jacobsen, 2016) on people's encounters with death due to the extreme mediatization and commercialization of images, explicit or, more frequently, implicit political and ideological agendas, and a structural limitation inherent in the visual nature of their scripts (Teodorescu & Jacobsen, 2020).

Indeed, flamboyant deaths (e.g., Tarantino's movies), abundances of shootings and killings, colorful reactions to loss mixed with impassive attitudes towards personal death, zombified and decomposed corpses cohabitate with romanticized deaths, luminous afterlives, beautiful or hidden corpses, simplified attitudes in the face of losing someone dear, and superficial pedagogies of living produced by epiphanies of personal mortality. While they may have little to do with the complexity and ambiguity of death, dying, and bereavement as experienced in a non-mediated environment, as well as with the ontological void brought by dead bodies into the world, they function as possible instruments of (safely) exploring death on various levels (personal, social, cultural), with various intensities and diverse consequences (e.g., producing knowledge, facilitating understanding of subjective experiences of loss, exorcising death anxiety, etc.).

A classic movie such as Ingmar Bergman's *The Seventh Seal* (1957), in which death comprises one of the main characters, playing chess with a young Max von Sydow – with a foreseeable winner – is emblematic for its aesthetic achievement both of death and of the entire movie as such. Although the aesthetic side of death prevailed, the film produced knowledge related to death through mimetic proximity, as the movie portrayed social and cultural aspects pertaining to how people perceived and experienced death and dying in the Middle Ages. Throughout the entire cinematographic history, movies or television series have not only fictionalized death, but sometimes over-aestheticized it, acquiring extravagant nuances and facilitating a detached, ironical, or critical perspective on commonplaces related to both movies and death without obnubilating a certain *memento mori* function.

For example, many films by Quentin Tarantino depict death somewhere between the absurd, the hilarious, and the ridiculous (e.g., *Reservoir Dogs*, 1992; *Pulp Fiction*, 1994; *Natural Born Killers*, 1994; *Inglorious Basterds*, 2009; or *The Hateful Eight*, 2015). Death does not come to the characters in any dignified way, and even the main characters die in

Tarantino's Movies

In the Coen brothers' films, such as *No Country for Old Men* (2007), death was excessively and transgressively brutal, but it was also simultaneously almost a mocking joke, something to laugh about – perhaps a fitting and merciful reminder to the (still) living audience that their own deaths were unlikely to be as brutal and absurd as those of the characters. In contrast, one television series, *The Fall of the House of Usher* (2023), seemed to dissolve a little bit of Tarantinesque spectacular and self-ironic death in a more sophisticated composition of macabre and decadence that subtly displays a moral pedagogy (death as moral punishment). In fact, death also abounds in horror movies and thrillers where the exaggerated aestheticism of death leads to a momentary exorcism of death to keep fearing mortality at bay (see Bruckner, 2011).

Products of an era that values knowledge and perhaps even more the idea of translating everything into information and, most of all, communication, documentaries, on the other hand, lack the aesthetic dimension in relation to death. Their relevance is situated within the mimetic proximity area, as they can re-present various dimensions and elements of death that are highly socially debatable (euthanasia, end-of-life care, life after death, suicide, etc.), as well as their possible implications on multiple levels. As such, exploring two American palliative care facilities, *End Game* (2018) focused on end-of-life care and highlighted the different approaches to what a good death could be, putting in the foreground the unnamed concept such of assisted suicide. Similarly, another short documentary, *Extremis* (2016), spotlighted end-of-life decisions and illustrated how values dear to our contemporary times – autonomy, agency, control – sometimes get jeopardized when people can no longer decide anymore by themselves on how they should live or die due to difficult medical conditions;

whereas other values – empathy, care, love – become ethically problematic with the blurring of the borders between living and dying.

For example, *The Suicide* (2007) explored how a man diagnosed with Amyotrophic Lateral Sclerosis tried to incorporate his decision into his life, also in relation to death and dying, identifying and questioning social limits to this endeavor. *Hope Frozen. A Quest to Live Twice* (2018) discussed the ethical controversies ignited by the decision of a Thai family to cryogenize their 2-year-old daughter who passed away due to brain cancer. Science, religion, medical intervention and discourse, care, personal beliefs, and responsibilities toward oneself and toward the community all participate in complexifying death and grief. Other documentary movies or series, unsatisfied with the idea of a strict symbolic continuity of the human being, explore the possibility, still not scientifically provable, of a death that is not the end of an individual through topics such as near-death experiences, communication with the dead, or reincarnation (e.g., *Surviving Death*, 2020; *Life after Death*, 2022).

Films such as *Whose Life is It Anyway* (1981), *Mar Adentro* (2004), or *Me before You* (2016) tackled euthanasia by using aesthetic means while aiming to transcend both aesthetic and mimetic approaches to death and to shed light on less explored meanings (the semiotic approach), from extremely personal perspectives. The three movies addressed living with severe physical limitations and considered the decision to resort to death as an alternative to an unacceptable life, revealing the limits of palliative care both formally and informally.

Similarly, movies dedicated to grief and loss, such as *A Monster Calls* (2016) – adapted for the screen from the homonym novel written by Patrick Ness in 2011 – went beyond documenting grief and explored how it could be expressed far from conventional, socially acknowledged forms, embracing ambivalence and complexity. Thus, the idea of a child secretly desiring the death of his mother to end both his and her sufferings became understandable and socially acceptable, a sort of symbolic exorcism of the monsters born at the intersection between interpersonal love and the very human personal limits of caring for others. Combining fantastic elements with drama, *Lovely Bones* (2009) presented the continuing bonds between the living and those departed from this life and can also be seen also as a story of grief from the perspective of the deceased. A television series, *After Life* (2019-2022), featuring Ricky Gervais, depicted the way in which the loss of a dear one transgresses social expectations of how grief and bereavement should manifest. Moreover, it discussed, in an aesthetic manner, how suicidal thoughts can function as a kind of personal strategy to cope with the absurdity brought by the untimely death.

The semiotic perspective on death is also present also in the many popular movies where death, portrayed as imminent – real or only perceived as such – has a pedagogical function, in the sense that it encourages self-awareness, gratitude toward the gift of life, decisional empowerment in relation to the time left to live, and, when possible, creates new roles not despite but exactly because the end is or seemed to be near. To mention only a few examples in this sense: *Terms of Endearment* (1983), *My Life without Me* (2003), *The Bucket List* (2007), *The Fault in Our Stars* (2014), and *Last Laugh* (2019).

Other times, the pedagogical function of death is exogenous, in the sense that it does not refer to sheer issues related to death and dying but to various social issues for which death appears to be the most visible side. Several Romanian movies produced after 2000 featured a prominent sentiment that corruption was rampant in Romanian society and becoming a mortal weapon in the hands of politicians, public institutions, and individuals playing their social roles. *The Death of Mr. Lăzărescu* (2005) is probably the most iconic movie in this direction. The plot was very simple: an older man encountered a series of obstacles in getting medical help for his health issues, being treated with indifference, shallowness, and inefficiency so that he died from otherwise treatable or manageable medical conditions. His death symbolized the failure of the Romanian medical system because of the lack of political reforms, systemic corruption, and medical communication skills. "Corruption kills" claimed the movie, gathering a chorus of voices criticizing Romanian thanatopolitics, while making dying a little bit less existential (see Toplean, 2019).

Death also encompasses a recurring feature of popular movie series often directed toward a teenage audience, such as *Lord of the Rings* or *Harry Potter*. Such films associate death with evil forces and sorcery and tend to be schematized as a negative consequence of fighting the dark or not making the right decisions. This kind of movie manifests a reduced interest in representing natural death or the normality of death, with killing being the most visible form of dying. In general, a strong aesthetic vein dictates how films represent death, especially in those targeting teenagers. However, this preference does not mean that this approach always prevails over other dimensions. For example, in the animated movie *Coco* (2017), produced by Pixar, everything revolves around death, and the central idea – functioning as a sort of manifesto for including death within the Western way of approaching existence – is that death and life, the dead and the living, this world and the afterlife are only artificially separated (for related works, see Nickels & Tenzek, 2022; Tenzek & Nickels, 2019).

Conclusion: For More Research on Death in Popular Culture

This chapter has provided an overview – and admittedly not an exhaustive or too systematic overview – of the cultural, social, and aesthetic logics, mechanisms and, to a lesser extent, the social implications of depicting and representing death and dying in popular culture. The first two sections, with a special interest in theoretical and historical issues, discussed how death's great disappearing act, apparently produced in the last century, is put into question by contemporary Western popular culture that situates death (as it does with sex) at the core of its strategies for attracting a large audience. Depicting and representing death in popular culture go, however, beyond the simple idea of selling and entertainment and can have, depending on multiple parameters (such as genre, artistic achievement, etc.), various functions, including educating and challenging stereotyped or narrow ways of approaching death and dying. Popular culture proves to be versatile enough to be able to capture the multi-dimensional, complex nature of death and dying, which does not mean that it cannot be shallow and inefficient in managing a personal and mature encounter with death and dying. The other two sections, dedicated to the representation of death and dying in literature and popular films, tried to analyze some features of death representation in relation to both literature and movies seen as significant segments of popular culture and pointed out, among other things, the great – and perhaps even unsettling – variability in terms of content, function, and proximity to reality.

For death scholars, but also for other scholars interested in death, popular culture provides an important tool for exploring how societies understand death, dying, and connected topics – grief, bereavement, afterlife, disposal of the body, communication during the end-of-life, etc. – including the meanings assigned to them, the ways they are experienced, practiced, conceptualized, and embedded in institutions. It offers complex occasions to test sociological theories related to death and dying and, the other way around, to build social theories by analyzing the interplay between death and dying as lived realities and, on the other side, death and dying as represented realities, between death and dying as triggers for social structures and meanings, and, on the other side, death and dying as products of social and cultural forces. Films, poems, television series, autobiographies, etc., could serve as imaginative resources for educating different groups of professionals working with death and dying (such as funeral directors, nurses, doctors, palliative care professionals, etc.) as well as "selling points" for students studying the topics of death and dying in disciplines such as sociology, anthropology, cultural studies, gerontology, or communication.

If the experience of death and dying provided by popular culture offers a vicarious experience, often embraced within the confines of one's home, that experience holds potential benefits for people all over the world. It can serve as a valuable instrument in various ways, starting with raising awareness about the reality of their own mortality and the incentive of living a more meaningful life exactly because it is always watched by the perpetual eye of death, continuing with acquiring knowledge on the social dimensions of death and dying, and nurturing a vital interest in these topics, and ending with improving communication skills related to health, well-being, and the many faces of mortality.

However, more research on the many faces of death in popular culture, the intricate aesthetic, social, and even economic mechanisms, and the stakes of how death, dying, and connected topics are depicted or put into representation is highly, if not urgently needed.

References

Adams, E. (1968). *Saigon execution* [Photograph]. Associated Press (AP) Archives. https://www.apimages.com/metadata/Index/Vietnam-Saigon Execution/0c6ba6df9fe64ecdbedb9f69450cc7b2

Ankersmit, F. R. (1996). *Aesthetic politics: Political philosophy beyond fact and value*. Stanford University Press.

Ariès, P. (1974). *Western attitudes toward death from the Middle Ages to the present*. Johns Hopkins University Press.

Ariès, P. (1985). *Images of man and death*. Harvard University Press.

Ariès, P. (2008). *The hour of our death: The classic history of Western attitudes toward death over the last one thousand year.* Vintage.

Bauman, Z. (1992). *Mortality, immortality and other life strategies*. Polity Press.

Berridge, K. (2002). *Vigor mortis – The end of the death taboo*. Profile Books.

Bruckner, P. (2011). *Le fanatisme de l'apocalypse [The fanaticism of the apocalypse]*. Editions Grasset & Fasquelle.

Buzzati, D. (1960/1967). *Larger than life*. Walker & Co.

Capa, R. (1936). *The falling soldier* [Photograph]. International Center of Photography (ICP) Collections. https://www.icp.org/browse/archive/objects/the-falling-soldier

Choron, J. (1963). *Death and Western thought*. The Macmillan Company.

Collins, J. (2010). *Bring on the books for everybody: How literary culture became popular culture*. Duke University Press.

de Beauvoir, S. (1946/1955). *All men are mortal*. World Publishing Company.

DeLillo, D. (1985). *White noise*. Viking Press.

Dell, H., & Hickey, H. (Eds.) (2017). *Singing death: Reflections on music and mortality*. Routledge.

Didion, J. (2005). *The year of magical thinking*. Knopf.

Dollimore, J. (1998). *Death, desire and loss in Western culture*. Routledge.

Doughty, C. (2019). *Will my cat eat my eyeballs? Big questions about death.* W. W. Norton & Company.

Durkin, K. F. (2003). Death, dying and the dead in popular culture. In C. D. Bryant (Ed.), *Handbook of death and dying – volume one: The presence of death* (pp. 43–49). SAGE.

Eagleman, D. (2009). *Sum: Forty tales from the afterlives*. Pantheon Books.

Elias, N. (1985). *The loneliness of the dying*. Continuum.

Flynn, G. (2012). *Gone girl*. Crown Publishing Group.

Foltyn, J. L. (2008). Dead famous and dead sexy: Popular culture, forensics and the rise of the corpse. *Mortality*, *13*(2), 153–173.

Freud, S. (1915/2001). Thoughts for the times on war and death. In S. Strachey (Ed.), *The standard edition of the complete psychological works of Sigmund Freud* (Vol. 14, pp. 273–302). Vintage Books.

Freud, S. (1919/2003). *The uncanny*. Penguin Books.

Gaiman, N. (1989-present). *The sandman*. DC Comics, Vertigo, DC Black Label.

Gorer, G. (1955, October). The pornography of death. *Encounter*, 49–52.

Graeber, L. (2023, April). At these exhibitions, death is a lively subject. *The New York Times*. https://www.nytimes.com/2023/04/26/arts/design/museums-death-afterlife.html

Haigg, M. (2017). *How to stop time*. Canongate Books.

Hawkins, P. (2017). *Into the water.* Doubleday.

Hills, P. C., & Hills, L. R. (1968). The eye of fiction. In P. C. Hills & L. R. Hills (Eds.), *How we live: Contemporary life in contemporary fiction* (pp. 891–895). Macmillan.

Homer (8th century BCE/2011). *Iliad & Odyssey*. Canterbury Classics.

Horkheimer, M., & Adorno T. W. (1947/2007). *Dialectic of enlightenment: Philosophical fragments*. Stanford University Press.

Jacobsen, M. H. (2016). "Spectacular death" – Proposing a new fifth phase to Philippe Ariès's admirable history of death. *Humanities*, 5(19), 1–20.

Jacobsen, M. H. (2017). Introduction: Towards a postmortal society. Paving the pathway for a sociology of immortality. In M. H. Jacobsen (Ed.), *Postmortal society. Towards a sociology of immortality* (pp. 1–13). Routledge.
Jacobsen, M. H., & Runge, N. (2020). Death in Don DeLillo's *White Noise*: A literary diagnosis of contemporary death culture. In A. Teodorescu & M. H. Jacobsen (Eds.), *Death in contemporary popular culture* (pp. 192–214). Routledge.
Jones, H. (1992). *The Epicurean tradition*. Routledge.
Kastenbaum, R. J. (2003). Arise, ye more than dead: Culture, music and death. In C. D. Bryant (Ed.), *Handbook of death and dying – volume two: The response to death* (pp. 1008–1018). SAGE.
Kastenbaum, R. J. (2007). *Death, society and human experience*. Pearson Education.
Kearl, M. C. (1989). *Endings: A sociology of death and dying*. Oxford University Press.
Kearl, M. C. (2015). The proliferation of skulls in popular culture: A case study of how the traditional symbol of mortality was rendered meaningless. *Mortality*, *20*(1), 1–18.
Keeley, M. P. (2016). Family communication at the end of life. *Journal of Family Communication*, *16*(3), 189–197. https://doi.org/10.1080/15267431.2016.1181070
Keeley, M. P., & Yingling, J. (2007). *Final conversations: Helping the living and the dying talk to each other*. VanderWyk & Burnham.
Llewellyn, N. (1997). *Art of death: Visual culture in the English death ritual c.1500 - c.1800.* Reaktion Books.
Magary, D. (2011). *The postmortal*. Penguin Group.
Mills, C. W. (1959/2000). *The sociological imagination*. Oxford University Press.
Mitroi, Ş. (2013). *Biblia pentru furnici.* [The bible for the ants]. Rao.
Ness, P. (2011). *A monster calls.* Walker Books.
Nickels, B. M., & Tenzek, K. E. (2022). Family communication at the end of life: Breaking
the taboo through entertainment media. In G. Luurs (Ed.), *Handbook of research on communication strategies for taboo topics* (pp. 241–260). Information Science Research. httsp://doi.org/10.4018/978-1-7998-9125-3.ch012
Pavel, T. G. (1989): *Fictional worlds*. Harvard University Press.
Penfold-Mounce, R. (2018). *Death, the dead and popular culture*. Emerald Publishing.
Picard, M. (1995). *La littérature et la mort [The literature and the death].* Presses Universitaires de France.
Poirier, P-A. (2001). *De la mort occultée au renouveau de la mort* [*From the hidden death to the revive of death]. Sociétés, 73*(3), 51–59.
Porterfield, M. (2020). *Lesson 04: Death and mourning in the prehistoric and ancient*. Digital Commons @ East Tennessee State University. https://dc.etsu.edu/cgi/viewcontent.cgi?article=1004&context=art-appreciation-oer
Robert, M., & Tradii, L. (2019). Do we deny death? I. A genealogy of death denial. *Mortality*, *24*(3), 247–260.
Saramago, J. (2005/2009). *Death at intervals*. Vintage.
Schmitt, É-E. (2002). *Lorsque j'étais une oeuvre d'art* [When I was a work of art]. Albin Michel.
Stewart, G. (1993). A valediction for bidding mourning: Death and narratee in Brontë's *Vilette*. In E. Bronfen & S. Webster Goodwin (Eds.), *Death and representation* (pp. 51–79). John Hopkins University Press.
Storey, J. (2003). *Inventing popular culture: From folklore to globalization.* Blackwell.
Suceavă, B. (2008). *Vincent nemuritorul* [Vincent, the immortal one]. Curtea Veche.
Sullivan, D., & Goldberg, J. (Eds.) (2013). *Death in classic and contemporary film: Fade to black.* Palgrave/Macmillan.
Tenzek, K. E., & Nickels, B. M. (2019). End-of-life in Disney and Pixar films: An opportunity for engaging in difficult conversation. *OMEGA-Journal of Death and Dying*, *80*(1), 49–68. https://doi.org/10.1177/0030222817726258
Teodorescu, A. (Ed.) (2015). *Death representations in literature: Forms and theories.* Cambridge Scholars Publishing.
Teodorescu, A. (2019). Facing death. A Sartrean perspective on the contemporary tendency to over-humanize death. In A. Teodorescu (Ed.), *Death within the text: Social, philosophical and aesthetic approaches to literature* (pp. 84–112). Cambridge Scholars Publishing.
Teodorescu, A., & Jacobsen, M. J. (Eds.) (2020). *Death in contemporary popular culture*. Routledge.
Tercier, J. (2013). The pornography of death. In H. Maes (Ed.), *Pornographic art and the aesthetics of pornography* (pp. 221–235). Palgrave/Macmillan.
Tolstoy, L. (1886). *The death of Ivan Ilyich.* William Heinemann.
Toplean, A. (2019). Sistemul morţii. După 1989 [Death system. After 1989]. *România literară*, 46–47. https://romanialiterara.com/2019/11/sistemul-mortii-dupa-1989/
Townsend, C. (2008). *Art and death.* I.B. Tauris.

Tsagaris, E. (2023). *Capital punishment in popular culture, toys, games, and nursery rhymes: Toying with death.* Cambridge Scholars Publishing.
United States Holocaust Memorial Museum. (1945). *The bodies of prisoners lie on the ground in the newly liberated Nordhausen concentration camp*. [Photograph]. USHMM Collections.
Vallejo, C. (1926/2022). *A murit eternitatea mea. Opera poetică* [My eternity died. The poetic work]. Pandora M.
Vovelle, M. (1983/2001). *La mort et l'Occident de 1300 à nos jours*. Gallimard.
Walter, T. (1994). *The revival of death*. Routledge.
Young, K. (Ed.) (2010). *The art of losing: Poems of grief and healing*. Bloomsbury.
Zusak, M. (2007). *The book thief.* Alfred A. Knopf.

PART II

Exploring Popular Culture Influences on Health Behaviors and Beliefs

10

HOLLYWOOD'S INTOXICATING EFFECTS

A Qualitative Analysis of Alcohol Use in 50 Popular College Fraternity Films

Alan D. DeSantis

Since its inception in 1888, film has remained one of the most beloved communication mediums around the world. This popularity has made the film industry in the U.S. (a.k.a., "Hollywood") worth an estimated $95 billion while provided $504 billion to the U.S. GDP (Gupta, 2023). While viewers screen some of Hollywood's films in traditional brick-and-mortar movie theaters, most have viewed them on one of the growing numbers of popular streaming services (e.g., Netflix, Apple, Amazon, Disney, etc.) that have become ubiquitous in the lives of Americans. According to Sangari (2022), over 85% of homes in the U.S. subscribe to at least one streaming service, or 109.4 million households. While this popularity has posed a continued threat to theater owners, it has also allowed many more films to entertain many more audiences than ever before.

As a Communication scholar of films, however, I am significantly less interested in film's ability to entertain and more concerned with its power to both a) persuade audiences to behave in certain ways and b) shape social reality for viewers. The study of these two outcomes gets complicated, given hidden consequences smuggled into the unsuspecting consciousnesses of audiences through the Trojan Horse of cinematic amusement. That is to say, while most audiences consciously turn to popular film to be entertained, many of these same viewers remain unaware of the potential "side effects" that often accompany these entertaining messages.

Film as a Public-Health Concern

The research on cigarette smoking has successfully contributed to the sharp decline of teen cigarette smoking in the United States. Its evidence-based findings have served as compelling sources of evidence in most of the influential governmental reports and legal arguments of the last 60 years (see U.S. Food and Drug Administration, n.d.; U.S. Department of Health, Education, and Welfare, 1964; U.S. Department of Health and Human Services, 2014).

The battle to regulate alcohol misuse and its representation in media, however, has not met with the same success. This difference, in part, has been attributed to both fewer governmental and industry regulations (Jackson et al., 2018), combined with the popularity of alcohol in society, as 63% of American adults over the last two decades report consuming alcohol, a number far greater than that

DOI: 10.4324/9781003436409-12

of cigarette smokers (Saad, 2023). Consequently, adolescent alcohol abuse has remained a plaguing public health issue for families, friends, researchers, and policymakers. Mokdad et al. (2004) estimated, for example, that alcohol use is responsible for over 75,000 deaths every year in the United States. Of these, adolescents have remained an exceptionally vulnerable segment of our society. According to Primack et al. (2009), alcohol use is now considered the leading cause of death for adolescents, since its misuse is also attributed to a substantial proportion of motor-vehicle, accidental, and violent deaths as well.

This body of research is part of a larger charge by public health and communication researchers investigating the deleterious and pro-social effects of health messaging in popular culture. This Handbook offers a wide-ranging survey of some of this research located at the intersection of Health Communication and popular culture. While the chapters in this volume investigate a myriad of communication media, health outcomes, and audiences, their scholarship is united by a common focus on understanding the profound influence of popular culture on health behaviors and attitudes.

Toward this shared goal, this chapter examines the role that popular films play in promoting alcohol use in adolescent audiences as an exemplar of popular culture and risky behaviors that can be consequential for health and wellness. Toward this end, I summarize the salient research on the depictions of alcohol use in film and the potential dangers these messages pose for young audiences. Adding to this body of literature, I then present my findings from my ongoing cinematic analysis of the drinking lessons taught to adolescent viewers by the 50 most popular college-fraternity films in America. Next, I discuss the possible implications of these lessons on pre-college adolescents (especially those interested in Greek affiliation) and the role such depictions may have in encouraging alcohol misuse on American college campuses. I close by considering what such mediated depictions of poor health and wellness decision-making mean for health communication and health communicators. While fraternity members comprise a small minority (approximately 5 to 10%) on most college campuses, members of these organizations have consistently been responsible for a disproportionate amount of campus harm, including property damage, public intoxication, assaults, and rapes. Not coincidentally, members of these college drinking clubs have also been found to drink more alcohol, more often, than their unaffiliated counterparts (Scott-Sheldon et al., 2007).

Discovering these hidden consequences has dominated research in media studies. For media scholars interested in public health, the primary focus has been on the role that popular entertainment has played in fostering tobacco and alcohol use by teens (Borzekowski & Strasburger, 2008; Kessler, 2001). Contributing to this line of investigation, this chapter focuses on one of the more popular film genres for adolescent males in the United States of America over the last five decades. Like many of the contributions found in this Handbook, my specific analysis will similarly explore the ways in which popular media influence audiences' at-risk health behaviors and attitudes. Within this larger framework, this study pays particular attention to the ways that American college fraternity films rely on a series of recurring narrative structures and character tropes that encourage binge drinking (i.e., consuming five or more drinks on an occasion) and anti-social behaviors and attitudes. Strengthening the persuasive nature of these messages, these same cinematic strategies also simultaneously minimize the myriad of negative consequences that often accompany excessive alcohol consumption (e.g., diminished academic performance, physical and sexual assaults, student-conduct suspensions and expulsions, civil and criminal prosecutions, etc.). When read collectively, this two-pronged approach in cinematic storytelling transforms these seemingly innocuous films into a series of entertainingly seductive messages that both celebrate and promote excessive alcohol use.

Research on Alcohol Use in Film

In examining film's relationship to alcohol use, scholars have primarily relied on four different, but often compatible, methodological approaches (i.e., cross-sectional, experimental, longitudinal, and content analysis). Collectively, they provide a significantly fuller, more complex understanding of the relationship between cinematic depictions of alcohol and audience alcohol consumption.

Dalton et al.'s (2002) *cross-sectional* analysis, for instance, investigated 4,544 students in grades 5 through 8 who attended middle schools in New England. They discovered that of those students with no viewing restrictions, 46% had consumed alcohol. In contrast, only 4% of the students from houses with R-rated restrictions had tried alcohol; 4 years later, Sargent et al. (2006) studied a similar cohort of 4,655 middle-school students and found that there was statistical evidence to support "a curvilinear association between higher exposure to movie alcohol use and increased risk of prevalent and incident alcohol use" (p. 61).

Studying the topic from an *experimental* perspective, Kulick and Rosenberg (2001) found that participants who viewed positive portrayals of alcohol consumption in films held more "positive alcohol expectancies" compared to the control group, but not compared to the negative portrayal group. Wasylkiw & Currie (2011), interested in films' power to change attitudes about both alcohol and higher education, concluded that watching a 15-minute clip of the college fraternity film, "*Animal House*," produced more positive views on alcohol consumption and more negative attitudes towards academics compared to those who watched a clip of the nature documentary, "*Planet Earth*."

Finally, Koordeman et al. (2011) created a semi-naturalistic home setting, offering their college participants free beverages (e.g., beer, wine, soda, or water) as they watched a popular Hollywood film. They found that participants imitated the timing and frequency of the drinking behaviors of on-screen characters. They also discovered that males were more likely to imitate male actors and that this imitation was more likely to occur at the beginning of the movie rather than at the end.

Expanding the focus from a single cause-and-effect event to tracking changes over time, *longitudinal* researchers Hanewinkel et al. (2014) examined the impact of alcohol in movies on 2,346 adolescent students from 6 European countries who reported that they would "definitely not" drink alcohol within the next year. After age, gender, family affluence, school performance, TV screen time, personality characteristics, and drinking behavior of peers, parents, and siblings were controlled for, researchers determined that the students who viewed the most films involving alcohol consumption were 30% more likely to try alcohol within the year and 20% more likely to binge drink than those who viewed fewer alcohol-themed films during the same period (p. 973).

In Wills et al.'s (2009) longitudinal study on alcohol depictions in film and alcohol-related problems, a direct relationship was found between viewing alcohol in popular movies and both an increase in alcohol use and an increase in associating with friends who consume alcohol. Both outcomes also had effects on subsequent alcohol-related problems (e.g., fighting, disciplinary problems, reduced academic performance, and rebelliousness) through several different pathways (p. 32). More importantly, when tracked from time 1 through time 4, this pathway of watching movies and drinking with friends led to alcohol-related problems as students got older. Such undesirable outcomes, however, could be attenuated if participants received parental warmth and responsiveness at home, especially from mothers. A "protective effect" was also found in students with moderately high self-control and good school performance.

The final methodological approach most often used in studying alcohol depictions in films comes from *content analysis*. In a prototypical example of this perspective, Thompson and Yokota (2001) analyzed all 81 G-rated films released in the USA from 1937 to 2000 to identify substance use in "family-friendly" cinema. The researchers concluded that 47% of these films, deemed "appropriate" entertainment for children of all ages, showed at least one scene involving alcohol consumption. On average, the use of alcohol in these films lasted for 42 seconds per film. Most disturbingly, none of the 38 films containing alcohol showed any long-term effects from its use or contained any anti-alcohol messaging in their narratives. With a similar focus on young audiences, Goldstein et al. (1999) found that half of the 50 most popular animated films (from 1937 through 1997) included at least one scene involving alcohol. The researchers also discovered that "good" characters were just as likely as "bad" ones to drink and that no negative consequences associated with alcohol use appeared in any of these 25 films. Finally, while researchers such as Thompson and Yokota (2001) and Stern and Morr (2013) strategically analyzed children and adolescents, most of the published works in this area used box-office earnings to define their datasets. Everett et al. (1998), for example, investigated the 110 biggest box-office hits between 1985 and 1995. They discovered that 98% of them made supporting references to tobacco and/or alcohol use and that "discouraging the use of these substances was uncommon" (p. 317). Additionally, they discovered that lead protagonists (i.e., "the good guys") were the characters consuming alcohol 79% of the time.

Alcohol Use in College-Frat Films: A Qualitative Case Study

Adding to the current body of research on alcohol use in film, I studied the 50 most popular college-frat films to understand their depictions of alcohol use. Unlike the quantitative content analysis summarized above, I approached this data set through the methodological lens of qualitative textual analysis. Specifically, I have incorporated a granular-level *qualitative content analysis* as a tool in a *rhetorical/literary* analysis of popular films. Together, the two approaches allow me not only measure the occurrences of on-screen substance abuse but also to interpret the pro-alcohol messages found in the narratives, tropes, and character dialogues of these films.

Why Study Frat Films?

My interest in this topic is a practical one, born out of over 30 years of serving as a professor and faculty adviser for dozens of male social fraternities at a large, public university. My institution, like many of its benchmark institutions, shares one plaguing problem in common: Greeks, especially fraternity members. As a segment of society, fraternity members drink far more than their unaffiliated counterparts. A 2001 Harvard School of Public Health national study of college drinking found that fraternity members were much more likely to engage in heavy drinking than their non-fraternity peers (75.1% versus 48.6%) (Wechsler et al., 2002). Seven years later, Wechsler et al. (2009) similarly found that 86% of men living in fraternities had indulged in binge drinking, compared to 45% of non-fraternity men.

These rates of fraternity alcohol misuse have been shown to be a consistent factor that both accompanies and exacerbates many of the other Greek transgressions found on many college campuses. Although fraternity members comprise a smaller portion of the student body (5 to 10%) on most campuses, they are responsible for a disproportionate rate of drinking-related problems. Research affirms that alcohol abuse and membership in a fraternity, for instance, negatively affect academic performance, with members being twice as likely to fall behind in academic work as their non-fraternity counterparts (Wechsler et al., 2009).

More troubling are the disruptive, abusive, and criminal behaviors that are often associated with fraternity affiliation. According to Wechsler et al. (2002), more than half of the 83% who report negative Greek behavior have, in fact, been the victims of crimes by Greeks. These transgressions range from physical assault and property damage to sexual assault and acquaintance rape. As disturbing as these findings are, they do not count the alcohol-related deaths within the Greek community. Investigative reporters John Hechinger and David Glovin (2014) identified over 60 deaths since 2005 in which alcohol played a role. In fact, after studying hundreds of Greek injury and death cases, another investigative reporter, Caitlin Flanagan, "couldn't find one in which alcohol did not play a role" (DiMaria, 2014, para. 21). Flanagan (2014, para. 7) wrote that those death rates are "dwarfed by the numbers of serious injuries, assaults, and sexual crimes that regularly take place in these houses."

Starting with both an understanding of the current state of frat life on American college campuses and an intimate familiarity with the frat-film genre, I argue that frat films do more than just entertain young audiences. These films constitute powerful lessons that inform viewers of the types of behaviors and attitudes that are popular and rewarded on college campuses. In doing so, these films sell frat life to pre-college teens with seductive promises of a) unlimited alcohol and unsupervised parties, b) wild, promiscuous coeds, c) minimal academic demands, and d) a consequence-free life for their misbehavior.

Identifying My Dataset

In selecting the films included in this study, I used the Internet Movie Database, or IMDb to help me identify the 50 most popular films that include some aspect of fraternity life. I began my search by identifying all feature-length English-language fiction films, from the non-silent era (post-1927), that included at least one identifiable term referencing fraternity life that appeared either in the film's title or anywhere in the IMDb description, including each film's "keywords," "plot summary," or "plot synopsis." From this initial list of over 580 English-speaking feature films, I selected the 50 most popular films based on the total number of votes each film received on the IMDb website.

A cursory review of these 50 popular films suggests that frat life varied in narrative importance from film to film. While all these films included some derivation of "fraternity life" in their IMDb description or key terms, not all of them placed Greek life at the center of their storyline or had frat brothers as primary antagonists or protagonists. Consequently, I classified each of the films into one of three narrative categories based on the importance of frat life in each film's storyline: *Primary, Secondary, and Tertiary.* Of the 50 films in this study, 24 comprise "***primary***" fraternity films, with some aspect of frat life placed at the center of the film's storyline. Ten films had a "***secondary***" emphasis, where the storyline included some aspect of frat life that was not essential to the overall narrative. In the remaining 16 "***tertiary***" films, Greek life plays an insignificant role in their overall storylines. Notably, even decades after many of these films premiered in theaters, 20% of the films in this study made it into IMDb's list of the "89 best teenage comedies of all time" (2012), while Complex's "The 50 best raunchy teen comedies" (2013) honored six films in this dataset.

Alcohol Use in these 50 Films

The one thing that united every film on this list, regardless of their target audiences or their moral evaluations of frat life, was the inclusion and celebration of alcohol in their storylines. Remarkably, all 50 films included scenes of alcohol consumption, with most showing multiple drinking scenes. Specifically, my sample featured 125 parties, or an average of 2.5 parties per film, that served alcohol, 20.6% (26) of which also supplied illicit drugs to their guests. In addition to these college "parties," a) 50% of these films also included scenes of students drinking at a "bar or nightclub," b) 70% showed students drinking alcohol while hanging out, and c) 42% had students engaging in recreational drug use while hanging out. Taken together, 206 scenes involved substance use in this dataset, with an average of 4.12 acts of alcohol or drug use per film.

When comparing these "social" scenes to their "academic" counterparts in the films, a collective narrative emerges that disproportionately teaches viewers that partying constitutes the primary objective of higher education. In contrast to this, 4.12 scenes per film involve substance use, and almost half (46%) of the films in this analysis contain no academic scenes involving students and their professors. Of the 27 films that include at least one pedagogical interaction, the average length of such "learning" moments lasted just 68 seconds.

These films also pack social scenes with other equally significant lessons about college life. In this chapter, I will discuss the five most recurring party lessons found in these films. Collectively, I argue, they contribute to the formation of one grand over-arching narrative about the importance of pledging a social fraternity to maximize one's social life (i.e., getting drunk), which is the key to making one's college experience memorable.

Five Lessons of College Fraternity Films

Lesson One: Frats Monopolize the Social Life on Most of these Cinematic Campuses

The totality of the films in this study creates a social reality for audiences in which five groups control the social life of colleges: fraternities, sororities, independent/unaffiliated students, the larger collective Greek community, and miscellaneous campus organizations. This controlling power, however, is not equally distributed. Instead, the films depict a clear social caste system that permeates most institutions of higher education.

Within this highly stratified structure, fraternities are presented as, far and away, the metaphoric "big dogs" on most of these campuses, hosting 73.55% (or 90) of the 125 parties in this dataset, four of which were co-hosted with sororities. Additionally, in 30 of these 50 movies (or 60%), fraternity brothers are the only students shown partying, monopolizing the entirety of their film's social life. In 10 other films, frats shared the party scene with unaffiliated-student partiers 9 times and with sororities once. Putting this social dominance in perspective, of the 45 films that included at least one party within their narrative, only five films (or 11.1%) did not show a frat roister. In comparison, 84% of the films exclude sorority parties, and 80% do not show independent bashes around campus.

This monopolizing power can also be seen in the number of films in which fraternities dominate the social life of their cinematic campuses. While 11 (or 22%) of the 50 films created campuses in which no single group controlled most or all the fun in their narratives, 28 others (or 56%) presented a college experience that was predominantly subjugated by fraternities. Eight others presented campuses where the collective Greek Community (i.e., fraternities and sororities) controlled social life. In stark contrast, independent or affiliate students only dominated three campuses. Each of these three campuses, however, was shown in films that gave screen time to two different colleges (e.g., *Accepted*, *Butterfly Effect*, *Road Trip*), and at these other three colleges, fraternities again were depicted as controlling the campus' social life, thus diminishing the scant social power of non-Greeks even more.

When considered collectively, I assert that audiences view such one-sided stories, especially young males with limited first-hand experiences of college life, as an imperative for the necessity of pledging. For while some competing counter-narratives exist in the bunch, the overwhelming majority of these films, including most of those that are openly critical of elite frat culture, show frats hosting most of the parties, and their brothers having most of the fun on their cinematic campuses. While filmmakers likely created such scenes to entertain audiences, they also unintentionally underscore the necessity of Greek membership, a lesson especially relevant to pre-college audiences.

Notably, frat life's social dominance in these films was not a foregone conclusion. For a film to be included in my study, it only needed a fraternity to appear somewhere. The fraternity did not need to be the primary focus of its narrative, nor play any meaningful role in its storyline. As such, fraternities comprised the "primary" focus in less than half of the 50 films (24) in this study. Ten other films placed frat life in less important "secondary" roles. Sixteen "tertiary" films used fraternities as little more than background props on their cinematic campuses. Additionally, 70% of these films (or 35 of 50) criticized their narrative's most selective and elite fraternities. Nonetheless, the majority of these secondary and tertiary anti-frat films still placed fraternities, commonly framed as class-conscious elitists, at the center of their films' social narrative, unwittingly undermining their editorial critiques of these private male social clubs.

Lesson Two: Fraternities Not Only Host Most of the Parties, But Also Host the Best Parties

The quantity of parties provides only one indicator in creating the perception of Greek social prominence in the minds of viewers. Perhaps a more important question is one of quality. In answering this query, I coded for the group or individual "*who hosted the best social event" in each of the 50 films.*

Again, fraternities either won, shared (in a tie), contributed (as half of the Greek Community), or split (in films with two campuses) the "best event" in 39 films. While not all the "best social event" winners served alcohol (*e.g., Monsters University's "Scare Games"*), all the best frat parties were very "wet."

The four university-sponsored "Greek events," involving their campuses' sorority and fraternity members (*e.g., Monsters University's Scare Games, Pumpkin's Greek Ball, Revenge of the Nerds' Greek Games, and Stomp the Yard's Step Show*), came in a distant second. The three films that celebrated sorority parties (*e.g., House Bunny, Neighbors 2, and Scream 2*), and the three films that spotlighted the social benefits of remaining unaffiliated (*i.e., Accepted, The Butterfly Effect, and Road Trip*) tied for third place.

Lesson Three: Fraternities Offer Six Significant Social Benefits

While the 90 frat parties portrayed in these films serve as powerful social incentives for membership, most of these parties also supply at least **eight** subsidiary advantages to "going Greek." These subordinate social benefits, while possibly overlooked by adult viewers, promise pre-college adolescents a utopian social lifestyle that is free from adult supervision and that encourages uninhibited hedonism.

Benefit One: Freedom from Adult Supervision

One of the first noticeable differences between the social lives experienced by most younger viewers and the fictional frat parties depicted in these films is the complete absence of adult supervision. The cinematic world of frat parties suggests no adult surveillance or behavioral monitoring, regardless of the size of the party or the amount of social disruption it produces. Instead, the only concern for these host organizations involves the possible threat that they may prematurely run out of beer or that their live band may arrive late for their first set.

Of the 90 different parties hosted by the 77 different fraternities in this study, adults did not interrupt a single social event, including the likes of deans of students, university presidents or provosts, Greek-housing administrators (charged with keeping the peace on frat row), or even angry visits from parents who pay for their child's room and board.

Benefit Two: The Parties Are Free (a.k.a., "Open Bar")

In this cinematic world of frat parties, not only do partygoers not worry about adult restrictions, they also never worry about finances. Of the hundreds of fraternity brothers that make appearances in these 50 films, none addressed, implicitly or explicitly, the thousands of dollars that they would realistically owe for their a) annual dues (paid to their corporate headquarters), b) insurance premiums, c) local chapter dues, d) semi-annual formal and semi-formal balls, and, most importantly, social dues needed to fund the seemingly endless array of parties that stretch from the first day of the fall semester to the last day of finals in the spring.

Mirroring the findings of Kendall's (2011) research on the depictions of the spending habits of young adult characters found in American TV, the young adults in this study also live free from any economic pressures or financial demands. Characters freely and readily spend with little to no concern for budget or debt, teaching audiences that the cost of an active social life is both invisible and inconsequential. Even in rare films, such as *The Skulls* or *Stomp the Yard*, that feature blue-collar brothers working their way through college, they always discuss their employment as a necessity to pay for their college tuition, never for the many expenses associated with frat membership.

Instead, they, as well as their more financially privileged brethren, binge drink an endless stream of beer, wine, and alcohol shots, and smoke, snort, and pop a constellation of illicit drugs without ever taking money out of their wallets, credit cards, or ATM accounts. When the parties appear as epic and extravagant as many of the blowouts in this study, the option of pledging a frat becomes a social and financial "no-brainer": It's all the fun without any of the pain or cost!

Benefit Three: Campus Females Love Frat Parties

Along with free beer, films showcase the presence of eager and inebriated female students as a necessary ingredient for any legitimate frat party. In fact, in the cinematically constructed world created by these films, campus coeds are as important in the iconography of this genre as are "kegs of beer," "pledges," and the "frat house" itself.

Of the 90 parties found in this dataset, only 12 (or 13.48%) did not include females. Of those films, 5 featured fraternity ritual parties, occasions typically reserved for official members only, including the Zeta Theta Psi "rush party" in *22 Jump Street*, the Chi Psi Beta's bizarre "hazing-day party" in *The Butterfly Effect*, *Monsters University*'s basement initiation, and *Animal House*'s "Bid-Day" party, an event made memorable by Bluto (played by John Belushi) singing "***Louie Louie***," as his inebriated Delta brothers drank, danced, and sprayed beer on the heads of their new pledges in joyous male-bonding celebration.

While most of the Greek rituals in this analysis encompassed binge drinking and male bonding, others highlighted the elite and class-conscious nature of frat life, such as *The Skulls*' fictionalized account of Yale's Skull and Bones initiation, a student organization that currently lists six US presidents as alumni brothers. That film depicts new members being secretly sequestered to the fraternity's private castle, located on their private island. After finding tailored tuxedos waiting for them in their private 4-star rooms, the secret society welcomed the pledges with a gift of $100,000, a token of their wealthy and powerful alumni's appreciation. Notably, not all ritual parties occur without females. During the next Skulls party, for example, the fraternity gifted brothers with beautiful and elegant high-priced escorts and rare sports cars, selected by the alumni to match their wildest fantasies.

This sample of films included 12 "rush" parties in this study, 11 of which supplied free alcohol to their naive, first-year visitors. The "dry rush" outlier of the bunch was hosted by the exaggeratedly snobby Omegas, *Animal House*'s despicable antagonists. This alcohol-free anomaly stands in stark contrast to one of the greatest (and wettest) cinematic frat parties of all time: The Deltas' recruiting party, marked by the appearance of Dean Wormer's intoxicated and promiscuous wife and the music of Otis Day and the Knights' "sing-along" version of "Shout!"

What makes these common depictions of rush parties noteworthy is that, for the last half-century, the Interfraternity Council (IFC), the governing body that oversees fraternity life in the U.S., has mandated that rush functions should be free of both alcohol and females, urging their chapters to keep their focus on brotherhood. The IFC affirms that the goal of rush events should be for fraternity members to get to know potential new members without the distractions of beer and females (Interfraternity Council, n.d.).

Benefit Four: No I.D. Check

For today's adolescents, restrictions on underage drinking have increasingly become more intense. According to the Centers for Disease Control and Prevention (CDC), when states increased the legal drinking age to 21, drinking during the previous month among persons aged 18 to 20 years declined by 19% (2022). In contrast to the increasingly restrictive and surveilled lives of real-world adolescents, the cinematic frat parties in this study present underage students getting served alcohol effortlessly and without the need for even fake IDs, given that hosts do not ask or seem to care about the age of their guests. Even the youngest looking, baby-faced undergrads can move freely, from party to party, without fear of scrutiny. After all, the host organizations in this study, like most real-world social fraternities, are aware that approximately 75% of their undergraduate attendees and approximately 99% of their pledges are younger than 21 years of age (Reyes, 2023).

None of the 90 cinematic frat parties in this study featured any college student, male or female, ever being asked to show their ID (i.e., "being carded") or questioned about their age. Remarkably, at least nine parties in six different films in this study showed high-school students visiting frat houses and being served alcohol, including *Animal House*'s Toga Party, all three parties in *College*, *Goat*'s summer rush party, two different parties in *The Naked Mile* (with the same three high-school students being served at a campus bar), *Old School*'s Mitchapalooza party, *Revenge of the Nerds 2* Spring Break Party, and *PCU* Funkadelic Party.

Of the 125 parties in this dataset, only a single "carding" scene took place. This lone independent (i.e., non-Greek) event happened during *Van Wilder*'s "Unity Coalition" festival (for minority and under-represented students) where the antagonist Delta Iota Kappa frat snuck a busload of elementary schoolers into the event for the strategic purpose of framing the film's titular protagonist. For adolescent audiences watching this seemingly endless array of unregulated frat parties, populated by unconcerned underaged undergrads, the fact that no college student, not even high school teens, are ever asked to produce ID must certainly register as a consequential benefit of Greek membership and involvement.

Benefit Five: Party Never Gets Broken Up

Many teens, as well as their slightly older college-aged cohorts, are all too familiar with parties being broken up by overly attentive police enforcing neighborhood noise ordinances. Students over the years have told me that this imminent threat has forced them to attempt to keep their parties small and to tightly monitor the volume of the stereo. Yet, such efforts almost always fail. Once word of a party typically gets out, uninvited peers inevitably show up, and the "small gathering" quickly grows in both size and volume.

However, this real-world concern becomes inconsequential in the world of cinematic frat parties. In this enticingly social world, fraternities are liberated from any restrictive standards that otherwise circumscribe the behavior of all non-Greeks. Of the 90 different parties in this study, only two got prematurely interrupted. *PCU*'s vindictive and petty college president pulled the proverbial plug on The Pit's "*Everybody Gets Laid*" party, but not before this mixed-race, mixed-gender group of stoned nihilists gave their attendees a live concert by the legendary George Clinton and his Parliament-Funkadelic band and raised enough money ($7,000) to save their historic frat house for future generations of stoners.

The second terminated frat party, unlike its predecessor, was not shut down by forces within its own campus structure, but outside of it. After six highly successful and rowdy frat parties, nefariously sneaky neighbors, Mac and Kelly Radner, targeted the seventh and final Delta Psi blowout. Hellbent on getting rid of this lovable collective of drunkards and stoners, the Radners conspired to have the city police arrive when they were most legally vulnerable. However, even in this case, where the brothers were obviously guilty of hosting an out-of-control "hot-house" pot party, fueled by 300 to 400 kilos of high-grade marijuana, openly displayed in wheelbarrows and garbage bags on their front porch, these undergrads still almost got away with it. If it was not for said neighbors desperately shooting fireworks into the departing police vehicle's window, this Delta Psi blowout would have continued, uninterrupted, until the morning, like all their other parties.

Benefit Six: No Limits, No Restrictions

Unlike the real adult world, where well-defined and punitive laws restrict any host, both private (i.e., social host liability laws) and public (i.e., dram shop laws), from serving alcohol to visitors/patrons who *appear* tipsy, buzzed, or inebriated, the cinematic frat world has no such limits. Indeed, far from embracing moderation or encouraging temperance, frat culture openly celebrates the overindulgence and immoderation of most societal vices. Of all these sinful transgressions, however, the most common depravity, consistently flaunted by almost every frat in this study, is alcoholic gluttony, or binge drinking.

As revealed through this study, films treat "binge drinking" as the acceptable and encouraged approach to alcohol consumption at these cinematic parties. Binge drinking constitutes their *raison d'etre*, the purpose of their existence, and the defining characteristic that unites almost every drunk gathering in this study. Scenes of brothers and their guests both chugging (or funneling) beer and shooting distilled liquor comprise much of the visual iconography associated with these fraternal gatherings. Their inclusion in their respective films serves as narrative shorthand, immediately conveying to audiences that the party is a success and that wild and often humorous debauchery will certainly follow. These scenes also serve as valuable lessons to the uninitiated, supplying future college students with models of appropriate and expected behaviors while on campus.

Benefit Seven: Free and Safe Drugs

Illicit drug use was surprisingly common in the lives of cinematic frat brothers. Drug use appeared in 22 of the 50 films (or 44%), including 8 of the top 10 most popular films in this study. While marijuana was by far the most popular on-screen drug, featured in 19 films, 7 other drugs also found screen time. On three occasions, for example, audiences witnessed on-screen protagonists popping illicit pharmaceutical pills (e.g., Painkillers/Opioids and Quaaludes/Methaqualone), while three other scenes celebrate students amusingly snorting (or inhaling) powdered cocaine into their nasal passages.

Additionally, in three large gatherings, masses of attendees collectively digested hallucinogenic psychoactive drugs. The first was the previously mentioned mushroom party at the Delta Psi Beta house in *Neighbors*. The second took place at *Van Wilder*'s campus "Rave Party" where a large cross-section of Coolidge College's undergrads "dosed" themselves with hits of herbal Ecstasy, a psychoactive "party drug" comprised of a combination of legal herbs and illicit ephedrine.

Yet, these two single events paled in comparison to the campus-wide, year-long popularity of a fictional synthetic drug called *WHY-PHY* on the campus of M.C. State University (in *22 Jump Street*). An acronym for "*Work hard? Yes. Play Hard? Yes*," partiers enthusiastically described this new designer drug as the greatest high ever, "like Adderall, Heroin, and Acid" mixed together. By spring break of the academic year, this synthetic psychoactive hallucinogen had become so widely abused that it became both a public-health epidemic and the focus of a major law-enforcement undercover sting operation. Notably, this storyline constitutes the only incident found in this 50-film dataset that framed substance abuse, in its many celebrated forms, as either a personal or societal problem requiring legal or public-health intervention.

Two other illicit substances found in this study involved, first, the relatively benign use of Viagra by three high-school visitors at a Beta Delta Xi house party in *The Naked Mile* and the collective inhalation of Nitrous Oxide (a.k.a., "laughing gas") by the Beta Phi Tau brothers in *College*. In the second case, the hard-partying Beta fraternity owned their own medical-grade Nitrous tank, a highly coveted possession by hard-core partiers, whose ownership is typically reserved for board-certified surgeons, dentists, and periodontists.

Besides the frequency of drug use in its multiple forms, it was also alarming to discover how common and popular drugs appeared on some of these cinematic campuses. Four of the 22 "drug films" portrayed getting "high" as equally valued and common as getting drunk (*e.g., College, Dead Man on Campus, Goat, Hell Night*). Even more surprisingly, eight films framed drug use as even more popular and celebrated than chugging beer or doing shots (*e.g., 22 Jump Street, Boo!, Goat, Neighbors 1 & 2, Revenge of the Nerds 1 & 2, and Van Wilder*).

Drugs also played a central and defining role in the storylines of many of these films, including the pot-loving Tri Lambda brothers of *The Revenge of the Nerds 1 and 2*, the epic "hot house" and hallucinogenic mushroom parties in *Neighbors 1*, and the ubiquitous presence of Van's party bong in *Van Wilder*. In *The Revenge of the Nerds*, for example, audiences nervously watch as the Tri Lambdas host their first "alcohol-free" party. As feared, this "dry" social gathering initially appears to be a social disaster. Saving the day at the 11th hour, as well as securing the future of the fledgling Tri Lambda frat, the crude and lewd Brother Booger (played by Curtis Armstrong) breaks out his cache of pot and miraculously transforms the gathering into one of this dataset's many legendary on-screen parties.

From a public-health perspective, perhaps the most disturbing aspect of drug use found in this study did not involve the quantity of on-screen use, but the positive, often euphoric, depictions of the effects of taking drugs. Such positive and inconsequential outcomes occurred with the pills consumed in *Dead Man on Campus* and in *Hell Night*, the cocaine snorted in *Goat* and *The Social Network*, the psychedelic mushrooms eaten in *Neighbors*, and the Ecstasy taken in *Van Wilder* all produced similar euphoric outcomes, heightening the overall cinematic impact of their host parties. Even *22 Jump Street's* hallucinogenic "WHY-PHY" generally got framed as an incredible high, a cross between "Adderall, Heroin, & Acid," all in one hit. When read collectively, the message is clear: Drug use on college campuses is popular, fun, and safe.

Lesson Four: Most of these Party-Hosting Frats Were Antagonists in Their Films

The single most interesting and perplexing finding to emerge from this analysis is that, while approximately two-thirds of the films in this study adopted an openly critical stance on frat life, many of these same films unintentionally sold the advantages of the institution's social life to pre-college heterosexual males. This hostility was even more pronounced when framing elite, wealthy, and highly selective fraternities; 71% of the films in which such bourgeois groups appeared depicted them as major sources of campus strife as well as the hosts of successful and exclusive social gatherings on their respective campuses.

Of the 19 frats that threw the 24 best parties in this study, antagonist frats hosted 57.90% (or 11) of them. This percentage increases to 60% when isolating the five different organizations that hosted the six most successful cinematic frat parties in this analysis (i.e., *College*'s Omega Theta Pi, *The Social Network*'s Phoenix – S.K Club, and *The Skulls*' Skull and Bones).

Furthermore, films more often presented antagonistic frats versus their protagonist counterparts, a) living in nicer houses, b) being more popular on campus, c) having greater access to females, d) throwing bigger and crazier parties, and e) benefiting more often from their professional connections with their influential alumni. Thus, even when many of the films in this study created narratives that criticized fraternities, their depictions of these antagonistic groups inadvertently stressed aspects of frat life that serve as highly seductive inducements for a certain type of pre-college heterosexual male.

From a script-writing perspective, granting such advantages and benefits to the "bad guys" is essential in constructing the three most recurring antagonistic character tropes of the genre: the "*frat bully,*" "*privileged jerk,*" and the "*Big (Arrogant) Man on Campus.*" In each case, the unlikeable characters must be framed as bigger, richer, more popular, and more privileged than their underdog protagonists. This moral and material dichotomy allows audiences to not only disdain the privileged ruthlessness and cruelty of the film's villain, but to also celebrate the eventual third-act triumphs of the "under-sized" hero with a big heart.

Lesson Five: Male Undergrads Must Become Brothers in Order to Gain Access to Most of These Campus Parties

While films rarely feature the specific rules for which characters can attend these parties, the basic guidelines for admittance can be easily deduced. They include the following:

1) ***Females who were framed as attractive within their film's narrative***, regardless of any sorority affiliation, will almost always gain entrance into any social gathering hosted by fraternities.
2) ***Females who were framed as unattractive within their film's narrative*** should avoid attending elite frat parties or run the risk of being subjected to cruel and humiliating treatment. This lesson is underscored in films such as *Sorority Boys*, where the Kappa Omicron Kappa brothers threw a dog-catcher's net over the heads of their "unattractive" visitors before discarding them on their front lawn. Similarly, audiences learned of the dangers of being an overweight coed as the Alpha Beta Brothers released a sounder of swine into the Omega Mu's party, yelling, "We thought you could use some more pigs for your party" in 1984's hit comedy, *The Revenge of the Nerds*.
3) ***Rival fraternity*** members rarely attend another fraternity's party. However, almost all the frats in this study hosted their own parties, leaving little need for brothers to look outside their own frat houses for entertainment.
4) ***Ethnic and racial minorities*** are also *persona non gratae*. While films do not incorporate many examples of minorities being overtly banned or rejected from predominantly white frat houses, the lesson is still clearly and resoundingly communicated to audiences through the near-total exclusion of lead minority characters in these films. While seven African American fraternities appeared in 5 of the 50 films in this study, these racially segregated groups inadvertently reinforce the rule of racial separation created, controlled, and maintained by their white counterparts.
5) ***Unaffiliated males***, especially first-year male students, have virtually no chance of gaining access to the myriad of frat parties that dominate the social landscape on American college campuses. Instead, these independent undergrads, as most of these films illustrate, will spend most of their weekends in dorm rooms with other lonely male students, coveting the social life that is most often monopolized by their Greek counterparts.

However, hope exists for many of these freshmen trapped in this latter group. As the majority of these films clearly instruct, all they have to do is sign up for "fraternity rush" during their first week on campus. Then, according to scripts in this study, they will have access to a seemingly endless supply of beer, brotherhood, and coeds. This final lesson also expands the power of these films to not only promote alcohol use, but to also sell frat life inadvertently to a certain segment of the viewing audience (i.e., pre-college, heterosexual, white, Christian males).

Conclusion

Along with uncovering these specific lessons taught to audiences about the importance of fraternity life on college campuses and the central role alcohol plays in the social lives of undergraduates, I seek to contribute a voice to the larger academic conversation surrounding popular culture and Health Communication. Toward this end, this chapter underscores the power of film to not only entertain but also to also inform and persuade. This insight is especially important to parents who may falsely believe that sending their children to a raunchy comedy that celebrates the social aspects of college life is a benign activity. For it is the Trojan-horse nature of not only film but also of most popular media that makes their seemingly harmless messages so potentially powerful and dangerous. When an entertained audience drops their guard, believing their need for critical thinking and evaluation is unwarranted, they become vulnerable to media's potentially harmful outcomes.

However, stakeholders beyond parents could benefit from rethinking the persuasive power of entertaining popular culture. Agencies, such as the Motion Picture Association of America (MPAA), responsible for determining the appropriateness of content based on an audience's age, could also learn from the research generated at the intersection between popular culture and health communication. Specifically, since its inception in 1968, the MPAA board, comprised almost exclusively of non-academic "lay" evaluators, primarily conducts numerical counts of the occurrences and durations of explicit sexual behavior, explicit violence, and profanity in deciding on a film's parental ranking (e.g., G, PG, PG13, R, & NC17).

While such monitoring is an honorable undertaking, empowering parents to make more informed decisions regarding their children's exposure to sex and violence, I assert that such groups, including the MPAA, fall short in their charge of protecting children from the harmful consequences of popular media by ignoring depictions of alcohol consumption and drug use.

In summarizing the salient research on alcohol use in film, it becomes clear that the depictions of alcohol consumption seem ubiquitous in film (Everett et al.,1998; Goldstein et al., 1999; Thompson & Yokota, 2001). Further, when viewed by adolescent audiences, exposure to these messages increases their 1) likelihood to take their first drink sooner (Sargent et al., 2006), 2) positive attitudes toward alcohol (Kulick & Rosenberg, 2001; Wasylkiw & Currie, 2011), 3) modeling of on-screen alcohol use (Koordeman et al., 2011), 4) likelihood of binge drinking (Hanewinkel et al., 2014), and 5) selection of at-risk peer groups who consume alcohol (Wills et al., 2009).

In closing, with the myriad of content-analysis studies that illuminate the omnipresence of alcohol use in popular media and the preponderance of social-scientific research supporting the strong causal relationship between viewing alcohol consumption and changes in the at-risk alcohol behaviors and attitudes of under-age audiences, it is long overdue for monitoring agencies, and the parents who trust the wisdom of such groups, to seriously consider Hollywood's intoxicating effects on children and adolescents in their evaluation process.

References

Borzekowski, D. L. G., & Strasburger, V. C. (2008). Adolescents and media messages about tobacco, alcohol, and drugs. In S. L. Calvert & B. J. Wilson (Eds.), *The handbook of children, media, and development* (pp. 432–452). Blackwell Publishing. https://doi.org/10.1002/9781444302752.ch19

Centers for Disease Control and Prevention. (2022, December 7). Age 21 minimum legal drinking age. https://www.cdc.gov/alcohol/fact-sheets/minimum-legal-drinking-age.htm

Dalton M. A., Ahrens M. B., Sargent J. D., Mott L. A., Beach M. L., Tickle J. J., & Heatherton, T. F. (2002). Relation between parental restrictions on movies and adolescent use of tobacco and alcohol. *Effective Clinical Practices*, *5*(1), 1–10.

DiMaria, F. (2014, July 25). Lawsuits against fraternities: Reveal risks and responsibilities. *Insurance Newsnet*. https://insurancenewsnet.com/oarticle/Lawsuits-Against-Fraternities-Reveal-Risks-and-Responsibilities-a-535697

Everett, S. A., Schnuth, R. L., & Tribble, J. L. (1998). Tobacco and alcohol use in top-grossing American films. *Journal of Community Health*, *23*(4), 317–324. https://doi.org/10.1023/a:1018727606500

Flanagan, C. (2014). The dark power of fraternities. *The Atlantic*. https://www.theatlantic.com/magazine/archive/2014/03/the-dark-power-of-fraternities/357580

Goldstein, A. O., Sobel, R. A., & Newman, G. R. (1999). Tobacco and alcohol use in G-rated children's animated films. *Journal of the American Medical Association*, *281*(12), 1131–1136. https://doi.org/10.1001/jama.281.12.1131

Gupta, M. (2023, March 17). Hollywood film industry statistics & facts 2023. *New Vision Blog*. https://www.newvisiontheatres.com/hollywood-film-industry-statistics

Hanewinkel, R., Sargent, J. D., Hunt, K., Sweeting, H., Engels, R. C., Scholte, R. H., Mathis, F., Florek, E., & Morgenstern, M. (2014). Portrayal of alcohol consumption in movies and drinking initiation in low-risk adolescents. *Pediatrics*, *133*(6), 973–982. https://doi.org/10.1542/peds.2013-3880

Hechinger, J., & Glovin, D. (2014). Fraternity bans recruits' initiation. *Bloomberg News*. https://www.bostonglobe.com/news/nation/2014/03/08/most-deadly-fraternity-scraps-initiation-for-newmembers/hWZwgntJOMGf4DjZWMmpyI/story.html

IMDb. (2012, July 25). Best teen comedies of all time. https://www.imdb.com/list/ls009988118/

Interfraternity Council. (n.d.). Recruitment officer guide. https://nicfraternity.org/wp-content/uploads/2019/02/IFC-Recruitment-Officer-Guide-1.pdf

Jackson, K. M., Janssen, T., & Gabrielli, J. (2018). Media/marketing influences on adolescent and young adult substance abuse. *Current Addiction Reports*, *5*(2), 146–157. https://doi.org/10.1007/s40429-018-0199-6

Kendall, D. E. (2011). *Framing class: Media representations of wealth and poverty in America*. Rowman & Littlefield.

Kessler D. A. (2001). *Question of intent: A great American battle with a deadly industry*. Public Affairs.

Koordeman, R., Kuntsche, E., Anschutz, D. J., van Baaren, R. B., & Engels, R. C. (2011). Do we act upon what we see? Direct effects of alcohol cues in movies on young adults' alcohol drinking. *Alcohol and Alcoholism*, *46*(4), 393–398. https://doi.org/10.1093/alcalc/agr028

Kulick, A. D., & Rosenberg H. (2001). Influence of positive and negative film portrayals of drinking on older adolescents' alcohol outcome expectancies. *Journal of Applied Social Psychology*, *31*(7), 1492–1499.

Mokdad, A., Marks, J., Stroup, D., & Gerberding, J. (2004). Actual causes of death in the United States, 2000. *Journal of the American Medical Association, 291*, 1238–1245.

Primack, B. A., Kraemer, K. L., Fine, M. J., & Dalton, M. A. (2009). Media exposure and marijuana and alcohol use among adolescents. *Substance Use & Misuse*, *44*(5), 722–739. https://doi.org/10.1080/10826080802490097

Reyes, A. (2023, August 25). What is the average age of college students? *CollegeRanker*. https://www.collegeranker.com/what-is-the-average-age-of-college-students/

Saad, L. (2023, June 6). What percentage of Americans drink alcohol? *Gallup.com*. https://news.gallup.com/poll/467507/percentage-americans-drink-alcohol.aspx

Sangari, N. (2022, January 26). 85% of US households have a video subscription service. *Kantar*. https://www.kantar.com/north-america/inspiration/technology/85-per-cent-of-us-households-have-a-video-subscription-service

Sargent, J. D., Wills, T. A., Stoolmiller, M., Gibson, J., & Gibbons, F. X. (2006). Alcohol use in motion pictures and its relationship with early-onset teen drinking. *Journal of Studies on Alcohol*, *67*(1), 54–65. https://doi.org/10.15288/jsa.2006.67.54

Scott-Sheldon, L. A., Carey, K. B., & Carey, M. P. (2007). Health behavior and college students: Does Greek affiliation matter? *Journal of Behavioral Medicine*, *31*(1), 61–70. https://doi.org/10.1007/s10865-007-9136-1

Stern, S., & Morr, L. (2013). Portrayals of teen smoking, drinking, and drug use in recent popular movies. *Journal of Health Communication*, *18*(2), 179–191. https://doi.org/10.1080/10810730.2012.688251

The 50 best raunch teen comedies. (2013, February 14). *Complex*. https://www.complex.com/pop-culture/a/complex/the-50-best-raunchy-teen-comedies-1

Thompson, K. M., & Yokota, F. (2001). Depiction of alcohol, tobacco, and other substances in G-rated animated feature films. *Pediatrics*, *107*(6), 1369–1374. https://doi.org/10.1542/peds.107.6.1369

U.S. Food and Drug Administration (n.d.). 2009 Family Smoking Prevention and Tobacco Control Act, Pub. L. No. 111-31. https://www.fda.gov/tobacco-products/rules-regulations-and-guidance/family-smoking-prevention-and-tobacco-control-act-overview#:~:text=To%20protect%20the%20public%20health,and%20marketing%20of%20tobacco%20products

U.S. Department of Health, Education, and Welfare. (1964). *Smoking and health: Report of the Advisory Committee to the Surgeon General of the Public Health Service*. (Public Health Service Publication No. 1103).

U.S. Department of Health and Human Services. (2014). *The health consequences of smoking: 50 years of progress: A report of the Surgeon General*. U.S. Department of Health and Human Services, Centers for Disease Control and Prevention, National Center for Chronic Disease Prevention and Health Promotion, Office on Smoking and Health.

Wasylkiw, L., & Currie, M. (2011). The *Animal House* effect: How university-themed comedy films affect students' attitudes. *Social Psychology of Education*, *15*, 25–40. https://doi.org/10.1007/s11218-011-9167-x

Wechsler, H., Eun Lee, J., Kuo, M., Seibring, M., Nelson, T. F., & Lee, H. (2002). Trends in college binge drinking during a period of increased prevention efforts: Findings from 4 Harvard School of Public Health College alcohol surveys: 1993–2001. *Journal of American College Health*, *50*, 203–217.

Wechsler, H., Kuh, G., & Davenport, A. E. (2009). Fraternities, sororities, and binge drinking: Results from a national study of American colleges. *National Association of Student Personnel Administrators Journal*, *46*(3), 395–416. https://doi.org/10.2202/1949-6605.5017

Wills, T. A., Sargent, J. D., Gibbons, F. X., Gerrard, M., & Stoolmiller, M. (2009). Movie exposure to alcohol cues and adolescent alcohol problems: A longitudinal analysis in a national sample. *Psychology of Addictive Behaviors*, *23*(1), 23–35. https://doi.org/10.1037/a0014137

11

MISINFORMATION ABOUT HEALTH IN POPULAR CULTURE

The Prevalence, Influence, and Mitigation of Health Misinformation

Weirui Wang and Yan Huang

Introduction

Health misinformation abounds in contemporary media. The declaration by the World Health Organization (WHO, 2023) provided a recent and concrete example of this phenomenon when it labeled the substantial volume of misinformation propagated regarding COVID-19 as an "info-demic." The false information about COVID-19, unintentionally or intentionally distributed online, eroded people's trust in health authorities and institutions and promoted behaviors that lead to harmful effects. At a collective level, according to the WHO, misinformation weakened public health responses and lengthened a public health crisis.

The fact that social media has been increasingly used as a major information source for health issues exacerbates the misinformation problem, including its spread and adverse effects. For instance, misinformation about the COVID-19 vaccine was well-detected on social media, particularly surging on Twitter and Facebook (Frenkel et al., 2020; Zhao et al., 2023). To demonstrate the effect, people were more likely to get vaccinated if they did not rely upon social media for virus information (Ruiz & Bell, 2021).

Public figures and celebrities also contributed to the infodemic by sharing their personal opinions and unverified claims on social media platforms (see also Chapter 15, this volume). For example, the foremost COVID-19 conspiracy theory revolved around "miracle cures," stemming from former President Trump's remarks during a press conference, suggesting the possibility of utilizing bleach or other disinfectants as remedies for coronavirus infection (Evanega et al., 2020). Nicki Minaj, "a Trinidadian-born rapper, singer, and songwriter" (https://en.wikipedia.org/wiki/Nicki_Minaj, para. 1), took to Twitter to express her disagreement with the Covid-19 vaccination mandate for attending the MET Gala. She tweeted that "[t]hey want you to get vaccinated for the Met. If I get vaccinated it won't be for the Met. It'll be once I feel I've done enough research." In another tweet, she shared an anecdote about her cousin's friend who allegedly became impotent after getting vaccinated. However, Dr. Anthony Fauci addressed this claim as misinformation during a CNN interview (The Associated Press, 2021). While Twitter functions as a social media platform where individuals express their personal reflections, the influence of celebrities' posts on Twitter extends beyond the realm of the

DOI: 10.4324/9781003436409-13

personal. Such personal claims, without ensuring accuracy and validity, can become widespread, highly influential, and mislead millions of people.

In this chapter, we discuss how health misinformation has emerged in various popular culture venues, including information popularized through public discourse and social media buzz, celebrity endorsements, and instances that arise in TV shows with a wide audience. We will also detail misinformation mitigation practices to the best of our knowledge and explain why these strategies may or may not be effective in battling health misinformation in popular culture.

Health Misinformation: Impacts and Mechanisms

Misinformation refers to information that contains erroneous arguments not supported by scientific evidence or the consensus of the scientific community (Swire-Thompson & Lazer, 2020). Researchers have diligently examined the factors that make people vulnerable to health misinformation (Ecker et al., 2022; Nan et al., 2022). Limited health knowledge and access to reliable health information certainly comprise contributing factors, but the landscape is far more complex. Healthcare providers no longer serve as the exclusive source of health information in today's digital age. Individuals are constantly bombarded with an overwhelming amount of information from various channels, including user-generated content that has not been vetted by medical professionals or scientists (Swire-Thompson & Lazer, 2020). This deluge makes the lack of adequate health literacy – specifically, the ability to accurately process, interpret, and critically evaluate health information – particularly problematic (Ecker et al., 2022). The situation is further exacerbated by declining public trust in science, governments, health institutions, medical professionals, and mainstream media (Nan et al., 2022).

The rapid spread of health misinformation has far-reaching and detrimental consequences. At the individual level, it can foster ill-informed beliefs and knowledge about critical health issues, leading to poor health decisions and behaviors (Tan et al., 2015). Both the theory of reasoned action (Fishbein & Ajzen, 2009) and the health belief model (Champion & Skinner, 2008) highlight that an array of beliefs and perceptions shape health behaviors regarding a health issue, including perceived risks, social norms, and perceived efficacy to cope with the risks. Exposure to misinformation can distort individuals' appraisals of these important aspects and lead them to act upon these misperceptions, resulting in negative health outcomes.

The adverse impacts of health misinformation can also extend beyond the personal sphere and have broader societal implications. For instance, during the COVID-19 pandemic, widespread misinformation about the coronavirus disease and vaccines contributed to public resistance to risk-mitigation measures and mass vaccination programs (Ferreira Caceres et al., 2022). As such, misinformation posed significant barriers to the effective management of a global public health crisis. Similarly, misinformation surrounding the link between childhood vaccines and autism has had lasting and harmful impacts on public health (Shelby & Ernst, 2013). Despite extensive intervention efforts, the misperceptions popularized by public figures like Andrew Wakefield and some celebrities gave rise to a significant decrease in vaccination rates for diseases like measles, mumps, and rubella (MMR). These inaccurate narratives have not only endangered unvaccinated children but also weakened herd immunity, increasing the chances of outbreaks of these diseases that are preventable and previously well-contained (Lewandowsky et al., 2012). These examples underscore the substantial obstacles presented by misinformation to the effective implementation of beneficial public health programs.

The harms of misinformation are further compounded by the challenges of correcting misbeliefs resulting from misinformation exposure (Huang & Wang, 2022). The social judgment theory emphasizes the profound influence of existing attitudes on audience responses to subsequent persuasive messages (Brehmer, 1988). Rather than forming judgments based on the merits of a persuasive message, individuals tend to compare the information and the advocated position to their pre-existing beliefs. This tendency explains why misinformation correction is often difficult. Individuals holding misbeliefs from misinformation exposure are predisposed to resist correction messages that contradict their views (Ecker et al., 2014). This tendency can be better understood through the lens of cognitive dissonance (Festinger, 1962), which suggests that individuals experience psychological discomfort when encountering inconsistent or conflicting ideas. Faced with correction messages that challenge their existing beliefs, individuals are motivated to either directly avoid these messages through selective exposure (Knobloch-Westerwick et al., 2017) or scrutinize them more critically through selective processing to alleviate their discomfort (Rollwage et al., 2020).

Moreover, literature has underscored another challenge – the "continued influence" of misinformation (Thorson, 2016; Walter & Tukachinsky, 2020). Researchers have found that the adverse effects of misinformation exposure can persist for a long time, even following correction interventions. This lingering influence extends from the cognitive biases stemming from pre-existing misbeliefs, as erasing misinformation stored in long-term memory and replacing it with accurate, factual information can be challenging (Hamby et al., 2020). These difficulties can be better understood through the concept of mental models – frameworks that people use to make sense of the world around them (Lewandowsky et al., 2012). When misinformation fills a part of these mental models, simply erasing it could leave an incomplete and unsettling gap in one's understanding. For example, when individuals believe that vaccines cause autism – a frequently corrected but persistent myth – simply presenting the correct information may not be sufficient to modify their overall mental models regarding childhood vaccines. Consequently, even after exposure to corrections, these mental models containing misinformation would be automatically retrieved when related topics come up again. This process undermines the efficacy of correction efforts and highlights the complex challenges in changing deeply rooted misbeliefs.

Health Misinformation Disseminated on Social Media

Social media has increasingly been used to disseminate health information, share resources and tips related to health, and normalize the experiences of living with certain health conditions (see, e.g., Chen & Wang, 2021). While social media opens the door for the public to become information creators and empowers ordinary individuals in health-related communication, who are often disadvantaged in the traditional hierarchical physician–patient structure, the entry of non-healthcare professionals into the authorship of health information also leads to a wide variation in the quality of health information that can be retrieved from social media platforms. For example, accumulated empirical evidence suggests that social media contributed significantly to the infodemic during the COVID-19 pandemic and vaccine hesitancy (Skafle et al., 2022), with widespread health misinformation on platforms such as Twitter, YouTube, and Facebook (Skafle et al., 2022; A. W. K. Yeung et al., 2022).

Recently, TikTok, a platform used to share short videos, has frequently spread health misinformation (Tam et al., 2022; Waterton & Lipner, 2023; A. Yeung et al., 2022). Using the same keywords to retrieve top videos about urinary tract infection on YouTube and TikTok, Tam categorized 94% of videos from YouTube as educational/informational as opposed to only 42% from TikTok. In contrast, Tam coded 4% from YouTube and 30% from TikTok as humor/entertainment. Notably, videos coded as humor/entertainment contained more misinformation than other categories. Waterton and Lipner echoed these concerns about TikTok health misinformation, and they suggested health professionals should advise their patients not to rely on TikTok for health recommendations.

Montag et al. (2021) characterized TikTok as a social media platform, particularly famous for its function allowing lip-sync videos – a type of short video where users can perform playback videos of diverse pop songs. According to Montag et al., typical TikTok users are young individuals who may not be concerned about the consequences of self-disclosure. Primary motivations for using TikTok include finding funny or entertaining videos and filling up spare time ("TikTok Usage Motivations according to U.S. and U.K. Users 2020, n.d.). We suggest that the widespread health misinformation on social media platforms might have emerged due to the variability of information creators with varying levels of health knowledge and motivations, coupled with the platforms' reluctance to detect and correct health misinformation. Of practical importance, users considering relying on health-related information on social media platforms need to understand the nature of these platforms and their fellow users as information sources.

Health Misinformation Conveyed through Memes

Among various forms of user-generated content circulated on social media, memes are worth discussing as they have become a popular way of spreading health misinformation. For instance, during the COVID-19 pandemic, a circulated meme derived from the music video for Canadian rapper Drake's "Hotline Bling" conveyed misinformation about the virus and the vaccine. The meme featured two images of Drake, one expressing disapproval and the other approval, arranged vertically on the left side. The accompanying text on the right criticized the idea of taking a vaccine for a virus with a 99.97% recovery rate. This claim was inaccurate as the recovery rate surpassed known statistics and failed to account for both short- and long-term COVID-19-associated morbidity. The meme also asserted that the vaccine was experimental and from a corrupt industry and that it would alter DNA without any liability, a claim contradictory to known scientific facts (Goodman & Carmichael, 2020). Another viral meme portrayed Bill Gates dressed as the Joker, embodying the well-known characteristics associated with a menacing appearance, evoking a sense of threat, coldness, and chaos. The image included green hair, pale skin, dark eyes, wide and bloody red lips, and a purple suit. He held a needle resembling a weapon, and at the bottom of the image, three computer keys – "Ctrl Alt Delete" – were labeled, suggesting an analogy between vaccines and a computer shutdown. According to Goodman and Carmichael, the meme included a red label reading "scaremongering."

To understand how memes work to spread health misinformation and influence individuals' beliefs and opinions, it is useful to start the inquiries about what memes are and what characteristics memes have. Memes refer to a form of colorful and concise communication, often involving short videos and images. They present symbols well-known in popular culture, indicating culturally shared interpretations through humor. According to Shifman (2013), memes were initially introduced as cultural units that may include catchphrases, melodies, and other forms, but through an analogy with genes. Shifman explained that, like genes, people spread memes through "copying or imitation" (p. 363), and memes that fit the sociocultural environment spread more widely while others that do not fit will gradually disappear. Imitation suggests that memes are repeated among a group with or without slight alterations. The repetition indicates how memes presenting misinformation may influence people. According to the illusory truth effect, repetition can increase the perceived truth of claims, regardless of their veracity (Morgan & Cappella, 2023; Udry & Barber, 2023), perhaps because repetition increases familiarity, and familiarity can be treated as an indicator of accuracy (Foster et al., 2012). Researchers have determined the effects of repetition as more pronounced for false than true information (Morgan & Cappella, 2023) and when the claims are not so well-known (Udry & Barber, 2023).

Not only does repetition influence the ease of retrieving the presented misinformation, but memes are also characterized by their deep roots in popular culture, further facilitating information retrieval and processing. As Milner (2013) defined, memes are "multimodal artifacts remixed by countless participants, employing popular culture for public commentary" (p. 2357). While memes can take various forms, contemporary memes often employ video and image formats. Molina (2023) stated that memes delivering misinformation may be easily believed as truth since the imagery activates the realism heuristic, making the information seem credible due to the realistic visual presentation.

In addition to the characteristics of memes that enable them to exert a profound influence on information retrieval and familiarity, facilitating judgment about the perceived truth of the information, memes also serve to solidify in-group cohesion (Harvey et al., 2019). Kahan et al. (2017) found that memes have a unique function of reinforcing in-group membership and stigmatizing another. An example could be the well-known contemptuous message associated with HPV vaccine mandates, stating, "They value your virginity more than your life," or the pro-vaccine meme featuring two women in tea party outfits, where one commented "I hate the term anti-vax. It is so negative," and the other responded, "How about pro-disease." These memes illustrate the dual functions of reinforcing an idea when circulated among like-minded individuals within the same membership and prejudicing against out-groups. As a result of consuming these memes, individuals will generate an identity-protective cognition regarding risks and benefits, fusing affect and identity (Kahan et al., 2017). This response appears to explain well how the information processing of memes and motivated reasoning are connected. Motivated reasoning, a cognitive process in which individuals tend to favorably process information that aligns with their preexisting beliefs while unfavorably processing conflicting views, often explains why people accept misinformation and persist in believing it even after being corrected (Lewandowsky et al., 2012).

While memes often spread rumors and misinformation, health professionals have also entered the realm of meme creation to compete for attention, aiming to promote accurate health beliefs. For example, the Baltimore City Health Department used exact images from Drake's Hotline Bling music video, as mentioned earlier, to disseminate information about social distancing during the COVID-19 pandemic ("Baltimore City Gets in the Meme Game with Drake's "Hotline Bling" to Encourage Social Distancing," 2020). Despite using the exact same images, the accompanying messages differed. Beside the disapproval image, where the rapper conveyed a negative stance in the music video, the message read "Having a cookout with all of your friends and relatives." In contrast, beside the approval image, where the rapper displayed pleasure and agreement, it stated "Having a cookout with just the people you live with." The effects of utilizing memes for disseminating accurate health information warrant further empirical investigations.

Health Misinformation in Media and Entertainment

Health information presented in media and entertainment has often been used by the public to understand health issues. Many individuals, for instance, acquire cancer information from television programs and consider it as trustworthy as information provided by physicians (Thomas et al., 2018). Due to their wide reach and profound impact, when these media deliver incorrect health information accidentally or purposefully, the consequences could be significant. For instance, *Catalyst*, a television program that aired in Australia, once questioned the link between high cholesterol levels and cardiovascular disease as well as the use of statins for treatment. Schaffer et al. (2015) determined a correlation between the program and a temporary increase in discontinuation and a sustained decrease in statins use. The controversial episodes were later removed due to violations against impartiality standards (Meade, 2014; Schaffer et al., 2015).

In addition to partial or inaccurate claims, health misinformation in media and entertainment may manifest through inappropriate or oversimplified metaphors. Many scholars have observed that epidemics of fictional viruses are increasingly popular in movies, TV shows, science fiction, and many other forms of popular media (Kendal, 2021; Schweitzer, 2019). This trend is evident in zombie narratives, where shows depict viruses as dehumanizing individuals into brainless monsters. Another common theme comprises the outbreak narrative, which typically tells a story about a virus introduced to the developed world from low- or middle-income countries (Kendal, 2021). While these narratives are fictional, the horror portrayed towards a health threat, combined with the depiction of the virus originating from a distant and underdeveloped world, creates an image of uncontrollable danger. Such an image could trigger anxiety when facing a public health threat. Moreover, it perpetuates stereotypes that further disadvantage poorer nations.

While some analyses have shown improvements in claim accuracy, indicating that the majority of the content in medical dramas is accurate within reasons (Ismail & Salama, 2023) or that exposure to medical dramas increases audience's topical knowledge (Sisson et al., 2021), fictional portrayals often overrepresent rare diseases or reduce the depiction of medical procedures that do not facilitate the narrative flow or increase audience enjoyment (see, e.g., Cowley et al., 2017). For instance, Cowley et al. determined that fictional health care providers only checked on a patient's allergy status 6% of the time when dispensing medication, which, in practice, should be a routine procedure. Analyzing patient profiles in *Grey's Anatomy* and comparing them with those from the National Trauma Databank (NTDB), Serrone et al. (2018) found higher rates of mortality on the show (22% vs. 7% NTDB) but hospital stays were much shorter for severely injured survivors (50% portrayed to have a stay of less than 1 week vs. 20% in NTDB). The data patterns explain well how sensational medical dramas can be in portraying injuries, illnesses, and diseases (see Chapter 12, this volume, on medical errors). To avoid potential mistakes that may perpetuate incorrect health information, credible organizations have established programs to provide quick facts and tips to scriptwriters (Hollywood, Health & Society, n.d.; see also Chapter 17, this volume). However, notably, for entertainment media programs to avoid communicating misinformation, it is not sufficient to merely back up each isolated claim with evidence. Shows must also present a comprehensive rather than a partial picture, including ensuring that representations of health conditions and patients correspond to the statistics of prevalence, incidence, morbidity, mortality, vulnerable groups, and other factual information associated with a health condition. It also entails avoiding misleading oversimplifications and providing appropriate health recommendations, including correct responsibility attributions.

Celebrity-Endorsed Health Misinformation

Celebrity-endorsed health misinformation is not only prevalent during epidemics, when people encounter greater uncertainty and tend to follow someone they admire, but also in industries closely related to celebrities' lives. Such misinformation occurs, for example, in celebrities' endorsement of detox tea, including Cardi B, Kylie Jenner, Nicki Minaj, Britney Spears, to name a few, which they label as magic, despite the products lacking support from scientific evidence (Tinker & Moulite, 2018). The same happens to elite athletes, such as baseball superstar Max Scherzer, advocating stem cell treatments while experts state that "there's really not much evidence that it's going to help … other than a psychological boost or as a placebo effect" (Szabo, 2019). Nevertheless, the endorsement of body-shape related products by celebrities and the promotion of injury treatments by athletes not only come across as personal anecdotes but also carry an air of authenticity and credibility.

We offer a few explanations of why celebrities often impact the public. Celebrity culture encompasses the extensive attention that celebrities receive from the public, primarily due to heightened media attention. As the theory of herd behavior suggests, people tend to imitate what others do in a similar situation (Hoffman & Tan, 2015). Celebrities, who are often the early adopters of technology and scientific advancement, create larger information cascades and influence a great many people's choices. In social media, celebrities function as the higher-level nodes in their social networks (Alatif et al., 2021). According to Alatif et al., their tweets, for example, likely receive more prominence on Twitter due to algorithms based on engagement metrics such as retweeting, liking, posting, and sharing, leading to a broader dissemination and the creation of larger information cascades. Such prominence may also flavor public perceptions of social norms, including injunctive norms, perceptions about what other people think we should do, and descriptive norms, perceptions about what other people important to us are actually engaged in doing (Myrick & Erlichman, 2020). Prior research suggests that bandwagon cues in social media posts, such as the aggregated positive ratings due to celebrities' popularity effects, prompt individuals to conform with the favorable evaluations by other social media users, causing individuals consider the posts credible even when the posts contain health misinformation (Shin et al., 2022; S. Wang et al., 2023). Of course, bandwagon cues, signaling social validation, can, in fact, outweigh individuals' initial skepticism about information and guide credibility evaluations (Mena et al., 2020).

Second, a halo effect associated with celebrity endorsement of health misinformation can emerge. Celebrities have "a huge culture footprint" (p. 383) that shapes their followers' identity packages (Caulfield, 2016). Many celebrity endorsements involve not-so-healthy foods or medical advice, such as energy-dense and nutrient-poor products (Bragg et al., 2013). Consumers, on the other hand, tend to perceive professional athletes as healthy and consider athlete-endorsed food and beverages as healthy too (Dixon et al., 2011). Audiences also extend their beliefs to arrive at an implausible sense of credibility, regardless of whether celebrities have any experience with the products or medical advice they are endorsing. A halo effect occurs when a person's exceptional ability in one domain influences perceptions of competence in other domains (Hoffman & Tan, 2015). For example, trusting COVID-19 vaccine information advocated by celebrities might be a good example of the halo effect, considering that most celebrities are not necessarily experts in infectious diseases and public health (Honora et al., 2022).

Third, celebrity influence may extend from identification with the celebrity or a perceived parasocial relationship (for related work, please see Beck, 2022; Beck et al., 2015; see also Chapter 15, this volume). Beck asserted in her analysis of celebrities and Covid-19 that, as audiences feel more involved with and connected to a celebrity, they may experience more emotional responses toward celebrity-endorsed misinformation. Emotional responses, ranging from inspiration as a natural response to celebrity involvement to negative emotions, often have a significant influence on (mis) information dissemination and biased processing (Nanath et al., 2022). Studies have documented that emotion-laden or emotion-evoking information is more likely to be disseminated regardless of its accuracy, possibly due to its ease of drawing attention and that emotional arousal increases people's willingness to share (mis)information (Lee et al., 2023; Lewandowsky et al., 2012; R. Wang et al., 2020; Weeks, 2015). Moreover, when people are driven by strong emotions such as anxiety and anger, they are more susceptible to the influence of disinformation and misinformation provided to them (Lee et al., 2023; Myrick & Erlichman, 2020; Weeks, 2015).

Importantly, celebrities do not always deliver or endorse health misinformation themselves, but others can employ celebrities as a persuasion tactic to promote health mis/disinformation due to the public attention they draw. Right after American football star Damar Hamlin's collapse on the field in the game between the Buffalo Bills and the Cincinnati Bengals, claims about the collapse spurred on the Internet, suggesting that Hamlin collapsed because of the COVID-19 vaccine (Fichera, 2023). For instance, former Newsmax correspondent Emerald Robinson tweeted that "[e]verybody knows what happened to Damar Hamlin because it's happened to too many athletes around the world since COVID vaccination was required in sports" (Zakrzewski & Weber, 2023, para. 4). Similarly, Georgia congresswoman Marjorie Taylor Greene tweeted that "[b]efore the covid vaccines we didn't see athletes dropping dead on the playing field like we do now … Time to investigate the covid vaccines" (Wendling & Schraer, 2023, para. 3). However, to date, doctors have never attributed Hamlin's incident to the COVID-19 vaccine (Merschel, 2023), and unexplained deaths caused by cardiac arrest certainly happened to athletes before the pandemic (Wendling & Schraer, 2023). However, such incidents gave misinformation spreaders opportunities to employ their misinformation rhetoric. Anti-vaccine activities have used pre-established narratives to create the noise while the scientific evidence often comes later than the misinformation has already prevailed (Hagen, 2023). Such misinformation could impact the public through many above-mentioned celebrity influence mechanisms due to celebrities' popularity effect, and the identification and connection people may feel with celebrities.

Current Efforts in Mitigating the Impact of Health Misinformation in Popular Culture

As misinformation becomes more prevalent, efforts to mitigate the adverse effects of misinformation have also received increased attention. In this section, we discuss several commonly employed strategies for mitigating misinformation, including fact-checking, using expert sources, algorithmic correction interventions, compelling narrative rebuttals, and educational programs focusing on literacy and inoculation. While empirical studies have examined these approaches, not all of them have been employed to counteract health misinformation in popular culture. We explore the unique opportunities that these strategies offer in mitigating the influence of health misinformation in popular culture.

Fact-Checking. Fact-checking refers to a rigorous process of verifying statements and claims against credible sources, data, and expert opinions to establish their accuracy and/or pinpoint their fallacies (Graves et al., 2016). It serves as an important tool for combating misinformation, serving as a way of quality control or gatekeeping of the information disseminated in public space. Social media users may accept popular claims they encounter as truth without further verification (Knoll & Matthes, 2016). A timely fact-check can reach social media users and offer an evidence-based counterargument, contrasting popular false claims with facts and scientific evidence.

When it comes to celebrity-endorsed misinformation, the potential for reputational damage could serve as a powerful incentive for celebrities to reconsider and possibly retract their false claims (Nyhan & Reifler, 2015). One notable example involves actress Jessica Biel, who faced public scrutiny after lobbying with Robert F. Kennedy Jr., a vocal critic of vaccine mandates, against a bill in California that would tighten medical exemptions for vaccines (Burke, 2019). Responding to widespread media coverage and international headlines, she clarified her position on Instagram, stating that she was "not against vaccination." Instead, she supported "children getting vaccinations" and "families having the right to make educated medical decisions for their children alongside their physicians."

Although scholarly research has presented mixed empirical evidence regarding the efficacy of fact-checking (Ma et al., 2022), particularly considering the influence of audience biases such as partisanship (Freiling et al., 2021), the value of fact-checking should not be underestimated. Public fact-checking can establish a norm of accountability and responsibility, sending a clear message that misleading statements are always under public scrutiny, regardless of who has made them. The reputational risk and cost can act as a warning signal, urging public figures and social media users to exercise greater caution in their public statements and discouraging them from spreading misinformation in the public sphere.

Leveraging Expert Sources. Health Communication research has paid considerable attention to the influence of different information sources on audiences' perceptions and reception of health messages (Hu & Sundar, 2009). Despite the increasingly diversified sources and fragmented channels for health information online, public health agencies and medical professionals continue to be viewed as the most trustworthy and authoritative sources of reliable health information (Huang & Liu, 2021). Medical authorities remain the go-to sources for the public seeking health guidance. Their credibility positions them uniquely in the efforts of misinformation correction. Scholarly research has supported this notion, demonstrating that correction messages from medical experts work effectively in reducing public misperceptions and susceptibility to health misinformation (Vraga & Bode, 2017).

Therefore, expert sources may play a significant role in combating health misinformation in popular culture. We should increase awareness among social media users that non-expert sources may not provide correct health recommendations. Additionally, it may be necessary to remind fans about the possibility that they don't accurately evaluate the credibility of celebrities' health-related claims due to the halo effect. Despite their popularity and massive influence, celebrities typically lack the expertise needed to convey medical information. When they spread false claims, an immediate and public rebuttal from a reputable medical source can provide a powerful counterpoint. The authoritative weight of these medical sources lends the correction a layer of credibility that is difficult to ignore. Consequently, the public could more likely consider the correction message, thereby curbing the spread of misbeliefs.

One example occurred during the COVID-19 pandemic: high-profile figures, like Elon Musk and former President Donald Trump, publicly endorsed hydroxychloroquine as an effective treatment for COVID-19 and a "game-changer," despite insufficient evidence to support its effectiveness (Liu et al., 2020). In response, authoritative medical organizations like the WHO, the U.S. Food and Drug Administration (FDA), and the National Institutes of Health (NIH) issued public statements cautioning against the use of hydroxychloroquine for treating COVID-19 outside of clinical trials or hospitals (Cathey, 2020). These warnings highlighted both the lack of substantial evidence for its efficacy and the potential for severe side effects. Prominent medical experts such as Dr. Anthony Fauci further clarified in media interviews that clinical trials had demonstrated hydroxychloroquine's ineffectiveness in treating COVID-19. These correction efforts from trusted medical sources were instrumental in countering the misinformation and guiding public opinion toward scientifically validated treatments and risk-mitigation measures.

While further empirical research is necessary to quantify the impact of medical experts' correction efforts, we argue that they offer a credible alternative to health misinformation in popular culture. By strategically leveraging expert sources and amplifying their voices in the public discourse, we can mitigate the undesirable influence of health misinformation in popular culture and foster a better-informed public.

Algorithmic Correction. Scholars have also examined the role of algorithms in misinformation correction. Specifically, algorithms can be employed to deliver correction messages to individuals' social media feeds (Bode & Vraga, 2018). These algorithms often label the corrective content with markers such as "people also liked" or "related stories." These labels may serve dual purposes: on the one hand, they imply a form of social consensus or norm by suggesting that many other users have viewed and approved the information (Huang & Wang, 2022); on the other hand, they imply an algorithmic recommendation, adding credibility to the corrective content by leveraging the presumed objectivity and the lack of ideological biases associated with technology (Sundar et al., 2015).

Although these psychological appeals of algorithmic correction have been well-documented, we need further research to assess its effectiveness, particularly in mitigating the impact of popularized misinformation. Considering the functionalities of algorithmic correction, it can be useful for the following reasons. First, misinformation that has been widely circulated and becomes viral often wields considerable influence due to large social media followings (Shin et al., 2022). Algorithms can be programmed to immediately identify and respond to this type of misinformation, acting as a real-time counterforce, and prioritize fact-checked content in the feeds of individuals who have engaged with false posts. Second, algorithms can also be used to target specific demographics or interest groups that are more influenced by accounts that often circulate false information (Betsch, 2014). By delivering tailored correction messages to the targeted audiences, algorithmic correction can enhance the effectiveness of intervention programs. This level of precision allows for a more efficient allocation of campaign resources.

Narrative Rebuttals. Stories or narratives have long been recognized as a fundamental way of human communication and a powerful device for persuasion (de Graaf et al., 2016; Fisher, 1984). Misinformation posts that gain wide acceptance often disseminate health misinformation by incorporating it into personal stories, adding emotional weight to the false claims and making them resonate strongly with the audience (Waszak et al., 2018). The engaging and affect-laden nature of these narratives can not only elicit strong emotional responses but also create lasting memories in the audience. As a countermeasure, researchers recommend employing narrative-based strategies to correct misinformation, proposing that a compelling story may serve as a strong defense against emotionally charged, misleading narratives (Shelby & Ernst, 2013).

The potential of narratives to counteract health misinformation from popular culture remains an area for future research, although existing literature has explored the general effectiveness of narratives in correcting misinformation (Ecker et al., 2020; Shelby & Ernst, 2013). Contrary to the idea that narratives are universally beneficial for correction, empirical findings suggest that their efficacy is influenced by various factors such as message features, correction mechanisms, and individual differences. For example, two-sided narratives are more impactful among individuals who have previous experience with the health issue in question, while one-sided narratives appear to resonate more with those who do not have such prior experience (W. Wang & Huang, 2021). Moreover, narratives delivered via social media algorithms tend to be more effective than those shared by peer users (Huang & Wang, 2022). Additionally, narratives that include a clear refutational statement (referred to as "refutational narratives") are more persuasive when used to preemptively counter misinformation ("prebunking"); whereas simple narratives without an explicit rebuttal are more effective for correction following misinformation exposure ("debunking") (W. Wang & Huang, 2023).

While further research is necessary to understand the nuanced effects of narratives in misinformation correction, narratives offer a promising direction for addressing the specific challenge of high-profile health misinformation from popular culture. By crafting compelling narratives that not only correct misinformation but also emotionally resonate with the target audience, health professionals may offer a more balanced perspective that fosters meaningful public engagement and contributes to more informed health decisions.

Education and Inoculation. The adverse effects of celebrity-endorsed misinformation may be linked to the public's misconception that celebrities are qualified or credible sources of health information (Besalú et al., 2021). The same applies to the incorrect judgment of user-generated health misinformation that is widely circulated on social media. As such, we should design and implement media literacy programs that educate individuals on how to evaluate sources, understand biases, and differentiate reliable health information from misinformation. These programs may specifically address the limitations and potential biases of relying on non-medical sources such as celebrities as credible health sources. They can also highlight the potential of celebrities to mislead the public by creating a strong sense of connection, trust, and social approval (Myrick & Erlichman, 2020). Such education can foster a healthy skepticism in the public, empowering them to challenge false claims spread by public figures or when these false claims are considered true by a great number of social media users. Ideally, these efforts will not only reduce the public's susceptibility to health misinformation but also encourage the responsible sharing of health information.

These education programs may also integrate an inoculation component. The inoculation theory suggests that preemptively exposing individuals to weakened forms of misinformation ahead of time can prepare them to resist its influence in future encounters (Traberg et al., 2022). In light of this notion, education programs may proactively inform individuals about the common types of misinformation that emerge in popular culture, including examples of logical fallacies or biased reasoning often employed to support false claims (Vraga et al., 2019). The ultimate goal of incorporating inoculation is to equip individuals with the critical thinking skills and necessary knowledge required to refute similar misinformation they may encounter in the future. While the efficacy of inoculation is not universal and can be conditioned by factors like timing, message design, and the characteristics of the target audience (Banas & Rains, 2010), this strategy can be a valuable addition to a comprehensive approach to combating health misinformation in popular culture.

Conclusion

Health misinformation in popular culture can yield significant adverse consequences due to its extensive dissemination and profound influence, often resulting in resistance when corrections are attempted. Nevertheless, as we delved into the discussion on health misinformation emerging in various venues of popular culture and its diverse formats, we hoped to gain a better understanding of how to curb the influence of such health misinformation. We explored several mitigation strategies that have undergone scrutiny for their efficacy and examined how they might provide insights into countering health misinformation in popular culture. We cautioned against a one-size-fits-all approach, considering the diverse types of misinformation in popular culture, their unique characteristics, and the underlying causes of their emergence. More empirical research is needed to examine the effectiveness of these misinformation mitigation strategies in reducing the impact of different types of health misinformation within popular culture.

Further Reading

Lewandowsky, S., Ecker, U. K. H., Seifert, C. M., Schwarz, N., & Cook, J. (2012). Misinformation and its correction: Continued influence and successful debiasing. *Psychological Science in the Public Interest, 13*(3), 106–131.

Walter, N., & Tukachinsky, R. (2020). A meta-analytic examination of the continued influence of misinformation in the face of correction: How powerful is it, why does it happen, and how to stop it? *Communication Research, 47*(2), 155–177.

References

Alatif, B., Su, J. T., Wang, M., & Xi, S. (2021). Are you spreading misinformation? Analyzing how influential Twitter users contribute to the spread of COVID-19 information. STEM Fellowship Undergraduate Big Data Challenge. https://xasayi.github.io/files/UnBDC2021.pdf

Baltimore city gets in the meme game with drake's "hotline bling" to encourage social distancing. (2020, May 11). *CBS Baltimore*. https://www.cbsnews.com/baltimore/news/baltimore-city-gets-in-the-meme-game-with-drakes-hotline-bling-to-encourage-social-distancing/

Banas, J. A., & Rains, S. A. (2010). A meta-analysis of research on inoculation theory. *Communication Monographs, 77*(3), 281–311.

Beck, C. S. (2022). *Celebrity in the time of Covid*. McFarland.

Beck, C. S., Chapman, S. A., Simmons, N., Tenzek, K., & Ruhl, S. (2015). *Celebrity health narratives and the public health*. McFarland.

Besalú, R., Pont-Sorribes, C., & Martí, A. (2021). Perceived credibility of tweets by opinion leaders during the COVID-19 pandemic in Spain. *International Journal of Communication Systems, 15*(0), 28.

Betsch, C. (2014). Social media targeting of health messages. A promising approach for research and practice [Review of *Social media targeting of health messages. A promising approach for research and practice*]. *Human Vaccines & Immunotherapeutics, 10*(9), 2636–2637.

Bode, L., & Vraga, E. K. (2018). See something, say something: Correction of global health misinformation on social media. *Health Communication, 33*(9), 1131–1140.

Bragg, M. A., Yanamadala, S., Roberto, C. A., Harris, J. L., & Brownell, K. D. (2013). Athlete endorsements in food marketing. *Pediatrics, 132*(5), 805–810.

Brehmer, B. (1988). The development of social judgment theory. In B. Brehmer & C. R. B. Joyce (Eds.), *Human judgment: The SJT view* (pp. 13–40). North-Holland.

Burke, M. (2019, June 13). Jessica Biel denies she's anti-vaccination after lobbying against California bill. *NBC News*. https://www.nbcnews.com/health/health-news/jessica-biel-denies-she-s-anti-vaccination-after-lobbying-against-n1017171

Cathey, L. (2020, August 8). Timeline: Tracking Trump alongside scientific developments on hydroxychloroquine. *ABC News*. https://abcnews.go.com/Health/timeline-tracking-trump-alongside-scientific-developments-hydroxychloroquine/story?id=72170553

Caulfield, T. (2016). From Kim Kardashian to Dr. Oz: The future relevance of popular culture to our health and health policy. *Ottawa Law Review, 47*(2), 371–392.

Champion, V. L., & Skinner, C. S. (2008). The health belief model. In K. Glanz, B. K. Rimer, & K. Viswanath (Eds.), *Health behaviour and health education: Theory, research, and practice* (4th ed., pp. 67–96). Jossey-Bass.

Chen, J., & Wang, Y. (2021). Social media use for health purposes: Systematic review. *Journal of Medical Internet Research, 23*(5), e17917. https://doi.org/10.2196/17917

Cowley, M., Naunton, M., Thomas, J., Waddington, F., & Peterson, G. M. (2017). Does the "script" need a rewrite? Is medication advice in television medical dramas appropriate? *Journal of Clinical Pharmacy and Therapeutics, 42*(6), 765–773.

de Graaf, A., Sanders, J., & Hoeken, H. (2016). Characteristics of narrative interventions and health effects: A review of the content, form, and context of narratives in health-related narrative persuasion research. *Review of Communication Research*, *4*, 88–131.

Dixon, H., Scully, M., Wakefield, M., Kelly, B., Chapman, K., & Donovan, R. (2011). Parent's responses to nutrient claims and sports celebrity endorsements on energy-dense and nutrient-poor foods: An experimental study. *Public Health Nutrition*, *14*(6), 1071–1079.

Ecker, U. K. H., Butler, L. H., & Hamby, A. (2020). You don't have to tell a story! A registered report testing the effectiveness of narrative versus non-narrative misinformation corrections. *Cognitive Research: Principles and Implications*, *5*, 64. https://doi.org/10.1186/s41235-020-00266-x

Ecker, U. K. H., Lewandowsky, S., Cook, J., Schmid, P., Fazio, L. K., Brashier, N., Kendeou, P., Vraga, E. K., & Amazeen, M. A. (2022). The psychological drivers of misinformation belief and its resistance to correction. *Nature Reviews Psychology*, *1*(1), 13–29.

Ecker, U. K. H., Lewandowsky, S., Fenton, O., & Martin, K. (2014). Do people keep believing because they want to? Preexisting attitudes and the continued influence of misinformation. *Memory & Cognition*, *42*(2), 292–304.

Evanega, S., Lynas, M., Adams, J., & Smolenyak, K. (2020). Coronavirus misinformation: Quantifying sources and themes in the COVID-19 "infodemic." *Alliance for Science*. https://allianceforscience.org/wp-content/uploads/2020/09/Evanega-et-al-Coronavirus-misinformationFINAL.pdf

Ferreira Caceres, M. M., Sosa, J. P., Lawrence, J. A., Sestacovschi, C., Tidd-Johnson, A., Rasool, M. H. U., Gadamidi, V. K., Ozair, S., Pandav, K., Cuevas-Lou, C., Parrish, M., Rodriguez, I., & Fernandez, J. P. (2022). The impact of misinformation on the COVID-19 pandemic. *AIMS Public Health*, *9*(2), 262–277.

Festinger, L. (1962). Cognitive dissonance. *Scientific American*, *207*, 93–102.

Fichera, A. (2023, January 18). CNN didn't publish story linking Damar Hamlin collapse to vaccine. *AP News*. https://apnews.com/article/fact-check-cnn-headline-damar-hamlin-covid-vaccine-715865760728

Fishbein, M., & Ajzen, I. (2009). *Predicting and changing behavior: The reasoned action approach*. Psychology Press.

Fisher, W. R. (1984). Narration as a human communication paradigm: The case of public moral argument. *Communication Monographs*, *51*, 122.

Foster, J. L., Huthwaite, T., Yesberg, J. A., Garry, M., & Loftus, E. F. (2012). Repetition, not number of sources, increases both susceptibility to misinformation and confidence in the accuracy of eyewitnesses. *Acta Psychologica*, *139*(2), 320–326.

Freiling, I., Krause, N. M., Scheufele, D. A., & Brossard, D. (2021). Believing and sharing misinformation, fact-checks, and accurate information on social media: The role of anxiety during COVID-19. *New Media & Society*, 25(1), 141–162. doi: 10.1177/14614448211011451

Frenkel, S., Alba, D., & Zhong, R. (2020, March 8). Surge of virus misinformation stumps facebook and twitter. *The New York Times*. https://www.nytimes.com/2020/03/08/technology/coronavirus-misinformation-social-media.html

Goodman, J., & Carmichael, F. (2020, November 29). Covid-19: What's the harm of "funny" anti-vaccine memes? *BBC News*. https://www.bbc.com/news/55101238

Graves, L., Nyhan, B., & Reifler, J. (2016). Understanding innovations in journalistic practice: A field experiment examining motivations for fact-checking. *The Journal of Communication*, *66*(1), 102–138.

Hagen, L. (2023, January 10). How Damar Hamlin's collapse fueled anti-vaccine conspiracy theories. *NPR*. https://www.npr.org/2023/01/10/1147969504/how-damar-hamlins-collapse-fueled-anti-vaccine-conspiracy-theories

Hamby, A., Ecker, U., & Brinberg, D. (2020). How stories in memory perpetuate the continued influence of false information. *Journal of Consumer Psychology*, *30*(2), 240–259.

Harvey, A. M., Thompson, S., Lac, A., & Coolidge, F. L. (2019). Fear and derision: A quantitative content analysis of provaccine and antivaccine internet memes. *Health Education & Behavior*, *46*(6), 1012–1023.

Hoffman, S. J., & Tan, C. (2015). Biological, psychological and social processes that explain celebrities' influence on patients' health-related behaviors. *Archives of Public Health*, *73*, 3. https://doi.org/10.1186/2049-3258-73-3

Hollywood, Health & Society (n.d.). Tip sheets. https://hollywoodhealthandsociety.org/tip-sheets/

Honora, A., Wang, K.-Y., & Chih, W.-H. (2022). How does information overload about COVID-19 vaccines influence individuals' vaccination intentions? The roles of cyberchondria, perceived risk, and vaccine skepticism. *Computers in Human Behavior*, *130*, 107176.

Huang, Y., & Liu, W. (2021). Promoting COVID-19 vaccination: The interplay of message framing, psychological uncertainty, and public agency as a message source. *Science Communication*, *44*(1), 3–29.

Huang, Y., & Wang, W. (2022). When a story contradicts: Correcting health misinformation on social media through different message formats and mechanisms. *Information, Communication and Society*, *25*(8), 1192–1209.

Hu, Y., & Sundar, S. (2009). Effects of online health sources on credibility and behavioral intentions. *Communication Research, 37*(1), 105–132.

Ismail, I. I., & Salama, S. (2023). Depiction of nervous system disorders in television medical drama: A content analysis of 18 seasons of Grey's Anatomy. *Clinical Neurology and Neurosurgery, 224*, 107569. https://doi.org/10.1016/j.clineuro.2022.107569

Kahan, D. M., Jamieson, K. H., Landrum, A., & Winneg, K. (2017). Culturally antagonistic memes and the Zika virus: An experimental test. *Journal of Risk Research, 20*(1), 1–40.

Kendal, E. (2021). Public health crises in popular media: How viral outbreak films affect the public's health literacy. *Medical Humanities, 47*(1), 11–19.

Knobloch-Westerwick, S., Mothes, C., & Polavin, N. (2017). Confirmation bias, ingroup bias, and negativity bias in selective exposure to political information. *Communication Research, 47*(1), 104–124.

Knoll, J., & Matthes, J. (2016). The effectiveness of celebrity endorsements: A meta-analysis. *Journal of the Academy of Marketing Science, 45*(1), 55–75.

Lee, J., Hameleers, M., & Shin, S. Y. (2023). The emotional effects of multimodal disinformation: How multimodality, issue relevance, and anxiety affect misperceptions about the flu vaccine. *New Media & Society, Online First*. https://doi.org/10.1177/14614448231153959

Lewandowsky, S., Ecker, U. K. H., Seifert, C. M., Schwarz, N., & Cook, J. (2012). Misinformation and its correction: Continued influence and successful debiasing. *Psychological Science in the Public Interest, 13*(3), 106–131.

Liu, M., Caputi, T. L., Dredze, M., Kesselheim, A. S., & Ayers, J. W. (2020). Internet searches for unproven COVID-19 therapies in the United States. *JAMA Internal Medicine, 180*(8), 1116–1118.

Ma, S., Bergan, D., Ahn, S., Carnahan, D., Gimby, N., McGraw, J., & Virtue, I. (2022). Fact-checking as a deterrent? A conceptual replication of the influence of fact-checking on the sharing of misinformation by political elites. *Human Communication Research, 49*(3), 321–338.

Meade, A. (2014, May 12). ABC takes down catalyst heart disease episodes after review criticism. *The Guardian*. https://www.theguardian.com/media/2014/may/12/abc-takes-down-catalyst-heart-disease-episodes-after-review-criticism

Mena, P., Barbe, D., & Chan-Olmsted, S. (2020). Misinformation on instagram: The impact of trusted endorsements on message credibility. *Social Media + Society, 6*(2), 2056305120935102. https://doi.org/10.1177/2056305120935102

Merschel, M. (2023, April 18). What is commotio cordis, which NFL player Damar Hamlin says stopped his heart? https://www.heart.org/en/news/2023/04/18/what-is-commotio-cordis-which-nfl-player-damar-hamlin-says-stopped-his-heart

Milner, R. M. (2013). Pop polyvocality: Internet memes, public participation, and the occupy wall street movement. *International Journal of Communication, 7*, 2357–2390.

Molina, M. D. (2023). Do people believe in misleading information disseminated via memes? The role of identity and anger. *New Media & Society, Online First*. https://doi.org/10.1177/14614448231186061

Montag, C., Yang, H., & Elhai, J. D. (2021). On the psychology of TikTok use: A first glimpse from empirical findings. *Frontiers in Public Health, 9*, 641673. https://doi.org/10.3389/fpubh.2021.641673

Morgan, J. C., & Cappella, J. N. (2023). The effect of repetition on the perceived truth of tobacco-related health misinformation among U.S. adults. *Journal of Health Communication, 28*(3), 182–189.

Myrick, J. G., & Erlichman, S. (2020). How audience involvement and social norms foster vulnerability to celebrity-based dietary misinformation. *Psychology of Popular Media, 9*(3), 367–379.

Nanath, K., Kaitheri, S., Malik, S., & Mustafa, S. (2022). Examination of fake news from a viral perspective: An interplay of emotions, resonance, and sentiments. *Journal of Systems and Information Technology, 24*(2), 131–155.

Nan, X., Wang, Y., & Thier, K. (2022). Why do people believe health misinformation and who is at risk? A systematic review of individual differences in susceptibility to health misinformation. *Social Science & Medicine, 314*, 115398. https://doi.org/10.1016/j.socscimed.2022.115398

Nyhan, B., & Reifler, J. (2015). The effect of fact-checking on elites: A field experiment on U.S. state legislators. *American Journal of Political Science, 59*(3), 628–640.

Rollwage, M., Loosen, A., Hauser, T. U., Moran, R., Dolan, R. J., & Fleming, S. M. (2020). Confidence drives a neural confirmation bias. *Nature Communications, 11*(1), 1–11.

Ruiz, J. B., & Bell, R. A. (2021). Predictors of intention to vaccinate against COVID-19: Results of a nationwide survey. *Vaccine, 39*(7), 1080–1086.

Schaffer, A. L., Buckley, N. A., Dobbins, T. A., Banks, E., & Pearson, S.-A. (2015). The crux of the matter: Did the ABC's catalyst program change statin use in Australia? *The Medical Journal of Australia, 202*(11), 591–595.

Schweitzer, D. (2019). *Going viral: Zombies, viruses, and the end of the world.* Rutgers University Press.
Serrone, R. O., Weinberg, J. A., Goslar, P. W., Wilkinson, E. P., Thompson, T. M., Dameworth, J. L., Dempsey, S. R., & Petersen, S. R. (2018). Grey's anatomy effect: Television portrayal of patients with trauma may cultivate unrealistic patient and family expectations after injury. *Trauma Surgery & Acute Care Open*, *3*(1), 1–4. https://doi.org/10.1136/tsaco-2017-000137
Shelby, A., & Ernst, K. (2013). Story and science: How providers and parents can utilize storytelling to combat anti-vaccine misinformation. *Human Vaccines & Immunotherapeutics*, *9*(8), 1795–1801.
Shifman, L. (2013). Memes in a digital world: Reconciling with a conceptual troublemaker. *Journal of Computer-Mediated Communication*, *18*(3), 362–377.
Shin, I., Wang, L., & Lu, Y.-T. (2022). Twitter and endorsed (fake) news: The influence of endorsement by strong ties, celebrities, and a user majority on credibility of fake news during the COVID-19 pandemic. *International Journal of Communication*, *16*, 2573–2595.
Sisson, G., Walter, N., Herold, S., & Brooks, J. J. (2021). Prime-time abortion on Grey's Anatomy: What do US viewers learn from fictional portrayals of abortion on television? *Perspectives on Sexual and Reproductive Health*, *53*(1–2), 13–22.
Skafle, I., Nordahl-Hansen, A., Quintana, D. S., Wynn, R., & Gabarron, E. (2022). Misinformation about COVID-19 vaccines on social media: Rapid review. *Journal of Medical Internet Research*, *24*(8), e37367. https://doi.org/10.2196/37367
Sundar, S., Jia, H., Franklin Waddell, T., & Huang, Y. (2015). Toward a theory of interactive media effects (TIME). In S. Sundar (Ed.), *The handbook of the psychology of communication technology* (pp. 47–86). John Wiley & Sons, Ltd.
Swire-Thompson, B., & Lazer, D. (2020). Public health and online misinformation: Challenges and recommendations. *Annual Review of Public Health*, *41*, 433–451.
Szabo, L. (2019, August 2). Superstar athletes popularize unproven stem cell procedures. *The Washington Post*. https://www.washingtonpost.com/health/2019/08/02/superstar-athletes-popularize-unproven-stem-cell-procedures/
Tam, J., Porter, E. K., & Lee, U. J. (2022). Examination of information and misinformation about urinary tract infections on TikTok and YouTube. *Urology*, *168*, 35–40.
Tan, A. S. L., Lee, C.-J., & Chae, J. (2015). Exposure to health (mis) information: Lagged effects on young adults' health behaviors and potential pathways. *Journal of Communication*, *65*(4), 674–698.
The Associated Press. (2021, September 16). The White House offered to answer Nicki Minaj's COVID vaccine questions, not a visit. *NPR*. https://www.npr.org/2021/09/16/1037832909/nicki-minaj-covid-vaccine-side-effects-white-house
Thomas, J., Peterson, G. M., Walker, E., Christenson, J. K., Cowley, M., Kosari, S., Baby, K. E., & Naunton, M. (2018). Fake news: Medicines misinformation by the media. *Clinical Pharmacology and Therapeutics*, *104*(6), 1059–1061.
Thorson, E. (2016). Belief echoes: The persistent effects of corrected misinformation. *Political Communication*, *33*(3), 460-480.
TikTok usage motivations according to U.S. and UK users 2020. (n.d.). Statista. https://www.statista.com/statistics/1179080/tiktok-reasons-use-app/
Tinker, B., & Moulite, M. (2018, August 14). Can "detox teas" like Teami help you lose weight? *CNN*. https://www.cnn.com/2018/08/14/health/detox-tea-explainer/index.html
Traberg, C. S., Roozenbeek, J., & van der Linden, S. (2022). Psychological inoculation against misinformation: Current evidence and future directions. *The Annals of the American Academy of Political and Social Science*, *700*(1), 136–151.
Udry, J., & Barber, S. J. (2023). The illusory truth effect: A review of how repetition increases belief in misinformation. *Current Opinion in Psychology*, *56*, 101736. https://doi.org/10.1016/j.copsyc.2023.101736
Vraga, E. K., & Bode, L. (2017). Using expert sources to correct health misinformation in social media. *Science Communication*, *39*(5), 621–645.
Vraga, E. K., Kim, S. C., & Cook, J. (2019). Testing logic-based and humor-based corrections for science, health, and political misinformation on social media. *Journal of Broadcasting & Electronic Media*, *63*(3), 393–414.
Walter, N., & Tukachinsky, R. (2020). A meta-analytic examination of the continued influence of misinformation in the face of correction: How powerful is it, why does it happen, and how to stop it? *Communication Research*, *47*(2), 155–177.
Wang, R., He, Y., Xu, J., & Zhang, H. (2020). Fake news or bad news? Toward an emotion-driven cognitive dissonance model of misinformation diffusion. *Asian Journal of Communication*, *30*(5), 317–342.
Wang, S., Chu, T. H., & Huang, G. (2023). Do bandwagon cues affect credibility perceptions? A meta-analysis of the experimental evidence. *Communication Research*, *50*(6), 720–744.

Wang, W., & Huang, Y. (2021). Countering the "harmless E-cigarette" myth: The interplay of message format, message sidedness, and prior experience with e-cigarette use in misinformation correction. *Science Communication, 43*(2), 170–198.

Wang, W., & Huang, Y. (2023). Comparing the effects of simple and refutational narratives in misinformation correction: The moderating roles of correction placement and issue involvement. *Public Understanding of Science, 32*(8), 985–1002.

Waszak, P. M., Kasprzycka-Waszak, W., & Kubanek, A. (2018). The spread of medical fake news in social media – The pilot quantitative study. *Health Policy and Technology, 7*(2), 115–118.

Waterton, K. A., & Lipner, S. R. (2023). Truth or trend–misinformation spreading fast on TikTok: A cross-sectional analysis of onychomycosis content. *Skin Appendage Disorders, 9*(6), 444–448.

Weeks, B. E. (2015). Emotions, partisanship, and misperceptions: How anger and anxiety moderate the effect of partisan bias on susceptibility to political misinformation. *The Journal of Communication, 65*(4), 699–719.

Wendling, M., & Schraer, R. (2023, January 4). Damar Hamlin: How anti-vaxxers exploited player's collapse. *BBC*. https://www.bbc.com/news/world-us-canada-64158202

World Health Organization (2023). Managing the COVID-19 infodemic: Promoting healthy behaviours and mitigating the harm from misinformation and disinformation. https://www.who.int/news/item/23-09-2020-managing-the-covid-19-infodemic-promoting-healthy-behaviours-and-mitigating-the-harm-from-misinformation-and-disinformation

Yeung, A., Ng, E., & Abi-Jaoude, E. (2022). TikTok and Attention-Deficit/Hyperactivity Disorder: A cross-sectional study of social media content quality. *Canadian Journal of Psychiatry, 67*(12), 899–906.

Yeung, A. W. K., Tosevska, A., Klager, E., Eibensteiner, F., Tsagkaris, C., Parvanov, E. D., Nawaz, F. A., Völkl-Kernstock, S., Schaden, E., Kletecka-Pulker, M., Willschke, H., & Atanasov, A. G. (2022). Medical and health-related misinformation on social media: Bibliometric study of the scientific literature. *Journal of Medical Internet Research, 24*(1), e28152. https://doi.org/10.2196/28152

Zakrzewski, C., & Weber, L. (2023, January 3). Covid misinformation spikes in wake of Damar Hamlin's on-field collapse. *The Washington Post*. https://www.washingtonpost.com/technology/2023/01/03/covid-misinfo-damar-hamlin-collapse/

Zhao, S., Hu, S., Zhou, X., Song, S., Wang, Q., Zheng, H., Zhang, Y., & Hou, Z. (2023). The prevalence, features, influencing factors, and solutions for COVID-19 vaccine misinformation: Systematic review. *JMIR Public Health and Surveillance, 9*, e40201. https://doi.org/10.2196/40201

12

POP CULTURE AND MEDICAL ERRORS

Heather J. Carmack

Patient safety focuses on the *misuse*, *underuse*, and/or *overuse* of medical care when treating patients (Carmack, 2022). Patient safety policies and practices typically focus on four major adverse events: falls and injuries, hospital-acquired infections, hospital readmissions, and the most prevalent event – the medical error. Medical error-related deaths account for approximately 250,000 patient deaths, or 10% of all deaths, in the United States (Makary & Daniel, 2016). Pre-COVID, medical error-related deaths comprised the third leading cause of death in the US (James, 2013). The Joint Commission (2012) estimated that approximately 80% of medical errors result from miscommunication or poor communication, making medical errors an important health communication phenomenon for communication scholars.

Communication research about medical errors is still a growing area, but the research that has been conducted mainly focuses on the patient-provider interaction and the disclosure of medical errors to patients and families. Providers who have been given the opportunity to disclose medical errors report positive feelings, seeing the disclosure and apology process as a cathartic learning experience (Carmack, 2010a, 2014). The disclosure and apology process shows patients that providers have empathy for them (Hannawa, 2017; Nazione & Pace, 2015). Patients' desire for providers to feel remorseful for the event is often even more meaningful than knowing about the error itself (Mazor et al., 2009). For providers, organizational policies, institutional guidelines, and legal rules complicate the process of disclosure and apology, impacting the communication experience (Carmack, 2010b, 2014, 2017; Hannawa, 2009).

To date, Communication scholars have yet to deeply explore how pop culture media present medical errors to consumers. Only one published communication study (Foss, 2011) examines mediated representations of medical errors on television medical dramas, leaving room for more examination of the different ways in which medical errors are part of popular culture conversations. In this chapter, I examine three of the major ways in which medical errors have entered popular culture conversations: representations of medical errors on television, popular press coverage of medical errors, and celebrity medical error stories.

Medical Errors: A Brief Primer

A medical error constitutes an "unintended act or one that does not achieve its intended outcome" (Leape, 1994, p. 1851). This definition includes errors of omission (caused by not doing a treatment

DOI: 10.4324/9781003436409-14

or procedure) and errors of commission (caused by performing an incorrect procedure or prescribing an incorrect treatment). Scholars generally accept Leape's definition of medical errors. However, some key elements remain hidden in this definition. First, Leape's definition of errors implies that someone is at fault and worthy of blame (Paget, 2004). Second, the definition includes therapeutic action "that does not achieve its intended outcome" (Leape, 1994, p. 1851), spanning all adverse events, including errors, known complications, and near misses. Known complications consist of bad outcomes of a procedure or pre-identified potential risks. A near miss entails a medical error that a health care provider prevented or corrected before it caused the patient physical harm (Aspden et al., 2004). Near misses are not always reported, but they account for between 2% and 6% of reported errors (Bari et al., 2016; Noland & Carmack, 2015). Finally, the definition only acknowledges physical harm and overlooks emotional harm or the harm caused by poor communication.

Numerous types of medical errors exist, ranging from small errors such as spelling a patient's name incorrectly to large errors like leaving medical equipment inside a body cavity. Most medical errors presented in popular culture can be grouped into four major categories (Wachter & Shojania, 2005). The first and most common major medical error is misdiagnosis, including giving the wrong diagnosis, prescribing the wrong medication, or suggesting the wrong treatment for a patient. The second major type of medical error involves the misinterpretation of physicians' handwriting on prescription and treatment orders, resulting in medication errors. The third major type of medical error, and perhaps the rarest type, is wrong-side/wrong-site surgery. This error encompasses performing a procedure on the wrong side of a patient (e.g., removing the wrong leg) or performing a procedure on the wrong site of the body (e.g., performing heart surgery on a patient who needs a brain aneurysm removed). The final type of medical error is the "retained sponge," when the surgical team inadvertently leaves surgical paraphernalia (e.g., sponges, towels, needles) in patients. The examples presented in the following sections feature these major errors.

"What's Up Doc?": Medical Errors on Television

Most people likely encounter medical error stories on television, especially if they enjoy medical dramas and comedies. Medical dramas have been a mainstay on network television since the 1960s and continue to be one of television's most popular genres (Alahmari, 2023) as well as now being readily available to binge-watch on streaming services. I can easily catch up on *Grey's Anatomy, The Resident, The Good Doctor, Chicago Med,* and *New Amsterdam,* or rewatch old favorites like *ER, House, M.D.,* and *Chicago Hope*. If medical dramas are not a favorite genre, medical dramedy offers an alternative, popularized by shows like *Scrubs* (considered to be the most realistic medical show on television, Weiss, 2009), *Royal Pains, Nurse Jackie,* and *Doogie Howser, M.D.* I can watch specialized shows such as *Nurses,* soapy dramas like *Private Practice,* or small-town medicine shows (e.g., *Northern Exposure* and *Hart of Dixie*). As a scholar interested in medical errors, I am not restricted to a few storylines on my favorite shows; in 2013, TNT aired the short-lived *Monday Mornings,* a medical drama dedicated exclusively to medical errors and a hallmark of patient safety practice: the morbidity and mortality conference (known as M&Ms) where staff talk through medical error cases.

No medical drama would be complete without a medical error storyline, and medical errors are the most remembered storylines watched by nursing, pre-medicine, and other health science/pre-professional health students (Cambra-Badii et al., 2021). Although a plethora of research exists on the mediated representations of physicians and nurses, limited research has been conducted on the mediated representation of medical errors on medical shows, and that scholarship has yielded somewhat contradictory findings. Communication scholar Foss (2011) examined the mediated representations of medical errors in 536 episodes of medical dramas. Foss identified only 52 errors across all 536 episodes, arguing that the genre rarely shows medical providers making errors. In her analysis, Foss noted that medical errors usually result from inexperience, performed by young and new providers, and typically get addressed in private away from patients, families, and other providers. Foss argued that these representations reinforce a dominant narrative of "silence" about medical errors, be it through storylines that discourage disclosure or through characters receiving nothing more than a stern warning from their supervisors.

More recently, Carney et al. (2020) presented a contradictory analysis of medical errors in medical dramas. The researchers identified 242 medical errors in the first 6 episodes of 8 medical dramas, for an average of 6.4 errors for every hour of television. These results likely differed because Carney et al. coded the shows using a robust typology of medical errors based on typologies created from the two largest medical error studies in the United States (e.g., Brennan et al., 1991; Thomas et al., 2000). Conversely, Foss, who did not explain how she identified medical errors, appeared to only include obvious surgical errors or errors that resulted in patient death. This approach makes sense as Carney et al. also found that medical dramas tend to depict operative/surgical errors instead of diagnostic errors. Finally, Carney et al. found that older, experienced, White, male attending physicians tended to commit most medical errors, in contrast to Foss' finding that younger, inexperienced providers made the errors. The differences between Carney et al.'s and Foss' studies highlight the complexity of medical error storylines in trying to capture the medical error experience.

What Medical Television Teach Us About Medical Errors

Medical error storylines, although often dramatized, provide insight for viewers into real-world issues patients and providers encounter when a medical error happens. When shows include medical errors as a storyline in their early seasons, they tend to highlight one of medicine's largest and longest-running tensions: doctors are god-like and do not care if they make mistakes versus doctors are human and make mistakes like everyone else (Carmack, 2016). *ER*, one of television's most popular medical dramas, often explored this tension in its early seasons with its young third-year medical students John Carter and Jing-Mei "Deb" Chen. Deb's experience with a medical error in season 1's episode "House of Cards" showcases this tension. Deb attempted to hook up a patient to an IV but could not do so because the patient had collapsed veins. Instead, Deb tried to insert a central line in the patient without supervision. As she said to the nurse, "I was just going to start it, but it seemed so easy." Deb lost the guide wire, and the patient began to bleed profusely, almost killing them. When Deb decided to quit, she told John, "I really didn't care about the patient. I just wanted the procedure." She explained to John that she "doesn't really like" medicine and taking care of patients; she just likes the science and research of medicine. Throughout the first season, the show set Deb and John as counterpoints to each other, Deb representing the technically proficient but rigid doctor and John representing the caring, empathetic doctor who learned from his mistakes. Medical dramas often set up characters to be these counterpoints (Carmack, 2016), and as *ER* shows, they can be used to demonstrate the insufficiency of technical proficiency when discussing medical errors.

A second common lesson in medical error storylines involves medical error disclosure, either through reporting errors to supervisors or patients. Medical dramas often have scenes dedicated to reporting and disclosure (Carney et al., 2020), showing viewers how these conversations could occur. Season 1 of *Grey's Anatomy* featured multiple instances of reporting and disclosures. Episode 5, "Shake Your Groove Thing," told the story of two major medical errors: a "retained sponge" event and a surgical mishap when first-year intern Dr. Meredith Grey accidentally punctured her glove during surgery and nicked a heart with her fingernail. The "retained sponge" event, where Dr. Preston Burke left a surgical towel in a patient, constitutes one of *Grey's* most famous medical error storylines. After waking from surgery to remove the towel, the patient recounted to Dr. George O'Malley that Dr. Weber, the chief of surgery, disclosed the error to her.

Patient:	There was a towel that somebody left last time.
O'Malley:	Yes m'am.
Patient:	Who would do that? That doesn't seem right does it?
O'Malley:	No m'am no. It doesn't.
Patient:	How can that happen?

In this case, the show presented a common patient response: frustration and disbelief.

When Dr. Grey's heart surgery patient began to experience distress, Dr. Grey accidentally disclosed the nick error to Dr. Burke in front of the patient's husband.

Burke:	What the hell went wrong?
Grey:	I popped the glove.
Burke:	What?
Grey:	In surgery, when I was holding it [the heart], I popped my glove with my fingernail. I think I may have nicked her heart.

Once in the OR, Dr. Burke chided Dr. Grey about not disclosing the error to him and instead, disclosing the error in front of the patient's husband.

Burke:	What were you thinking about? You had every opportunity to speak up before I closed her chest. Every opportunity.
Grey:	I'm sorry.
Burke:	And then you go and confess in front of her husband? You don't even know if you were the cause. You have no idea.

Later in the surgery, Dr. Burke said, "I'm going to go back and talk to the husband, review the history, apologize profusely." The interaction between Drs. Grey and Burke illustrated a common concern with medical error disclosure: disclosing errors to patients means admitting guilt and liability. This concern is not just for television; health care providers worry about medical malpractice and how what they say could be used in malpractice lawsuits, resulting in strategic communication disclosure choices (Noland & Carl, 2006).

Medical dramas tend to center their stories on providers' experiences after medical errors occur, especially when a medical error is only featured in one episode. *Grey's Anatomy has* presented multiple medical errors across its 20 (and counting) seasons, exposing viewers to how providers handle medical errors. In a particularly poignant episode, "I Saw What I Saw" exemplified how facilities attempt to identify the root cause of an error when officials questioned the interns and residents after the death of a burn victim. The episode walked through the event from each provider's point of view, revealing new pieces of information, much like a traditional medical error event review. Ultimately, investigators determined that Dr. April Kepner committed the error. Distracted by an axe in the patient's chest, Kepner forgot to check the patient's airway. The episode ends with Dr. Kepner being fired and the providers making sense of the event. This episode portrayed the different emotional responses of providers after an error happens and highlighted the emotional struggle that they may experience after the death of a patient.

Occasionally, a medical error storyline extends into a detailed storyline, such as Dr. Alex Corday's medical malpractice trial on *ER*. In such a case, viewers gain a glimpse into how patients and families negotiate the aftermath of errors. Dr. Corday committed several medical errors on the show. Season 7 devoted multiple episodes to one of Corday's medical errors – the paralysis of a patient during an outpatient procedure – and the subsequent malpractice trial. During the trial, viewers heard the patient recount the physical and emotional impact of the medical error on his life.

Television representations of medical errors present viewers with an uneven and sometimes unrealistic explanation of medical errors by using extreme and sensationalized errors in storylines. Looking past the types of errors, viewers can learn about the communication interactions associated with reporting, disclosing, and talking about medical errors. These storylines also depict the emotional struggles that patients and providers go through when dealing with the aftermath of medical errors.

"If It Bleeds, It Leads": Popular Press Coverage of Medical Errors

In 1999, the Institute of Medicine (IOM) released its groundbreaking report, *To Err is Human*, which documented that between 44,000 and 98,000 patients die every year in the U.S. because of a medical error (Kohn et al., 1999). The report also called for a culture change in medicine to adopt transparent reporting structures and encouraged providers and facilities to engage in open and honest communication with patients and families. The IOM report comprised one of the first national reports on medical errors released to the public and served as the turning point moment for patient safety conversations in the United States. Before the IOM report, the news rarely covered medical errors. The IOM report introduced the general public to the statistics of medical errors, numbers that hospitals and clinics had previously often kept private. Since the release of the IOM report, scholars have examined worldwide news coverage of medical errors to identify what information the general public receives about medical errors and the framing of medical errors. Most medical errors news stories reported on individual patient errors (Stebbing et al., 2006), including medication errors, misdiagnosis, radiation errors, and surgical errors (Hinchcliff et al., 2012; Li et al., 2015). Articles occasionally offered recommendations or solutions for how to prevent medical errors (Hinchcliff et al., 2012); however, many of these recommendations focused on individual policy changes, rather than cultural changes to address systemic underlying issues (Carmack, 2010c).

Popular press coverage of medical errors often relies on certain narrative tropes to tell their stories to readers. In her framing analysis of 10 years of medical error news stories in U.S. newspapers, Carmack (2010c) identified an overarching narrative of blaming, shaming, and naming – a narrative that places blame on individual providers and is designed to shame providers, hospitals, and facilities for making errors. Carmack argued that news coverage almost always presented the medical error story as one of victim (patient) vs. villain (physicians; hospitals). Li et al. (2015) found something similar in their analysis of U.S. and non-U.S. medical error coverage, with responsibility placed almost exclusively on physicians. News coverage typically included patient statements but rarely encompassed statements from physicians or patient safety experts (Li et al., 2015). Both analyses placed little to no emphasis on facilities' systems-based approaches to errors, which positioned systems and cultural breakdowns as the reasons for errors. Additionally, news coverage of medical errors often leaned heavily into reporting severe and fatal errors over smaller, non-fatal errors (Li et al., 2015), contributing to an "over-sensationalization" of medical errors meant to shock the general public (Carmack, 2010c). Covering stories of severe or fatal errors means the general public receives an incomplete picture of medical errors.

Two cases stand apart as exemplars of popular press coverage of medical errors: the 2003 Jesica Santillan transplant error and the 2006 Methodist Hospital neonatal heparin overdose. Both cases received national and international news coverage, and they perfectly illustrated the way in which news outlets frame medical errors in a sensational manner meant to shock readers. These cases also contributed to patient safety changes across the US.

"The Worst Ordeal a Family Can Face": The Story of Jesica Santillan

Doctors diagnosed Jesica with a heart condition called restrictive cardiomyopathy and secondary nonreactive pulmonary hypertension, which caused her heart and lungs to not receive enough blood.

The Santillan family did not feel that Jesica could receive the necessary care in their native Mexico, and the family reportedly paid a coyote to help them cross the border into the U.S., where they traveled to North Carolina (Wailoo et al., 2006). The family lived and worked in and around the Durham area as undocumented workers, and they partnered with a local businessman to raise money for a heart-lung transplant (Hopkins Tanne, 2003). Jesica was placed on a transplant list in 2002, and, in 2003, at age 17, she received the news that every transplant patient hopes to hear: We've found a match.

Jesica's first surgery took place on February 7, 2003, where she received a heart and lungs. However, the transplant was doomed from the start because the organ donor had type A blood. Given that Jesica had type O blood, the organs were not compatible with her body (Archibold, 2003). Unfortunately, health care providers did not discover this error before the surgery started. Hopkins Tanne (2003) reported that the surgeon, Dr. James Jaggers, became aware of the mismatch as he was completing the surgery. Upon discovery of the error, the transplant team gave Jesica immunosuppressant drugs to prevent immediate organ failure and kept her on life support until they could find replacement organs. Amazingly, they found new donor organs, and, on February 20, she underwent a second heart and lung transplant (Gettleman & Altman, 2003). Although the new organs matched Jesica's blood type, the damage to her body from the first transplant proved to be too much, and she was declared brain dead on February 22, 2003. Jesica's family tried to redonate the organs; however, they were told that the organs were too damaged from being on life support and receiving antirejection medications (AP, 2003).

Media coverage of Jesica's ordeal showcased several hallmark frames of medical error coverage and served as an entry for larger conversations about organ donation in the United States. First, the coverage highlighted the sensational nature of the case. Jesica's ordeal clearly exemplified a wrong site/wrong side medical error – in her case, Jesica was the "wrong site" because of incompatibility. Morgan et al. (2006) identified several examples of sensational language used to cover the case, including "botched," "hunting for organs," and "tragedy."

Second, media coverage quickly identified the victims and villains of the story – Jesica and Dr. Jaggers. Early media coverage framed Jesica as "a 'mediagenic' individual – and these accounts quickly cast her as a young, pretty, 'innocent,' and sympathic figure" (Morgan et al., 2006, p. 24). Conversely, the media framed Dr. Jaggers and Duke University Hospital as the villains. A review of the case identified two causes for the error: (1) Dr. Jaggers failed to check the lab results for compatibility, assuming that had already been done, and (2) he failed to confirm compatibility with the donor agency (Kher & Cuadros, 2003). In a *60 Minutes* story about Jesica's case, journalist Ed Bradley asked, "How did an operation performed by a team of expert surgeons go so wrong? What it came down to was a failure to communicate basic information" (Hopkins Tanne, 2003, para. 8). These errors presented Dr. Jaggers as an incompetent surgeon who was incapable of doing the most basic checks, engaging in basic communication, before surgery.

"Our Hearts Go Out to the Families": Overdose in the NICU

On September 16, 2006, six families heard the four words that no patient or family wants to hear: There's been a mistake. The families all had babies in the newborn intensive care unit (NICU) at Methodist Hospital in Indianapolis, Indiana. That Saturday, doctors told parents that six babies had received accidental overdoses of heparin, a popular anti-clotting medication, causing the babies to bleed uncontrollably. Two babies – two-day-old Emmery Miller and five-day-old D'myia Sabrina Nelson – died ("2 babies," 2006). Medical officials listed three babies in critical but stable condition and transferred the fourth baby to Riley Hospital for Children to undergo surgery ("Premature babies," 2006). A third baby, Thursday-Dawn Jeffers, died several days later. The hospital swiftly determined that a pharmacy technician accidentally took doses from the adult version of heparin and placed them in the NICU drug cabinet. None of the nurses checked the label to confirm versions when retrieving the drug from the cabinet (Wilson, 2006). How did no one notice? The adult and child versions of heparin look identical, except one has a dark blue label and one has a light blue label. The hospital offered an apology for the error; however, families did not feel that was adequate. As Lena Nelson, D'myia's grandmother, said, "They couldn't give me enough apologies for what they have done. She was just taken away from us" ("Premature babies," 2006, para. 5). Two years after the error, the families of Emmery Miller and Thursday-Dawn Jeffers, along with the families of two of the surviving infants, sued Methodist Hospital and drugmaker Baxter Health care for malpractice, arguing that both bore responsibility for the error – the hospital for the pharmacy technician and nursing errors and Baxter Health care for labeling the adult and child versions in an almost identical fashion, which could lead to errors (Higgins, 2008).

News coverage of the death of three babies and serious injury to three others painted a picture of a domino effect: Baxter Healthcare's problematic labels led to the pharmacy technician's error, which led to the nursing error. Although it did offer an apology, the hospital's response shifted from a systems approach, calling it a "procedural" error ("2 babies," 2006), to a blaming approach, calling it a "human" error (Wilson, 2006), which framed the pharmacy technician and the nurses as villains. This shift created space to question provider competency and ability, with parents wondering how this situation could happen, as did Whitney Alexander, D'myia's mother: "They may apologize but it didn't help. It didn't help, because I feel like whoever the nurse was on call, they should know what they are doing and how much my baby should have" (Wilson, 2006, para. 9). The media further enforced this victim/villain narrative in stories that emphasized the families' losses, as evidenced in the opening of the *Los Angeles Times'* article: "Lena Nelson had looked forward to buying dolls and other presents for her first granddaughter, who was born prematurely last week. Instead, she was planning Monday for the girl's funeral" ("Premature babies," 2006, para. 1). Additionally, the media further positioned the hospital as a villain after including statements from Sam Odle, chief executive officer at Methodist, that seemed to imply that Miller's and Nelson's deaths may have been precipitated by being "very, very, small babies" who were extremely premature at 25 and 26 weeks (Wilson, 2006, para. 4).

Coverage of the Methodist heparin case, along with a similar case involving actor Dennis Quaid's newborn twins, did lead to patient safety practice changes, most notably in Baxter's packaging of adult and infant heparin (Higgins, 2008). Methodist, along with the other two hospitals in its health care system, adopted stricter policies related to the entrance and delivery of drugs by the pharmacy, as well as a new double-check system for nurses ("Premature babies," 2006). Additionally, according to Higgins, Methodist Hospital began buying its heparin from a different manufacturer, which used distinct labels. Interestingly, most mentions of practice changes were listed at the bottom of news articles, mirroring previous research that popular press emphasizes practice changes over culture changes (Hinchcliff et al., 2012).

Popular Press's Impact on How We See Medical Errors

We lack clarity about the kind of impact that press coverage about medical errors has on the general public's understanding of medical errors, expectations for care, or decisions to seek care at certain facilities. In their examination of news reports of medical errors at Veterans Health Administration facilities in the 1990s, Weeks and Mills (2003) found that when news outlets reported a major medical error, the hospitals named experienced a decrease in patient visits. Conversely, Fukuda (2021) concluded that news coverage of medical errors did not impact patient enrollment in Japanese facilities. Several factors could explain these differences, including cultural expectations and the ability to go to other local facilities. Clearly, news coverage of medical errors raised general awareness of medical errors and introduced patient safety language into the public discourse about health care. Millenson

(2002) argued that journalists covering medical errors, whether in reporting cases or presenting information about legislation and organizational changes, helped the general public "remember" patient safety as something important to their health experiences. Millenson cautioned journalists, however, about the impact of their stories on how the general public thinks and talks about medical errors. Past journalists have also contributed to the culture of shaming and blaming that still permeates patient safety, and they have a professional responsibility to help the general public think differently about medical errors (Millenson, 2002).

"A Spoon Full of Sugar": Celebrities, Medical Errors, and Accidental Advocacy

Communication scholars agree that celebrities' impact on the public's understanding and actions related to a specific health issue stems from the public's perceived identification and parasocial involvement with specific celebrities (Brown & Chaván de Matviuk, 2010; Kosenko et al., 2016; Myrick et al., 2013; see also Chapter 15, this volume). As Myrick et al. concluded, a direct connection exists between celebrity identification and their influence on individuals' information-seeking and communication with others about health issues. Kosenko and colleagues referred to the "Angelina Effect" in their study of the impact of Angelina Jolie's communication about her BRCA gene mutation-driven decision to undergo prophylactic surgeries to prevent future cancer diagnoses. According to Kosenko et al., women who identified with Jolie expressed more interest in getting the BRCA gene test than those who did not identify with her. Advocating for health issues or openly talking about their personal health struggles creates a parasocial involvement cycle: the more celebrities share personal health connections with us, the more we become personal stakeholders in their lives (Beck, 2022; Beck et al., 2015). However, we know little about how fans or the general public connect with celebrities because of their medical error stories or the impact their error stories and advocacy have on changing others' behaviors or health practices. Yet, their public stories do provide insight into patients' often-silenced experiences with errors.

Learning from Public Stories: Julie Andrews

Celebrity stories related to medical errors tend to begin with similar language – "it was a routine procedure," "a simple operation," or "a normal surgery." This language has been used to begin many celebrities' medical error stories, such as Andy Warhol's "routine" gallstone and hernia surgery, Dick Schaap's "routine" hip replacement surgery, or Joan Rivers' "routine" gastric endoscopy. The use of the word "routine" here matters because it communicates to people reading or listening to celebrity stories that their errors did not result from some experimental or high-tech procedure; they happened during procedures that the everyday reader could also have done. Julie Andrews' story highlighted the importance of talking about medical errors and how medical errors can impact people's professional and personal lives.

In 1997, Julie Andrews – famous for her roles in *Mary Poppins, The Sound of Music,* and originating the role of Eliza Doolittle in *My Fair Lady* on Broadway – received a diagnosis of non-cancerous nodules in her throat (Moyer, 2015). Andrews' nodules required a "minor, routine" surgery to remove them. The doctor "botched" the surgery, leaving Andrews with persistent hoarseness and damaged vocal cords. The damage to her vocal cords meant Andrews could no longer sing. She said at the time, "Singing has been a cherished gift, and my inability to sing has been a devastating blow" (Jones, 2000, para. 5). Andrews sued Mt. Sinai Hospital in 1999, and the hospital settled with the performer in 2000.

In 1999, after filing the malpractice lawsuit, Andrews sat down with Barbara Walters in a *20/20* interview to talk about her experiences with the medical error and its impact on her life. Andrews' narrative centered on her identity as a performer and how the error fundamentally altered how she saw herself. She told Walters:

> To not sing with an orchestra, to not be able to communicate through my voice which I've done all my life and not to be able to phrase lyrics and give people that kind of joy, I think I would be totally devastated.
>
> *(Jones, 2000)*

At the time, Andrews hoped that she would regain her singing voice and underwent rehabilitation therapy to restore her vocal cords. Unfortunately, her singing voice never returned, although she has been able to "speak-sing," as she did in *The Princess Diaries 2*. The transition to "speak-sing" required Andrews to rethink her professional identity as a performer and transition to other areas:

> Andrews says in a strange way that she feels fortunate that she no longer can sing because it pushed her to find a "different way" of using her voice. Paraphrasing a line from her Sound of Music character Maria von Trapp, Andrews noted that "When one door closes another window opens."
>
> *(AP, 2015, para. 8)*

Julie Andrews' experience provided rare insights into how patients who survive medical errors make sense of those experiences, yet limited research on the topic has underscored emotional and physical harm and disruption of their everyday lives (Mazor et al., 2009). Andrews' story highlighted how medical errors can create ruptures in our identities as survivors seek to understand who they are after an error.

Accidental Advocacy: Dennis Quaid

Celebrities, because of their constant media exposure, possess a communicative bullhorn – when they talk about a specific health issue, they can raise the public's awareness of that issue, increase media exposure, and influence attitudes and behavioral intentions (Beck, 2022; Beck et al., 2015; Brown et al., 2003; see also Chapter 15, this volume). Celebrities' level of involvement or connection to the health issue only increases this awareness and action, and many – such as Mark McGwire, Michael J. Fox, and Angelina Jolie – have used their personal connections to a health issue to become advocates (Beck, 2022; Beck et al., 2014; Brown et al., 2003; Kosenko et al., 2016). Even when the media associate celebrities with health issues – such as steroid use, alcohol abuse, or type-II diabetes – they influence the public's understanding, conversations, and actions about health issues (Beck et al., 2015; Brown & Chaván de Matviuk, 2010; Brown et al., 2003). Medical errors offer a similar trajectory for celebrities to advocate for change, with a few slight differences. Rather than promoting individual behavioral change, celebrities who become activists for medical error reform can target institutional practices and cultural changes.

Perhaps the most famous celebrity patient safety advocate is Dennis Quaid. Approximately a year after the Methodist Hospital NICU heparin overdose, in November 2007, Quaid's newborn twins experienced the same error at Cedars-Sinai Hospital in Los Angeles. A staff member gave the twins, along with another baby, an overdose of heparin more than 1,000 times the proper dosage (Ornstein, 2007). The babies' blood turned the "consistency of water" (AP, 2008, para. 5), and it took the twins' blood 41 hours to begin to clot again (Rubin, 2010). Quaid recounted the harrowing scene in a *60 Minutes* interview:

> They were working on (my son) Boone, whose belly button would not stop bleeding, and while they were trying to … clamp it, blood squirted across the room about six feet and landed on the wall. It was blood everywhere.
>
> *(AP, 2008, para. 2)*

The hospital's statement about how the error occurred eerily mirrors what happened at Methodist – a pharmacy technician accidentally put the adult-dose heparin in the pharmacy delivery for pediatrics, and no one checked to make sure the medication was correct (Ornstein, 2007). Baxter Healthcare had yet to change the labels on the bottles, even though the Methodist NICU babies had died almost a year prior because of the label color mistake.

Quaid and his wife sued Baxter Healthcare for negligence and product defects, arguing that Baxter knew the vial mix-ups were an issue because of previous errors (Ornstein, 2007). Rather than stop at a lawsuit, Quaid emerged as a patient safety advocate, creating the Quaid Foundation to raise awareness and change practices to improve patient care. According to Ornstein, he became a "self-described 'frontman' for a campaign to improve patient care with the implementation of 'safe practices' as simple as hand-washing and the use of technologies such as bar codes to match medications to patients" (para. 1). In 2008, Quaid spoke to Congress in opposition to a Bush administration initiative to protect companies, like Baxter Healthcare, from malpractice suits if they had Food and Drug Administration (FDA) approval (Rockoff, 2008). Quaid told Congress about his experiences as a father watching his twins bleed uncontrollably and how he later wondered why this error kept happening if Baxter Healthcare knew that it was a problem. Quaid also worked to produce the popular documentary *Chasing Zero: Winning the War on Healthcare Harm* (Rubin, 2010). Unfortunately, this activism was short-lived; the Quaid Foundation merged with the Texas Medical Institute of Technology in 2010, and Quaid stepped away from his advocacy role (Hurley, 2023).

Celebrity stories of medical errors demonstrate the powerful impact that celebrities can have on helping others make sense of their own medical error experiences and advocating for patient safety change. Dennis Quaid's story exemplified the potential of celebrity clout to try to make real change to improve patients' health care experiences. Not every celebrity wants to talk about their medical errors or can talk about the errors; likewise, celebrity family members may not be able to talk publicly about the grief. Medical errors constitute normally private experiences, so celebrities being open about their errors and how they fight to redress the error can provide average patients with tools to negotiate their medical errors.

Conclusion

This chapter begins a much-needed conversation about medical errors in popular culture. The medical errors presented across all three major areas of popular culture all have one constant current: consumers tend to see severe and hyper-sensationalized medical errors, not the average, everyday medical errors we might normally encounter. However, these representations of medical errors also underscore one of our biggest fears about health care: being vulnerable and unable to stop something bad from happening. Understanding how medical errors are presented to audiences through television shows, popular press and media coverage, and advocating in the halls of Congress is just part of the puzzle presented to communication researchers. We next need to explore how these presentations impact patients' expectations of care and communication when they find themselves dealing with a medical error. We can learn from how medical errors are portrayed in popular culture if we peel back the layers to understand the complexity of medical error experiences.

References

2 babies at Methodist die of overdose: 4 others also get wrong dosage of anti-clotting drug. (2006, September 18). *Indianapolis Star*, 1A.

Alahmari, A. A. (2023). Professionalism, ethics, and realism of television medical dramas as perceived by Saudi medical students. *Journal of Medical Education and Curricular Development, 10*(1), 1–6. https://doi.org/10.1177/23821205231175037

Archibold, R. C. (2003, February 23). Girl in transplant mix-up dies after two weeks. *The New York Times*. https://www.nytimes.com/2003/02/23/us/girl-in-transplant-mix-up-dies-after-two-weeks.html

Aspden, P., Corrigan, J. M., Wolcott, J., & Erickson, S. M. (Eds.). (2004). *Patient safety: Achieving a new standard for care*. Committee on Data Standards for Patient Safety. Institute of Medicine.

Associated Press. (2003, February 25). Organ donation got too emotional. *The Commercial Appeal (Memphis, TN)*, A5.

Associated Press. (2008, March 14). Quaid opens up about near-death of twins. *Today Show*. https://www.today.com/popculture/quaid-opens-about-near-death-twins-1C9425939

Associated Press. (2015, February 23). Julie Andrews' famous singing voice ruined by throat operation. *The (London) Telegraph.* https://www.telegraph.co.uk/news/celebritynews/9725893/Julie-Andrews-famous-singing-voice-ruined-by-throat-operation.html

Bari, A., Khan, R. A., & Rathore, A. W. (2016). Medical errors: Causes, consequences, emotional response and resulting behavior change. *Pakistan Journal of Medical Sciences, 32*(3), 523–528. https://doi.org/10.12669/pjms.323.9701

Beck, C. S. (2022). *Celebrity in the time of COVID: Fandom and the influence of pandemic messaging.* McFarland.

Beck, C. S., Aubuchon, S. M., McKenna, T. P., Ruhl, S., & Simmons, N. (2014). Blurring personal health and public priorities: An analysis of celebrity health narratives in the public sphere. *Health Communication, 29*(3), 244–256. https://doi.org/10.1080/10410236.2012.741668

Beck, C. S., Chapman, S. M. A., Simmons, N., Tenzek. K. E., & Ruhl, S. M. (2015). *Celebrity health narratives and the public health.* McFarland.

Brennan, T. A., Leape, L. L., Laird, N. M., Hebert, L., Localio, A. R., Lawthers, A. G., Newhouse, J. P., Weiler, P. C., & Hiatt, H. H. (1991). Incidence of adverse events and negligence in hospitalized patients—Results of the Harvard medical practice study I. *The New England Journal of Medicine, 324*(6), 370–376. https://dx.doi.org/10.1056/NEJM199102073240604

Brown, W. J., Basil, M. D., & Bocarnea, M. A. (2003). The influence of famous athletes on health beliefs and practices: Mark McGwire, child abuse prevention, and androstenedione. *Journal of Health Communication, 8*(1), 41–57. https://doi.org/10.1080/10810730305733

Brown, W. J., & Chaván de Matviuk, M. A. (2010). Sports celebrities and public health: Diego Maradona's influence on drug use prevention. *Journal of Health Communication, 15*(4), 358–378. https://doi.org/10.1080/10810730903460575

Cambra-Badii, I., Moyano, E., Ortega, I., Baños, J-E., & Sentí, M. (2021). TV medical dramas: Health sciences students' viewing habits and potential for teaching issues related to bioethics and professionalism. *BMC Medical Education, 21*, Article 509. https://doi.org/10.1186/s12909-021-02947-7

Carmack, H. J. (2010a). Bearing witness to the ethics of practice: Storying physicians' medical mistake narratives. *Health Communication, 25*(5), 449–458. https://doi.org/10.1080/10410236.2010.484876

Carmack, H. J. (2010b). Structuring and disciplining apology: A structurational analysis of health care benevolence laws. *Qualitative Research Reports in Communication, 11*(1), 6–13. https://doi.org/10.1080/17459430903413432

Carmack, H. J. (2010c, April). The hidden health epidemic: Narrative constructions of medical mistakes in public discourse [Paper presentation]. Kentucky Conference on Health Communication, Lexington, KY, United States.

Carmack, H. J. (2014). A cycle of redemption in a medical error disclosure and apology program. *Qualitative Health Research, 24*(6), 860–869. https://doi.org/10.1177/1049732314536285

Carmack, H. J. (2016). Defining "doctor": Constructing a representative anecdote of physician ethos on television medical dramas. *Texas Speech Communication Journal, 40*(1), 20–33. https://www.etsca.com/journal.asp

Carmack, H. J. (2017). Crafting a culture of patient safety: Structuring physicians' medical error disclosure and apology. *Ohio Communication Journal*, 55(1), 29–42. https://www.ohiocomm.org/wp-content/uploads/2017/01/Carmack-OCJ-2017.pdf

Carmack, H. J. (2022). Patient safety and quality. In E. Y. Ho, C. L. Bylund, & J. C. M. van Weert (Eds.), *Wiley international encyclopedia of health communication*. Wiley. https://doi.org/10.1002/9781119678816.iehc0708

Carney, M., King, T. S., Yumen, A., Harnish-Cruz, C., Scales, R., & Olympia, R. P. (2020). The depiction of medical errors in a sample of medical television shows. *Cureus, 12*(12), e11994. https://doi.org/10.7759/cureus.11994

Foss, K. A. (2011). "When we make mistakes, people die!": Constructions of responsibility for medical errors in televised medical dramas, 1994-2007. *Communication Quarterly, 59*(4), 484–506. https://doi.org/10.1080/01463373.2011.597350

Fukuda, H. (2021). Changes in hospital inpatient volume after newspaper reporting of medical errors. *Journal of Patient Safety, 17*(5), e401–e405. https://doi.org/10.1097/pts.0000000000000349

Gettleman, J., & Altman, L. K. (2003, February 21). New organs give Jesica another chance at life. *Milwaukee Sentinel Journal,* 1A.

Hannawa, A. F. (2009). Negotiating medical virtues: Toward the development of a physician mistake disclosure model. *Health Communication, 24*(5), 391–399. https://doi.org/10.1080/10410230903023279

Hannawa, A. F. (2017). What constitutes "competent error disclosure"?: Insights from a national focus group in Switzerland. *Swiss Medical Weekly, 147*, e14427. https://doi.org/10.4414/smw.2017.14427

Higgins, W. (2008, September 13). Babies' overdoses prompt lawsuit: Infants were given too much heparin at Methodist Hospital. *Indianapolis Star,* A1.

Hinchcliff, R., Westbrook, J., Greenfield, D., Baysari, M., Moldovan, M., & Braithwaite, J. (2012). Analysis of Australian newspaper coverage of medication errors. *International Journal for Quality in Health Care, 24*(1), 1–8. https://doi.org/10.1093/intqhc/mzr067

Hurley, C. (2023). The philanthropy of Dennis Quaid. *Arts Management Magazine.* https://www.artsmanagementmagazine.com/article/the-philanthropy-of-dennis-quaid/

Hopkins Tanne, J. (2003). When Jesica died. *British Medical Journal, 326*(7391), 717. PMCID: PMC1125622.

James, J. T. (2013). A new, evidence-based estimate of patient harms associated with hospital care. *Journal of Patient Safety, 9*(3), 122–128. https://doi.org/10.1097/pts.0b013e3182948a69

Jones, K. (2000, September 8). Julie Andrews settled malpractice lawsuit over loss of the sound of her music. *Playbill.* https://playbill.com/article/julie-andrews-settles-malpractice-lawsuit-over-loss-of-the-sound-of-her-music-com-91729

Kher, U., & Cuadros, P. (2003, February 23). A miracle denied. *Time, 161*(9), 61.

Kohn, L. T., Corrigen, J. M., & Donaldson, M. S. (Eds.). (1999). *To err is human: Building a safer health system. Committee on Quality of Health Care in America.* National Academy Press.

Kosenko, K. A., Binder, A. R., & Hurley, R. (2016). Celebrity influence and identification: A test of the Angelina effect. *Journal of Health Communication, 21*(3), 318–326. https://doi.org/10.1080/10810730.2015.1064498

Leape, L. L. (1994). Error in medicine. *JAMA: The Journal of the American Medical Association, 272*(23), 1851–1857. PMID: 7503827

Li, J. W. Morway, L., Velasquez, A., Weingart, S. N., & Stuver, S. O. (2015). Perceptions of medical errors in cancer care: An analysis of how the news media describe sentinel events. *Journal of Patient Safety, 11*(1), 42–51. https://doi.org/10.1097/pts.0000000000000039

Makary, M. A., & Daniel, M. (2016). Medical error—the third leading cause of death in the US. *British Medical Journal, 353*, i2139. https://doi.org/10.1136/bmj.i2139

Mazor, K. M., Goff, S. L., Dodd, K., & Alper, E. J. (2009). Understanding patients' perceptions of medical errors. *Journal of Communication in Healthcare, 2*(1), 34–46. https://doi.org/10.1179/cih.2009.2.1.34

Millenson, M. L. (2002). Pushing the profession: How the news media turned patient safety into a priority. *Quality & Safety in Health Care, 11*(1), 57–63. https://doi.org/10.1136/qhc.11.1.57

Morgan, S. E., Harrison, T. R., Volk Chewing, L., & Habib, J. G. (2006). America's angel or thieving immigrant? Media coverage, the Santillan story, and publicized ambivalence toward donation and transplantation. In K. Wailoo, J. Livingston, & P. Guarnaccia (Eds.), *A death retold: Jesica Santillan, the bungled transplant, and paradoxes of medical citizenship* (pp. 19–45). University of North Carolina Press.

Moyer, J. W. (2015, March 19). How Julie Andrews's voice was stolen by a medical disaster. *The Washington Post.* https://www.washingtonpost.com/news/morning-mix/wp/2015/03/19/how-julie-andrewss-voice-was-stolen-by-a-medical-disaster/

Myrick, J. G., Willoughby, J. F., Noar, S. M., & Brown, J. (2013). Reactions of young adults to the death of Apple CEO Steve Jobs: Implications for cancer communication. *Communication Research Reports, 30*(2), 115–126. https://doi.org/10.1080/08824096.2012.762906

Nazione, S., & Pace, K. (2015). An experimental study of medical error explanations: Do apology, empathy, corrective action, and compensation alter intentions and attitudes? *Journal of Health Communication, 20*(12), 1422–1432. https://doi.org/10.1080/10810730.2015.1018646

Noland, C. M., & Carl, W. J. (2006). "It's not our ass": Medical residents' sense-making regarding lawsuits. *Health Communication, 20*(1), 81–89. https://doi.org/10.1207/s15327027hc2001_8

Noland, C. M., & Carmack, H. J. (2015). "You never forget your first mistake": Nursing socialization, memorable messages, and communication about medical errors. *Health Communication, 30*(12), 1234–1244. https://doi.org/10.1080/10410236.2014.930397

Ornstein, C. (2007, December 5). Actor files suit in drug mishap; Dennis Quaid and wife fault maker of heparin in their twins' overdose. *Los Angeles Times,* B1.

Paget, M.A. (2004). *The unity of mistakes.* Temple University Press.

Premature babies die after blood thinner overdose. (2006, September 19). *Los Angeles Times,* A23.

Rockoff, J. D. (2008, May 15). Actor backs right to sue companies: Quaid tells Congress of twins' overdose. *The (Baltimore, MD) Sun,* A10.

Rubin, R. (2010, April 13). Dennis Quaid takes aim at health care mistakes: Actor's newborn twins nearly died from error. *USA Today,* B11.

Stebbing, C., Kaushal, R., & Bates, D. W. (2006). Pediatric medication safety and the media: What does the public see? *Pediatrics, 117*(6), 1907–1914. https://doi.org/10.1542/peds.2005-2017

The Joint Commission. (2012). Joint Commission Center for Transforming Healthcare releases targeted solutions tool for hand-off communication. https://www.jointcommission.org/assets/1/6/tst_hoc_persp_08_12.pdf

Thomas, E. J., Studdert, D. M., Burstin, H. R., Orav, E. J., Zeena, T., Williams, E. J., Howard, K. M., Weiler, P. C., & Brennan, T. A. (2000). Incidence and types of adverse events and negligent care in Utah and Colorado. *Medical Care, 38*(3), 261–271. https://dx.doi.org/10.1097/00005650-200003000-00003

Wailoo, K., Livingston, J., & Guarnaccia, P. (2006). Introduction. In K. Wailoo, J. Livingston, & P. Guarnaccia (Eds.), *A death retold: Jesica Santillan, the bungled transplant, and paradoxes of medical citizenship* (pp. 1–16). University of North Carolina Press.

Wachter, R. M., & Shojania, K. G. (2005). *Internal bleeding: The truth behinds America's terrifying epidemic of medical mistake*s. Rugged Land.

Weeks, W. B., & Mills, P. D. (2003). Reduction in patient enrollment in the Veterans Health Administration after media coverage of adverse medical events. *Joint Commission Journal on Quality and Safety, 29*(12), 652–658. https://doi.org/10.1016/s1549-3741(03)29077-8

Weiss, J. (2009, May 6). Scrubs: Goofy, cartoonish, and the most accurate portrayal of the medical profession on television. *Slate.* https://slate.com/culture/2009/05/the-most-accurate-television-show-about-the-medical-profession-scrubs.html

Wilson, C. (2006, September 18). Overdose kills 2 premature infants; Indianapolis hospital admits error in 6 cases. *Chicago Tribune,* 5.

13

POPULAR CULTURE AND PRO-HEALTH CHOICES

Diane B. Francis and Marian Jaitto-Jeffrey

Introduction

Through various mediums such as television shows (e.g., *The Biggest Loser*), social media platforms (e.g., *Instagram*), and video games (e.g., *Animal Crossing*), popular culture can significantly influence pro-health choices. As we detail in this chapter, pro-health choices mean decisions, actions, and behaviors that aim to promote and support one's health and overall well-being. These choices are made to improve the quality of life and maintain good health. Pro-health choices can take many forms, including maintaining a balanced and nutritious diet, engaging in regular physical activity, getting sufficient rest and sleep, avoiding harmful substances, managing stress, seeking medical care, maintaining a healthy weight, practicing safe behavior, building supportive relationships, and taking care of one's mental health. Interest in the effects of popular culture messaging and content has increased tremendously over the last few decades, as it has become clear that popular culture channels and platforms, and more generally mass-mediated content, shape how people make decisions about their own and others' choices and behaviors (Gollust et al., 2019). In this chapter, we discuss the affordances of specific popular culture platforms and how they influence pro-health choices. We focus primarily on mediated popular culture genres (e.g., print media, entertainment channels, and digital and social media). We then examine how popular culture has influenced pro-health outcomes across health domains such as cancer, mental health, sexual health, nutrition, and physical activity.

Popular Culture Platforms and Pro-Health Choices

News Media and Magazines and Pro-Health Choices

Print media (e.g., newspapers, magazines, and leaflets) have long been important sources of information about health and wellness, helping readers make informed pro-health choices. In the 19th century, British newspapers reported on Florence Nightingale's nursing interventions during the Crimean War and thereafter, educating the public about Nightingale and her nurses' efforts to tend to wounded soldiers (Rhodes, 2023). Some newspaper reports about Nightingale made their way to the United States and influenced nursing there (McHugh, 2022). Starting in 1918, the Spanish press began reporting on a deadly flu outbreak ravaging the country. Soon after, European and American press started printing stories about what would become the Spanish flu pandemic (Wills, 2018, January 15). Even during World War II, print media, such as posters and leaflets, were utilized to educate American service

DOI: 10.4324/9781003436409-15

members about venereal diseases, emphasizing the importance of protection for themselves and their partners, and, by extension, the military (Kennedy, 2017, July 12).

The influence of print media on health-related matters continues to be evident in modern times (Favaro, 2017). We note this influence in the continued interest in advice columns that offer people the opportunity to tell their stories (about sex and romance, friendships, illnesses, recovery, etc.) and receive ways to help themselves, whether it's *Dear Abby* (US) or *Ask Phillipa* (UK). Magazines such as *O: The Oprah Magazine*, *Men's Health*, *Women's Health*, and *AARP: The Magazine* provide readers with valuable information and advice to make informed decisions about their health and well-being. Moreover, a growing emphasis exists on representation and diversity in print media, particularly in magazines like *British Vogue.* By featuring individuals from diverse backgrounds, including people with disabilities and supermodels from various racial and ethnic groups, these magazines are helping to improve the conversation about representation and inclusivity in the health and wellness space.

The May 2023 cover of *British Vogue* featured several prominent people with disabilities. The magazine's September 2023 cover featured four supermodels from diverse racial/ethnic backgrounds in their 50s and 60s. In sum, researchers have taken a keen interest in examining the representation and portrayal of pro-health content in print media, recognizing its potential impact on shaping public perceptions and behaviors related to health. Print media continues to be a valuable source of information and inspiration for individuals seeking to lead healthier lives.

Entertainment Media and Pro-Health Choices

Entertainment media has also long been a source of pro-social and positive messages about physical and mental health. For example, a 1972 episode of the U.S.-based television show *Maude* featured the title character talking about and getting an abortion. In 1983, at the early stages of what would become the HIV/AIDS epidemic, the medical drama *St. Elsewhere* aired an episode titled "AIDS and Comfort," where it provided facts and countered misconceptions about the disease. Additionally, the 1948 American film *The Snake Pit* explored mental illness by chronicling one woman's stay in a psychiatric hospital. These examples illustrate how popular culture intersects with pro-health choices and how it can potentially influence our knowledge about health topics, attitudes toward diseases and preventive behaviors, and our beliefs about what causes diseases and how to cure them, mainly through mass, social, and digital media. We now turn to a broader description of pro-health messaging in television, movies, and films.

Television. The range of television shows that have included positive messages about health is astounding, from children's programming such as *Doc McStuffins* and *Daniel Tiger's Neighborhood* to teen-focused shows, including *Degrassi* and *Sex Education,* to more general audience programs such as *One Day at a Time* and *Insecure* (see also Chapter 24, this volume). These television shows and others have addressed issues such issues as literacy, social and emotional development, age-appropriate health discussions, and significant public health issues, including addiction, cancer, mental health, sexual violence, obesity, and organ donation (Francis & Finn, 2022; Morgan et al., 2010; Valente et al., 2007). We have also witnessed an increase in the diversity of body image representation in soap operas, sitcoms, and even Hallmark and Lifetime Christmas movies (see Chapter 5, this volume). Additionally, those networks show many romance movies made-for-television audiences that feature female leads from Black or other racial/ethnic minority groups year-round. For example, Tatyana Ali, best known for her role in the TV show *The Fresh Prince of Bel Air*, appeared in several Hallmark movies, including *Christmas Everlasting*.

In popular culture in the United States and globally, programming from the television channel MTV has further influenced young people's health through social and behavior change programming. MTV's *Shuga* underscored the significance of promoting pro-health choices among young people through television shows. *Shuga* combines drama, romance, and social commentary to draw its audience toward sexual health messages (see also Chapter 6, this volume). The show originated in Kenya but has since expanded to Nigeria and South Africa. In a series of studies, Banerjee and colleagues found that *Shuga* improved knowledge and attitudes about HIV and risky sexual behaviors, increased the likelihood of testing for HIV, and reduced sexually transmitted diseases and domestic violence (Banerjee et al., 2019a; Banerjee et al., 2019b). Different studies focused on MTV's American reality TV show *16 and Pregnant*. In the 18 months following the start of the show, teen births in the United States reduced by 4.3%, while Google Trends and Twitter data indicated increased Internet searches and tweeting behavior about contraceptive use and abortion (Kearney & Levine, 2015). In another study, researchers found that girls who watched a teen pregnancy narrative with their mothers and then discussed the issue endorsed more favorable attitudes toward pregnancy prevention (Moyer-Gusé et al., 2019).

Movies and Film. Like television, pro-health messages have also been prevalent in movies and films. Media producers commonly embed pro-health messages in the United States within commercially made entertainment programming. Movies and film can be a powerful medium for addressing mental, physical, and sexual health themes and helping to promote positive health choices and actions (see also Chapters 3 and 6, this volume). While some movies address sensitive or taboo topics, these movies can also foster understanding, empathy, and informed decision-making among audiences and viewers. The 1993 movie *Philadelphia* explored stigma and discrimination against people living with HIV/AIDS and raised awareness and public consciousness about this issue. *Precious*, a 2009 movie, told the story of an overweight teenager who suffered sexual abuse and teen pregnancy and delved into the importance of social and emotional support and environment for young mothers. The 2021 Disney animated musical film *Encanto* comprises one such example. *Encanto* tells the story of the Madrigal family from Colombia, who were blessed with a miracle following the traumatic events of conflict and death. The movie features Mirabel, who accepted and communicated with her Uncle Bruno despite his isolation from the family. *Encanto* sheds light on intergenerational trauma, and it has been used to discuss trauma, mental health, and healing with children (Conroy, 2022; Knox & Leshen, 2023). The famous song from the film, "We Don't Talk About Bruno," describes how Bruno was shunned by his family because he had strange and troubling visions. Yet, his niece, Mirabel, decided to seek him out and talk to him, thus modeling the importance of support in addressing social isolation and alienation.

In Nigeria, Ajayi (2018) described film "as an important form, a source of popular entertainment, and a powerful medium for educating or indoctrinating citizens" (p. 9). Ajayi focused her analysis on *Jenifa's Diary*, a Nigerian television show designed to entertain and educate Nigerian youth and that highlighted widespread social issues. Ajayi sought to raise awareness and prompt relevant social agencies to intervene, ultimately addressing and alleviating the challenges affected individuals and communities face. *Jenifa's Diary* has explored various themes, including health, human trafficking, and sex trafficking, shedding light on the societal repercussions of these issues. The protagonist, Jenifa, served as a voice and advocate, urging her friends to prioritize medical check-ups before marriage because, despite societal advancements, some couples continue to marry without assessing their genotypes, blood groups, or HIV status. The series premiered in 2015 and continues to be broadcast on TV and social media platforms as of 2024.

Social and Digital Media and Pro-Health Choices

In recent years, social and digital media platforms have emerged as powerful tools for disseminating information and promoting pro-health choices. With the widespread use of platforms such as Facebook, Twitter, Instagram, and YouTube, as well as mobile apps, and video games, individuals have unprecedented access to various health-related content, including articles, videos, and discussions on topics ranging from nutrition and fitness to mental health and well-being. Influencers and experts use these platforms to share their knowledge and experiences, providing followers with valuable insights and practical tips for making healthier lifestyle choices (see also Chapter 16, this volume). Moreover, social media campaigns and challenges often encourage individuals to adopt positive health behaviors, such as practicing mindfulness, exercising regularly, eating nutritious foods, reducing sugar intake, and practicing mindfulness. When used for pro-social and pro-health outcomes, social and digital media can empower individuals to prioritize their health and well-being. In this section, we give examples of how social media platforms, podcasts, video and digital games, and virtual reality are harnessed for pro-health choices.

Social Media. Positive health content is prevalent across the Internet and social and digital media platforms, from #SelfCareSunday to Wellness Wednesdays to posts by doctors and other healthcare providers, workout videos by physical trainers, and inspirational quotes of the day. A plethora of social media content exists across various platforms that can help individuals make pro-health decisions. YouTube is a platform where content creators often share videos and channels promoting positive health, self-care, and well-being. On TikTok, users create and share short video content, and it has become a space for promoting positive mental and physical health. Users can find content related to positive health, well-being, and self-care on Instagram. Facebook users can locate various health content, communities, and resources, especially health-related support groups and positive psychology and well-being pages sharing content related to happiness, resilience, and personal growth. Stakeholders have employed social media platforms such as Twitter (or X) to engage viewers and audiences with conversations about taboo topics.

Hashtag campaigns exemplify the positive influence of social media. Hashtag campaigns are popular on social media, and they have been harnessed across various health topics (Francis, 2021; Jackson et al., 2020). A set of studies has examined the use of Twitter to engage male audiences in prostate cancer awareness (Bravo & Hoffman-Goetz, 2015, 2016). Mental health also entails a popular topic of discussion on social media and an active area of research (McClellan et al., 2016). Berry et al. (2017) examined why people use social media for mental health by evaluating the hashtag #WhyWeTweetMH. Their study revealed four main reasons for tweeting: A sense of community, raising awareness and combatting stigma, a safe space for expression, and coping and empowerment. In 2020, many people joined a Twitter conversation to discuss sexual violence, police-involved trauma, and mental health in the Black community (Francis & Finn, 2022). The Twitter chat was produced by the creators of the television show *Queen Sugar* and occurred the day an episode on the topic aired.

Podcasts. *The Psychology of Your 20s*, *Therapy for Black Girls*, *Ten Percent Happier*, *Food Medic*, and *Just One Thing*. *Salud* exemplified podcasts that focus on health and well-being, aiming to help people and audiences make more informed pro-health choices. Podcasts are music or talk programs made available for download over the Internet (Merriam-Webster) and first emerged in 2003 (International Podcast Day). Like social media, podcasts are promising, intentional ways of reaching the public with positive health messages. While podcasts were initially primarily audio formats, more recent podcasts can be audio or video. Medicine, health, and well-being constitute one of the more popular genres for podcast topics, often ranking in the top 10 (Edison Research, 2023).

The *Defining Moments* podcast, hosted by Dr. Lynn Harter (2019–2022), has drawn on articles published in *Health Communication* and elsewhere. The CDC's Division of Communication Science and Services (Centers for Disease Control and Prevention, 2023) created a podcast series, *Listen UP!* To date, the podcast has centered on contemporary topics and incorporates perspectives from academics, innovators, practitioners, and other experts. One episode, "The Psychology and Impact of Digital Influence and Manipulation," included segments on being protected from manipulation and negative digital influence.

Another illustrative example of podcasting that enables pro-health choices is 'Chasing Life' with Sanjay Gupta (2020–present). As CNN's Chief Medical Correspondent, Dr. Sanjay Gupta draws upon his extensive experience as a neurosurgeon to delve into the diverse states of the brain and their impact on our overall health. Through engaging episodes featuring experienced guest speakers and interviews, he imparts insights that resonate with everyday experiences. Listeners can access these episodes conveniently on the CNN website.

Video and Digital Games. Like much of popular culture, the links between video/digital game playing and adverse outcomes have been the focus of decades of research (Bean et al., 2017; Elson & Ferguson, 2014). Yet, studies have demonstrated that video game playing can improve mood and psychological functioning, the ability to hold attention, and impact cognitive function (Granic et al., 2014; Johannes et al., 2021). Playing casual video games can help improve memory and aid in mental decline. Accordingly, organizations, such as the British children's charity Barnardo's (n.d.), now pointedly assert that video games are suitable for young people.

Among the public, playing games such as Wordle and Pokémon Go has grown even more popular since the coronavirus pandemic. Wordle, released in October 2021 when some people remained shuttered because of the pandemic, became a global sensation due to much social media hype (Hall, 2022). The web-based game Wordle has a simple premise: Players get six chances to guess a 5-letter word. The company has published a new puzzle each day. At its height, more than 2 million people played Wordle daily, and it seemed that nearly everyone was playing Wordle. Queen Camilla of England (then Camilla, Duchess of Cornwall) reported being obsessed with the game and playing with her granddaughter (Burack, 2022). Actress Carol Burnett said she played Wordle with other actor friends, including Allison Janney, Charlize Theron, and David Crane (Brockington, 2023, April 26). Actor Ben Affleck was also reportedly part of a celebrity Wordle group (Calvario, 2023, March 16). These examples illustrate one of the many pro-health benefits of playing video games: Social connection and community (Comello et al., 2019; Francis et al., 2016).

Virtual Reality Platforms. Pokémon Go was also a big hit during the pandemic. The game uses augmented and virtual reality to engage audiences. With Pokémon Go, players find objects in the real world using digital maps; players engage in physical activity such as walking to capture the Pokémon creatures. Harry Potter: Wizards Unite used similar location-based, role-playing augmented reality technology to get players up and moving during gameplay. Virtual reality (VR), augmented reality (AR), and extended reality (XR) can provide immersive experiences and involvement that allow people to imagine and even simulate various settings, including being in good health. Virtual reality technology involves using headsets to demonstrate a particular environment and replicate a user's physical existence in a virtual or imaginary setting (Fertleman et al., 2018). Within such a setting, avatars (virtual characters with whom the user interacts) are designed to express emotions, thus providing the user with a greater sense of reality, facilitating meaningful interaction (Kim et al., 2017) and a safe environment to learn and reflect (Fertleman et al., 2018). Virtual reality has been effective in curbing public speaking anxiety (Bellido Rivas et al., 2021; North et al., 1998), promoting VR-based psychology therapy (Freeman et al., 2017), and enhancing relaxation and stress reduction (Pizzoli et al., 2019). Bellido Rivas et al. further revealed that, through virtual reality, people see a life-sized body instead of their own, which gives them the illusion of body ownership as the virtual body moves with their movements. From the viewer's perspective, this illusion confirms that the influence of embodiment in a cartoon character can lead to a high level of body ownership, which is crucial to the viewer's experience.

Popular culture plays a significant role in shaping societal attitudes and behaviors towards various aspects of health, including cancer outcomes, mental health, sexual health, diet, and exercise. Through mediums such as television, movies, music, and social media, popular culture can positively influence individuals' perceptions and actions regarding their health. These platforms can be used to raise awareness about cancer prevention, mental health stigma reduction, safe sexual practices, and the importance of maintaining a balanced diet and a regular exercise regimen.

Popular Culture and Pro-Health Outcomes

In this section of the chapter, we briefly outline some of the outcomes associated with exposure to pro-health messaging across popular culture. As we documented, pro-health messaging and content are prevalent across various popular culture domains. However, what effect does exposure to such messaging have on individuals? Specifically, is exposure to positive and pro-social messages across popular culture associated with pro-health choices? Extensive research across multiple health domains such as cancer, diabetes, obesity, mental health, sexual health, and others affirms a multitude of benefits to having pro-health messages in popular media and culture (Francis & Finn, 2022; Len-Ríos et al., 2010; Moyer-Gusé et al., 2019; Quick et al., 2013; Valente et al., 2007; Wright, 2020).

Outcomes such as awareness of health issues, information seeking, interpersonal communication, attitudes and beliefs, role modeling, normative perceptions, and behavioral actions are explained by communication and persuasion theories including McGuire's information processing model (McGuire, 1984), Bandura's social cognitive theory (Bandura, 1986, 2001), and the elaboration likelihood model (Petty & Cacioppo, 1986; Slater & Rouner, 2002). Other theories of behavior prediction, such as the stages of change (Prochaska & DiClemente, 2005; Prochaska et al., 1992) and the reasoned action approach (Fishbein & Ajzen, 1975; Fishbein & Ajzen, 2010) have also helped to predict the effects of popular culture on pro-health choices. Additionally, theoretical models, such as the self-determination theory (Ryan & Deci, 2000) and a values-based approach (Schwartz, 1994), have helped to understand the relationship between exposure to and use of cultural formats such as video games on psychological and health outcomes.

One of the most studied domains at the intersection of popular culture and pro-health choices involves cancer-related outcomes. Researchers have studied the reporting of cancer information in the media and found that readers pay attention to such information and gain knowledge and understanding about various cancers (Len-Ríos et al., 2010). Knowing this information, researchers have also conducted interventions to place cancer information in select newspapers in the United States through the *Ozioma* News Service project. Intervention communities that received cancer information were more likely to localize the stories and make them relevant to their readers (Caburnay et al., 2012). Readers also gained culturally specific cancer information from those stories (Cohen et al., 2014). Evidence also attests that exposure to cancer information through social media can improve cancer screening, early diagnosis, and behavior change (Plackett et al., 2020). For cancer patients, social media platforms allow young adult patients to connect with their peers, share cancer treatment experiences and life concerns, and create a space for mutual validation (Lazard et al., 2021). Finally, other studies have examined whether playing casual video games such as World of Warcraft and Words with Friends benefited cancer survivors (Comello et al., 2019; Comello et al., 2016; Francis et al., 2016). The researchers found that, not only did playing such games align with players' values, but more than half of the study participants used the game playing for social connection and community (Comello et al., 2019; Francis et al., 2016).

Researchers have also studied the benefits of popular culture on mental health outcomes (Francis, 2021; Oliver, 2022). In the study of cancer survivors who played video games, many participants said they played games as an escape from their emotionally difficult situations; others played to avoid loneliness and isolation (Comello et al., 2019). In essence, playing video games was good for their mental well-being. An emerging argument exists for healthcare providers to prescribe casual video game play to specific populations (Fish et al., 2014). Besides video games, websites, news and entertainment media, and social media channels offer mental health information, support, advice, help-seeking, and care (Francis, 2018; To et al., 2023; Vargas et al., 2021). Podcasts are another genre that seems to benefit listeners greatly; motivations for listening to podcasts include parasocial relationships with podcast hosts and social engagement (Tobin & Guadagno, 2022). One study found that podcast hosts and listeners were able to use the platform to process thoughts and feelings about sexual abuse after viewing the documentary "Surviving R. Kelly" (Barner, 2023). Interest in the benefits of podcasting is growing, as evidenced by the increase in studies on podcast interventions (Rogers et al., 2020; Turner-McGrievy et al., 2009). Researchers from Australia developed a podcast to reduce stigma against people with complex mental health issues. Surveys of listeners indicated a high willingness to listen to the podcast and gain knowledge of the lived experiences of people with such illnesses (Carrotte et al., 2023).

Despite much concern about the impact of popular culture on sexual health and sexuality, growing evidence attests that not all the effects are adverse (Moyer-Gusé et al., 2011). According to Moyer-Gusé, teen pregnancy and sexually transmitted diseases remain critical issues across popular culture. However, in many instances, television shows, films, and even social media such as TikTok or YouTube videos provide positive sexual scripts that foster conversations about the potential health risks of unprotected sex, sexual initiation, contraception, and responsible sexual behaviors (White et al., 2023). For example, the television show *East Los High*, aired on the online platform Hulu and marketed primarily to Hispanic youths, featured several episodes where young people discuss sexual health, contraception, and teen pregnancy (Wang & Singhal, 2016; see also Chapter 17, this volume).

Like the positive health messaging about sex and sexuality, popular culture can positively affect people's knowledge and choices regarding food, nutrition, and physical activity. Research has shown that the media, Internet, and popular culture can teach children about healthy food and nutrition choices (Binder et al., 2021; Dixon et al., 2017). Dixon et al. found that children had more positive ratings of more nutritious meals if movie tie-in premiums accompanied the meals compared to when the healthier meals did not have such tie-ins. However, positive outcomes can emerge even without movie tie-ins; kids who watch Sesame Street make better food choices than those who do not (Kotler et al., 2012; see also Chapters 4 and 24, this volume).

Conclusions and Future Directions

This chapter focuses on the linkages between popular culture and pro-health choices. The chapter explores the complex interplay between popular culture, mass media, social media, and digital media, and positive health outcomes, considering the positive impacts that media and societal trends can have on individual decision-making and public health. As Health Communication and media effects scholars have pointed out, popular culture can influence positive health at personal and public levels (Brown & Walsh-Childers, 2002). Furthermore, the positive effects of popular culture on individuals and the public can be intended and unintended. The impact of popular culture may be *intended*, such as when people learn about long-acting reversible birth control after seeing it on a television show, or may be *unintended*, such as when people talk about intergenerational trauma with children after watching the Disney movie *Encanto*. These outcomes are generally positive from a public health perspective. We focus on such outcomes in this chapter.

Over the past 25 years, intense interest in the effects of popular culture on health has been expressed by non-governmental organizations, federal agencies, and departments, all of which have realized the significant power of traditional and emerging media and technology to shift cultural norms and help people make healthy decisions (Institute of Medicine (U.S.) Committee on Assuring the Health of the Public in the 21st Century, 2002; Jenkins et al., n.d.; The White House, 2021). For example, the Bill and Melinda Gates Foundation (2023) called for proposals on "Entertainment Media Content Analysis and Monitoring" to generate data on how multimedia platforms influence gender norms and behaviors among adolescent girls and young women in developing countries. Another example includes a call for proposals from the United Kingdom-based Wellcome Trust, focusing on the effects of digital mental health interventions (Wellcome, 2022).

We call for more work on children, young people, and people with neurodivergent experiences or varying abilities. This work should take on a more global perspective, given differences in how various cultures think of and understand the impact and influence of popular culture, media, and technologies on people and society. For example, the Global Kids Online (n.d.) project has provided data and evidence on children's well-being and rights in the digital age. Growing out of this research is an increasing need for digital literacy and digital citizenship across the life course. Digital literacy encompasses the ability to utilize digital media critically. A strong line of research shows the positive effects of media literacy programs on essential health choices and outcomes (Geraee et al., 2015; Scull et al., 2022). This research needs to be further expanded across diverse population segments.

In the digital age, another significant development entails the role of artificial intelligence in popular culture. As we write this chapter, meaningful discussions occur across personal and public domains about the impact of artificial intelligence (AI) on societal trends (West & Allen, 2018, April 24). Future research on popular culture's effects on pro-health choices will have to consider the role of AI across domains such as content and audience response. Some emerging studies suggest AI may be a powerful tool for positive health promotion (Goh et al., 2022). AI, for example, could be used to develop tailored messages for audiences (Huang & Rust, 2021; Kreps & Neuhauser, 2013).

Along with AI, virtual, augmented, or extended reality programs and their impact on pro-health choices deserve more attention. The field of virtual reality first came to light decades ago; however, recent technological advances have made it an exciting and emerging area. Its applications are vast, ranging from military training to gaming. In health, the technology has been trialed for uses such as cognitive rehabilitation post-stroke (De Luca et al., 2019), improving reaction times in children with cerebral palsy (Pourazar et al., 2018), and aiding the diagnosis of psychiatric conditions (van Bennekom et al., 2017). Individual responses to virtual reality experiences can vary, so what works well for one person may not be as effective for another.

Accordingly, some people need clarification about virtual reality technology's ability to reflect patients' diversity and complexity in a typical healthcare setting. Fertleman et al. (2018) outlined geographical and cultural factors, personality traits, and the type of healthcare setting that contribute to this concern. While virtual reality has many potential benefits in healthcare, its application should be used as a complementary tool under healthcare professionals' guidance when appropriate. Although virtual reality shows relevant potential in improving and regulating emotional well-being, Pizzoli et al. (2019) advocated that a new approach – personalized virtual reality – is needed to provide the user with more adequate and person-adapted techniques through distinctive features picked by users' memories of relevant life events, and on adaptive virtual reality to manipulate the emotional experience of people positively. They proposed that personalized virtual reality will be a user-centered approach to designing and implementing the virtual reality setting itself.

A long-standing concern for researchers has been how to measure exposure to media and popular culture artifacts. What counts as exposure in the current context of platform-shifting and multiscreen engagement? We know that media and technology companies are collecting vast amounts of exposure-related data on audiences, but how do communication scholars capture such data to make claims about the effects of exposure on pro-health choices? Such data could also be used to facilitate answering another critical question. The extant research has solid correlational data, but a need exists for more longitudinal data, especially as some of these popular culture contexts lend themselves to multiple exposures. Researchers and practitioners must take advantage of new ways of measuring media and popular culture exposure, such as real-time data and multiscreen viewing. The intersection of popular culture and pro-health choices is an exciting area of Health Communication and health humanities research that holds considerable promise for pro-health choices and positive health outcomes.

Further Reading

Alper, M. (2023). *Kids across the spectrum: Growing up autistic in the digital age*. MIT Press. This book examines the role of media, technology, and popular culture in children's everyday lives.

Hornik, R. C. (2013). *Why can't we sell human rights like we sell soap*? SAGE. This book contains an argument for positive marketing of pro-social issues.

Jackson, S. J. et al. (2020). *#hashtagactivism: Networks of Race and Gender Justice*. MIT Press. La Ferrara, E. (2016). *Mass media and social change: Can we use television to fight poverty*? Oxford University Press. This book asks and answers another thought-provoking question.

Livingstone, S. (2002). *Young people and new media. SAGE.* This book is a ground-breaking work providing rich empirical and theoretical insights.

References

Ajayi, A. O. (2018). *Critical discourse analysis of Nigerian TV series, Jẹnifa's Diary*. Federal University Oye-Ekiti.

Bandura, A. (1986). *Social foundations of thought and action: A social cognitive theory*. Prentice Hall.

Bandura, A. (2001). Social cognitive theory of mass communication. *Media Psychology*, *3*(3), 265–299. https://doi.org/10.1207/S1532785XMEP0303_03

Banerjee, A., La Ferrara, E., & Orozco, V. (2019a). Entertainment, education, and attitudes toward domestic violence. *AEA Papers and Proceedings*, *109*, 133–137. https://doi.org/10.1257/pandp.20191073

Banerjee, A., La Ferrara, E., & Orozco-Olvera, V. H. (2019b, July). The entertaining way to behavioral change: Fighting HIV with MTV. National Bureau of Economic Research, *26096*. https://doi.org/10.3386/w26096

Barner, B. (2023). 'Our pain prioritized for once': Survivor-centred Black podcasts reckoning with Surviving R. Kelly. *Radio Journal: International Studies in Broadcast & Audio Media*, *21*(1), 83–98. https://doi.org/10.1386/rjao_00074_1

Bean, A. M., Nielsen, R. K. L., Van Rooij, A. J., & Ferguson, C. J. (2017). Video game addiction: The push to pathologize video games. *Professional Psychology: Research and Practice*, *48*(5), 378–389. https://doi.org/10.1037/pro0000150

Bellido Rivas, A. I., Navarro, X., Banakou, D., Oliva, R., Orvalho, V., & Slater, M. (2021). The influence of embodiment as a cartoon character on public speaking anxiety. *Frontiers in Virtual Reality*, *2*, 695673. https://doi.org/10.3389/frvir.2021.695673

Bernado's (n.d.). *Pesky gNATs*. https://www.barnardos.org.uk/ready-player-b/pesky-gnats

Berry, N., Lobban, F., Belousov, M., Emsley, R., Nenadic, G., & Bucci, S. (2017). #WhyWeTweetMH: Understanding why people use Twitter to discuss mental health problems. *Journal of Medical Internet Research*, *19*(4), e107, 154–166. https://doi.org/10.2196/jmir.6173

Bill & Melinda Gates Foundation. (2023). *Adolescents & social norms*. https://www.gatesfoundation.org/our-work/programs/gender-equality/adolescents-and-social-norms

Binder, A., Naderer, B., & Matthes, J. (2021). Shaping healthy eating habits in children with persuasive strategies: Toward a typology. *Frontiers in Public Health*, *9*, 676127. https://doi.org/10.3389/fpubh.2021.676127

Bravo, C. A., & Hoffman-Goetz, L. (2015). Social media and men's health: A content analysis of Twitter conversations during the 2013 movember campaigns in the United States, Canada, and the United Kingdom. *American Journal of Men's Health*, *11*(6), 1627–1641. https://doi.org/10.1177/1557988315617826

Bravo, C. A., & Hoffman-Goetz, L. (2016). Tweeting about prostate and testicular cancers: Do Twitter conversations and the 2013 movember Canada campaign objectives align? *Journal of Cancer Education*, *31*(2), 236–243. https://doi.org/10.1007/s13187-015-0796-1

Brockington, A. (2023, April 26). Carol Burnett says she plays Wordle every day with this celebrity. *Today*. https://www.today.com/popculture/news/ben-affleck-part-celebrity-wordle-group-guess-else-rcna75360

Brown, J. D., & Walsh-Childers, K. (2002). Effects of media on personal and public health. In J. Bryant & D. Zillmann (Eds.), *Media effects: Advances in theory and research (*2nd ed.). (pp. 453–488). Erlbaum.

Burack, E. (2022). Camilla, Duchess of Cornwall, is also obsessed with Wordle. *Hearst*. https://www.townandcountrymag.com/society/tradition/a40363964/camilla-duchess-of-cornwall-wordle/

Caburnay, C. A., Luke, D. A., Cameron, G. T., Cohen, E. L., Fu, Q., Lai, C. L., Stemmle, J. T., Paulen, M., Jackson, L., & Kreuter, M. W. (2012). Evaluating the Ozioma cancer news service: A community randomized trial in 24 U.S. cities. *Preventive Medicine*, *54*(6), 425–430. https://doi.org/10.1016/j.ypmed.2012.04.010

Calvario, L. (2023, March 16). Ben Affleck is part of a celebrity Wordle group — guess who else is in it. *Today*. https://www.today.com/popculture/news/ben-affleck-part-celebrity-wordle-group-guess-else-rcna75360

Carrotte, E., Hopgood, F., Blanchard, M., Groot, C., & Phillips, L. (2023). A new podcast for reducing stigma against people living with complex mental health issues: Co-design study. *JMIR Formative Research*, *7*, e44412. https://doi.org/10.2196/44412

Centers for Disease Control and Prevention. (2023). *Listen UP! Podcast Series*. https://www.cdc.gov/healthcommunication/podcast.html

Cohen, E., Caburnay, C. A., Stemmle, J. T., Len-Rios, M. E., Poor, T., Powe, B. D., Rath, S., Robinson, E., Semenkovich, K., Cameron, G. T., Luke, D. A., & Kreuter, M. W. (2014). The Ozioma news service: Targeting cancer communication to African American communities. In M. J. Dutta & G. L. Kreps (Eds.), *Reducing health disparities: Communication interventions* (pp. 259–277). Peter Lang.

Comello, M. L., Francis, D. B., Hursting, L., Swarner, E., & Marshall, L. H. (2019). Values of cancer survivors and the supportive role of recreational video games. *Journal of Health Psychology*, Advanced online publication. https://doi.org/10.1177/1359105319871663

Comello, M. L., Francis, D. B., Marshall, L. H., & Puglia, D. R. (2016). Cancer survivors who play recreational computer games: Motivations for playing and associations with beneficial psychological outcomes. *Games for Health Journal*, *5*(4), 286–292. https://doi.org/10.1089/g4h.2016.0003

Conroy, S. (2022). Narrative matters: Encanto and intergenerational trauma. *Child and Adolescent Mental Health*, *27*(3), 309–311. https://doi.org/10.1111/camh.12563

De Luca, R., Lo Buono, V., Leo, A., Russo, M., Aragona, B., Leonardi, S., Buda, A., Naro, A., & Calabrò, R. S. (2019). Use of virtual reality in improving poststroke neglect: Promising neuropsychological and neurophysiological findings from a case study. *Applied Neuropsychology: Adult*, *26*(1), 96–100. https://doi.org/10.1080/23279095.2017.1363040

Dixon, H., Niven, P., Scully, M., & Wakefield, M. (2017). Food marketing with movie character toys: Effects on young children's preferences for unhealthy and healthier fast food meals. *Appetite*, *117*, 342–350. https://doi.org/10.1016/j.appet.2017.07.014

Edison Research. (2023). *Top podcast genres in the U.S. Q4 2022 – Q1 2023*. Edison Research. https://www.edisonresearch.com/top-podcast-genres-in-the-u-s-q4-2022-q1-2023/

Elson, M., & Ferguson, C. J. (2014). Twenty-five years of research on violence in digital games and aggression: Empirical evidence, perspectives, and a debate gone astray. *European Psychologist*, *19*(1), 33–46. https://doi.org/10.1027/1016-9040/a000147

Favaro, L. (2017). Mediating intimacy online: Authenticity, magazines and chasing the clicks. *Journal of Gender Studies*, *26*(3), 321–334. https://doi.org/10.1080/09589236.2017.1280385

Fertleman, C., Aubugeau-Williams, P., Sher, C., Lim, A.-N., Lumley, S., Delacroix, S., & Pan, X. (2018). A discussion of virtual reality as a new tool for training healthcare professionals. *Frontiers in Public Health*, *6*, 44. https://doi.org/10.3389/fpubh.2018.00044

Fish, M. T., Russoniello, C. V., & O'Brien, K. (2014). The efficacy of prescribed casual videogame play in reducing symptoms of anxiety: A randomized controlled study. *Games for Health Journal*, *3*(5), 291–295. https://doi.org/10.1089/g4h.2013.0092

Fishbein, M., & Ajzen, I. (1975). *Belief, attitude, intention and behavior: An introduction to theory and research*. Addison-Wesley.

Fishbein, M., & Ajzen, I. (2010). *Predicting and changing behavior: The reasoned action approach*. Psychology Press.

Francis, D. B. (2018). Young Black men's information seeking following celebrity depression disclosure: Implications for mental health communication. *Journal of Health Communication*, *23*(7), 687–694. https://doi.org/10.1080/10810730.2018.1506837

Francis, D. B. (2021). "Twitter is really therapeutic at times": Examination of Black men's Twitter conversations following Hip-Hop Artist Kid Cudi's depression disclosure. *Health Communication*, *36*(4), 448–456. https://doi.org/10.1080/10410236.2019.1700436

Francis, D. B., Comello, M. L., & Marshall, L. H. (2016). How does game playing support values and psychological well-being among cancer survivors? *Games for Health Journal*, *5*(2), 128–134. https://doi.org/10.1089/g4h.2015.0044

Francis, D. B., & Finn, L. (2022). A theoretically based analysis of Twitter conversations about trauma and mental health: Examining responses to storylines on the television show Queen Sugar. *Health Communication*, *37*(9), 1104–1112. https://doi.org/10.1080/10410236.2021.1888454

Freeman, D., Reeve, S., Robinson, A., Ehlers, A., Clark, D., Spanlang, B., & Slater, M. (2017). Virtual reality in the assessment, understanding, and treatment of mental health disorders. *Psychological Medicine*, *47*(14), 2393–2400. https://doi.org/10.1017/S003329171700040X

Geraee, N., Kaveh, M. H., Shojaeizadeh, D., & Tabatabaee, H. R. (2015). Impact of media literacy education on knowledge and behavioral intention of adolescents in dealing with media messages according to stages of change. *Journal of Advances in Medical Education & Professionalism*, *3*(1), 9–14.

Global Kids Online. (n.d.). Children's rights in the digital age. http://globalkidsonline.net/

Goh, Y. S., Ow Yong, J. Q. Y., Chee, B. Q. H., Kuek, J. H. L., & Ho, C. S. H. (2022). Machine learning in health promotion and behavioral change: Scoping review. *Journal of Medical Internet Research*, *24*(6), e35831. https://doi.org/10.2196/35831

Gollust, S. E., Fowler, E. F., & Niederdeppe, J. (2019). Television news coverage of public health issues and implications for public health policy and practice. *Annual Review of Public Health*, *40*, 167–185. https://doi.org/10.1146/annurev-publhealth-040218-044017

Granic, I., Lobel, A., & Engels, R. C. (2014). The benefits of playing video games. *American Psychologist*, *69*(1), 66–78. https://doi.org/10.1037/a0034857

Gupta, S. H. (2020-present). Chasing life with Dr. Sanjay Gupta. *CNN*. https://www.cnn.com/audio/podcasts/chasing-life

Hall, R. (2022, January 11). Wordle creator overwhelmed by global success of hit puzzle. *The Guardian (UK)*. https://www.theguardian.com/games/2022/jan/11/wordle-creator-overwhelmed-by-global-success-of-hit-puzzle

Harter, L. H. (2019-2022). *Defining moments*. https://www.npr.org/podcasts/727287962/defining-moments

Huang, M.-H., & Rust, R. T. (2021). A strategic framework for artificial intelligence in marketing. *Journal of the Academy of Marketing Science*, *49*(1), 30–50. https://doi.org/10.1007/s11747-020-00749-9

Institute of Medicine (U.S.) Committee on assuring the health of the public in the 21st century. (2002). The future of the public's health in the 21st century. National Academies Press (U.S.). https://doi.org/10.17226/10548

International Podcast Day (n.d.). International Podcast Day. https://internationalpodcastday.com/podcasting-history/

Jackson, S. J., Bailey, M., & Welles, B. F. (2020). *# HashtagActivism: Networks of race and gender justice*. MIT Press.

Jenkins, H., Clinton, K., Purushotma, R., Robison, A. J., & Weigel, M. (n.d.). *Confronting the challenges of participatory culture: Media education for the 21st century*. The MacArthur Foundation. https://www.macfound.org/media/article_pdfs/jenkins_white_paper.pdf

Johannes, N., Vuorre, M., & Przybylski, A. K. (2021). Video game play is positively correlated with well-being. *Royal Society Open Science*, *8*(2), 202049. https://doi.org/10.1098/rsos.202049

Kearney, M. S., & Levine, P. B. (2015). Media influences on social outcomes: The impact of MTV's 16 and Pregnant on teen childbearing. *The American Economic Review*, *105*(12), 3597–3632. https://doi.org/10.1257/aer.20140012

Kennedy, K. (2017, July 12). The wartime posters that tried to shame soldiers away from STDs. *Atlas Obscura*. https://www.atlasobscura.com/articles/venereal-disease-posters-sti-world-war-ii-sex-shame#

Kim, M., Jeon, C., & Kim, J. (2017). A study on immersion and presence of a portable hand haptic system for immersive virtual reality. *Sensors*, *17*(5), 1141. https://doi.org/10.3390/s17051141

Knox, D., & Leshen, G. (2023). Let's talk about Bruno: Encanto as a medium to teach psychodynamic theory. *Psychiatry*, *86*(1), 70–74. https://doi.org/10.1080/00332747.2022.2113318

Kotler, J. A., Schiffman, J. M., & Hanson, K. G. (2012). The influence of media characters on children's food choices. *Journal of Health Communication*, *17*(8), 886–898. https://doi.org/10.1080/10810730.2011.650822

Kreps, G. L., & Neuhauser, L. (2013). Artificial intelligence and immediacy: Designing health communication to personally engage consumers and providers. *Patient Education and Counseling*, *92*(2), 205–210. https://doi.org/10.1016/j.pec.2013.04.014

Lazard, A. J., Collins, M. K. R., Hedrick, A., Varma, T., Love, B., Valle, C. G., Brooks, E., & Benedict, C. (2021). Using social media for peer-to-peer cancer support: Interviews with young adults with cancer. *JMIR Cancer*, *7*(3), e28234. https://doi.org/10.2196/28234

Len-Ríos, M. E., Cohen, E., & Caburnay, C. (2010). Readers use Black newspapers for health/cancer information. *Newspaper Research Journal*, *31*(1), 20–35. https://doi.org/10.1177/073953291003100103

McClellan, C., Ali, M. M., Mutter, R., Kroutil, L., & Landwehr, J. (2016). Using social media to monitor mental health discussions - evidence from Twitter. *Journal of the American Medical Informatics Association*, *24*(3), 496–502. https://doi.org/10.1093/jamia/ocw133

McGuire, W. J. (1984). Public communication as a strategy for inducing health-promoting behavioral change. *Preventive Medicine*, *13*(3), 299–319. https://doi.org/10.1016/0091-7435(84)90086-0

McHugh, J. (2022). A war with Russia led Florence Nightingale to revolutionize nursing. *The Washington Post*. https://www.washingtonpost.com/history/2022/05/08/florence-nightingale-nursing-covid/

Merriam-Webster (n.d.). Podcast. https://www.merriam-webster.com/dictionary/podcast

Morgan, S. E., King, A. J., Smith, J. R., & Ivic, R. (2010). A kernel of truth? The impact of television storylines exploiting myths about organ donation on the public's willingness to donate. *Journal of Communication*, *60*(4), 778–796. https://doi.org/10.1111/j.1460-2466.2010.01523.x

Moyer-Gusé, E., Chung, A. H., & Jain, P. (2011). Identification with characters and discussion of taboo topics after exposure to an entertainment narrative about sexual health. *Journal of Communication*, *61*(3), 387–406. https://doi.org/10.1111/j.1460-2466.2011.01551.x

Moyer-Gusé, E., Woods, K., Rader, K., & Luong, K. T. (2019). Talking about TV: Mother-daughter viewing and discussion of an entertainment narrative about teen pregnancy. *Health Communication, 35*, 1–10. https://doi.org/10.1080/10410236.2019.1623642

North, M. M., North, S. M., & Coble, J. R. (1998). Virtual reality therapy: An effective treatment for the fear of public speaking. *International Journal of Virtual Reality, 3*(3), 1–6.

Oliver, M. B. (2022). Social media use and eudaimonic well-being. *Current Opinion in Psychology, 45*, 101307. https://doi.org/10.1016/j.copsyc.2022.101307

Petty, R. E., & Cacioppo, J. T. (1986). The elaboration likelihood model of persuasion. In R. E. Petty & J. T. Cacioppo (Eds.), *Communication and persuasion: Central and peripheral routes to attitude change* (Vol. 19, pp. 123–205). Springer-Verlag. https://doi.org/https://doi.org/10.1007/978-1-4612-4964-1

Pizzoli, S. F. M., Mazzocco, K., Triberti, S., Monzani, D., Alcañiz Raya, M. L., & Pravettoni, G. (2019). User-centered virtual reality for promoting relaxation: An innovative approach. *Frontiers in Psychology, 10*, 479. https://doi.org/10.3389/fpsyg.2019.00479

Plackett, R., Kaushal, A., Kassianos, A. P., Cross, A., Lewins, D., Sheringham, J., Waller, J., & von Wagner, C. (2020). Use of social media to promote cancer screening and early diagnosis: Scoping review. *Journal of Medical Internet Research, 22*(11), e21582. https://doi.org/10.2196/21582

Pourazar, M., Mirakhori, F., Hemayattalab, R., & Bagherzadeh, F. (2018). Use of virtual reality intervention to improve reaction time in children with cerebral palsy: A randomized controlled trial. *Developmental Neurorehabilitation, 21*(8), 515–520. https://doi.org/10.1080/17518423.2017.1368730

Prochaska, J. O., & DiClemente, C. C. (2005). The transtheoretical approach. In Norcross, J. C., & Goldfried, M. R. (Eds.), *Handbook of psychotherapy integration* (2nd ed., pp. 147–171). Oxford.

Prochaska, J. O., DiClemente, C. C., & Norcross, J. C. (1992). In search of how people change: Applications to addictive behaviors. *American Psychologist, 47*(9), 1102–1114. https://doi.org/10.1037/10248-026

Quick, B. L., Morgan, S. E., LaVoie, N. R., & Bosch, D. (2013). Grey's Anatomy viewing and organ donation attitude formation: Examining mediators bridging this relationship among African Americans, Caucasians, and Latinos. *Communication Research, 41*(5), 690–716. https://doi.org/10.1177/0093650213475476

Rhodes, C. (2023). How a fiery newspaper article took Florence Nightingale into the Crimean War and sparked her crusade for hospital reform. https://www.workingnurse.com/articles/nightingale-in-crimea/

Rogers, D., Herbert, M., Whitzman, C., McCann, E., Maginn, P. J., Watts, B., Alam, A., Pill, M., Keil, R., Dreher, T., Novacevski, M., Byrne, J., Osborne, N., Büdenbender, M., Alizadeh, T., Murray, K., Dombroski, K., Prasad, D., Connolly, C., Kaa, A., Dale, E., Murray, C., & Caldis, S. (2020). The city under COVID-19: Podcasting as digital methodology. *Journal of Economic and Human Geography, 111*(3), 434–450. https://doi.org/10.1111/tesg.12426

Ryan, R. M., & Deci, E. I. (2000). Self-determination theory and the facilitation of intrinsic motivation, social development, and well-being. *American Psychologist, 55*(1), 68–78. https://doi.org/10.1037/0003-066X.55.1.68

Schwartz, S. H. (1994). Are there universal aspects in the structure and contents of human values? *Journal of Social Issues, 50*(4), 19–45. https://doi.org/10.1111/j.1540-4560.1994.tb01196.x

Scull, T. M., Dodson, C. V., Geller, J. G., Reeder, L. C., & Stump, K. N. (2022). A media literacy education approach to high school sexual health education: Immediate effects of media aware on adolescents' media, sexual health, and communication outcomes. *Journal of Youth Adolescence, 51*(4), 708–723. https://doi.org/10.1007/s10964-021-01567-0

Slater, M. D., & Rouner, D. (2002). Entertainment—education and elaboration likelihood: Understanding the processing of narrative persuasion. *Communication Theory, 12*(2), 173–191. https://doi.org/10.1111/j.1468-2885.2002.tb00265.x

The White House. (2021). Advancing equity and racial justice through the federal government. https://www.whitehouse.gov/equity/#health-equity

To, S. B., Gray, J., Jain, P., Porter, J. H., & Comello, M. L. G. (2023). Advocating, unlearning, tearing it all down? How BIPOC young adults with mental health concerns perceive and engage with the media. *Health Communication*, 1–13. Advanced online publication. https://doi.org/10.1080/10410236.2023.2290882

Tobin, S. J., & Guadagno, R. E. (2022). Why people listen: Motivations and outcomes of podcast listening. *PLoS One, 17*(4), e0265806. https://doi.org/10.1371/journal.pone.0265806

Turner-McGrievy, G. M., Campbell, M. K., Tate, D. F., Truesdale, K. P., Bowling, J. M., & Crosby, L. (2009). Pounds off digitally study: A randomized podcasting weight-loss intervention. *American Journal of Preventive Medicine, 37*(4), 263–269. https://doi.org/10.1016/j.amepre.2009.06.010

Valente, T. W., Murphy, S., Huang, G., Gusek, J., Greene, J., & Beck, V. (2007). Evaluating a minor storyline on ER about teen obesity, hypertension, and 5 a day. *Journal of Health Communication, 12*(6), 551–566. https://doi.org/10.1080/10810730701508385

van Bennekom, M. J., de Koning, P. P., & Denys, D. (2017). Virtual reality objectifies the diagnosis of psychiatric disorders:
A literature review. *Frontiers in Psychiatry*, *8*, 163. https://doi.org/10.3389/fpsyt.2017.00163
Vargas, L. C., Comello, M. L. G., & Porter, J. H. (2021). The Web's potential to provide depression literacy resources to Latinx teens: A missed opportunity? *Howard Journal of Communications*, *32*(4), 366–381. https://doi.org/10.1080/10646175.2020.1819480
Wang, H., & Singhal, A. (2016). East Los High: Transmedia edutainment to promote the sexual and reproductive health of young Latina/o Americans. *American Journal of Public Health*, *106*(6), 1002–1010. https://doi.org/10.2105/ajph.2016.303072
Wellcome. (2022). Mental health award: Looking backwards, moving forward – understanding how interventions for anxiety, depression, and psychosis work. *Wellcome*. https://wellcome.org/grant-funding/schemes/mental-health-award-interventions-anxiety-depression-psychosis
West, D. M., & Allen, J. R. (2018, April 24). How artificial intelligence is transforming the world. *Brookings*. https://www.brookings.edu/articles/how-artificial-intelligence-is-transforming-the-world/
White, A., Boehm, M., Glackin, E., & Bleakley, A. (2023). How sexual information sources are related to emerging adults' sex-positive scripts and sexual communication. *Sexuality & Culture*, *27*, 1224–1245. https://doi.org/10.1007/s12119-022-10061-z
Wills, M. (2018, January 15). The flu pandemic of 1918, as reported in 1918. *JSTOR Daily*. https://daily.jstor.org/the-flu-pandemic-of-1918-as-reported-in-1918/
Wright, K. (2020). *Dear media: Tell more stories about health disparities*. National Communication Association. https://www.natcom.org/spectra/dear-media-tell-more-stories-about-health-disparities

14

SPORTS AND HEALTH ADVOCACY

Jimmy Sanderson

Introduction

Sport is a popular activity for many people worldwide. People come together to consume sport mega events such as the Olympics, World Cup, and Super Bowl (Fan et al., 2020; Lever, 2023). More regionally, people gather together in community settings (Mastromartino et al., 2022) to watch local sporting events such as college football, high school basketball games, and youth league (community) soccer matches. Sport is globally popular and serves as a significant identity mechanism for many individuals (Seaton et al., 2022). That is, sport is an enterprise that many people consistently follow and consume, seeking to satiate informational needs to better strategize their fantasy football draft or simply to be in the "know" of what is going on in the sports world at a given moment in time (Dwyer et al., 2019; Ruihley et al., 2022). Sport fans are passionately invested in the performance of sport organizations, which largely rests on the performance of athletes (Sanderson et al., 2020).

While sport is immensely popular, oftentimes, costs associated with sport remain hidden and unseen. Indeed, many athletes experience significant physical and mental health challenges resulting from their participation in sport (Poucher et al., 2023). For instance, basketball players who tear their anterior cruciate ligament (ACL) are often sidelined for 12–18 months as they rehabilitate. The accompanying loss of playing time has a considerable impact on athletic identity, as many athletes' identity validation is connected to sport competition (Cassilo & Sanderson, 2019). Additionally, losing playing time also impacts their ability to compete for additional playing time in the future, as other players get more practice and game experience (Sanderson et al., 2017). Consequently, according to Sanderson et al., some athletes seek to rush back or hastily rehabilitate to return to competition before they are fully healed. Other examples that have been documented include athletes failing to report or seeking to hastily return from head injuries (concussions) (White et al., 2022), and baseball pitchers overusing their arm, leading to "Tommy John" surgery, wherein the ulterior collateral ligament must be repaired, with rehabilitation taking 12–18 months (Savoie III & O'Brien, 2023). Hyman (2009) discussed how children as young as 9–10 years old were having Tommy John surgery due to playing baseball, often pitching and throwing year-round.

Fans also have an interest in health issues that arise in sport. For example, sport fans can be exposed to injuries through sport broadcasts, and their interpretations of health and injury can be shaped by how sport media companies and journalists discuss and frame these topics (Bell & Applequist, 2022). Some sport fans also have dual roles as parents with children who play sports, and media narratives

 DOI: 10.4324/9781003436409-16

about health can potentially influence their decisions about what sports their children will play, such as tackle football (Cassilo & Sanderson, 2018; Tallapradaga & Cranmer, 2022). Sport fans also interact with others via social media platforms such as Twitter (X) and use these channels to converse about health and safety topics in sport (Cox et al., 2023). Social media allows sport fans to consume health advocacy content, including athletes' disclosures of their mental health challenges (Cassilo, 2022a). Exposure to such messages can help destigmatize perceptions about seeking help for mental health issues (Chen & Kwak, 2023).

Accordingly, this chapter will take up health advocacy by examining factors that contribute to physical and mental health issues in sport. Within each section, I will discuss how advocacy can help to address physical and mental health challenges in sport. I hope that this structure will help parents, practitioners, researchers, and others to advocate for stronger and more robust health practices and policies in sport, along with helping to increase health awareness and literacy among sport fans as they consume sport broadcasts and news.

Physical Health Issues in Sport

A number of factors influence physical health issues in sport (Sanderson & Weathers, 2022). Some of these are inherent to sport cultural ideology (e.g., playing through pain), while others may vary based on individual, familial, and social factors. For example, some families view sport as an activity to obtain physical exercise and to be "for fun." Yet, other families may envision sport as "serious business," a mechanism for child(ren) to obtain a college scholarship and, perhaps, eventually ascend to the professional ranks. The children in each of these family contexts will have vastly different experiences with sport. These family dynamics also influence how parents approach health and safety issues with their children's sport participation (McGlynn et al., 2022).

For example, with tackle football, some families equate participation as a family tradition and ritual (Boneau et al., 2020). These parents may be less likely to hold children out of tackle football or may be more willing to have their children play through pain or injury. Conversely, other parents who consider sport to be more for leisure and recreation may withhold their children from participating in high-contact sports and take preventative approaches to injury and rehabilitation. Importantly, in some cases, parents, coaches, or others involved in sport may be unaware that certain practices or behaviors could induce health issues for their children, or they may employ cognitive dissonance to rationalize or avoid thinking that their actions could harm the child's health. Unfortunately, an injury or health issue could occur before the child athlete or a family member recognizes that changes need to be made. To illustrate, I share a personal, major "wake up" moment.

Parent Identification

Given that I am writing a chapter on sport, not surprisingly, I am a big sports fan. As a child, I dreamed of playing professional sports, and I followed sport religiously, particularly baseball. I soon realized that professional baseball was not in my future, and, while I still followed it, I forgot about my love for the game as a young child. Fast forward a decade or so and my second son was four years old. My wife and I felt that having our kids involved in sport would be a good thing, so we signed my son up to play tee-ball. My son thoroughly enjoyed playing tee-ball and possessed good enough hand-eye coordination to be able to hit the ball pretty far for a child his age. My son also carried his bat around the house and imitated professional players' batting stances when we had baseball games on the living room television – in short, he loved the game! After the next baseball season, someone told me that I should get my son enrolled in private lessons with a hitting coach – keep in mind that he was five years old! So, I enrolled him in hitting lessons (much to my wife's chagrin), and we were on our way to being "all in" with baseball.

As my son continued to develop and practice, he displayed pitching aptitude. For those unfamiliar with youth baseball, very few kids can pitch with accuracy before 9–10 years old. So, when my son displayed this capability, he often pitched for his teams. Being "all in" with baseball, we played both competitive travel baseball and Little League Baseball. Thus, at about eight years old, my son began playing baseball year-round. I enjoyed watching him play and experience success on the field. As a 9-year-old, in a fall baseball league, our team made it to the championship game, and my son pitched the entire game. After the game, he started complaining about his arm hurting. I remember simply putting ice on his arm and not worrying too much about it. Over the next couple of seasons, his arm continued to hurt while he pitched, and I continued to ice it afterward. I just treated this pain as part of the game and I figured that, eventually, it would stop hurting. Also, during this time, we were working out/practicing most every day, including taking infield and throwing across the baseball diamond.

In my son's 7th grade year (13 years old), we were playing on a summer team, and his arm started to hurt more than usual. We took him to a doctor who took an x-ray, and we were told our son needed to rest from throwing, as it appeared his elbow was inflamed. Thus, while he could continue to bat in games, he could no longer play the field. Over the next year, we continued to practice hitting and eventually went back to throwing, using a throwing care program provided by the physician. In the summer of his 8th grade year (14 years old), in our last travel tournament of the summer, he ended up pitching. As he pitched, I noticed he was in visible pain and was trying not to cry. Eventually, he asked the coach to take him out. After the game, his right arm at the elbow was visibly swollen, and he was in significant pain. I realized that something was "wrong" and that we needed to get him to a specialist.

We were fortunate to be living in a city with an excellent sports medicine clinic, where his doctor had experience working with, among others, the United States national ski team. At the meeting with the physician and after an MRI procedure, the doctor informed us that our son had an osteochondral lesion in his right arm. The doctor told us that we could opt for surgery but that we also could try to rehabilitate without surgery. However, a 5% chance loomed that our son would never be able to throw a baseball again. As a parent, sitting in the medical office and being told that my child might never be able to play the game that he loved again was heart-wrenching. I was flooded with immense guilt, and even now, five years after the fact, I struggle to express how utterly horrible I felt. We were lucky that we were able to treat our son's injury without surgery, and, while he could not use his right arm for about nine months (not even to brush his teeth), his doctor eventually cleared him to play.

When he was cleared to play, I resolved that we would prioritize arm care, and we ensured that we took both intermittent and extended time off from throwing. We were blessed that our son's injury has never flared up since that time, and he enjoyed his high school and travel baseball experience. He is now playing junior college baseball. *However, we were lucky*. For every story like ours, other families confront the end of a child's sport career. While I will always carry guilt with me because of my decisions (akin to the Marley brothers in Dickens' *Christmas Carol* who tell Scrooge they wear chains as spirits because of their deeds in mortality), I am hopeful that my experience can help others recognize the importance of advocating for athlete health, especially at younger ages. Parents can easily get blinded, particularly when a child shows potential early in life (Witt & Dangi, 2018). However, some safeguards can help prevent other children from experiencing what my son and other young athletes have gone through.

As my story depicts, a significant factor that contributes to health challenges for young athletes involves parent identity. That is, parents may derive significant social capital from their child's athletic performance, particularly if the child shows aptitude. Early talent identification can blur boundaries with managing and, indeed, prioritizing, children's health in sport. For example, Boneau et al. (2020) discovered that identity comprised a central factor for some parents in having their child participate in tackle football. Notably, some parents reported that they were "football families," and this identity was quite salient and prioritized, even leading some parents to minimize or avoid thinking about concussion risk. Boneau et al.'s study vividly demonstrated identity through some parental comments:

> [T]hey don't know anything else. They just know football. They know every sport, but we didn't give them a choice. We made them do it. It helps build character, it helps them grow up and believe in their selves. We made them play. But they wanted to play.
>
> *(p. 34)*

And:

> I was named after a football player. My daddy played football. I was at a football game when I was 10 days old watching my dad play. He played college football. My dad was a coach my whole life. Then I married a coach … I mean, I can actually say that … little league football, we've probably done it since … my son was … seven or eight years old.
>
> *(p. 34)*

Boneau et al. (2020) noted that, for families with a strong football identity orientation, "any sort of cost-benefit analysis used for their football decisions was skewed heavily towards the benefits" (p. 35). In related work, McGlynn et al. (2020) concluded that community pressure motivated families to enroll their children in tackle football.

This research provides compelling findings that demonstrate how identity influences parental approaches to sport and health. Even the phrase, "we made them do it," could influence the ways in which parents handle health issues with their children. Anecdotally, both my sons played youth tackle football, and I remember many times when a child got hurt, and parents (me included) initially responded with "shake it off," "rub some dirt on it," and/or "get up!" Although children should not be encouraged to avoid any adversity or not work through difficulty in sport, such a parental perspective may influence how parents navigate the injury process. Could parents underestimate the severity of their child's injury? If so, what are the short-term and long-term consequences of such a decision? It seems plausible that parents who handle a child's physical injuries in this manner may: (1) fail to report future, perhaps more serious injuries, (2) see their child(ren) drop out from sport, and/or (3) have their child(ren) develop resentment toward their parents and/or sport, which could influence how they manage their own children's athletic participation. I remember a family with a player on one of our 9-10U baseball teams. The father got injured through pitching overuse as a child, and the arm injury still impacted him at that later point in life. Consequently, he refused to allow his son to pitch.

Sport Culture – Valorizing Playing through Pain

As demonstrated in the prior section, sport culture affirms that athletes must play through pain (Sabo, 2004) or refrain from showing weakness, an ideology that can influence the health decisions of sport participants (Berg et al., 2023). Sanderson et al. (2017) interviewed athletes who had sustained concussions during athletic participation and who did not report these injuries. Sanderson et al. determined that athletes choose to not report concussions due to conformance to sport cultural norms, such as playing through pain and wanting to show allegiance to their team. Comments from participants included, "You just play through it," "I sucked it up and continued to play," and "I knew if I informed my coach of how I was feeling, he would either be disappointed in me or take me out of the game" (p. 278). With respect to team loyalty, participants disclosed that, "I had to play because it was a high stakes game in which the outcome affected our overall team rankings," and, "I was our best option most of the time, so coming out wasn't really a choice" (p. 279).

In another study, Wilson et al. (2021) interviewed adult, female competitive rowers who experienced lower back pain (LBP) and failed to report it. According to Wilson et al., athletes commented that, within rowing, a culture existed of concealing pain from coaches and teammates. They also expressed concern about being perceived as "weak" for reporting LBP. Wilson et al. noted that athletes and support staff should be educated about the benefits of early reporting and emphasized the need for these organizational personnel (e.g., coaches) to support athletes who disclose injury without negatively judging them. Other researchers have observed the importance that coaches play in athletes' health decision-making (Cranmer et al., 2022). Additionally, athletic training staff or other medical personnel may be pressured by coaches to clear athletes before they fully recover (Buckley et al., 2023). Given that sports constitute a massive and lucrative enterprise (see, e.g., Gregory, 2017), coaches' ability to earn money could be tied to the performance of their teams. As such, financial motivations could enhance the pressure for medical personnel to clear athletes before they are fully rehabilitated from injury.

Moreover, in some sport organizations, trainers and medical personnel report directly to the head coach. In such arrangements, a trainer resisting coach pressure to clear an athlete could ultimately impact their employment. For example, one trainer for a college football program reported, "They [coaches] would always, you know, tend to put pressure on you to get players back" (Fitzgerald, 2016, para. 4). Lacy et al. (2020) noted that, for some trainers, this pressure is a job expectation and can be a significant source of conflict. Additionally, in a 2019 survey by the National Collegiate Athletic Association (NCAA), Lavigne (2019) determined that 19% of college athletic trainers reported that coaches had played athletes who had been deemed, "medically out of participation" (para. 1). As these studies illustrate, clear structural barriers within sport constrain athletes' willingness or ability to report injuries, or what could be termed "self-advocacy."

Youth Sports Injuries

A significant area of concern for physical health in sport pertains to injuries experienced by young athletes. As discussed above, one of the contributing factors to this situation entails the high levels of identification that parents place on their children's sporting success. One of the chief strategies involves honest and transparent assessments by parents about their child(ren)'s participation in sports. Although potentially difficult, such a process may help parents get on the "same page" with their child(ren) about goals and motivations for sport participation and keep participation within age-appropriate boundaries. Parents can certainly desire their child(ren) to be successful in sport; however, such desires need to be tempered and balanced with the child(ren)'s agency as well. These assessments are also important as participation in competitive youth travel or select sports requires significant financial and time investments from parents (Gregory, 2017). Thus, while a parent may desire their child(ren) to be a star athlete, the financial and time commitments required may make this goal impractical for some families.

To further illustrate, Boneau et al. (2020) found that some parents did not give their children a choice to play tackle football. Certainly, parents may guide children at ages 4–5 in what sports they play, decisions that may be based on factors such as convenience and the family's other obligations. However, as children develop, more informed, age-appropriate conversations can be held to discuss injury risks in sports, and children can decide if they wish to incur those risks. Parents also may need to account for their child's body type and how that compares with other age cohort children playing high-contact sports (Flack, 2015). In some cases, it may be more beneficial to delay a child playing a sport such as hockey or tackle football until they have developed a bit more physically. Evaluating these factors may help parents and children make more informed choices about sport participation, which ultimately may help reduce injury.

Parents also need to consider the importance of giving their children breaks from sports. Many children are now playing one sport year-round, leading to an enhanced risk of overuse injuries, such as with Tommy John surgery in baseball. Parents can enroll their children in multiple sports, which can help offset some of the injury risks, as certain sports require repetitive use of different muscles. For example, a child who plays baseball can take time off and play a sport like soccer, which allows for different body parts to be used and reduces strain on the arm. Additionally, parents might suggest breaks from playing sports altogether. Such encouragement may help to avoid the burnout that has become prevalent among youth sport participants (Jayanthi et al., 2019). Considering that over 70% of children will quit playing sports before age 13 ("Uncovering the Reasons," n.d.), encouraging children to participate in other activities or allowing them to simply be a kid and hang out with their friends can help alleviate both physical and mental health issues. Nevertheless, some children very much enjoy working out and engaging in sport-related activities, so parents should be mindful of children who fall into this category, as it may be more challenging to get these young athletes to take time off. Speaking from personal experience, such a balanced approach can be challenging for a parent, as parents (and players) often receive clear messages about "other kids working" and those kids getting ahead and positioning themselves better for college scholarships. While children who put in more work generally may reap more athletic rewards, and while such messages can be quite persuasive, parents (and players) may need to temper their expectations and desires.

Physical Health Advocacy

Sport organizations provide athletes with an abundance of training on topics related to alcohol use, organizational culture, and team policies (Jussim, 2018). Some sport organizations have also have started to enact health programming and policies to better support athletes who experience injury. Admittedly, some of this work, such as with the NFL, appears to have arisen after public concerns manifested about the NFL being less than transparent with players about health risks, including concussions (Castonguay & Lowes, 2022; see also Chapters 15 and 22, this volume). Some sport leagues, including the NFL, have also made it challenging for reporters to cover health issues as very little information was provided to journalists (Cassilo, 2021). In 2022, the NFL revised its concussion protocol to include motor instability (Battista, 2022). Ironically, this revision was announced after Miami Dolphins quarterback Tua Tagovailoa was taken off the field on a stretcher. According to Battista, Tagovailoa remained in a game the previous week after taking a substantial hit that appeared to impact his motor stability.

The NCAA has a comprehensive concussion protocol that was revised for 2024 to include enhanced evaluation and assessment tools, and it strengthened recommendations for return-to-learn and return-to-play ("Concussion Safety Protocol Management," n.d.). In 2016, the Ivy League conference enacted a policy eliminating tackling from football practices for all member schools (Cranmer & Sanderson, 2018). The National Hockey League's (NHL) policy includes the mandatory removal of a player if a concussion is spotted, and staff members responsible for concussion spotting are instructed to look for symptoms such as players lying motionless on the ice, players having motor or balance problems, and players displaying blank or vacant looks (Murphy, 2023). Youth sport organizations also have enacted policies to promote health and reduce injury. For example, Pop Warner, a youth tackle football organization, eliminated kickoffs in its youngest divisions (Sanderson & Cassilo, 2019). The National Federation of High Schools (NFHS) policy requires that any athlete (in any sport) who displays signs or symptoms associated with a concussion is to be immediately removed from competition ("NIAA and NFHS Guidelines," 2012).

Such programming and policies represent a sport cultural shift (Cranmer & Sanderson, 2018; Sanderson & Cassilo, 2019). Certainly, changing sport culture is difficult (Spaaij et al., 2020), but advocacy is never guaranteed to be easy! As efforts are made to prioritize athletes' physical and mental well-being, sport culture can transform into one where health is prioritized and valued (Cranmer & Sanderson, 2018). The culture around sport and health can be changed, perhaps slowly, to be more supportive of athletes who are injured. This shift enables athletes to be valued for their holistic identity and worth, rather than solely as commodities who only have value on a field or court (Cassilo, 2022b).

Mental Health Issues in Sport

Social Media

Mental health has been consistently stigmatized in sport (Cassilo & Kluch, 2023). Historically, mental health conversations have been trivialized, and athletes who voice mental health concerns have often been marginalized and framed in unfavorable ways (Cassilo, 2022a). Consequently, many athletes appear to have been reticent about voicing their mental health concerns, and structural organizational barriers have contributed to this silence (Parrott et al., 2020). However, in recent years, a shift has occurred where more athletes are willing to speak out and disclose their mental health struggles via social media (Chen & Kwak, 2023). For example, women's tennis player Naomi Osaka used Twitter to announce that she was withdrawing from the 2021 French Open to focus on her mental health (Kumble et al., 2022). Kumble et al. observed how this social media post by Osaka helped to destigmatize mental health disclosures. Additionally, sport media seem to have become more empathetic in how they report stories about athletes' mental health challenges, which can help to change norms in sport and society about expressing mental health concerns (Parrott, 2023; see also Chapter 3, this volume). Athletes also collectively can come together, such as the U.S. Women's National Soccer Team (USWNT) using the World Cup exposure to launch a mental health initiative aimed at underserved communities (Frandino, 2023).

Whereas social media provides a vehicle for athletes to discuss mental health concerns, it also can be a triggering agent for them (Sanderson, 2018). Many athletes remain subject to online abuse via social and digital media for diverse reasons ranging from poor athletic performance to issues in their private lives, such as taking mental health breaks (Kavanagh et al., 2021, 2022). For instance, Doehler (2023) observed that, after U.S. Olympic gymnast Simone Biles withdrew from several events during the 2020 Olympics, comments on social media framed her as someone who quit on her team on the biggest stage. The following sections illustrate how abusive behavior on social media can exacerbate mental health issues for athletes.

Social Media and Athlete Abuse

Some athletes encounter extremely hostile behavior on social media (MacPherson & Kerr, 2023; MacPherson et al., 2022). Indeed, early research in social media examined the presence of death threats and other abusive messages directed toward athletes (Browning & Sanderson, 2012; Sanderson & Truax, 2014). Unfortunately, athletes receiving hostile messages via social media seem to have become normalized, and athletes are routine targets of cyberbullying behavior (MacPherson & Kerr, 2023). For instance, Purdum (2023) chronicled how college basketball players received abusive messages, including death threats, from people engaging in sports betting. Purdum also noted how unnamed Pepperdine University men's basketball players endured messages such as, "Your throat will be severed with a dull knife" (para. 12). McCarthy (2022) analyzed YouTube comments directed at women participating in street skating competitions and found that comments centered on gender roles, such as women's place being in the kitchen, along with comments questioning the legitimacy of women's sport. Female athletes also tend to be at higher risk for expressions of gender-based violence on social media (Phipps, 2023).

The work of Kavanagh and colleagues has been instrumental in raising awareness about the abusive behavior to which athletes have been subjected via digital and social media platforms (Kavanagh

& Jones, 2017; Kavanagh et al., 2021, 2022). Kavanagh et al. (2016) classified such abuse into the following categories: (a) physical; (b) sexual; (c) emotional/psychological; and (d) discriminatory based on categories such as gender, race, sexual orientation, religion, and/or disability. Researchers have employed this framework to better understand the ways that athletes encounter abuse in digital/social media domains (Litchfield et al., 2018; MacPherson & Kerr, 2020). Litchfield et al. examined comments on Facebook and Twitter directed at tennis player Serena Williams. They found that user comments included questioning Williams' gender, accusing her of using performance-enhancing drugs, and making racist remarks. Litchfield et al. noted that "gendered hostility, sexualised threats of violence and racially charged invective are part of a dark narrative of human behaviour within a particular virtual space" (p. 166).

As noted earlier, fans are often very invested in the outcome of sporting events, and this investment can fuel aggressive behavior towards athletes when they and/or the team do not perform up to expectations. For example, during the 2023 NCAA Men's College Basketball Tournament, University of Michigan player Terrence Williams II received messages expressing hope that Williams would end up in a ditch (Pells, 2023). Similarly, Krammer (2023) chronicled how Minnesota Vikings player Alexander Mattison dealt with death threats and racial slurs on Instagram following the Vikings' loss in Week 2 of the 2023 NFL season. During the 2023 World Cup, The Fédération Internationale de football association (FIFA) reported that one in five players received abusive, discriminatory, or threatening messages (Women's World Cup, 2023). Given the nature of such messages, and with the stress/pressure that many athletes self-inflict, these messages seem likely to exacerbate mental health issues.

Social Media and Sexual Harassment/Abuse of Young Athletes

Another problematic area to consider with technology, and one which is rising in frequency, involves young athletes being targeted and sexually groomed by adult coaches/teachers via social media platforms, most notably Snapchat. Sanderson and Weathers (2020) examined news articles reporting on coaches/teachers who had been arrested for sending sexual messages to minors via Snapchat. They revealed that these perpetrators enacted a variety of abusive tactics that led to sexualized messages on Snapchat, some of which evolved into actual physical, sexual abuse. Examples included coaches posing as teenagers to solicit nude photos from minor athletes, then upon receipt of such photos, threatening to publicly reveal them unless the minor engaged in sex, using the geo-location on Snapchat to track minor athletes in the community and approach them, along with sending sexual photos and videos including fully nude photos and videos that included coaches masturbating. Sanderson and Weathers argued for the importance of developing safeguards to protect minor athletes in these spaces, including educational programs and policy. Such measures certainly comprise an important area for sport and health advocacy to address. As further evidence of the need for such work, a recent Internet search with the term, "Coaches arrested for Snapchat" yielded the following results: "Sioux Falls dance coach arrested for allegedly sending illicit Snapchat photos to minor" (Todd, 2023), and "Ohio high school coach posed as teen to get child porn over Snapchat, prosecutor says" (Feurborn, 2023)

Social Media Safeguards as Advocacy

Social and digital media spaces have introduced challenges for sport organizations (Weathers & Sanderson, 2021). Indeed, digital domains subject athletes to abuse of all kinds and provide a vehicle for perpetrators to harm minor athletes (Sanderson & Weathers, 2020). Thus, sport organizations and other governing bodies must prioritize athlete safeguarding, particularly with social and digital media. Sport organizations can provide athletes with comprehensive training and education on social media (Sanderson et al., 2015). Such training can include specific components on recognizing and reporting abusive behavior, including threats to one's or one's family members' safety. As one example, in 2023, the NCAA announced a partnership with several technology providers to help the organization respond to issues of online athlete abuse ("NCAA Launches Ground Breaking Initiative," 2023). The International Olympic Committee (IOC) also has created an online training module devoted to online harassment and abuse ("Safeguarding Athletes," n.d.).

Additionally, sport organizations can also offer dedicated mental health counseling resources to support athletes who experience abusive social media behavior, including encouraging athletes to take a social media "break" along with utilizing functions within social media platforms to report abuse. Sport organizations can also can identify times when athletes may be more likely to experience social media abuse (e.g., after an important game, after a poor performance) and develop solutions to help safeguard athletes from abusive behavior (e.g., encouraging athletes to not look at social media after a subpar athletic performance). Sport organizations should proactively disseminate messaging to fans and other stakeholders, notifying them that the organization does not tolerate abusive behavior on social media directed at athletes. Such efforts can promote expectations for acceptable fan behavior and may help people associate being a "good fan" with avoiding abusive behavior (Sanderson & Truax, 2014).

With respect to minor athletes and sexualized messages on social media from coaches, sport organizations must develop very clear policies around such behavior. These policies and expectations also must be consistently communicated to coaches and other personnel who will be around young athletes. For instance, in my own consulting work with sport organizations in this area, I have recommended that sport organizations restrict coaches from engaging in any private, 1:1 messaging with minor athletes and to instead, only use group messaging applications for digital communication tasks (e.g., GroupMe). Some youth sport organizations utilize such approaches. For example, the Potomac Soccer Association in Maryland has a policy that, among other things, prohibits coaches from having any private or 1:1 conversation with any athletes on any social media platform ("Social Media and Electronic Communication Policy," n.d.).

Importantly, organizations should share these policies with parents and athletes to help them understand the expectations and boundaries for coaches and other staff members. These educational sessions can equip parents and athletes with confidential reporting mechanisms should they feel inappropriate contact has been initiated. These meetings can occur at regular intervals, such as the beginning of each school year or the beginning of each sport season, to help promote consistency around the expectations for athlete welfare with digital and social media channels. Such advocacy measures can help lower incident rates and better safeguard minor athletes as they participate in sport.

Sport and Mental Health Advocacy

Given the significance of mental health issues in sport, sport organizations are initiating more programming that encourages mental health advocacy (Rugg, 2022). In addition to organizationally driven campaigns, athletes have collectively come together to promote mental health awareness. For instance, after James Madison University softball player Lauren Bernett took her life, college softball players rallied by wearing purple ribbons in their hair to honor Bernett and raise awareness for mental health (Carlson, 2022). As another example, Oklahoma University softball player Alex Storako wore a green ribbon in her hair every time she pitched to promote mental health awareness and its importance to her (Carlson, 2023).

Campaigns also help sport organizations visibly advocate for mental health. Sport organizations have a high profile and can be instrumental in health advocacy (Rugg, 2022). For instance, the NCAA has engaged in campaigns to promote mental health among college athletes, such as #MentalHealthMonday, where college athletes share their efforts to promote mental health ("Mental Health Social Media Campaign," n.d.). As an additional example, Major League Baseball (MLB) created a campaign in May 2023 entitled, "MentalHealthisMainstream" ("Mental Health Awareness Month," n.d.), in an effort to normalize mental health. Specifically, "this month-long initiative aims to normalize mental health as a vital component to our general, physical health that touches people in all walks of life, including athletes" (para. 1). According to Rugg, whether internally focused or externally targeted at public messaging, campaigns constitute important advocacy measures that sport organizations can undertake to both support their athletes and be a positive force in their communities.

Professional athletes have spoken publicly about their personal mental health challenges and advocated for enhanced support. For example, in 2018, NBA players Kevin Love and DeMar DeRozan both publicly discussed their mental health challenges (Parrott et al., 2020). According to Parrott et al., these revelations generated a positive public response, which helped create a culture of acceptance, rather than rejection, around mental health disclosures. Additionally, in 2021, a *Time* magazine article featured tennis star Naomi Osaka, titled, "It's OK to Not Be OK" (Osaka, 2021), wherein she discussed her mental health challenges. Osaka wrote her article after she withdrew from the 2021 French Open (one of the four Grand Slam tournaments in tennis) to focus on her mental health, a move that generated significant media attention and controversy (Futterman, 2021).

Osaka's (2021) article also came in response to pressure by the media to disclose specifics related to her mental health challenges after she requested to be excused from tournament press conferences. In her *Time* article, Osaka defended her actions by stating, "I communicated that I wanted to skip press conferences at Roland Garros [French Open venue] to exercise self-care and preservation of my mental health. I stand by that. Athletes are humans" (para. 6). In the subsequent years since this incident, Osaka has continued to be a vocal advocate for mental health, and her advocacy raises some important questions about expectations for athletes and how we may better advocate for them. Is giving athletes the ability to opt out of some media availability a strategy that can help them better manage mental health? Can accommodations be provided for athletes to engage with the media in alternative formats? Osaka's advocacy illustrates that we may need to begin re-thinking and re-conceptualizing certain sport practices.

Conclusion

Sport and health advocacy is a vital topic that must be addressed by multiple sport stakeholders. Researchers interested in this area can take up future work in a number of important directions. For example, how do parents communicate and manage their child(ren)'s athletic injuries? What role do variables such as identity, gender roles, and sport experience play in these interactions? While we know that many children play sports, we know very little about the communication and decision-making process parents utilize when enrolling children into sports. Looking at the ways in which parents decide what sports their children participate in will help provide more understanding about the considerations parents give to sport and health. It also would be helpful to study the dynamics of the competitive youth sport landscape (e.g., travel/select sports). How do parents and children manage burnout? What are the implications for family members' mental health, given the significant financial and travel commitments associated with sport participation at this level?

Additionally, researchers can interview athletes to better understand their lived experiences with online abuse. Most of the research to date has taken content analytic approaches, which have been helpful for building this literature. However, athletes' voices and learning about their lived experiences would greatly enhance our knowledge about the effects of online abuse on athlete mental health.

We would also benefit from research about athletes taking health positions that run counter to public health recommendations (for related work, see Chapter 16, this volume). For example, NFL player Aaron Rodgers and NBA player Kyrie Irving have both been vocal about resisting COVID-19 vaccination (see, e.g., Morik, 2024; Oshin, 2022). These stances opened up a floodgate of media reports about their views, and perhaps offer an intriguing way to conceptualize health advocacy. That is, what are the impacts of athletes' individual health advocacy when it runs contrary to public health policy?

These possibilities comprise just a few of the exciting directions that await researchers. It is my hope that this chapter illustrates how vitally important sport and health are as a site for advocacy. Sport and health are a space where researchers and practitioners must work together. These collaborations will hopefully build on existing momentum around topics like mental health, while also providing continued advocacy for the health and well-being of sport participants.

References

Battista, J., (2022, October 2). Changes coming to NFL concussion protocol a needed step for player safety. *NFL.* https://www.nfl.com/news/changes-coming-to-nfl-concussion-protocol-a-needed-step-for-player-safety

Bell, T. R., & Applequist, J. (2022). Media framing, sport, and public health. In J. Sanderson & M. Weathers (Eds.), *Health communication and sport: Connections, applications, and opportunities* (pp. 15–30). Lexington.

Berg, A., Duffy, D., & DuBois, S. (2023). Elegant violence: The promise and peril of a new 'feminine' sport ethic. *Sport in Society, 26*(2), 335–349.

Boneau, R. D., Richardson, B. K., & McGlynn, J. (2020). "We are a football family": Making sense of parents' decisions to allow their children to play tackle football. *Communication & Sport, 8*(1), 26–49.

Browning, B., & Sanderson, J. (2012). The positives and negatives of Twitter: Exploring how student-athletes use Twitter and respond to critical tweets. *International Journal of Sport Communication, 5*(4), 503–521.

Buckley, T. A., Bryk, K. N., Hunzinger, K. J., & Costantini, K. (2023). National CollegiateAthletic Association athletic trainers' response to the Arrington settlement: Management, compliance, and practice patterns. *The Physician and Sportsmedicine, 51*(5), 427–433.

Carlson, J. (2022, May 9). How JMU catcher Lauren Bernett's death rocked college softball and pushed it to action on mental health. *USAToday.* https://www.usatoday.com/story/sports/college/softball/2022/05/09/lauren-bernett-suicide-jmu-college-softball-world-mental-health/9703602002/

Carlson, J., (2023, May 18). Why does OU pitcher Alex Storako wear a green ribbon? Mental health awareness 'hits home.' *The Oklahoman.* https://www.oklahoman.com/story/sports/college/sooners/2023/05/18/ou-softball-pitcher-alex-storako-wears-green-ribbon-for-mental-health-awareness/70226814007/

Cassilo, D. (2021). Shifting the coverage: Understanding why reporting and attitudes changed about the NFL and player safety. *Journal of Sports Media, 16*(2), 41–64.

Cassilo, D. (2022a). Royce White, DeMar DeRozan and the media framing of mental health in the NBA. *Communication & Sport, 10*(1), 97–123.

Cassilo, D. (2022b). Media framing and athlete mental health. In J. Sanderson & M. Weathers (Eds.). *Health communication and sport: Connections, applications, and opportunities* (pp. 1–14). Lexington.

Cassilo, D., & Kluch, Y. (2023). Mental health, college athletics, and the media framing of D.J. Carton's announcement to step away from his team. *Communication & Sport, 11*(3), 462–488.

Cassilo, D., & Sanderson, J. (2018). "I don't think it's worth the risk": Media framing of the Chris Borland retirement in digital and print media. *Communication and Sport, 6*(1), 86–110.

Cassilo, D., & Sanderson, J. (2019). From social isolation to becoming an advocate: Exploring athletes' grief discourse about lived concussion experiences in online forums. *Communication and Sport, 7*(5), 678–696.

Castonguay, S., & Lowes, M. (2022). Situational crisis communication theory and the National Football League: A case study of the NFL's response strategies to its concussion crisis. *International Journal of Sport Communication, 15*(4), 366–376.

Chen, Z., & Kwak, D. H. (2023). It's okay to not be okay: An analysis of Twitter responses to Naomi Osaka's withdrawal due to mental health concerns. *Communication & Sport, 11*(3), 439–461.

Concussion Safety Protocol Management (n.d.). NCAA. https://www.ncaa.org/sports/2016/7/20/concussion-safety-protocol-management.aspx

Cox, E. G., Cranmer, G. A., & Boatwright, B. (2023). "Why can't we play on grass?" An investigation into discourse on Sterling Shepard's ACL tear. *Communication & Sport.* Advance online publication. https://doi.org/10.1177/21674795231182903

Cranmer, G. A., Rey, R. T., & Mikkilineni, S. D. (2022). Coach-athlete communication and implications for health. In J. Sanderson & M. Weathers (Eds.). *Health communication and sport: Connections, applications, and opportunities* (pp. 79–94). Lexington.

Cranmer, G. A., & Sanderson, J. (2018). "Rough week for testosterone": Public commentary around the Ivy League's decision to restrict tackle football in practice. *Western Journal of Communication, 82(5)*, 631–647.
Doehler, S. (2023). Role model or quitter? Social media's response to Simone Biles at Tokyo2020. *International Journal of Sport Communication, 16*(1), 64–79.
Dwyer, B., Larkin, B., & Goebert, C. (2019). Measuring fantasy team and favorite team interactivity through implicit association. *Communication & Sport, 7*(6), 811–838.
Fan, M., Billings, A., Zhu, X., & Yu, P. (2020). Twitter-based BIRGing: Big data analysis of English national team fans during the 2018 FIFA World Cup. *Communication & Sport, 8*(3), 317–345
Feurborn, M. (2023, June 23). Ohio high school coach posed as teen to get child porn over Snapchat, prosecutor says. *NBC4i*. https://www.nbc4i.com/news/local-news/perry-county/ohio-high-school-coach-posed-as-teen-to-get-child-porn-over-snapchat-prosecutor-says/
Fitzgerald, M. (2016, January 26). Former Texas A&M trainer says coaches pressured him to clear injured players. *BleacherReport*. https://bleacherreport.com/articles/2611364-former-texas-am-trainer-claims-coaches-pressured-him-to-clear-injured-players
Flack, E. (2015, September 21). Weighty debate: Are some players too big for youth football? *Wave3*. https://www.wave3.com/story/30078785/too-big-for-football-doctor-wants-restrictions-on-some-youth-players/
Frandino, N. (2023, July 19). US players harness World Cup spotlight for mental health initiative. *Reuters*. https://www.reuters.com/sports/soccer/us-players-harness-world-cup-spotlight-mental-health-initiative-2023-07-19/
Futterman, M. (2021, July 27). Naomi Osaka quits the French Open after news conference dispute. *New York Times*. https://www.nytimes.com/2021/05/31/sports/tennis/naomi-osaka-quits-french-open-depression.html#:~:text=313-,Naomi%20Osaka%20Quits%20the%20French%20Open%20After%20News%20Conference%20Dispute,away%20from%20the%20tennis%20court
Gregory, S. (2017, August 24). How kids' sports became a $15 billion dollar industry. *Time*. https://time.com/magazine/us/4913681/september-4th-2017-vol-190-no-9-u-s/
Hyman, M. (2009). *Unit it hurts: America's obsession with youth sports and how it harms our kids*. Beacon.
Jayanthi, N. A., Post, E. G., Laury, T. C., & Fabricant, P. D. (2019). Health consequences of youth sport specialization. *Journal of Athletic Training, 54*(10), 1040–1049.
Jussim, M. (2018, October 1). How the NBA rookie transition program helps players become pros. *MensJournal*. https://www.mensjournal.com/sports/how-the-nba-rookie-transition-program-helps-players-become-pros
Kavanagh, E., & Jones, I. (2017). Understanding the cyber-enabled abuse in sport. In D. McGillivray, G. McPherson, & S. Carnicelli (Eds.). *Digital leisure cultures: Critical perspectives* (pp. 20–34). Routledge.
Kavanagh, E., Jones, I., & Sheppard-Marks, L. (2016). Towards typologies of virtual maltreatment: Sport, digital cultures and dark leisure. *Leisure Studies, 35*(6), 783–796.
Kavanagh, E., Litchfield, C., & Osborne, J. (2021). Virtual technologies as tools of maltreatment: Safeguarding in digital spaces. In M. Lang (Ed.). *Routledge handbook of athlete welfare* (pp. 221–230). Routledge.
Kavanagh, E., Litchfield, C., & Osborne, J. (2022). Social media, digital technology, and athlete abuse. In J. Sanderson (Ed.). *Sport, social media, and digital technology: Sociological approaches* (pp. 185–204). Emerald.
Krammer, A. (2023, September 23). When the hate hits on social media, Vikings players face difficult decisions. *StarTribune*. https://www.startribune.com/minnesota-vikings-nfl-players-abusive-messages-alexander-mattison/600307001/
Kumble, S., Diddi, P., & Bien-Amié, S. (2022). 'Your strength is inspirational': How Namoi Osaka's Twitter announcement destigmatizes mental health disclosures. *Communication & Sport*. Advance online publication. https://doi.org/10.1177/21674795221124584
Lacy, A. M. P., Singe, S. M., & Bowman, T. G. (2020). Collegiate athletic trainers' experiences with external pressures faced during decision making. *Journal of Athletic Training, 55*(4), 409–415.
Lavigne, P. (2019, June 25). Survey: NCAA coaches' clout concerns athletic trainers. *ESPN*. https://www.espn.com/espn/otl/story/_/id/27048906/survey-ncaa-coaches-clout-concerns-trainers
Lever, K. (2023). "Dabo wears male rompers": Examining expressions of hegemonic masculinity in ESPN's College GameDay. *Communication & Sport, 11*(4), 667–687.
Litchfield, C., Kavanagh, E., Osborne, J., & Jones, I. (2018). Social media and the politics of gender, race, and identity: The case of Serena Williams. *European Journal for Sport and Society, 15*(2), 154–170.
MacPherson, E., & Kerr, G. (2020). Sport fans' perspectives of public shaming of professional athletes on social media. *Qualitative Research in Sport, Exercise, and Health, 13*(1), 146–165.
MacPherson, E., & Kerr, G. (2023). Cyberbullying in sport. *International Journal of Sport Communication, 16*(3), 266–273.

MacPherson, E., Willson, E., & Kerr, G. (2022). Athletes, social media, and health. In J. Sanderson & M. Weathers (Eds.), *Health communication and sport: Connections, applications, and opportunities* (pp. 155–170). Lexington.

Mastromartino, B., Wang, J. J., Suggs, D. W., Hollenbeck, C. R., & Zhang, J. J. (2022). Dimensions of sense of membership in a sport fan community: Factors, outcomes, and social capital implications. *Communication & Sport, 10*(6), 1229–1256.

McCarthy, B. (2022). 'Who unlocked the kitchen': Online misogyny, YouTube comments and women's professional street skateboarding. *International Review for the Sociology of Sport, 57*(3), 362–380.

McGlynn, J., Boneau, R. D., & Richardson, B. K. (2020). "It might also be good for your brain:" Cognitive and social benefits that motivate parents to permit youth tackle football. *Journal of Sport and Social Issues, 44*(3), 261–282.

McGlynn, J., Richardson, B. K., & Boneau, R. D. (2022). Factors that reduce parental concern for concussion risks in youth tackle football. *Sociology of Sport Journal, 40*(3), 321–329.

Mental Health Awareness Month. (n.d.). MLBPlayers. https://www.mlbplayers.com/mental-health-awareness-month-2023

Mental Health Social Media Campaign. (n.d.). NCAA. https://www.ncaa.org/sports/2020/3/27/mental-health-social-media-campaign.aspx

Morik, R. (2024, February 8). Aaron Rodgers says he has 'important responsibility' to speak out against COVID, vaccines. *Fox News*. https://www.foxnews.com/sports/aaron-rodgers-important-responsibility-speak-out-against-covid-vaccines

Murphy, B. (2023, June 10). How does the NHL's concussion protocol work? Explaining the process for return to play in hockey. *SportingNews*. https://www.sportingnews.com/us/nhl/news/nhl-concussion-protocol-process-return/fjmsr0uwqlelys53gag6grrj

NCAA Launches Ground-Breaking Initiative to Study and Understand Online Abuse in College Sports. (2023, December 11). *NCAA*. https://www.ncaa.org/news/2023/12/11/media-center-ncaa-launches-ground-breaking-initiative-to-study-and-understand-online-abuse-in-college-sports.aspx

NIAA and NFHS Guidelines on Management of Concussions. (2012, August 30). *NIAA*. https://www.niaa.com/sports/niaa_releases/concussion_policy#:~:text=NFHS%20Suggested%20Concussion%20Management%20by%20Health%20Care%20Professionals,by%20an%20appropriate%20health-care%20professional%20that%20day.%203

Osaka, N. (2021, July 8). Naomi Osaka: 'It's OK to not be OK.' *Time*. https://time.com/6077128/naomi-osaka-essay-tokyo-olympics/

Oshin, O. (2022, September 20). Nets star Kyrie Irving says vaccine mandates among 'biggest violations' in human rights in history. *The Hill*. https://thehill.com/homenews/3652458-nets-star-kyrie-irving-says-vaccine-mandates-one-the-biggest-violations-of-human-rights-in-history/

Parrott, S. (2023). "This isn't a sports story…This is a life story": Elite athletes and myths about mental illness in sport. *International Journal of Sport Communication, 16*(4), 423–434.

Parrott, S., Billings, A. C., Hakim, S. D., & Gentile, P. (2020). From #endthestigma to #realman: Stigma-challenging social media responses to NBA players' mental health disclosures. *Communication & Sport, 33*(3), 148–160.

Pells, E. (2023, March 29). 'They don't even know': NCAA athletes grapple with hate on social media. *NBCBayArea*. https://www.nbcbayarea.com/news/sports/a-different-march-madness-online-hate-for-the-athletes/3193196/

Phipps, C. (2023). "You belong in the kitchen:" Social media, virtual manhood acts, and women strength sport athletes' experiences of gender-based violence online. *Feminist Media Studies, 23*(8), 4221–4337.

Poucher, Z. A., Tamminen, K. A., & Kerr, G. (2023). Olympic and Paralympic athletes' perceptions of the Canadian sport environment and mental health. *Qualitative Research in Sport, Exercise, and Health, 15*(5), 636–653.

Purdum, D. (2023, March 30). How college athletes face social media abuse from gamblers. *ESPN*. https://www.espn.com/mens-college-basketball/story/_/id/35983485/social-media-abuse-gamblers-concern-college-athletes

Rugg, A. (2022). Corporate social responsibility and health promotion campaigns among major U.S. professional sporting leagues. In J. Sanderson & M. Weathers (Eds.). *Health communication and sport: Connections, applications, and opportunities* (pp. 47–62). Lexington.

Ruihley, B. J., Buzzelli, N., & Billings, A. (2022). The fantasy sport context: Altering the uses and gratifications of sports fandom. *Journal of Sports Media, 17*(1), 1–23.

Sabo, D. (2004). The politics of sport injury: Hierarchy, power and the pain principle. In K. Young (Ed.), *Sporting bodies, damaged selves: Sociological studies of sports-related injuries* (pp. 59–80). Emerald

Safeguarding Athletes from Harassment and Abuse. (n.d.). Olympics. https://olympics.com/athlete365/courses/safeguarding/

Sanderson, J. (2018). Think twice before you post: Issues student-athletes face on social media. *New Directions for Student Services, 163,* 81–92.

Sanderson, J., Browning, B., & Schmittel, A. (2015). Education on the digital terrain: A case study exploring college athletes' perceptions of social media education. *International Journal of Sport Communication, 8*(1), 103–124.

Sanderson, J., & Cassilo, D. (2019). "I'm glad I played when the country still had gonads": Bottom-up framing around Pop Warner's kickoff policy change. *Journal of Sports Media, 14(1–2),* 1–22.

Sanderson, J., & Truax, C. (2014). "I hate you man!": Exploring maladaptive parasocial interaction expressions to college athletes via Twitter. *Journal of Issues in Intercollegiate Athletics, 7,* 333–351.

Sanderson, J., & Weathers M. (2020). Snapchat and child sexual abuse in sport: Protecting child athletes in the social media age. *Sport Management Review, 23,* 81–94.

Sanderson, J., & Weathers, M. (Eds.) (2022). *Health communication and sport: Connections, applications, and opportunities*. Lexington.

Sanderson, J., Weathers, M., Snedaker, K., & Gramlich, K. (2017). "I was able to do my job on the field and keep playing:" A case study investigating female and male athletes' experiences with (not)reporting concussions. *Communication & Sport, 5*(3), 267–287.

Sanderson, J., Zimmerman, M., Stokowski, S., & Fridley, A. (2020). "You had one job!": A case study of maladaptive parasocial interaction and athlete maltreatment in virtual spaces. *International Journal of Sport Communication, 13(2),* 221–238.

Savoie III, F. H., & O' Brien, J. (2023). Medial elbow injuries in the throwing athlete: Youth to professional. *Journal of Shoulder and Elbow Surgery*. Advance online publication. https://doi.org/10.1016/j.jse.2023.09.012

Seaton, W., Cranmer, G. A., White, C., Bober, J., Humphrey, K., & Obeng, A. (2022). "That's it. i'm done with this team!" Public reactions to NFL teams' racial activism as a function of social identity management. *Communication Quarterly, 70*(5), 585–607.

Social Media and Electronic Communication Policy. (n.d.). Potomacsoccer. https://potomacsoccer.org/policies/social-media-and-electronic-communication-policy/#:~:text=Internet%20and%20Communication%20Policies%20for%20Coaches%201%20All,provided%20through%20social%20media%20sites.%20...%20More%20items

Spaaij, R., Knoppers, A., & Jeanes, R. (2020). "We want more diversity but…:" Resisting diversity in recreational sports clubs. *Sport Management Review, 23*(3), 363–373.

Tallapradaga, M., & Cranmer, G. A. (2022). Media narratives about concussions: Effects on parents' intention to inform their children about concussions. *Communication & Sport, 10*(3), 517–540.

Todd, A. (2023, September 28). Sioux Falls dance coach arrested for allegedly sending illicit Snapchat photos to minor. " *Argus Leader*. https://www.argusleader.com/story/news/crime/2023/09/28/sioux-falls-dance-coach-arrested-for-sending-illicit-photos-to-minor-snapchat/70993133007/

Uncovering the Reasons Kids Drop out of Youth Sports. (n.d.). https://www.jerseywatch.com/blog/reasons-kids-drop-out-of-youth-sports

Weathers, M., & Sanderson, J. (2021). Social media, social and legal issues. In N. O'Reilly, G. Abeza. J. Sanderson, & E. Frederick (Eds.) *Social media and sport: Theory and practice* (pp. 313–344). World Science Publishing.

White, A. J. D., Parry, K., Humphries, C., Phelan, S., Batten, J., & Magrath, R. (2022). Duty of Karius: Media framing of concussion following the 2018 UEFA Champions league final. *Communication & Sport, 10*(3), 541–563.

Wilson, F., Ng, L., O' Sullivan, K., Caneiro, J. P., O' Sullivan, P. P. B., Horgan A., Thornton, J. S., Wilkie, K., & Timonen, V. (2021). "You're the best liar in the world': A grounded theory of rowing athletes' experiences of lower back pain. *British Journal of Sports Medicine*, *55*(6), 327–335.

Witt, P. A., & Dangi, T. B. (2018). Why children/youth drop out of sports. *Journal of Park and Recreation Administration, 36,* 191–199.

Women's World Cup (2023). One in five players received social media abuse, says Fifa report. *BBC*. https://www.bbc.com/sport/football/67686209

15

CELEBRITY HEALTH NARRATIVES AND IMPLICATIONS FOR PUBLIC CONVERSATIONS ABOUT HEALTH

Christina S. Beck

The image of Jimmy and Rosalynn Carter etched in my mind features both in work clothes, holding a hammer or other construction tool and working to build another house for Habitat for Humanity. As a Baptist Sunday School teacher until well into his 90s (Poole, 2023), Jimmy and his wife of over 70 years epitomized people with a "servant's heart" (Heilman, 2023; Martin, 2023; "Reactions to the death … ", 2023).

As individuals in the public eye for decades, both promoted a variety of causes, even as they experienced declining health due to their advancing age (see, e.g., Baker, 2023; Bartash, 2023; Ijaz & Jacobson, 2023). In February 2023, Jimmy announced that he would be entering hospice care. Notably, Parker (2023, para. 5) reminded readers that "[h]ospice is indelible to Carter's legacy as president. The federal payment model demonstration that led to the founding of the Medicare Hospice Benefit began during his tenure in the White House."

Decades after his term as President, Jimmy's announcement about choosing hospice care fostered end-of-life discussions and awareness of hospice as an option (see, e.g., Associated Press, 2024; Choi, 2023; Parker, 2023). As Choi reported,

"I don't think we can understate the significance of someone as prominent and well-respected as Jimmy Carter … openly and publicly making that decision," said Davis Baird, director of government affairs for hospice at the National Association for Home Care & Hospice.

Parker quoted the president and CEO of Delaware Hospice, Susan Lloyd:

> Even with the growth of hospice care, only half of eligible Medicare beneficiaries are taking advantage of this option. I think that it's due in part to the lack of awareness, and in part due to misconceptions about hospice … Increasing awareness and addressing these misconceptions takes open conversations. By choosing hospice care and sharing that choice with the American public, President Carter and his family are helping to educate people, and shedding light on the hospice experience.
>
> *(para. 15–16)*

Three months after former President Carter entered hospice care, the Carter Center (2023, para. 3) revealed that the 96-year-old former First Lady had been diagnosed with dementia, noting that "[w]e

 DOI: 10.4324/9781003436409-17

hope sharing our family's news will increase important conversations at kitchen tables and in doctor's offices around the country."

Years earlier, Rosalynn recalled being affected by conversations with constituents about mental health concerns while campaigning for Jimmy's gubernatorial campaign (Carter, 2010). Those interactions inspired her to urge Jimmy to prioritize mental health care in his administration (Bartash, 2023). Bartash reported that "Jimmy Carter promised to help—when he was elected president, he named his wife as the active honorary chair of the President's Commission on Mental Health during his White House tenure" (para. 8). She continued that advocacy work through the Carter Center (co-established with Jimmy), and her nearly life-long commitment to destigmatizing mental illness likely factored into the family's choice to confide otherwise personal health information with the public. Sadly, former President Carter lost his wife six months after the dementia disclosure and only a few days after she joined him in hospice care (Weiner, 2023).

President and Mrs. Carter exemplified the power of prominent individuals bringing visibility to a cause in two important but distinct ways. First, both engaged in advocacy work, and, obviously, their service made a difference across the globe (see, e.g., Ijan & Jacobson, 2023). Second, their personal health narratives have contributed to public and private conversations about hospice and dementia. Thomas (2023, para. 3) asserted:

> Increasingly we are seeing celebrities use their platforms to share their own deeply personal health stories, lifting the lid on topics previously regarded as taboo … [These stories] show that, like us, they are human, and like us, they are not immune to disease and ill-health.

Indeed, celebrity health narratives have attracted considerable attention from scholars over the past three decades (see, e.g., Basil & Brown, 1994; Beck, 2022; Beck et al., 2015; Cram et al., 2003; Hoffman et al., 2017; Hoffman & Tan, 2013; Kresovich & Noar, 2020; Lerner, 2006; Sabel & Cin, 2016; Sillence & Martin, 2020; Troiano et al., 2017; Vafeiadis et al., 2022). In this chapter, I examine how celebrity health narratives uniquely fuel public dialogues about health and wellness. I begin by defining *celebrity health narratives* and providing foundational information about narrative theorizing, celebrity studies, and parasocial experiences necessary for understanding the persuasive potential of these narratives. I then discuss the health-related implications of celebrity health disclosures as well as ethical challenges integral to the public co-telling/re-telling of these otherwise private narratives. I conclude by proposing next steps for scholars seeking to understand this increasingly prevalent part of popular culture and Health Communication.

Defining *Celebrity Health Narratives*

On myriad popular culture platforms, celebrities share health-related tips and perspectives, make product recommendations, and support health-related causes, and, clearly, such actions can be powerful, especially for those who follow them on social media or benefit from their philanthropic efforts (see, e.g., Aleti et al., 2019; Coffie et al., 2023; Hinnant & Hendrickson, 2014; Zhou & Kraak, 2022). Even though some of the theoretical and conceptual issues that I address in this chapter can apply broadly to such celebrity discourse, in this chapter, I focus on celebrity health narratives.

Celebrity health narratives constitute public health disclosures by a celebrity (or celebrity's family) about a personal health issue (see Beck, 2022; Beck et al., 2014; Beck et al., 2015). This sort of communication differs from other forms of celebrity health-related interactions in two central ways. First, celebrity health narratives entail the disclosure of a health challenge experienced personally by a prominent person or a member of that person's family. Beck et al. (2015, p. 6) explained:

> When a celebrity decides to disclose a diagnosis to a reporter (or update a Facebook status, send a tweet, or post an Instagram photo about it), especially in this era of social media, s/he initiates a very public and multi-faceted communicative firestorm, instantly propelling a previously private situation into a public discussion about everything from medical alternatives to motivations for sharing.

Thus, even though Rosalynn Carter certainly advocated passionately for mental health issues throughout her life, that work differed from public reactions to her family's revelation that she had been diagnosed with dementia near the end of her life.

Second, as argued by Beck et al. (2014), generally, celebrity health narratives involve a celebrity speaking out about a health-related situation without compensation for doing so. In other words, the person does not promote a health-related product or company solely as a paid spokesperson without a personal connection to the health issue.

For example, Brittany Mahomes, wife of Kansas City Chiefs quarterback Patrick Mahomes, has worked to raise awareness about food allergies (see, e.g., Halkidis, 2024; Roy, 2024; Smith, 2024). According to Kappes (2024, para. 2), "Brittany Mahomes has been aware of her daughter Sterling's mild nut allergies … However, a frightening incident last summer involving her son Bronze being rushed to the hospital after a severe reaction to nuts has heightened Mahomes's vigilance." According to Roy, Mahomes has employed "her massive platform to educate and empower parents of young children about allergies, including life-threatening signs and symptoms among infants and toddlers" (para. 3).

As Smith (2024, para. 4) noted, "Brittany began her allergy advocacy by leading a fundraising campaign for FARE, the food allergy non-profit. (This included her own contribution of $100,000.) Now, she is raising awareness of using epinephrine through a partnership with AUVI-Q, the compact epinephrine auto-injector," including endorsing "the first and only FDA-approved epinephrine auto-injector for infants and toddlers 16.5 to 33 pounds" (Roy, 2024, para. 1).

Smith's (2024) publication, *Allergic Living*, praised Mahomes for "using her voice to help raise awareness of food allergies. She is getting across the messages that these allergies can be life-threatening and the importance of having and using epinephrine" (para. 13). Mahomes' personal connection to this matter as a mom of two children with food allergies and her encouragement of the only approved medication of its kind fits as a *celebrity health narrative*. As this chapter documents, celebrity health narratives pack considerable persuasive potential, given the powerful combination of celebrity testimony as well as audience investment in the celebrity's emergent narrative (for related theoretical work on the persuasive power of narratives, please see, e.g., Miller-Day & Hecht, 2013; Shen & Edwards, 2023).

Persuasive Power of a Personal Celebrity Narrative

We weren't with Brittany and Patrick Mahomes as doctors treated their young son in the ER. As a mom, I can't imagine how difficult that experience must have been for their family. That life-changing hospital visit launched their journey as parents of a child with a potentially life-threatening condition, one requiring significant modification of food and awareness of risks. They could not have envisioned how their story would change with that revelation. As Frank (1995) would suggest, they encountered a disruption in what had been before and what could be possible moving forward.

Narratives as Personal and Social

I have no idea *how* that twist shifted and shaped the Mahomes' emergent family story, but the communicative choices about how to handle the food allergy within their immediate family unit – and even who to tell and when – necessarily impacted the unfolding narrative. Indeed, Fisher (1989) advanced the narrative paradigm, proposing "a reconceptualization of humankind as *Homo narrans*" and arguing that "all forms of human communication need to be seen fundamentally as stories—symbolic interpretations of aspects of the world occurring in time and shaped by history, culture, and character" (p. xiii). Fisher continued to assert that " symbols are created and communicated ultimately as stories meant to give order to the human experience" (p. 63).

Scholars contend that narratives concurrently and reflexively mold our sense of self (see, e.g., Gergen, 1991, 1994; Grodin & Lindlof, 1996; Holstein & Gubrium, 2000) as the moments and experiences of life affect us and how we orient to the world and to those around us. Health-related narratives can prove especially impactful for our sense of self and the master narrative of our lives and those of others who care about us (or even who learn about our story) (see, e.g., Frank, 1995; Harter et al., 2005a, 2005b; Harter et al., 2021; Langellier, 2001; Langellier & Peterson, 2004; Ma et al., 2023). Frank argued:

> All of these stories—health and illness stories together—constitute a formless but formative framework of interpretive effects that structures people's sense of what events and actions are worth telling stories about and how these stories are to be understood, including what actions follow from them.
>
> *(p. xi)*

Notably, as Frank asserted, "The ill body's articulation in stories is a personal task, but the stories told by the ill are also *social*" (p. 3).

In her work on Communication Privacy Management Theory, Sandra Petronio (2002) explained that we own private information, such as a health diagnosis, and we choose how (or if) we want to expand our *privacy boundaries* by disclosing that information to someone else. Sharing that information with another person necessarily means expanding the privacy boundary and entrusting that individual as a "co-owner" of what has been disclosed (see, e.g., Petronio & Child, 2020, p. 76). That act of confiding one's story to another matters. Garro and Mattingly (2000, p. 11) argued:

> "A story … not only is about something but also *does* something … If they have power as actions, this only comes through developing a particular kind of relationship between teller (or text) and audience, one in which the listener comes to care about the events recounted."

Extending from Petronio and Childs (2020), the move from protecting privacy to revealing information, even if "just" to one other person, reflexively and rhetorically shifts that narrative from personal to shared.

Celebrity Narratives as Relational

Disclosing personal information by anyone to chosen confidants certainly impacts the original owner of the information as well as those to whom disclosures have been made (see, e.g., Petronio, 2002; Petronio & Childs, 2020). However, the choice by prominent individuals to share what would otherwise be private health details on a public platform (e.g., social media, television interview, newspaper article) greatly expands privacy boundaries and transforms a personal health narrative into a public one. As such, although that prominent person still experiences the health situation as an individual (and, likely, along with close friends and family members), the original personal health narrative morphs with myriad others as now co-owners (see, e.g., Beck, 2022; Beck et al., 2015).

Of course, celebrities do not always want to blur the boundaries of their personal lives and professional persona (see, e.g., York, 2018). The late Princess Diana eventually acknowledged her battle with bulimia to a BBC reporter (Harvey-Jenner, 2020; Rotondi, 2023; Taylor, 2020). According to

Taylor, "Her raw, candid confession sent shockwaves through the world at the time [1995]—eating disorders were rarely talked about openly. To have a global superstar do so, on such a stage, challenged a major societal stigma" (para. 9). Yet, despite that rare disclosure, she still coveted her privacy and, sadly, died in a car crash two years later while trying to get away from the hounding paparazzi (Samuelson, 2017).

The case of Princess Diana underscores two key points. First, as I detail more in the next section, disclosures of celebrity health issues raise awareness of and encourage advocacy regarding a wide array of health-related concerns. Second, as I address in this section, their fans and followers fervently (and, I would argue, increasingly) want to—and almost feel a *right*—to know about such personal matters.

In her work on celebrity culture and gender influences, Suparsad (2023, p. 144) noted that "the role celebrities play in contemporary society now goes beyond just their work" (for related arguments about celebrities and political and/or economic influence, see Gunter, 2014; Harvey, 2017; Ribke, 2018; Wheeler, 2013; Wright, 2020). The proliferation of social media has cracked the "fourth wall" between those in the public eye and fans who follow them on social media, giving at least an illusion of more direct access (see, e.g., Elliott, 2018; Frost, 2023; Jerslev & Mortensen, 2018; Marwick & boyd, 2011; Nemer, 2016; for related arguments, please see Baym, 2010; Masur et al., 2023; Van Dijck, 2013). As Jerslev and Mortensen acknowledged, "The breakdown of rigid barriers between the private and the public [has] already started in the mid-50s and increased with television and other cultural changes" (p. 171). Meyrowitz (1985, p. 179) echoed that observation:

> "The presumption of intimacy" created by electronic media has affected not only the print interview, but biographies and memoirs as well. It now seems more acceptable to write books about the very personal lives of great people … Indeed, memoirs *without* such intimate revelations about the writer or others now seem stuffy and unrealistic.

I argue that the contemporary hypermediated era (see Gergen, 1991) intensifies what Horton and Wahl (1956) labeled as "para-social" interaction. In his work on electronic (pre-social) media, Meyrowitz (1985) explained that "[v]iewers come to feel they 'know' the people they 'meet' on television in the same way they know their friends and associates … Paradoxically, the para-social performer is able to establish 'intimacy with millions'" (p. 119). Over 30 years since Meyrowitz wrote his classic book (and since the evolution of social media), Jerslev and Mortensen (2018) asserted that "[w]hat is new is the ubiquity of exposure, the extent to which potentially everyone, including celebrities, offers parts of their selves for public scrutiny" (p. 171). As Frost (2023, p. 7) argued, "One of the most significant effects of parasocial interaction is the blurring of boundaries between public and private lives. As people form emotional attachments to media figures, they often feel entitled to know intimate details about their lives."

As Petronio (2002) theorized, celebrity decisions to disclose information to fans (and expand their privacy boundaries) foster deeper connections between those with whom information has been shared – or, in the case of celebrities and their fans, at least the perception of a personal bond. (For related research on parasocial interactions and social media, please see Frost, 2023; Hoffner & Cohen, 2023; Jarzyna, 2021; Kowert & Daniel, 2021; Lacap et al., 2024; Lotun et al., 2022; Rasmussen, 2018; Xu et al., 2022). Indeed, Frost argued:

> Today, we can engage with celebrities, influencers, and content creators in ways that were once unimaginable. The lines between reality and fiction have become increasingly blurred, as individuals curate their online personnas and share intimate details of their lives with millions of followers. This unprecedented level of access has led to a new era of parasocial relationships characterized by a sense of intimacy and connection that rivals those of real-life friendships.
>
> *(p. 9)*

Thus, if we feel that we "know" a celebrity and that celebrity reveals some sort of health challenge, that disclosure might resonate with us or prompt us to feel empathy because we care about that person (see, e.g., Calhoun & Gold, 2020; Vafeiadis et al., 2022; Van Den Bulck, 2017). For example, Cohen and Hoffner (2016) referenced perceived parasocial relationships as fans experienced grief and a sense of loss after learning about Robin Williams's suicide.

Beyond prompting fan reactions of "oh that's too bad" or "that's so sad," celebrity health narratives have inspired donations for health-related research, as in the case of late basketball coach and sports broadcaster Jim Valvano and ESPN, who co-founded the V Foundation just prior to Valvano's death from cancer in 1993. The V Foundation website reported that, "[s]ince its inception in 1993, the V Foundation has allocated over $353 million in grants for cancer research across the nation, solidifying its position as a leading advocate for cutting-edge cancer research" (n.d., para. 2; for additional information and examples about advocacy of health-related causes and social support, see Beck et al., 2014; Beck et al., 2015). The next section details how celebrity health narratives also raise awareness about health risks and preventive care.

Raising Awareness through Celebrity Health Narratives

According to an article in *The New York Times*, "actress Olivia Munn shared that she was diagnosed with and treated for breast cancer … 'Ask your doctor to calculate your Breast Cancer Risk Assessment Score,' Ms. Munn urged the public in her [Instagram] post" (Sheihk & Gupta, 2024, paras. 1–2). Sheikh and Gupta acknowledged that "[m]edical experts are enthusiastic about the spotlight on risk calculators, but they caution that the results are only rough estimates and need to be interpreted with the help of a doctor" (para. 3).

Multi-case or meta-analyses of celebrity health narratives affirm the potential positive value of celebrities speaking out about their personal health experiences (see, e.g., Beck, 2022; Beck et al., 2014; Beck et al., 2015; Hoffman et al., 2017; Hoffman & Tan, 2013; Kresovich & Noar, 2020; Wood & Bollinger, 2020; see also related work by Hoffner & Cohen, 2023). For example, in their longitudinal study, Wood and Bollinger argued that "celebrity influence in health care may often be driven by the ability of the celebrity to keep health issues top of mind through news coverage" (p. 309). As Wood and Bollinger noted, "We observe a significant generalized celebrity cancer effect in which celebrity breast cancer diagnoses can contribute to increased screening, but that is through the number of news stories that result" (p. 309).

Kresovich and Noar (2020), however, pointed to a connection between the level of parasocial interaction or identification with specific celebrities and their fans regarding the response. According to Kresovich and Noar, "These findings revealed that those who had higher PSI with the celebrity had greater behavioral intentions to engage in the health behavior that was the subject of the celebrity health event" (p. 508).

Whether because of sheer visibility or parasocial connection, celebrity health narratives have inspired action by those who learn about the celebrity health situation (see, e.g., Appleford, 2016; Bute et al., 2016; Curran & Larkin, 2023; Francis et al., 2019; Pavelko et al., 2017; Selberg, 2017). For example, when actress Nathalie Richardson passed away from a head injury after a ski accident, hospitals in Canada, New York, and New Jersey experienced spikes in pediatric ER visits for possible head injuries, with as much as "a 73% increase in visits for head trauma during the 10 days following the event" in the New York area hospitals, even though the number of head injury diagnoses remained near the baseline (Keays, 2010, p. 117).

Even more prominently, Cram et al. (2003) pointed to the "Couric effect" of then NBC anchor Katie Couric undergoing a colonoscopy on U.S. national television to emphasize the importance of colon screening. (She did so after losing her first husband to colon cancer in his early 40s.) According to Cram et al., "The significant increase in the number of colonoscopies performed by the CORI gastroenterologists was immediate and persisted at a higher rate for nearly a year after the campaign" (p. 1604). In this section, I highlight two cases that have received considerable media and scholarly attention concerning celebrity health narratives and impacts on raising awareness about health risks and preventive steps: Magic Johnson's HIV disclosure and Angelina Jolie's editorial in *The New York Times*.

Magic Johnson

In 1991, Earvin "Magic" Johnson, then-star basketball player for the Los Angeles Lakers, made the shocking announcement that he had been diagnosed with HIV. Now over 30 years later, I struggle to adequately describe the significance of this disclosure, given the vast difference between that historical moment and contemporary understandings of and perspectives on HIV and AIDS. As Cardazzi et al. (2023, p. 2047) explained, in the early 1990s, "[a]s [HIV/AIDS] became increasingly prevalent throughout the world, scientific understanding of its origins, causes, and consequences rapidly increased, while the general public understanding lagged." Cardazzi et al. asserted that "[t]here were few (if any) shocks to those beliefs which were greater than when" Johnson disclosed this news (p. 2047).

In their review of research about reactions to Johnson's disclosure, Cardazzi et al. (2023) determined that the news proved especially impactful because it underscored that heterosexual men could contract the disease and worked to destigmatize a positive diagnosis (for related studies, please see Basil & Brown, 1994, 1997; W. J. Brown & Basil, 1995; B. R. Brown et al., 1996; Casey et al., 2003; Kalichman & Hunter, 1992; Kalichman et al., 1993). Brown and Basil concluded that "emotional involvement with Johnson—not his message per se—produced changes in respondents' attitudes and intended/reported behaviors. Johnson was not simply the source of the message, or a spokesperson; he was the personification of the message." (p. 364).

In their meta-analysis of studies about this celebrity case, Casey et al. (2003) determined that "[t]he net effect of Magic's disclosure was most marked by a sharp increase in the number of individuals obtaining HIV tests immediately following the announcement of Magic Johnson's HIV status" (p. 260). Mirroring this finding, Cohn et al. (1992) found:

> In the 20 working days following the announcement, the number of clients at our HIV counseling and testing site increased 203% over the same period in 1990, and 151% over the 20 days preceding the announcement… The most dramatic increase (279%) occurred at the HIV counseling site, in the number of heterosexuals with no identified risk for HIV infection.
>
> *(p. 1692)*

As Laughland (2021) noted, Jordan's announcement comprised "a seismic moment, not only in the history of basketball, but in the continuing war on HIV and AIDS, as an athlete of Johnson's stature vowed in public to raise awareness about the virus" (para. 7). Three decades later, according to Laughland, Johnson "is one of those rare public figures who has redefined his purpose at different stages in life: first as an athlete, then as a public health advocate, and later as a successful businessman and philanthropist" (para. 5). In that interview, Johnson told Laughland that "[a]s we talk today, right now, I'm thinking, 'Wow' – it's been 30 years and I'm still here, healthy. Everything has gone right. There was one drug then, now we have 30-something drugs" (para. 6).

Angelina Jolie

On May 13, 2013, actress Angelina Jolie published an op-ed column in *The New York Times*, confiding with the publication's readers (and the rest of the world) about both her medical history and subsequent decision to undergo BRCA testing and, ultimately, a double mastectomy. As Jolie stressed in the column, "For any woman reading this, I hope it helps you to know that you have options" (p.

A25). She shared that "I chose not to keep my story private because there are many women who do not know that they might be living under the shadow of cancer" (p. A25). Jolie wrote that "[i]t is my hope that they, too, will be able to get gene testing" (p. A25).

Jolie's op-ed column thrust the possibility of genetic testing as a preventive measure for breast cancer into the spotlight worldwide (see, e.g., Al-Hussaini et al., 2019; Dean, 2016; Drizin et al., 2018; Emmers-Sommer & Terán, 2019; Freedman et al., 2017; Juthe et al., 2015; Lee et al., 2017; Ložar et al., 2021; Roberts & Dusetzina, 2017; Sillence & Martin, 2020; Troiano et al., 2017; Zimovjanova et al., 2023). Notably, as Sabel and Cin (2016) discussed in their review, Jolie was not the first celebrity to share a journey involving breast cancer; indeed, they situated Jolie's disclosure in the context of actress Christina Applegate's bilateral mastectomies a few years earlier and the breast cancer announcement by Australian singer-songwriter Kylie Minogue two weeks afterward.

Juthe et al. (2015) "observed a profound effect on Internet traffic to NCI's [National Cancer Institute] cancer genetics and risk reduction resources, most notably the Preventive Mastectomy fact sheet, after the publication of Jolie's op-ed piece on 14 May 2013" (p. 551). Beyond the United States, scholars have credited the "Angelina effect" with upward trends, for example, in BRCA testing in Jordan (Al-Hussaini et al., 2019), Australia (Freedman et al., 2017), and Korea (Lee et al., 2017) as well as RRMs (risk-reducing mastectomy) in Slovenia (Ložar et al., 2021) and the Czech Republic (Zimovjanova et al., 2023).

As with the case of Olivia Munn that I mentioned at the outset of this section, most scholars acknowledged Jolie's important work in raising awareness about genetic testing. However, they also stressed the need for health professionals to provide additional information in such cases so that individuals can assess their own risks and weigh the benefits of possible preventive measures, in consultation with their doctor (see, e.g., Juthe et al., 2015). Indeed, as I discuss in the next section, celebrity contributions to public dialogues about health should prompt critical reflection—by fans as well as Health Communication scholars and practitioners.

Future Considerations for Celebrity Health Narratives

Soap opera actor Maurice Benard has openly discussed his bipolar diagnosis, including in his best-selling book (2020) and on his podcast, *State of Mind* (see also Chapter 19, this volume). The podcast series boasts over 100,000 subscribers, with a goal of mental health advocacy (https://mbstateofmind.com/). Benard is not alone. Other celebrities – including Demi Lovato, Selena Gomez, Lady Gaga, Scott Mescudi, Naomi Osaka, and Simone Biles – have embraced their prominent platform and personal experiences to promote mental health and well-being (Calhoun & Gold, 2020; Francis, 2018; Franssen, 2020; Thelandersson, 2023). Francis pointed to the potential power of these narratives, noting that, in her study participants, "half reported seeking information about depression after prominent hip-hop artist Scott Mescudi disclosed his depression diagnosis and treatment" (p. 692).

This chapter has highlighted research about celebrity health narratives, especially in terms of raising awareness about important health-related issues. However, even though this form of discourse about health and wellness has prompted considerable scholarship over the past three decades, I encourage future researchers to explore and consider the following issues.

Pressing Privacy Boundaries

As Frost (2023) asserted, the advent of social media and pressures to share more and more intimate information have intensified expectations for celebrity disclosures. Yet, to what extent *should* prominent individuals yield to such pressure?

In a recent opinion piece, I made the case that public figures shouldn't *have* to disclose private health information if they don't want to do so (Beck, 2024). Yet, as I finished this chapter in March

2024, the Internet buzzed with theories about Catherine, Princess of Wales, amid her absence from the public stage following abdominal surgery in January 2024 (and the decision to issue an edited family photo three months later) (see Grady, 2024; Judkis et al., 2024). After the brief, initial announcement about the surgery, the palace asked for privacy. As time passed, a media frenzy ensued, spiked by spiraling speculation that filled the void. Dubbed as "Kategate," memes and rumors launched a wide range of alternate narratives, from a possible royal breakup to the potential reveal of Princess Kate as the "Masked Singer" (see, e.g., Judkis et al., 2024; Wanshel, 2024).

On March 22, 2024, Catherine broke her silence, explaining in a short video that she had been diagnosed with cancer (Judkis et al., 2024). She quietly confided that "William and I have been doing everything we can to process and manage this privately for the sake of our young family" (Sanchez, 2024, para. 4). As Judkis et al. (2024, para. 5) observed:

> *Yikes*, replied all the social media jokesters who had been posting about her getting a Brazilian butt lift. *Oof*, went all the people who, 24 hours earlier, had been absolutely certain that Prince William was leaving her for the Marchioness of Cholmondeley.

Frayer (2024, para. 1) put public response to Catherine's disclosure well: "The initial reaction was shock, then concern—soon followed by shame."

As the case of Princess Diana illustrated, celebrities have long sought to preserve privacy, even before social media. However, in this era of myriad would-be co-tellers creating memes and posts on their cell phones without regulation, celebrities face an even more daunting challenge of controlling their own stories at the hint of something amiss. As adoring fans, or perhaps even just amused others, pose questions, press for details, or speculate amid silence, how do celebrities manage expectations about what should and should not be disclosed by them? Moreover, although eventual disclosures, like the one made by Princess Kate, squash rumors, they also reward public pressure (and reinforce contemporary expectations about public disclosures of personal information; see Masur et al., 2023).

Navigating Expanded Boundaries

Relatedly, how do families manage those expectations? I began this chapter with the examples of Rosalynn and Jimmy Carter. I presume that President Carter consented to information being released about his move to hospice, and, certainly, given the former First Lady's advocacy in this area, it makes sense that the family would assume her support of disclosure about her dementia as well. However, how do (or should) families of celebrities make such decisions?

The families of actor Bruce Willis and television personality Jack Hanna decided to share some information with the public when the men started to decline from dementia. In 2023, the Willis family provided an update through a public statement. Acknowledging the diagnosis of frontotemporal dementia, the family stated:

> As Bruce's condition advances, we hope that any media attention can be focused on shining a light on this disease that needs far more awareness and research. Bruce always believed in using his voice in the world to help others, and to raise awareness about important issues both publicly and privately. We know in our hearts that – if he could today – he would want to respond by bringing global attention and a connectedness with those who are also dealing with this debilitating disease and how it impacts so many individuals and their families.
>
> *(Association for Frontotemporal Degeneration, 2023, para. 3-4)*

Jack Hanna's family also affirmed their belief that Jack would want to help people through the disclosures (France, 2023). France wrote:

> Hanna's family said they are sharing their story now because "they want other families to know they are not alone when the struggle with Alzheimer's feels overwhelming. "If this helps even one other family, it's more than worth sharing dad's story," Hanna's eldest daughter, Kathaleen, said. "He spent a lifetime helping everyone he could. He will never know it or understand it, but he is still doing it now."
>
> *(para. 14–15)*

I appreciate these altruistic sentiments, and hearing their stories may well be helpful for other families going through the same trials. Yet, extending from Masur et al. (2023), such disclosures might also yield the unintended consequence of implying that celebrity families (and, perhaps, even non-celebrity families too) *should* make such disclosures for "the greater good." I encourage researchers to explore the implications of such disclosures by family members on behalf of celebrity loved ones in terms of confiding personal health information in a public space. Moreover, this sort of issue merits discussion by all families, even those not in the public eye, in this era of social media. How do loved ones want to be represented on social media (or other platforms), particularly if they can't articulate their own preferences? Especially given the pervasiveness of social media, these types of conversations would be valuable.

Complications for Public Health Messaging

Fifty years ago (and well before social media), then First Lady Betty Ford's 1974

> brave decision to make her [breast cancer] diagnosis public broke the silence around the disease and prompted millions of women to go for screening. And, as they did, detection rates in the USA rose sharply. Researchers called it the 'Betty Ford blip.'
>
> *("The Breast Cancer Conundrum," 2013, para. 1)*

Certainly, public health officials recognized the persuasive potential of celebrity advocacy during the Covid-19 pandemic, especially regarding wearing masks or obtaining a Covid-19 vaccination (see, e.g., Beck, 2022; Kaminski et al., 2021; for related arguments, see Cohen, 2020). However, myriad prominent people communicated a wide array of public positions on Covid-19 as they shared their own symptoms or personal remedies and/or displayed concern about their own risk (or lack thereof) – some perspectives and experiences consistent with public health recommendations and others in direct contrast with them (for related work, please see, e.g., Beck, 2022; Field-Springer et al., 2024; Martinez-Berman et al., 2021; Myrick & Chen, 2022; see also Chapters 11 and 25, this volume).

Given the plethora of mediated platforms and personalities permeating the public sphere, how can public health officials best disseminate health recommendations, especially as highly visible (and perhaps even well-meaning) people concurrently share their "truth" with thousands or millions of followers? How can media consumers sort through conflicting messages to determine how to best proceed, especially when they feel connected to a given celebrity or official? How can public health campaigns persuade admiring supporters who opt to believe a public figure whose perspectives or practices clash with recommended guidelines (see, e.g, Myrick & Chen, 2022; Willson et al., 2019)? How do health care consumers weigh public health messages when they also encounter potentially conflicting (and personally compelling) celebrity health narratives? How do they juxtapose celebrity voices with friends, family, and other mediated sources?

References

Aleti, T., Pallant, J. I., Tuan, A., & van Laer, T. (2019). Tweeting with the stars: Automated text analysis of celebrity social media communications on consumer word of mouth. *Journal of Interactive Marketing*, *48*, 17–32.

Al-Hussaini, M., Ammar, K., Kasasbeh, N., Sultan, H., & Al-Omari, A. (2019). Global celebrities' effect on health awareness among Jordanians: A study using the case of Angelina Jolie. *Journal of Genetic Counseling*, *28*, 1021–1028.

Appleford, K. (2016). "This big bum thing has taken over the world:" Considering Black women's changing views on body image and the role of celebrity. *Critical Studies in Fashion & Beauty*, *7*(2), 193–214.

Associated Press (2024, February 18). Advocates hope Jimmy Carter's endurance in hospice care drives awareness. *Politico*. https://www.politico.com/news/2024/02/18/advocates-hope-jimmy-carters-endurance-in-hospice-care-drives-awareness

Association for Frontotemporal Degeneration (2023, February 16). A statement from the Willis family. https://www.theaftd.org/mnlstatement23/

Baker, P. (2023, February 18). Jimmy Carter, 98, opts for hospice care. *The New York Times*. https://www.nytimes.com/2023/02/18/us/politics/jimmy-carter-hospice

Bartash, C. (2023, November 22). How Rosalynn Carter became a champion for mental health. *ABC News*. https://abcnews.go.com/Politics/remembering-rosalyn-carter-tireless-mental-health-advocate/story

Basil, M. D., & Brown, W. J. (1994). Interpersonal communication in news diffusion: A study of "Magic" Johnson's announcement. *Journalism & Mass Communication Quarterly*, *71*(2), 305–320.

Basil, M. D., & Brown, W. J. (1997). Marketing AIDS prevention: The differential impact hypothesis versus identification effects. *Journal of Consumer Psychology*, *6*(4), 389–411.

Baym, N. K. (2010). *Personal connections in the digital age*. Polity.

Beck, C. S. (2022). *Celebrity in the time of Covid: Fandom and the influence of pandemic messaging*. McFarland.

Beck, C. S. (2024, February 12). How much personal information does King Charles owe the public? *Stat*. https://www.statnew/2024/02/12/king-charles-lloyd-austin-celebrities-health-disclosure

Beck, C. S., Aubuchon, S., McKenna, T., Ruhl, S., & Simmons, N. (2014). Blurring personal health and public priorities: An analysis of celebrity health narratives in the public sphere. *Health Communication*, *29*(3), 244–256.

Beck, C. S., Chapman, S. M. A., Simmons, N., Tenzek, K. E., & Ruhl, S. M. (2015). *Celebrity health narratives and the public health*. McFarland.

Benard, M. (2020). *Nothing general about it: How love (and lithium) saved me on and off General Hospital*. William Morrow.

Brown, B. R., Baranowski, M. D., Kulig, J. W., Stephenson, J. N., & Perry, B. (1996). Searching for the Magic Johnson effect: AIDS, adolescents, and celebrity disclosure. *Adolescence*, *31*(122), 253–264.

Brown, W. J., & Basil, M. D. (1995). Media celebrities and public health: Responses to "Magic" Johnson's HIV disclosure and its impact on AIDS risk and high-risk behaviors. *Health Communication*, *7*(4), 345–370.

Bute, J., Quinlan, M. M., & Quandt, L. K. (2016). Informing or exploiting? Public responses to Giuliana Rancic's health narrative. *Health Communication*, *31*(8), 1008–1018.

Calhoun, A. J., & Gold, J. A. (2020). "I feel like I know them:" The positive effect of celebrity self-disclosure of mental illness. *Academic Psychiatry*, *44*, 237–241.

Cardazzi, A., Martin, J. C., & Rodriguez, Z. (2023). Information shocks and celebrity exposure: The effect of "Magic" Johnson on AIDS diagnoses and mortality in the U.S. *Health Economics*, *32*, 2047–2079.

Carter, R. (2010). *Within our reach: Ending the mental health crisis*. Rodale Books.

Carter Center (2023, May 30). Carter family statement about health of First Lady Rosalynn Carter. www.cartercenter.org/news/pr/2023/statement-on-rosalynn-carter-health

Casey, M. K., Allen, M., Emmers-Sommer, T., Sahlstein, E., DeGooyer, D., Winters, A. M., Wagner, A. E., & Dun, T. (2003). When a celebrity contracts a disease: The example of Earvin "Magic" Johnson's announcement that he was HIV positive. *Journal of Health Communication*, *8*, 249–265.

Choi, J. (2023, July 21). How Jimmy Carter has changed the conversation around hospice. *The Hill*. https://thehill.com/policy/healthcare/4108943-how-jimmy-carter-has-changed-the-conversation-around-hospice

Coffie, I. S., Tweneboah-Koduah, E. Y., Ocloo, E. C., & Mann, V. (2023). The moderating influence of celebrity endorsement on intention to engage in infection prevention behaviours. *Health Promotion International*, *38*, 1–15.

Cohen, E. L. (2020). Stars—they're sick like us! The effects of a celebrity exemplar on COVID-19-related risk cognitions, emotions, and preventative behavioral intentions. *Science Communication*, *42*(5), 724–741.

Cohen, E. L., & Hoffner, C. (2016). Finding meaning in a celebrity's death: The relationship between parasocial attachment, grief, and sharing educational health information related to Robin Williams on social network sites. *Computers in Human Behavior*, *65*, 643–650.

Cohn, D. L., Miller, L. A., Yamaguchi, K. J., & Douglas, J. M. (1992). Denver's increase in HIV counseling after Magic Johnson's disclosure. *American Journal of Public Health*, *82*(12), 1692.

Cram, P., Fendick, A. M., & Inadomi, J. (2003). The impact of a celebrity promotional campaign on the use of colon cancer screening. *Archives of Internal Medicine*, *163*(13), 1601–1605.

Curran, M. G., & Larkin, M. A. (2023). "The Bird effect:" Positive impact of celebrity health disclosure on public awareness and soaring interest in motor neurone disease. *Irish Journal of Medical Science*, *193*(2), 973–974. https://doi.org/10.1007/s11845-023-03552-x

Dean, M. (2016). Celebrity health announcements and online health information seeking: An analysis of Angelina Jolie's preventative health decision. *Health Communication*, *31*(6), 752–761.

Drizin, J. H., Malcarne, V. L., Schiaffino, M. K., & Wells, K. J. (2018). College women's responses to a celebrity health disclosure. *Health Communication*, *33*(10), 1302–1307.

Elliott, A. (Ed.) (2018). *Routledge handbook of celebrity studies*. Routledge.

Emmers-Sommer, T. M., & Terán, L. (2020). The "Angelina effect" and audience response to celebrity vs. medical expert health messages: An examination of source credibility, message elaboration, and behavioral intentions. *Sexuality Research and Social Policy*, *17*, 149–161.

Field-Springer, K., Striley, K., Byerly, J., Simmons, N., Ferrell, T., & Quigley, S. (2024, February 29). "Are you vaccinated? Yeah, I'm immunized": A risk orders theory analysis of celebrity COVID-19 misinformation. *Journal of Communication in Healthcare*. https://doi.org/10.1080/17538068.2024.2320984

Fisher, W. (1989). *Human communication as narration: Toward a philosophy of reason, value, and action*. University of South Carolina Press.

France, L. R. (2023, June 22). Jack Hanna's Alzheimer's has progressed to the point he no longer recognizes most family members. *CNN*. https://www.cnn.com/2023/06/22/entertainment/jack-hanna-alzheimers/index.html

Francis, D. B. (2018). Young Black men's information seeking following celebrity depression disclosure: Implications for mental health communication. *Journal of Health Communication*, *23*, 687–694.

Francis, D. B., Stevens, E. M., Noar, S. M., & Widman, L. (2019). Public reactions to and impact of celebrity health announcements: Understanding the Charlie Sheen effect. *Howard Journal of Communications*, *30*(5), 479–494.

Frank, A. (1995). *The wounded storyteller: Body, illness, and ethics*. The University of Chicago Press.

Franssen, G. (2020). The celebritization of self-care: The celebrity health narrative of Demi Lovato and the sickscape of mental illness. *European Journal of Cultural Studies*, *23*(1), 89–111.

Frayer, L. (2024, March 23). Princess Kate's cancer triggers public shock, sympathy—and shame on the tabloids. *Wisconsin Public Radio*. https://www.wpr.org/news/princess-kates-cancer-triggers-public-shock-sympathy-and-shame-on-the-tabloids

Freedman, R., Mountain, H., Karina, D., & Schofield, L. (2017). A retrospective exploration of the impact of the "Angelina Jolie effect" on the single state-wide familial cancer program in Perth, Western Australia. *Journal of Genetic Counseling*, *26*, 52–62.

Frost, K. (2023). *The power of parasocial interaction: Exploring the psychology, media, and technology behind celebrities, influencers, and our unseen relationships*. Book Bound Studios.

Garro, L. C., & Mattingly, C. (2000). Narrative as construct and construction. In C. Mattingly & L. C. Garro (Eds.), *Narrative and the cultural construction of illness and healing* (pp. 1–49). University of California Press.

Gergen, K. J. (1991). *The saturated self: Dilemmas of identity in contemporary life*. Basic Books.

Gergen, K. J. (1994). *Realities and relationships: Soundings in social construction*. Harvard University Press.

Grady, C. (2024, March 14). Who is the British royal family willing to protect? *Vox*. https://www.vox.com/culture/24099969/kate-middleton-missing-controversy-meghan-markle-british-royal-family

Grodin, D., & Lindlof, T. R. (Eds.) (1996). *Constructing the self in a mediated world*. SAGE.

Gunter, B. (2014). *Celebrity capital: Assessing the value of fame*. Bloomsbury.

Halkidis, A. (2024, February 8). Brittany Mahomes shares her tips for other parents who have kids with food allergies. *Parents*. https://www.parents.com/brittany-mahomes-kids-food-allergies-8567809

Harter, L. M., Japp, P. M., & Beck, C. S. (2005a). Vital problematics of narrative theorizing about health and healing. In L. M. Harter, P. M. Japp, & C. S. Beck (Eds.), *Narrative, health, and healing: Communication theory, research, and practice* (pp. 7–30). Erlbaum.

Harter, L. M., Japp, P. M., & Beck, C. S. (Eds.) (2005b). *Narrative, health, and healing: Communication theory, research, and practice*. Erlbaum.

Harter, L. M., Yamasaki, J., & Kerr, A. M. (2021). Narrative features, forms, and functions: Telling stories to foster well-being, humanize healthcare, and catalyze change. In T. Thompson & N. G. Harrington (Eds.), *Routledge handbook of health communication* (3rd ed., pp. 47–60). Routledge.

Harvey, M. (2017). *Celebrity influence: Politics, persuasion, and issue-based advocacy*. University Press of Kansas.

Harvey-Jenner, C. (2020, November 11). The important reason Princess Diana's bulimia battle was included in The Crown. *Cosmopolitan.* https://www.cosmopolitan.com/uk/reports/a34640078/princess-diana-bulimia-eating-disorder/

Heilman, G. (2023, February 20). Online tributes and well-wishes for Jimmy Carter posted by fellow politicians and celebrities. *AS.* https://en.as.com/latest_news/online-tributes-and-well-wishes-for-jimmy-carter-posted-by-fellow-politicians-and-celebrities-n/

Hinnant, A., & Hendrickson, E. M. (2014). Negotiating normalcy in celebrity health behavior A focus group analysis. *Journal of Magazine & New Media Research, 15*(2), 1–20.

Hoffman, S. J., Mansoor, Y., Natt, N., Sritharan, L., Belluz, J., Caulfield, T., Freedhoff, Y., Lavis, J. N., & Sharma, A. M. (2017). Celebrities' impact on health-related knowledge, attitudes, behaviors, and status outcomes: Protocol for a systematic review, meta-analysis, and meta-regression analysis. *Systematic Reviews, 6,* Article number 13. https://doi.org/10.1186/s13643-016-0395-1

Hoffman, S. J., & Tan, C. (2013). Following celebrities' medical advice: Meta-narrative analysis. *British Medical Journal, 347.* https://doi.org/10.1136/bmj.f7151

Hoffner, C. A., & Cohen, E. L. (2023). Effects of parasocial experiences on health outcomes. In *The Oxford handbook of parasocial experiences* (pp. 309–334). Oxford University Press.

Holstein, J. A., & Gubrium, J. F. (2000). *The self we live by: Narrative identity in a postmodern world.* Oxford University Press.

Horton, D., & Wahl, R. R. (1956). Mass communication and parasocial interaction. *Psychiatry, 19*(3), 215–229.

Ijaz, K., & Jacobson, J. (2023, October). A tribute to the global health legacy of Jimmy and Rosalynn Carter. *The American Journal of Tropical Medicine and Hygiene, 109*(4), 713–714.

Jarzyna, C. L. (2021). Parasocial interaction, the COVID-19 quarantine, and digital age media. *Human Arenas, 4*(3), 413–429.

Jerslev, A., & Mortensen, M. (2018). Celebrity in the social media age: Renegotiating the public and the private. In A. Elliott (Ed.), *Routledge handbook of celebrity studies* (pp. 157–174). Routledge.

Jolie, A. (2013, May 14). My medical choice. *The New York Times.* A25.

Judkis, M., O'Neill, S., Andrews, T. M., & Maloy, A. F. (2024, March 22). They obsessed over Catherine. Now they're hit with a sobering truth. *The Washington Post.* https://www.washingtonpost.com/style/of-interest/2024/03/22/kate-middleton-ashamed-regret/

Juthe, R. H., Zaharchuk, A., & Wang, C. (2015). Celebrity disclosures and information seeking: The case of Angelina Jolie. *Genetics in Medicine, 17*(7), 545–553.

Kalichman, S. C., & Hunter, T. L. (1992). The disclosure of celebrity HIV infection: Its effects on public attitudes. *American Journal of Public Health, 82*(10), 1374–1376.

Kalichman, S. C., Russell, R. L., Hunter, T. L., & Sarwer, D. B. (1993). Earvin "Magic" Johnson's HIV serostatus disclosure: Effects on men's perceptions of AIDS. *Journal of Consulting and Clinical Psychology, 61*(5), 887–891.

Kaminski, M., Szymariska, C., & Nowak, J. K. (2021). Whose tweets on COVID-19 gain the most attention: Celebrities, political, or scientific authorities? *Cyberpsychology, Behavior, and Social Networking, 24*(2), 123–128. https://doi.org/10.1089/cyber.2020.0336

Kappes, W. (2024, February 8). Exclusive: Brittany Mahomes on game day rules and diaper bag go-tos. *The Bump.* https://www.thebump.com/news/brittany-mahomes-game-day-kids

Keays, G. (2010, March/April). Impact of a celebrity death on children's injury-related emergency room visits. *Canadian Journal of Public Health, 101*(2), 115–118.

Kowert, R., & Daniel, Jr., E. (2021, August-December). The one-and-a-half sided parasocial relationship: The curious case of live streaming. *Computers in Human Behavior Reports, 4.*

Kresovich, A., & Noar, S. M. (2020). The power of celebrity health events: Meta-analysis of the relationship between audience involvement and behavioral intentions. *Journal of Health Communication, 25,* 501–513.

Lacap, J. P. G., Cruz, M. R. M., Bayson, A. J., Molano, R., & Garcia, J. G. (2024). Parasocial relationships and social media interactions: Building brand credibility and loyalty. *Spanish Journal of Marketing, 28*(1), 77–97.

Langellier, K. M. (2001). 'You're marked:' Breast cancer, tattoo, and the narrative performance of identity. In J. Brockmeier & D. Carbaugh (Eds.), *Narrative and identity: Studies in autobiography, self, and culture* (pp. 145–186). John Benjamins.

Langellier, K. M., & Peterson, E. E. (2004). *Storytelling in daily life.* Temple University Press.

Laughland, O. (2021, June 24). Magic Johnson: The NBA superstar who smashed HIV stigma—then built a huge fortune. *The Guardian.* https://www.theguardian.com/society/2021/jun/24/magic-johnson-the-nba-superstar-who-smashed-hiv-stigma-then-built-a-huge-fortune

Lee, J., Kim, S., Kang, E., Park, S., Kim, Z., & Lee, M. H. (2017). Influence of the Angelina Jolie announcement and insurance reimbursement on practice patterns for hereditary breast cancer. *Journal of Breast Cancer, 20*(2), 203–207.

Lerner, B. H. (2006). *When illness goes public: Celebrity patients and how we look at medicine*. Johns Hopkins University Press.

Lotun, S., Lamarche, V. M., Samothrakis, S., Sandstrom, G. M., & Matran-Fernandez, A. (2022). Parasocial relationships on YouTube reduce prejudice towards mental health issues. *Scientific Reports, 12*.

Ložar, T., Žgajnar, J., Perhavec, A., Blatnik, A., Novaković, S., & Krajc, M. (2021). Trends and timing of risk-reducing mastectomy uptake in unaffected BRCA1 and BRCA2 carriers in Slovenia. *European Journal of Surgical Oncology, 47*, 1900–1906.

Ma, Z., Ma., R., Zhao, X., & Wang, X. (2023). Stories that engage the audience: An investigation of popular breast cancer narratives on social media. *Telematics and Informatics, 85*. https://doi.org/10.1016/j.tele.2023.102048

Martin, J. (2023, February 23). A peanut farmer with a servant's heart. *The Montgomery Independent*. https://www.montgomeryindependent.com/opinion/a-peanut-farmer-with-a-servant-s-heart/article_c9ea5f00-b394-11ed-9877-3fc1c0806211.html

Martinez-Berman, L., McCutheon, L., & Huynh, H. P. (2021). Is the worship of celebrities associated with resistance to vaccinations? Relationships between celebrity admiration, anti-vaccination attitudes, and beliefs in conspiracy. *Psychology, Health, & Medicine, 26*(9), 1063–1072.

Marwick, A., & boyd, D. (2011). To see and be seen: Celebrity practice on Twitter. *Convergence: The International Journal of Research into New Media Technologies, 17*, 139–158.

Masur, P., Bazarova, N. N., & DiFranzo, D. (2023). The impact of what others do, approve of, and expect you to do: An in-depth analysis of social norms and self-disclosure on social media. *Social Media+Society, 9*(1). https://doi.org/10.1177/20563051231156401

Meyrowitz, J. (1985). *No sense of place: The impact of electronic media on social behavior*. Oxford University Press.

Miller-Day, M., & Hecht, M. L. (2013). Narrative means to preventative ends: A narrative engagement framework for designing prevention interventions. *Health Communication, 28*(7), 657–670.

Myrick, J. G., & Chen, J. (2022). Schadenfreude after watching the news: How audiences respond to media coverage of partisans disclosing illness. *Journalism & Mass Communication Quarterly, 99*(1), 135–155.

Nemer, D. (2016). Celebrities acting up: A speech act analysis in tweets of famous people. *Social Networking, 5*, 1–10.

Parker, J. (2023, August 17). How former President Carter helped shape hospice care. *Hospice News*. https://hospicenews.com/2023/08/17/how-former-president-carter-helped-shape-hospice-care

Pavelko, R. L., Myrick, J. G., Verghese, R. S., & Hester, J. B. (2017). Public reactions to celebrity cancer disclosures via social media: Implications for campaign message design and strategy. *Health Education Journal, 76*(4), 492–506.

Petronio, S. (2002). *Boundaries of privacy: Dialectics of disclosure*. SUNY Press.

Petronio, S., & Child, J. (2020). Conceptualization and operationalization: Utility of communication privacy management theory. *Current Opinion in Psychology, 31*, 76–82.

Poole, S. (2023, December 30). Jimmy Carter's Sunday school lessons still a draw. *The Atlanta Journal-Constitution*. https://www.columbian.com/news/2023/dec/30/jimmy-carters-sunday-school-lessons-still-a-draw/

Rasmussen, L. (2018). Parasocial interaction in the digital age: An examination of relationship building and the effectiveness of YouTube celebrities. *The Journal of Social Media in Society, 7*(1), 280–294.

"Reactions to the death of Rosalynn Carter, former first lady and global humanitarian" (2023, November 19). *AP*. https://apnews.com/article/rosalynn-carter-obit-death-reaction-6d13e96cc89924a08895b200c10090c2

Ribke, N. (2018). Celebrity and power in South America. In A. Elliott (Ed.), *Routledge handbook of celebrity studies* (pp. 215–226). Routledge.

Roberts, M. C., & Dusetzina, S. B. (2017). The effect of a celebrity health disclosure on demand for health care: Trends in BRCA testing and subsequent health services use. *Journal of Community Genetics, 8*, 141–146.

Rotondi, J. P. (2023, August 29). Why Princess Diana's 1995 BBC interview shocked the world. *History*. https://www.history.com/news/princess-diana-bbc-interview-martin-bashir

Roy, L. (2024, January 31). Brittany Mahomes shares her son's health scare. *Forbes*. https://www.forbes.com/sites/lipiroy/2024/01/31/brittany-mahomes-shares-her-sons-health-scare/?sh=3f3d1c09504d

Sabel, M. S., & Cin, S. D. (2016). Trends in media reports of celebrities' breast cancer treatment decisions. *Annals of Surgical Oncology, 23*, 2795–2801.

Samuelson, K. (2017, August 27). The princess and the paparazzi: How Diana's death changed the British media. *Time*. https://time.com/4914324/princess-diana-anniversary-paparazzi-tabloid-media/

Sanchez, R. (2024, March 23). Prince William and Princess Kate release their first joint statement following her cancer diagnosis. *Harper's Bazaar*. https://www.harpersbazaar.com/celebrity/latest/a60281887/prince-william-reacts-kate-middleton-cancer-diagnosis/

Selberg, S. (2017). Rhinestone cowboy: Alzheimer's, celebrity, and the collusions of self. *American Quarterly, 69*(4), 883–901.

Sheihk, K., & Gupta, A. H. (2024, March 15). What a breast cancer risk calculator can and can't tell you. *The New York Times*. https://www.nytimes.com/2024/03/15/well/live/breast-cancer-risk-assessment.html

Shen, F., & Edwards, H. H. (Eds.) (2023). *Narratives in public communication*. Routledge.

Sillence, E., & Martin, R. (2020). Talking about decisions: The facilitating effect of a celebrity health announcement on the communication of online personal experiences about decision-making. *Health Communication, 35*(12), 1447–1454.

Smith, G. (2024, January 29). Brittany Mahomes on life after son's scary food allergy reaction. *Allergic Living*. https://www.allergicliving.com/2024/01/29/brittany-mahome-on-life-after-sons-scary-food-allergy-reaction/

Suparsad, V. (2023). *Being Bollywood: Postfeminism, celebrity culture and femininity in the Global South*. Palgrave MacMillan.

Taylor, E. (2020, November 15). Princess Diana's real-life battle with bulimia. *Vogue*. https://www.vogue.com/article/princess-diana-real-life-battle-with-bulimia

The breast cancer conundrum. (2013). *Bulletin of the World Health Organization, 91*, 626–627.

Thelandersson, F. (2023). *21st century media and female mental health: Profitable vulnerability and sad girl culture*. Palgrave Macmillan.

Thomas, E. (2023, June 28). Lewis Capaldi to Sarah Ferguson—How celebrities are driving health awareness. *PR Week*. https://www.prweek.com/article/1828118/lewis-capaldi-sarah-ferguson-%E2%80%93-celebrities-driving-health-awareness

Troiano, G., Nante, N., & Cozzolino, M. (2017). The Angelina Jolie effect: Impact on breast and ovarian cancer prevention: A systematic review of effects after the public announcement in May 2013. *Health Education Journal, 76*(6), 707–715.

V Foundation (n.d.). Our story. https://www.v.org/about-us/

Vafeiadis, M., Wang, W., Baker, M., & Shen, F. (2022). Examining the effects of celebrity (vs. noncelebrity) narratives on opioid addiction prevention: Identification, transportation, and the moderating role of personal relevance. *Journal of Health Communication, 27*, 271–280.

Van Den Bulck, H. (2017). "She died of a mother's broken heart:" Media and audiences' framing of health narratives of heart-related celebrity deaths. *International Journal of Communication, 11*, 4965–4987.

Van Dijck, J. (2013). *The culture of connectivity: A critical history of social media*. Oxford University Press.

Wanshel, E. (2024, March 13). Hilarious Kate Middleton conspiracy theory jokes are the reigning trend on Twitter. *Huffpost*. https://www.huffpost.com/entry/kate-middleton-conspiracy-theory-jokes_n_65f0d9b9e4b0bd5228d5e57d

Weiner, C. (2023, November 19). Rosalynn Carter, transformative former first lady and mental health advocate dies. *NPR*. https://www.npr.org/2023/11/19/1019825478/former-first-ladyrosalynn-carter-dies

Wheeler, M. (2013). *Celebrity politics: Image and identity in contemporary political communications*. Polity.

Willson, S. F., Perelman, A., & Goldman, K. N. (2019). "Age is just a number": How celebrity-driven magazines misrepresent fertility at advanced reproductive ages. *Journal of Women's Health, 28*(10), 1338–1343.

Wood, S., & Bollinger, B. (2020). Predicting changes in patient choice of preventive health care after celebrity diagnoses. *Journal of the Association for Consumer Research, 5*(3), 302–310.

Wright, L. (2020). *Star power: American democracy in the age of the celebrity candidate*. Routledge.

Xu, Y., Abeele, M. V., Hou, M., & Antheunis, M. (2022). Do parasocial relationships with micro- and mainstream celebrities differ? An empirical study testing four attributes of the parasocial relationships. *Celebrity Studies, 14*(3), 366–386.

York, L. (2018). *Reluctant celebrity: Affect and privilege in contemporary stardom*. Palgrave MacMillan.

Zhou, M., & Kraak, V. (2022). A mixed-methods study of American millennials' views about celebrity endorsement of foods and beverages. *Health Promotion International, 37*(1), 1–12.

Zimovjanova, M., Bielcikova, Z., Miskovicova, M., Vocka, M., Zimovjanova, A., Rybar, M., Novotny, J., & Petruzelka, L. (2023). Uptake and effectiveness of risk-reducing surgeries in unaffected female BRCA1 and BRCA2 carriers. A single institution experience in the Czech Republic. *Cancers, 5*. https://doi.org/10.3390/cancers15041072

16

SOCIAL MEDIA INFLUENCERS AND PUBLIC HEALTH NARRATIVES

Leandra Hinojosa Hernández and Stevie Munz

Introduction/Definitions

In the 2010s and 2020s, rates of social media accounts have skyrocketed across the world. An estimated 50 million social media influencers worldwide post on accounts spanning platforms such as Instagram, YouTube, and TikTok, resulting in more than $5 billion of investments into the creator space between 2021 and 2022 (Gagliese, 2022). Further estimates of the value of social media influencers suggest that the total creator economy market size is over $20 billion (Ismail, 2023), thus highlighting the mediated, cultural, and social significance of social media influencers (and, by extension, their messages). Put simply, one cannot underestimate the power wielded by social media influencers in shaping the perceptions, experiences, and actions of social media consumers and followers.

In this chapter, we dive deeper into one angle of the social media influencer sphere: social media influencers in bodybuilding, weightlifting, and exercise science contexts. With around 50,000 social media influencers on Instagram alone to date, academic and popular culture scholarship emphasize how social media influencers are doing more harm than good (Friedman, 2023). As many writers have illustrated, social media influencers in health and weight contexts claim to have plans, tips, and tricks to assist individuals with attaining a healthy lifestyle, more muscles, and stronger, better bodies; however, critiques of social media influencers argue that they utilize incomplete or inaccurate information, focus on "thinspiration" as opposed to other more holistic and biopsychosocial approaches to health, and promote unhealthy health messages to millions of consumers every day (Curtis et al., 2023; Friedman, 2023). Thus, we organize the chapter accordingly. First, we discuss some of the critical issues associated with social media health influencers related to fitspiration, thinspiration, and problematic messaging. Second, we consider current concepts related to social media health influencers through the lens of health consumerism, relatability, authenticity, and the role of pedagogies of the body in mediated spaces. Finally, we preview future directions for this topic, focusing on the role of ethics in mediated influencer contexts.

Current Contributions and Research

Given the proliferation of social media platforms throughout the past decade, the phenomenon of "digital guru media" has exploded across YouTube, Instagram, and TikTok. The concept of "digital guru media" (hereinafter referred to as DGM) refers to the self-styled and self-promoted experts,

DOI: 10.4324/9781003436409-18

entrepreneurs, influencers, and coaches who have developed online personas and businesses focusing on health, fitness, and wellness. With topical areas ranging from healthy eating and weight loss to bodybuilding and weightlifting, the DGM influence space has become highly popular and profitable. Social media influencers – beauty and food bloggers, fitness gurus, weightlifting and bodybuilding experts, and general fashionistas – often function as the face of brand advertising efforts by sharing their endorsed opinions about products across social media platforms in return for compensation and future branding opportunities (Kay et al., 2020; Khamis et al., 2017; Pedroni, 2016). They also make an attractive partnership for various corporations and brands because of their ability to develop high levels of trust with their followers and their ability to produce profit-related results (Clark, 2022). Described as a new type of opinion leader (Zou et al., 2021), their posts serve two fundamental purposes: to increase their followers' purchase intentions and behaviors, and to enhance product attractiveness and knowledge (Kay et al., 2020; Lou & Yuan, 2019).

Social media influencers can be split into five categories: mega-influencers, macro-influencers, mid-tier influencers, micro-influencers, and nano-influencers. Nano-influencers have less than 1,000 followers, micro-influencers have between 1,000 and 100,000 followers, mid-tier influencers have between 50,000 and 500,000 followers, macro-influencers have between 100,000 and 1 million followers, and mega-influencers have over 1 million followers (Clark, 2022; Ismail, 2023). In terms of parasocial relationship building and cultural impact, macro and mega-influencers amass diverse audiences with wide-ranging interests and preferences (Ismail, 2023). As Ismail argued, macro and mega-influencers are highly influential and can attain celebrity status, with mega-influencers being the highest-ranking category of influencer.

Critical Issues and Topics

In this section, we provide an overview of critical issues and topics shaping current social media health influencer trends, such as health consumerism and consciousness, health influencer self-branding, and considerations related to authenticity and relatability. Foundationally, social media has both positive and negative impacts on public health in ethical, professional, and social contexts (Kanchan & Gaidhane, 2023). On the more positive end of the spectrum of impact, social media can connect individuals to important health-related information and organizations. According to Kanchan and Gaidhane, social media use can also impact health behavior change in positive ways, and it can significantly shape policy influence. On the more negative end of the health impact spectrum, social media use can lead individuals to access misinformation from self-appointed "experts," contribute to excessive or compulsory media use and behaviors, and negatively impact consumers' mental health and body image perceptions (Kanchan & Gaidhane, 2023). For the purposes of this chapter, we focus on health influencers, those who emphasize health-related topics for political, financial, and/or educational purposes (Zou et al., 2021). More specifically, we feature health influencers whose channels and accounts utilize a variety of lenses to frame their bodybuilding and weightlifting content, including research in health sciences and exercise sciences contexts.

Health Consumerism and Consciousness

Health influencers can fit into several categories. On the one hand, health influencers can be those with credibility and topic expertise (such as medical doctors, academics, and healthcare providers) (Wellman, 2022); on the other hand, they can also be categorized as those who seek to sell health-related products and programs or those who can "affect relevant social norms and provide emotional peer support" (Pöyry et al., 2022, p. 481). According to Wellman, health influencers often use a variety of messaging techniques to reach their followers, such as anecdotal narratives, medical information, and even a blending of theory and practice. As public health and Health Communication scholars have observed, health influencers have gained prominence because of the intersecting impacts of health consumerism and the rise of digital technologies (Albalawi & Sixsmith, 2017; Arriagada & Bishop, 2021; Greenhalgh & Wessely, 2004; Hudders et al., 2021; Lutkenhaus et al., 2019). Originating in the 1960s and 1970s, health consumerism focused on developing health systems and services that prioritized individual needs and demands (Latimer et al., 2017; Weijs et al., 2022). Through a neoliberal lens, health consumerism prioritizes both individual responsibility and market solutions, as opposed to government intervention in one's health decision-making (Ayo, 2012; Weijs et al., 2022). It also frames inequality as a consequence of choice (Ayo, 2012). Weijs et al. asserted:

> Empowerment and individual responsibility for health decisions (Latimer et al., 2017) rely on liberal access to health information alongside opportunities for meaningful discussion to facilitate understanding and consent around health decisions for individuals and communities (e.g., the clinical consultation; shared decision-making models; citizen and community engagement in setting health priorities) (Schiavo, 2013; Taylor, 2009).
>
> *(p. 218)*

Thus, health consumerism incites "the desire within autonomous individuals to choose to follow the imperatives set out by health-promoting agencies, and thus, take on the responsibility of changing their own behaviors accordingly" (Ayo, 2012, p. 100). As a related outcome of health consumerism, health promotion has become intricately woven into the fabric of our contemporary social media moment, wherein influencers capitalize upon social media users' health consciousness. Health consumerism and health consciousness directly facilitate business models as influencers capitalize upon direct advertising, monetized channels, branding efforts, and the dissemination of (sometimes inaccurate and problematic) health information (Zou et al., 2021). Healthism, or the assumption that individuals should strive to maximize their health (Ayo, 2012; Petersen & Lupton, 1996), has become one of the most significant ideologies alongside health consumerism and health consciousness to support the ongoing success of health influencers worldwide.

> Thus, the enormous amount of personal resources invested into healthy living, be it in time, money, physical effort or a range of aesthetic regimes, is not seen as a narcissistic obsession with the self (Rose 1990), nor is it considered to be frivolous. Rather such personal investment is deemed as a willful obedience to the duties and obligations imposed by citizenship.
>
> *(Ayo, 2012, p. 101)*

In the era of the evolution of digital media and social media technologies, health influencers develop trusting relationships with followers, disseminate information about products and health behavior changes, and aid in their health journey.

Social Influencer Self-Branding

Social media health influencers develop relationships and trust with consumers as a means of self-branding. Khamis et al. (2017, p. 191) defined self-branding as the process that individuals undergo to develop "a distinctive public image for commercial gain and/or cultural capital." An individual's or company's brand signifies an idea, quality, or product that is associated with a commodity that aids in encouraging individuals to purchase said commodity (Keller, 2007; Khamis et al., 2017).

In social media health influencer contexts, the branding process could encompass an ideology or a phrase, a tangible product (such as protein powder, supplements, diet and nutrition plans, and apparel), or even an outcome related to the influencer's body or physique. In today's highly saturated media world, the brand must be seen as favorable, unique, and relevant in order to distinguish the product from other influencer offerings, thus imbuing a certain personality onto the product to increase the commodity's effectiveness and demand (Keller, 2007; Khamis et al., 2017).

Thus, the brand represents the commodity's identity, and in health influencer contexts, the commodity could include a tangible product or even the influencer's body directly. In other words, through the lens of neoliberalism, self-branding and monetization rest upon the commodification of the self, and health influencers (and influencers across a variety of contexts) become almost permanently visible and constantly self-promoting in order to sell products, increase viewers and followers, and thus increase self-worth (Hearn, 2008; Khamis et al., 2017), especially through discourses that highlight how they took their health into their own hands and, by watching their channels and purchasing their products, viewers can too. In YouTuber context, this process is represented by the necessity to create and publish a multitude of videos on various topics with both embedded and direct messages that encourage viewers to use influencer promotional codes to purchase products. Additionally, viewers are encouraged to "liking and subscribe" to the channel to increase monetization outcomes.

In order to effectively self-brand, individuals must have a unique selling point, a public identity that is charismatic, energetic, and able to respond to the preferences, needs, and interests of social media followers (Khamis et al., 2017). According to Khamis et al., through the use of attention, narrative, musical soundtracks, guest speakers, collaborations with other influencers, and eye-catching graphics, health influencers craft a personality that sells a product (or multiple), develop a sizable following throughout social media accounts, and extend the potential of developing fame or a celebrity persona. Influencers must also be relatable to develop meaningful connections with audiences. Khamis et al. defined relatability as the process of giving a commodity a human-like quality with certain values that encourage consumers to develop connections with the commodity (p. 192). One influencer who is well known for his relatability and effective branding is Will Tennyson.

At the time of this writing, 28-year-old Canadian social media health influencer Will Tennyson, for example, has 2.14 million subscribers on YouTube and 388 videos that can fall into the following categories: weight training and exercise (such as the videos *Training W/ 7x Mr. Olympia Phil Heath*, *Can I Survive 24 Hours with the World's Strongest Man*, and *I Tested World's Strangest Fitness Classes*), exercise science (such as the video *How to Fix Knee Pain for Life! Ft. Kneesovertoesguy*), and eating and consumption (such as the videos *I Created a Bodybuilder Fast Food Secret Menu*, *I Spent 50 Hours Only Eating Weight Loss Foods*, and *I Went to Fat Camp*). He started his YouTube channel in 2019 and has since become a very popular health, fitness, and weightlifting influencer.

On his website, Tennyson is described as a YouTuber with passions for fitness, motivating others, and cooking. Further, his "About" page revealed his own struggles with fitness and body image issues:

> Although I live a healthy, balanced lifestyle, I've struggled with body image, weight loss, and low self-esteem in the past. As a young adult, I was unhappy with myself both physically and mentally. I was unhealthy and unmotivated, but I felt stuck – afraid of failure. When I discovered lifting and how strong it made me feel, a fire lit from within, and I began my quest to be the best possible me.
>
> *("About – Will Tennyson," n.d., para. 1)*

As an energetic and relatable social media character, Will Tennyson has developed an online brand that features his sarcastic and quippy banter, his forthcoming perspectives on weightlifting and food, and his love for his dog and donuts. Part of his relatability stems from his bodybuilding journey and the process he underwent to add more muscle to his physique (Ellis, 2022), such as losing 60 pounds in his youth "through dedication, disciplined workout routines, and a healthy diet" ("Who Is Will Tennyson: A Fitness YouTuber, Food Enthusiast, and Much More," n.d., para. 3). One article characterized Tennyson as a "beacon of motivation for thousands looking to embark upon their fitness journey" – an influencer with determination and perseverance ("Who Is Will Tennyson: A Fitness YouTuber, Food Enthusiast, and Much More," n.d., para. 3). The same article stressed his relatability, mostly because of the ways in which he communicates about fitness to general audiences (see, e.g., "Who Is Will Tennyson: A Fitness YouTuber, Food Enthusiast, and Much More," n.d.). Although Will Tennyson might not have advanced degrees in exercise science (such as Dr. Mike Isratel or Jeff Nippard, discussed later in the chapter), his branding affirms that if he can go from a thin teenager to a muscle-packed bodybuilder, then he can assist his social media followers with undergoing the same transformation.

To add more dimensions to his brand, Will Tennyson has featured a variety of individuals on his channel, including his fiancée, sister, and mom, as well as professional weightlifters and everyday individuals who might be at various filming scenes (such as the gym, the beach, or various restaurants). Will Tennyson has created a brand, WILLPWR, inspired by the mantra that "we are all in control of our own lives, and that sometimes we just need that growth mindset" ("About – Will Tennyson," n.d., para. 2). WILLPWR features athletic t-shirts, shorts, hats, and hoodies, and several of his YouTube videos include discount codes for Gymshark athletic apparel and other athletic products. Estimates suggest that his net worth stands at around $1 million, which includes income from his YouTube channel, brand partnerships, and cookbook/apparel sales ("Who Is Will Tennyson: A Fitness YouTuber, Food Enthusiast, and Much More," n.d.).

Dr. Mike Israetel is another popular health influencer on both YouTube and Instagram. Two key factors distinguish Israetel from Tennyson. First, Israetel holds a PhD in Sport Physiology, works as a professor in a strength and hypertrophy master's program, and, thus, possesses more formal exercise science credentials than Tennyson. Second, Israetel co-founded Renaissance Periodization, an organization that offers physique training, sports performance training, and a strength and fitness phone application ("Meet the Team," 2024). Israetel's YouTube channel, Renaissance Periodization, has offered over 1,400 videos featuring content such as interviews with other bodybuilders and weightlifters, workout critiques, injury prevention, and muscle growth specialization. At the beginning of most videos, Israetel reminds viewers of his exercise science qualifications, which heightens the perceived credibility of the information presented in the videos and contributes to his personal brand as a health influencer with both doctoral-level knowledge of the topics and a professional bodybuilding career.

On the surface, self-branding presents itself as a straightforward marketing tool to assist individuals in developing a brand and in selling products. However, scholars have identified some of the issues associated with branding, such as how it raises "conceptual, practical, and ethical issues" that are either not acknowledged or outright avoided (Khamis et al., 2017, p. 192). First, questions arise about products' authenticity and consistency, particularly in contexts when individuals might commit a cultural, social, or public transgression that disrupts or thwarts the branding process. Second, questions arise about the relationship between commoditization and relatability. For the purposes of this study, ideologically, we will continue to interrogate the concept of relatability, particularly when considering how to make a health influencer commodity relatable, to whom, and at what cost?

Health Influencers, Mediated Messages, and Rawness

Another strategy often used in conjunction with self-branding involves the creation and dissemination of "raw" messages. Centrally located within the notion of "rawness" is the relationship among other characteristics such as authenticity and relatability. In health influencer contexts, "rawness" includes practices such as posting unedited or realistic body visuals; engaging in honest, open, and authentic conversations with viewers that include influencers' personal self-disclosures about their health, experiences, and struggles; and ultimately highlighting "real talk," not the traditional, scripted branding conversations that occupy most influencer programming (Reade, 2021). Rawness functions as a counter-discourse to traditional health influencer "fitspiration discourses" because the former highlights the flaws, wrinkles, struggles, and imperfections, as opposed to the picture-perfect aesthetics and bodies commonly featured and consumed in health influencer content. Authenticity in health influencer contexts, by extension, relies less on false binaries of personal and professional selves (Jurgenson, 2011) and depends more on the understanding that authenticity is "reflected in choices users make to appear 'real' to others" (Reade, 2021, p. 537).

Reade (2021) further explained that authenticity in health influencer-mediated contexts can be reflected by an individual disclosing information and intimate details about one's life. An influencer's understanding of their followers' context, audience, and preferences often informs such performative choices (Marwick & boyd, 2010). Authenticity, then, does not constitute a static state of being or a static component of representation, but, according to Reade, rather a communicative process "enacted through negotiations between producers of content and audience members" (p. 537). Raw discourses in health influencer contexts can cultivate what Reade referred to as digital intimacies between health influencers and their followers, or the mediated connections developed through digital technologies. Building upon work by Dobson et al. (2018), Reade asserted that such intimacies

> "are socially productive in that they facilitate a shared sense of belonging and trust, and economically productive in that they assist established or aspirational influencers to successfully promote products, brands and services through personal recommendations and endorsements."
> *(p. 537)*

However, we question the assertion that digital intimacies are socially productive, particularly when considering the potential physical and mental health outcomes of digital rawness in health influencer contexts. One health influencer – Stephanie Buttermore – recently went raw and "all in," and her public experience of "going all in with weight gain" to address her hunger satiation issues garnered both positive and negative responses from influencers, followers, and online chat boards, specifically related to concerns about eating disorder behaviors and discourses.

Dr. Stephanie Buttermore is a cancer research scientist with a Ph.D. in pathology and cell biology. Her research focuses on molecular mechanisms that drive ovarian cancer progression ("About – Stephanie Buttermore," 2022). She has active channels on both YouTube and Instagram. According to her personal website, she "transitioned from the world of academia to a world of sharing [her] life and passion for the things [she] loves" ("About – Stephanie Buttermore," para. 1). Under the website banner "from cancer research scientist to fitness educator," her website detailed her process of educating followers on the "scientific principles of training and nutrition" (para. 1). It further stated that "I've taken my many years of experience reading and writing scientific literature to understanding the fundamentals of exercise science" (para. 1). Her website has promoted her eight training programs available for purchase, which range from quick and effective women's training programs to at-home training guides, women's foundational programs, specialization programs, and optimization programs. Her website (www.stephaniebuttermore.com) has also spotlighted her phone application, which features her weight program structures, video demos, exercise cues, and a banner that describes the app as "a wealth of information about the scientific principles used to create the program" ("Science-Based Fitness Programs for All Experience Levels," 2022).

As of 2023, her Instagram account had over 612,000 followers and over 1,400 posts, with various content clusters organized around her research, fitness journey, cheat days, food guilt, and doctoral research. Her YouTube channel boasts over 1.22 million subscribers and 128 videos, and the pinned video comprises a 41-minute deep dive into her all-in food journey. Other videos include content that highlights her "new life" and her "new body" after going "all in." She also featured videos that focus on cheat day eating, weight loss fears, the problem with fat shaming, intuitive eating, and how her weight running has evolved over the past several years. Her channel also included videos that she recorded with her fiancé, Jeff Nippard, a professional bodybuilder, weightlifter, and health influencer.

To date, Nippard's YouTube channel has attracted over 3 million subscribers, and his brand has featured exercise science-informed journal articles and contemporary research to assist his followers with "building muscle, losing fat, and getting healthier" ("About Jeff Nippard Fitness," 2023, para. 1). Nippard was Mr. Junior Canada for natural bodybuilding in 2012 and has frequently presented lectures about weight training, nutrition, and bodybuilding at various institutions ("About Jeff Nippard Fitness," 2023). Thus, Buttermore has capitalized upon her research credentials and those of her partner, Nippard, to enhance her channel's perceived credibility and impact. Fellow influencers and social media questioned her credibility, however, when she decided to go "all in" in 2019. Going "all in" means that individuals allow themselves to eat until they are full and respond to hunger, not track calories or follow a meal plan, not weigh oneself or measure bodies, and ultimately allow bodies to rest from physical activity (Cecchele, 2021).

Similar to Will Tennyson, Stephanie Buttermore is a popular and relatable influencer because of her personality and passion for fitness, which is evidenced by her follower counts on her social media profiles. Her enthusiastic, relatable, and bubbly personality resonates throughout her video catalog. Fans have noted, for example, that Buttermore taught them important lessons about their body and eating habits (Clara, 2020). An easily recognizable component of her brand entailed her cheat day videos, where she paused her fitness regimen momentarily to indulge her sweet tooth and eat a variety of foods traditionally considered to be unhealthy. Her channel playlist entitled "Fantasy Cheat Days" spotlighted 14 videos with titles ranging from "Unrestricted CHEAT DAY Ep 2. (My New Experiment)" to "I Ate As Much As I WANTED … (+10,000 Calories CHEAT DAY) Ft. AlwaysHungry" and "FANTASY CHEAT DAY | Unlimited Donuts, Cheesecake, Ice Cream, Tacos & More." In these videos, she invited channel followers and viewers alike to indulge with her and participate in her cheat day journey, where she sampled donuts, tacos, ice cream, and other foods to satiate her sweet tooth. As her videos progressed and as definitions of rawness evolved (from watching her eat 10,000 calories to hearing her struggles with her weight and her eating), channel followers witnessed Buttermore's authenticity and rawness come to light.

One of her other channel playlists, entitled "All In," chronicled why she decided to stop restricting her diet, the challenges of dealing with her insatiable hunger cues, and the implications of gaining 40 pounds in a viscerally public digital space for her physique, mental health, as well as subsequent critiques about her brand and her ability to train others. By going "all in," she decided to stop restricting her eating and eat a minimum of 2500 calories daily. Further, she did not set a maximum caloric intake limit for herself, thus eating as much as she wanted every day with no cap. In her YouTube all-in announcement video, she stated, "I want to wake up and eat at every single meal, and I want to eat to the point that I actually feel satiated, regardless of how many calories it actually takes" (Buttermore, 2019).

Other videos in the "All In" playlist revealed a raw and emotional Buttermore as she shared fears, tears, and concerns about her changing body, metabolism, and weight training plans. Her decision to go "all in" resulted in several trending discourses on platforms such as YouTube, Reddit, and a variety of websites about eating disorders, body dysmorphia, and related concerns. One conversation on the Eating Disorder Support Forum website discussed how her process proved triggering for many individuals who struggle with eating disorders, particularly because it re-ignited their wishes to be skinny. Others critiqued how they perceive most health influencers to have complicated and distorted relationships with food and weight training, which occurs in very public spaces on their social media channels and accounts. Some Reddit users discussing Buttermore's "All In" journey asserted that her journey ruined the "All In" journey for the Internet, led to weight gain of 50 pounds or more for certain users, and used faulty science to justify her food actions. On the other end of the debate spectrum, writers described how Buttermore's public decision to go "all in" inspired followers to improve their health and to be more mindful of their struggles with eating and fitness (Clara, 2020; Nazarewich, 2021). In this moment, Buttermore has inspired others through a certain kind of "health talk" that has resulted in a variety of opinions. As Ratwatte and Mattacola (2021) illustrated, followers of "fitspiration" influencers often report body appearance dissatisfaction and internalization of the thin ideal in relation to viewing content. This response highlights the dual, complex relationship individuals can have with health influencers: in the same digitally intimate relationship, individuals can find influencers both authentic and relatable while struggling with their internalized responses to the influencers' content.

Ideologically, the concept of relatability holds important considerations for how health influencers make their mediated brand accessible. A digital guru who presents as relatable garners a type of spectacle status symbolically (Debord, 2010) through the continued commodification and consumption of their brand, knowledge, and workout plans. Through the process of representing visible behaviors related to health and fitness, a digital guru creates a type of materiality associated with power, commodification, and capitalism. Thus, the digital guru becomes a type of spectacle capable of seducing mediated audience members into claims specifically related to health, fitness, and broadly mental health concerns. When the spectacle (the influencer, their bodies, and their behaviors) is public and mediated, then the digital guru invites the audience into latent conversations about that person's health behaviors, body image, eating disorders/disordered eating, and/or mental health. For example, Stephanie Buttermore's symbolic status as an influencer has worked to engage her audience in conversations about her disordered eating, body image, and mental health. However, questions remain about the concentration of her power and the ethics associated with her mediated spectacle status.

As we further interrogate the ethics of a digital guru as a spectacle in the mediated sphere, we must consider the bonding of relatability as reliability. For digital gurus, a multifaceted image advances both the "everyday/lay person" and "expert authority." Through re-packaging graduate degrees (see Mike Israetel and Stephanie Buttermore) or certifications in training/exercise programming (see Mike Israetel and Stephanie Buttermore) or presenting as the "accessible" fitness influencer (see Will Tennyson), attributes become associated with reliability or fixed to the (perceived) stability of western biomedical and exercise science. For example, comments on Dr. Mike Israetel's Renaissance Periodization YouTube video entitled "Work SMARTER: Build Bigger Quads with Lighter Weights!" focus on the effectiveness of the workout program, the clarity of his instructions and communication, and the motivation and inspiration rooted within Dr. Mike's comments. Similarly, comments on Jeff Nippard's YouTube video "How to Train for Pure Muscle Growth" praise Nippard's exercise science and hypertrophy prowess, the creativity and comprehension that inspire future workout plans, and the clarity of instructions.

Through a process of fixing or stabilizing such behaviors or qualities, the digital guru engages audience members in the symbolic meaning-making process. Audience members are seduced into the spectacle and into the permanence associated with the digital guru, which includes commodification of health/wellness and fitness. In many ways, the digital guru is the center of "influencer pedagogy" or "the indirect, mediated processes of education produced through relatable interactions between influencers and their followers on social media platforms" (Hendry et al., 2022, p. 427). A DGM appropriates the power of stability from their constructed spectacle, which gets bolstered through all of the attributes of science with little consideration for questions related to bioethics, especially related to power, knowledge, and human nature.

Ultimately, as Wellman (2022) illustrated, "perceived authenticity and credibility are important for influencers to maintain through their engagement with other online users, as those norms result in influencers maintaining their status as popular users" (p. 58). For health influencers with advanced degrees in their channel or account's topical area, they must utilize a blend of both their professional education and their authentic selves and personalities to 1) connect with their followers and 2) encourage followers to accept their information and products.

Recommendations for Practice

Given the ubiquity of social media influencers' content across a variety of platforms, it is not surprisingly, media literacy can be a difficult task for individuals to practice, even for researchers and media experts. It is necessary, however, to ensure that social media audiences are not engaging in ill-informed or dangerous health practices (see also Chapter 11, this volume). As Moreno et al. (2023) argued, audience members should be equipped to discern whether digital gurus are suitably educated and trained to provide fitness and nutrition recommendations. Further, family members, friends, and schools play a significant role as both facilitators and evaluators of online health information. Balaban et al. (2022) asserted that school media literacy programs should incorporate social media influencer pedagogy components that emphasize critical perspectives, information literacy, and social media user agency. Additionally, van Dam and van Reijmersdal (2019) recommended that media literacy programs include a unit describing revenue models underlying influencers' sponsored content, which will assist audience members in understanding the underlying principles of influencer marketing (see also Chapter 20, this volume).

Further, Friedman (2023) provided four tips that individuals can use to assess health messages and information found on social media accounts. First, building upon advice from Stephanie Roth-Goldberg, a clinical social worker and therapist in New York, consumers should pause and ask themselves, "Does this fitness influencer make you feel good in your own skin?" (Friedman, para. 8). If accounts lead an individual to experience pain, shame, anxiety, or disapproval of their bodies, then individuals should consider unfollowing them. Second, social media consumers should search for accounts that focus on exercise through the lens of mobility, functionality, strength, and mental health, as opposed to those which promulgate "fitfluencer" messages that emphasize fat loss and dieting coupled with edited images of bodies or body parts. Third, social media consumers should take extra steps to verify influencers' credentials before practicing what they proverbially preach and ensure that the influencers' credentials align with their programming. Finally, social media consumers should seek influencer content that features a variety of body types, ages, abilities, and topics. In doing so, consumers can collectively shape discourses that feature the diversity of bodies and experiences in healthcare, weightlifting, bodybuilding, and healthy lifestyle contexts, as opposed to supporting and uplifting accounts that focus on disseminating messages about extreme dieting, extreme weight loss, and the sexualization and objectification of thin bodies.

Future Directions

Social media health influencers occupy one space among many in our increasingly complex digital media cultures. Through the micro-case study approach utilized here, focusing on health influencers such as Will Tennyson, Dr. Stephanie Buttermore, and Dr. Mike Israetel, social media health influencers practice authenticity and relatability in different ways with different outcomes. They utilize a variety of appeals, both appealing to personality and science-backed information, to develop and sustain their personal brands. Moreover, through pedagogies of the body, mediated health influencers develop and perform authentic rawness by sharing personal narratives and stories, humanizing bodybuilding and weightlifting performance plans, and even radically changing their bodies in front of millions of individuals. Future research in Health Communication should continue to explore the ethical concerns associated with embodied pedagogies in mediated contexts, particularly the "blurred politics of knowledge" (Hendry et al., 2022, p. 437) that characterize digitally intimate relationships between influencers and followers and the role of larger health education programs in this mediated sphere.

Further Reading

Curtis, R. G., Prichard, I., Gosse, G., Stankevicius, A., & Maher, C. A. (2023). Hashtag fitspiration: Credibility screening and content analysis of Instagram fitness accounts. *BioMed Central (BMC) Public Health*, *23*(1), 1–7.

Hendry, N. A., Hartung, C., & Welch, R. (2022). Health education, social media, and tensions of authenticity in the 'influencer pedagogy' of health influencer Ashy Bines. *Learning, Media and Technology*, *47*(4), 427–439.

Lawrence, S. (2022). *Digital wellness, health and fitness influencers* (1st ed., Vol. 1). Routledge. https://doi.org/10.4324/9781003256021

References

About. (2023). Will Tennyson. https://willtennyson.ca/pages/about#:~:text=My%20name's%20Will%20Tennyson%2C%20and,myself%20both%20physically%20and%20mentally

About. (2022). Stephanie Buttermore. https://www.stephaniebuttermore.com/app/

About Jeff Nippard Fitness. (2023). Jeff Nippard Fitness. https://jeffnippard.com/pages/about

About Will Tennyson. (2024). Will Tennyson. https://www.willtennyson.ca/pages/about

Albalawi, Y., & Sixsmith, J. (2017). Agenda setting for health promotion: Exploring an adapted model for the social media era. *Journal of Medical Internet Research (JMIR) Public Health and Surveillance*, *1*(2), e5014.

Arriagada, A., & Bishop, S. (2021). Between commerciality and authenticity: The imaginary of social media influencers in the platform economy. *Communication, Culture and Critique*, *14*(4), 568–586.

Ayo, N. (2012). Understanding health promotion in a neoliberal climate and the making of health conscious citizens. *Critical Public Health, 22*(1), 99–105. https://doi.org/10.1080/09581596.2010.520692

Balaban, D. C., Mucundorfeanu, M., & Mureşan, L. I. (2022). Adolescents' understanding of the model of sponsored content of social media influencer instagram stories. *Media and Communication, 10*(1), 305–316.

Buttermore, S. (2019, June 5). I'm going ALL IN | Why am I so Hungry? (Day 1) [Video]. *YouTube*. https://www.youtube.com/watch?v=DotlyWhBhak&list=PLfSsah8UsndTTurTjXGRY3klE0KGRl3hn

Cecchele, T. (2021, August 18). Going "all in" for eating disorder recovery. https://www.taliacecchele.com/post/all-in-eating-disorder

Clara. (2020, June 6). Lessons from Stephanie Buttermore's "all in" journey. *Medium.* https://medium.com/@claranah/lessons-from-stephanie-buttermores-all-in-journey-994dda3c82cc

Clark, S. (2022, September 9). Why your brand should care about influencer marketing. *CMSWire.* https://www.cmswire.com/digital-marketing/why-your-brand-should-care-about-influencer-marketing/

Curtis, R. G., Prichard, I., Gosse, G., Stankevicius, A., & Maher, C. A. (2023). Hashtag fitspiration: Credibility screening and content analysis of Instagram fitness accounts. *BioMed Central (BMC) Public Health*, *23*(1), 1–7.

Debord, G. (2010). *The society of the spectacle* (Reprint). Black & Red.

Dobson, A. S., Carah, N., & Robards, B. (2018). "Digital intimate publics and social media: Towards theorising public lives on private platforms." In A. S Dobson, B. Robards & N. Carah (Eds.) *Digital intimate publics and social media* (pp. 3–27). Palgrave.

Ellis, P. (2022, May 28). Bodybuilder Will Tennyson detailed his 'skinny to muscle' body transformation. *Yahoo.* https://www.yahoo.com/lifestyle/bodybuilder-tennyson-detailed-skinny-muscle-133000822.html?guccounter=1&guce_referrer=aHR0cHM6Ly93d3cuZ29vZ2xlLmNvbS8&guce_referrer_sig=AQAAAHMurl_Ljzgm2xu2qxPgEf-hdTz9ru5c58wT7QqpBurlFKkNAuTmqRvl771jw1pSyziS-YTEIk0oQZppxyYCxyiiELuHSvruSDXflgpY9hl9qblfqBQoB-ym-vkcGjfMgLBk4rtvJz4hOITpI0_GwHqe-B4qqGtccTgsSVb22dyL

Friedman, D. (2023, May 10). Most fitness influencers are doing more harm than good. *The New York Times.* https://www.nytimes.com/2023/05/10/well/move/fitness-influencers.html#:~:text=According%20to%20some%20estimates%2C%20Instagram,best%20and%20dangerous%20at%20worst

Gagliese, J. (2022, July 8). The rise of the influencer: Predictions for ways they'll change the world. *Forbes.* https://www.forbes.com/sites/theyec/2022/07/08/the-rise-of-the-influencer-predictions-for-ways-theyll-change-the-world/?sh=4e9d751d43a7

Greenhalgh, T., & Wessely, S. (2004). 'Health for me': a sociocultural analysis of healthism in the middle classes. *British Medical Bulletin, 69*(1), 197–213.
Hearn, A. (2008). "Meat, mask, burden": Probing the contours of the branded "self."' *Journal of Consumer Culture, 8*(2), 197–217.
Hendry, N. A., Hartung, C., & Welch, R. (2022). Health education, social media, and tensions of authenticity in the 'influencer pedagogy' of health influencer Ashy Bines. *Learning, Media and Technology, 47*(4), 427–439.
Hudders, L., De Jans, S., & De Veirman, M. (2021). The commercialization of social media stars: A literature review and conceptual framework on the strategic use of social media influencers. *International Journal of Advertising, 40*(3), 327–375.
Ismail, K. (2023, June 21). Types of social media influencers: Mega, macro, micro or nano. *CMSWire*. https://www.cmswire.com/digital-marketing/social-media-influencers-mega-macro-micro-or-nano/
Jurgenson, N. (2011). Digital dualism versus augmented reality. *The Society Pages*. https://thesocietypages.org/cyborgology/2011/02/24/digital-dualism-versus- augmented-reality/
Kanchan, S., & Gaidhane, A. (2023). Social media role and its impact on public health: A narrative review. *Cureus, 15*(1), 1–10.
Kay, S., Mulcahy, R., & Parkinson, J. (2020). When less is more: The impact of macro and micro social media influencers' disclosure. *Journal of Marketing Management, 36*(3–4), 248–278.
Keller, K. L. (2007). *Strategic brand management: Building, measuring, and managing brand equity*. Pearson Education.
Khamis, S., Ang, L., & Welling, R. (2017). Self-branding,'micro-celebrity' and the rise of social media influencers. *Celebrity Studies, 8*(2), 191–208.
Latimer, T., Roscamp, J., & Papanikitas, A. (2017). Patient-centredness and consumerism in healthcare: An ideological mess. *Journal of the Royal Society of Medicine, 110*(11), 425–427. https://doi.org/10.1177/0141076817731905
Lawrence. (2022). *Digital wellness, health and fitness influencers* (1st ed., Vol. 1). Routledge. https://doi.org/10.4324/9781003256021
Lou, C., & Yuan, S. (2019). Influencer marketing: How message value and credibility affect consumer trust of branded content on social media. *Journal of Interactive Advertising, 19*(1), 58–73.
Lutkenhaus, R. O., Jansz, J., & Bouman, M. P. (2019). Tailoring in the digital era: Stimulating dialogues on health topics in collaboration with social media influencers. *Digital Health, 5*, 1–11.
Marwick, A. E., & boyd, d. (2010). I tweet honestly, I tweet passionately: Twitter users, context collapse, and the imagined audience. *New Media & Society, 13*(1): 114–133.
Meet the Team. (2024). *Team FULLROM.* https://teamfullrom.com/pages/meet-the-team
Moreno, D. R., Quintana, J. G., & Riaño, E. R. (2023). Impact and engagement of sport & fitness influencers: A challenge for health education media literacy. *Online Journal of Communication and Media Technologies, 13*(3), 1–25.
Nazarewich, O. (2021, September 8). A fitness vlogger gained 40lbs to curb her extreme hunger and people are inspired. *Diply*. https://diply.com/63189/a-fitness-vlogger-gained-40lbs-to-curb-her-extreme-hunger-and-p
Pedroni, M. (2016). Meso-celebrities, fashion and the media: How digital influencers struggle for visibility. *Film, Fashion & Consumption, 5*(1), 103–121.
Petersen, A. R., & Lupton, D. (1996). *The new public health: Health and self in the age of risk*. Allen & Unwin.
Pöyry, E., Reinikainen, H., & Luoma-Aho, V. (2022). The role of social media influencers in public health communication: Case COVID-19 pandemic. *International Journal of Strategic Communication, 16*(3), 469–484.
Ratwatte, P., & Mattacola, E. (2021). An exploration of 'fitspiration' content on YouTube and its impacts on consumers. *Journal of Health Psychology, 26*(6), 935–946.
Reade, J. (2021). Keeping it raw on the 'gram: Authenticity, relatability and digital intimacy in fitness cultures on Instagram. *New Media & Society, 23*(3), 535–553.
Rose, N. (1990). *Governing the soul: The shaping of the private self.* Routledge.
Schiavo, R. (2013). *Health communication: From theory to practice*. John Wiley & Sons.
Science-Based Fitness Programs for All Experience Levels. (2022). https://www.stephaniebuttermore.com/app/
Taylor, K. (2009). Paternalism, participation, and partnership—the evolution of patient centeredness in the consultation. *Patient Education and Counseling, 74*(2), 150–155.
van Dam, S., & van Reijmersdal, E. (2019). Insights in adolescents' advertising literacy, perceptions and responses regarding sponsored influencer videos and disclosures. *Cyberpsychology: Journal of Psychosocial Research on Cyberspace*, 13(2), 1–18.
Weijs, C., Thawer, S., Fundytus, K., & McLaren, L. (2022). Advancing public health communication in the era of empowered health consumerism: Insights from dental hygienist-client interactions around community

water fluoridation. *Critical Public Health, 32*(2), 217–229. https://doi-org.ezproxy.lib.utah.edu/10.1080/09581596.2020.1791315

Wellman, M. L. (2022). Social media influencer rhetoric and the domestication of health at every size on Instagram. *Rhetoric of Health & Medicine*, *5*(1), 38–65.

Who Is Will Tennyson: A fitness youtuber, food enthusiast, and much more." (n.d.) *Influencer Agency*. https://us.gymfluencers.com/who-is-will-tennyson/

Zou, W., Zhang, W. J., & Tang, L. (2021). What do social media influencers say about health? A theory-driven content analysis of top ten health influencers' posts on Sina Weibo. *Journal of Health Communication*, *26*(1), 1–11.

PART III

Considering Pro-Social Public Health Interventions in Popular Culture

17

ENTERTAINMENT-EDUCATION AND HEALTH ISSUES

Suruchi Sood and Farren Rodrigues

Introduction to Entertainment Education

"Anyone who makes a distinction between entertainment and education doesn't know the first thing about either." Logan (2011) attributed this statement on the inextricable link between entertainment and education to Marshall McLuhan, a renowned Canadian philosopher whose work is considered one of the cornerstones of communication theorizing (p. 27). As much as we would like to assume that entertainment-education (EE) came into being when academicians in the Global North began to study the effects of combining entertainment with education, the reality is that using entertainment as a tool for education goes back centuries, with oral cultures, written texts, traditional and new media using storytelling to impart knowledge, skills, morals, and values to future generations (Riley et al., 2017). Aesop's Fables, The Upanishads, or the Analects of Confucius comprise examples of "morality texts" or guides to social behaviors that have been passed down through generations.

As a little girl, I remember begging my grandmother to tell us a story every night before bed. My grandmother, who migrated to India in 1947 as a refugee had never been to school, so she did not "read" to us at bedtime. She had a unique way of spinning tall tales about magical places and people. Her stories were about princes and princesses, demons and dragons, but this nightly ritual entailed more than just tall tales. These stories enabled her to pass down family history and preserve a lost cultural heritage. Her stories did not teach me the alphabet and numbers; instead, they taught me ways to understand the world and my place in the larger scheme of things.

While books impart knowledge and skills, true learning often happens outside of a classroom, through stories that tell us what was, what is, and what could be. Walter Fisher (1984) famously labeled the human species as "homo narrans" or creatures that can make up stories, hence labeling all forms of human communication as stories or symbolic interpretations of aspects of the world occurring in time and shaped by history and culture.

To understand the role of popular culture in shaping us as individuals and social beings, this chapter provides an overview of EE, a theory-driven and evidence-based communication approach promoting individual and social change, before discussing factors that make EE unique and concluding with some challenges associated with EE programming in public health.

DOI: 10.4324/9781003436409-20

Types of Entertainment Education

To explore the link between popular culture and public health communication, we must consider all communication programming that educates. In this sense, any form of communication that entertains and educates audiences concurrently can broadly be considered as EE (Global Population Speak Out, n.d.). Based on the objectives, design, and evaluation of effects in addressing public health issues, we outline three types of EE in this chapter. The first category can be considered accidental EE, referring to popular media that unknowingly performs a social function (Das et al., 2017). Modern-day academic study of EE stems from one such accidental program. The second category encompasses what practitioners label as social impact entertainment (SIE), which involves incorporating educational content into existing or under-development popular programs designed for mass audience entertainment (Social Impact Entertainment Society, n.d.). The third category involves public health communication interventions planned, implemented, and evaluated expressly for social and behavior change purposes (Singhal & Rogers, 1989).

Accidental EE

Accidental EE refers to acquiring knowledge unintentionally in entertainment (Singhal & Rogers, 1989). For example, popular media: Radio, television, print, or increasingly social media, designed with the purpose of entertainment, might result in prosocial change by happenchance. As a word of caution, the Communication literature is replete with examples of programs which inadvertently promote negative stereotypes. For example, Communication scholars have likened the lack of racial and ethnic representation in popular television and films to a form of symbolic annihilation (Means Coleman, 2008). Cultivation theory, a concept introduced by George Gerbner (1972), suggested that representation in a fictional world signifies social existence. Omissions cultivate dominant assumptions about how the world works and, as a result, where power resides. In 1976, Gerbner and Gross, using TV as an example, clarified that even though entertainment programming on TV is fiction, the ubiquity of TV as a source of information results in viewers adopting a "TV answer" to represent social reality. Although the negative impacts of mass media exposure on society are indisputable, in this chapter, we examine the positive effects of entertainment in educating around public health issues.

Regardless of suspected negative or positive outcomes, all Communication scholars who believe that the media are influenced by and, in turn, influence popular culture tacitly agree that media audiences constitute active consumers of information, who use media to achieve specific gratifications. Moreover, the media play an important agenda-setting function by interacting with and shaping both public and political agendas (Shaw & Martin, 1992). As B. C. Cohen (1963) famously claimed, the media do not tell us what to think, but they are spectacularly successful in telling us what to think about. Much of the literature on accidental EE involves post-hoc study rather than a planned effort at motivating individual and social change (Singhal et al., 2004; Singhal & Rogers, 1989). Communication scholars have documented the impact of multiple popular programs in promoting after-the-fact prosocial behaviors. A global example of such accidental EE comes from a wildly popular Peruvian telenovela *Simplemente Mariá*, often credited as being a precursor of the organized efforts to use EE as a strategy in public health communication. *Simplemente Mariá* essentially entailed a typical Cinderella story. It told the story of Maria, a simple housemaid who was taken advantage of by a wealthy medical student, Roberto, and she subsequently had his child. As the storyline progressed, Maria enrolled in adult literacy classes, with Maestro Esteban as her tutor, and she also learned how to sew and became a seamstress. As the telenovela ended, her dedication and hard work made Maria a successful fashion designer on her way to Paris. Along the way, Maria and Maestro Esteban fell in love and married in a grand wedding (Shefner-Rogers & Rogers, 1998). A retrospective qualitative study of *Simplemente Maria* found that young women signed up for adult literacy classes in the countries where the program aired. Thus, EE researchers concluded audience exposure to the program and subsequent social change (Singhal et al., 1995).

Another key lesson from *Simplemente Maria* revolved around the transcendent nature of popular entertainment in crossing national and cultural borders, evidenced by the fact that the telenovela was not just popular in Peru but achieved record-high ratings in other Latin American countries. The trajectory of mass media adoption in the Global South aligned with the development goals of previously colonized nations. The popularity and retrospective analysis of *Simplemente Maria* laid the foundation for employing EE to meet growth and development goals.

In countries like the U.S., a clear separation often exists between educational or public media and entertainment media. This distinction fosters a divide between educational and entertainment media. *Sesame Street* exemplifies the former. First broadcast in the U.S. in 1969, *Sesame Street* was not the first television program based on pedagogical ideas on stimulating children who did not yet attend school. However, its central idea of using television for systematic education emphasized the idea that children's television could (and should) be used for teaching skills to preschool children. A meta-analysis on the effects of *Sesame Street*, synthesizing the results of 24 studies conducted with over 10,000 children in 15 countries, illustrated significant positive effects of exposure to the program, including cognitive outcomes such as literacy and numeracy; learning about the world, including health and safety knowledge; and social reasoning and attitudes toward out-groups (Mares & Pan, 2013; see also Chapter 24, this volume).

Scholars have also examined popular media in the U.S. as a means for achieving prosocial outcomes. For example, a summary of known media effects on four adolescent health issues – violence and aggression; sex; obesity, nutrition, and eating disorders; and alcohol and tobacco use – includes entertainment-education as an approach with potential for helping turn the media into more positive forces for adolescents' health (Brown & Witherspoon, 2002).

A specific example of an entertainment program that resulted in positive effects was one of the most popular shows on NBC's Thursday line-up during its run. A medical drama set in a busy fictional emergency room in Chicago, *ER* amassed huge audiences. Between 1998 and 1999, the show drew an average audience of 25 million (Petrozzello, 1999). A study sponsored by the Kaiser Family Foundation found that 53% of *ER* viewers reported learning about important health care issues from the show and that 12% reported having contacted their physician because of something they saw on *ER* (Kaiser Family Foundation, 1997). The show also comprised one of the earlier attempts at codifying the second type of EE, now labeled as SIE. Intrigued by the popularity of *ER*, the Johns Hopkins Bloomberg School of Public Health collaborated with WBAL, the NBC affiliate in Baltimore, to develop a nationally syndicated news series called *Following ER* to highlight health topics featured in *ER*. *Following ER* attempted to take advantage of interest stimulated by *ER* to disseminate accurate public health information and supplement *ER*s fictional narratives with a real-world perspective (Kaiser Family Foundation, 2004). An experimental study analyzing the effects of *Following ER* found that, when the storyline covered a well-known topic, the *ER* tie-in enhanced the attention and satisfaction of viewers by elevating the importance and relevance of the health issue (Cooper et al., 2000). The researchers did not discover the same effect when pairing the tie-in with a novel topic. Cooper et al. concluded that framing news stories about familiar health concerns in the context of a television drama was a viable and timely public health strategy.

Social Impact Entertainment

As mentioned above, though an example of accidental EE, *ER* contributed to an already burgeoning interest in the idea that entertainment narratives could be harnessed to improve health. The Centers for Disease Control (CDC, 2023), through its Health Communication Gateway, reported that many Americans learn about health issues from popular media, making primarily entertainment programs great outlets for disseminating health messages. As such, the CDC provided multiple resources including examples of campaigns, trainings, tools, and templates, as well as educational and expert consulting resources for writers to develop their scripts. Additionally, organizations such as Hollywood, Health, and Society (HH&S), a center based in the Norman Lear Center at Annenberg School of Communication at the University of Southern California, have also harnessed the power of entertainment media for educational purposes. For more than 20 years, the HH&S has sponsored "Sentinel Awards" to recognize exemplary achievements in TV storylines that inform, educate, and motivate viewers to make choices for healthier and safer lives (Hollywood, Health, & Society, 2023; see also Chapter 25, this volume).

Recently codified as SIE, this strategy has gained popularity in the U.S. by assuming that the power and popularity of entertainment programs can be leveraged for educational purposes by incorporating socially conscious and responsible messages within existing media designed for entertainment (Riley & Chattoo, 2019). SIE programs, which currently tend to be concentrated in the Global North, may be funded by private donors and non-profits with a prosocial mission, contrasting with traditional EE (discussed next), which international development organizations largely fund. In other cases, SIE programs may have a for-profit mission with partners, including studios, networks, and distributors. Therefore, according to Riley and Chattoo, SIE producers may or may not know the global history surrounding EE but are highly interested in the "entertainment" part of entertainment-education.

Notably, the SIE Society, a loosely organized global alliance, described its mission as educating, connecting, and empowering entertainment, non-profit, and business professionals to harness storytelling for greater social good and measurable impact (Social Impact Entertainment Society, n.d.). A collaboration of *Cinema of Change* and Producers Guild of America (PGA) launched the SIE Society (Social Impact Entertainment Society, n.d.). *Cinema of Change* comprises an online magazine and podcast that focused on the effectiveness of films and provided a library of resources on how films can lead to change (Deml & Rippberger, 2014). The PGA aims to educate its members by organizing events for producers working on SIE projects in both traditional media and gaming and interactive media (Producers Guild of America, n.d.). The SIE Society represents individuals and organizations across the entire spectrum, including private enterprises, NGOs, governmental initiatives, and educational institutions.

Apart from utilizing traditional media including film, TV, radio, and theater, SIE increasingly leverages new media technologies including video games, virtual reality, and artificial intelligence (AI). An example of SIE is the Producers Guild of America Social Impact Entertainment Task Force (PGA SIETF), which focusses on how storytelling, the arts, and media have the power to create social change on an individual, local, national, and global level (SIE Society, n.d.). Some examples shared by the PGA SIETF include stories of human rights violations, race, and gender, such as *Just Mercy* (2019) and *Hidden Figures* (2016).

SIE also includes traditional television and over-the-top (OTT) content. OTT content refers to the delivery of media through the internet, such as streaming platforms (Netflix, Hulu, Disney+, etc.), where viewers can access an array of available and even original content on demand (Endavo, n.d.). SIE content has aired on traditional media and then been distributed through an OTT platform, making it available to a wider audience, including popular U.S. TV shows such as *Grey's Anatomy*, *Law and Order*, and *Scrubs*. For example, *Grey's Anatomy* originally debuted on ABC in 2005 and, in 2009, started streaming on Netflix (Maher, 2009).

The Kaiser Family Foundation worked with the director of medical research and writers of *Grey's Anatomy* to develop an episode (that aired in 2008) that highlighted the moderately low risk of mother-to-child transmission of HIV when the mother received proper medical care during her pregnancy (the risk is less than 2%). However, this information was not widespread, contributing to the stigma faced by some HIV-positive women who chose to have children (Rideout, 2008). Overall, according to Rideout, the percentage of viewers who expressed awareness that an HIV-positive woman would likely deliver a healthy baby when receiving proper medical treatment increased by 46% after the episode aired (from 15% to 61%).

Furthermore, some OTT platforms have created original content that incorporates SIE. *Reservation Dogs* premiered on Hulu on August 9, 2021 (International Day of the World's Indigenous Peoples). The show followed four Indigenous teenagers living on a reservation in rural Oklahoma. The creators of the show wanted to showcase the issues that Native youth face and focus on the struggles and inequalities of Native American life. Additionally, the show had an all-Indigenous writers' room, crew, and recurring cast members (Kemp, 2022).

The SIE has also been adapted and mainstreamed into popular entertainment programs for specific audiences. For example, *Vencer el Miedo* (https://www.populationmedia.org/the-latest/the-impact-of-pmes-vencer-el-miedo), a social impact telenovela with 47 episodes, centered around four Latina female protagonists who faced issues such as teen pregnancy, domestic violence, parent-teen communication challenges, and gender inequality. The show originally aired in Mexico and, due to its record of almost four million views, subsequently debuted in the U.S. The telenovela inspired viewers to make choices to improve the health and well-being of themselves and those around them, as seen by the increased number of calls to a reproductive health hotline and discussions around the use of contraceptive methods (Population Media Center, 2020). Increasingly, SIE has expanded beyond being just a media strategy, spanning the use of video games, VR, and AI technologies.

Video Games

- Developed in collaboration with Alaska Native storytellers, *Never Alone*, also known as *Kisima Inŋitchuŋa*, explored and preserved indigenous cultures and traditions (Bierman, 2015).
- *Sea of Solitude* focused on loneliness and its impact on mental health by following a young woman embarking on a journey of self-reflection (Sukkersudha, 2023).

Virtual Reality

- The United Nations Virtual Reality Series targeted decision-makers and provided them with an experience to gain an understanding of the realities faced by those who are in danger and marginalized (UN SDG Action Campaign, 2015).
- Developed by researchers at the University of Pennsylvania, VR Narcan Training features a nine-minute simulation on how to administer naloxone in the case of an opioid overdose (Yount, 2020).

Artificial Intelligence

Artificial intelligence is being integrated into everyday life more and more, including entertainment media (Nader et al., 2022). AI can enhance the creation and distribution of SIE content through personalization, predictive analytics, production assistance, audience engagement, data collection, analysis, measurement, recommendations, and global reach (Dhumal, 2023; Takyar, n.d.). Producers employ AI to create a more interactive and personalized experience through its ability to analyze data in real-time, making it a useful tool to enhance personal learning platforms utilizing entertainment education such as Duolingo (Wodzak, 2023) and Minecraft: Education Edition (Mojang AB, n.d.).

The primary distinction between SIE and our third category of EE is that stakeholders describe the former as media designed, first and foremost, to be entertaining and to make a profit. Although SIE embeds accurate health content into existing entertainment programs, the story comes first, with impact issues and the goal of positively impacting society as secondary concerns (Tikhonova, 2022).

In the latter, or more traditional EE, the "impact issue" usually comes first, and writers build characters and stories around the issue.

Planned Entertainment-Education

The third kind of EE refers to planned health interventions or programs that communicate messages to their audiences (Kaiser Family Foundation, 2004), with the specific objective of achieving behavior and social change with an increasing emphasis on the social determinants of health. This third category of entertainment education has been frequently used in the field of development communication. Singhal and Rogers (1989) provided an early academic definition of EE, focused on its efficacy as a mass media strategy, and positioned entertainment-education as the process of purposely designing and implementing a media message to both entertain and educate, to increase audience members' knowledge about an educational issue, create favorable attitudes, and change overt behavior.

However, this definition of EE has evolved over time (Riley et al., 2023; Wang & Singhal, 2021a). With an increased reliance on multidisciplinary perspectives and a focus on methodological innovation to design EE programs and unpack their effectiveness, scholars now consider EE to be a theory-driven, social, and evidence-based SBCC strategy that combines entertainment and education to address real-world issues across the social ecological model (SEM), including new and emerging health priorities. Wang and Singhal advanced a more recent definition:

> Entertainment-education is a social and behavioral change communication strategy that leverages the power of storytelling in entertainment and wisdom from theories in different disciplines—with deliberate intention and collaborative efforts throughout the process of content production, program implementation, monitoring, and evaluation—to address critical issues in the real world and create enabling conditions for desirable and sustainable change across micro-, meso-, and macro-levels.
>
> *(p. 227)*

The Sabido-led television programs in Latin America encompassed some of the first theoretically grounded examples of modern EE (Riley, Rodrigues, et al., 2021). In India, the soap opera *Hum Log* comprised an early replication of the EE format outside of Spanish-speaking countries and included educational information on family planning, gender equality, and social norms (Singhal & Rogers, 1988). The intentional use of EE as a health communication strategy has been studied in countries around the world for over half a century (Singhal & Rogers, 2004). In lower- and middle-income countries (LMICs), public health officials typically develop and implement EE programs as standalone health communication efforts to promote social and behavior change across a wide range of health-enhancing behaviors, including contraceptive use, condom promotion, addressing sexual violence, optimal maternal and child health practices, and habits such as diet and exercise.

Shen and Han (2018) conducted a meta-analysis to examine the effects of EE on health outcomes and explored significant moderator variables to determine if they are affecting the impact of EE. These moderating variables include types of health behaviors, channel differences, research design and locations, amount of time spent viewing EE content, and gender of the participant. Shen and Han found that gender (using males only resulted in larger effect sizes), research design (field experiments resulted in larger effect sizes), and amount of time spent viewing EE content (being exposed to multiple episodes leads to larger effect sizes) had significant effects. Overall, Shen and Han concluded that EE can be a successful platform to deliver health-related information. Moreover, in a meta-analysis, Orozco-Olvera et al. (2019) determined that EE narratives were successful in promoting HIV testing and reducing risky sex among 15–24-year-olds while also advocating for further experimental research.

As a key public health communication strategy, more recent applications of EE have addressed a host of other development issues across the Sustainable Development Goals (SDGs) (United Nations, n.d.), including girls' education, gender equity, healthy social norms, livelihood and income generation, peacebuilding, and climate change (Sood et al., 2017). Initially using channels like radio, TV, theater, and public service announcements (PSAs), current-day EE programs have embraced new and emerging media while still relying on these traditional channels. EE programs range from streaming online videos, video games, interactive social media, to smartphone applications. The use of multiple media channels and formats has also evolved to share messaging through transmedia storytelling (Wang et al., 2019).

Crosscutting Example: Climate Change

Despite our attempt to describe three discrete categories of EE, it is important to keep in mind that issues of global concern make their way into the public and political agenda through messaging across the three categories of EE. Messaging around climate change illustrates this point. Sood et al. (in press) provided numerous examples of programs from all three categories that emphasized the gravity of climate change and brought it front and center on the public and policy agenda.

More traditional and planned EE programs utilizing a long-running format on climate change tend to be implemented in the Global South. Creators specifically design these EE programs dealing with climate change to be entertaining while also educating, and they weave global warming and climate change into the storyline as one of several development concerns. Uniquely, these programs explore the links between climate change and human and planetary health by situating climate change as an urgent priority rather than a distant possibility. Producers of these EE efforts include organizations with long histories of working in LMICs on climate change communication, such as PCI Media (Cheung et al., 2018; PCI Media, 2020), Population Media Center (Barker et al., 2013; Population Media Center, 2020), BBC Media Action (BBC, n.d.; Whitehead, 2017), and the Johns Hopkins Center for Communication Programs (Johns Hopkins Center for Communication Programs, 2020, n.d.). The main motivation driving their decision to implement these global climate change-focused EE projects likely extended from donor interest in a particular outcome (such as increasing people's participation in adapting to climate change on the ground), combined with the salience of the issues (Bauck, 2023). Some examples of these EE efforts include *Bienvenida Salud* (Welcome Health) in the Peruvian Amazon, an intercultural radio program which has been on-air for 20 years and dealt with a variety of social issues including biocultural preservation (Durá et al., 2013). Minga, the organization that spearheaded *Bienvenida Salud*, works in rural indigenous communities in the Pacaya Samiria National Reserve to deepen local understanding and action to conserve local plant species, reconnect with indigenous languages and values, and increase food security while protecting the environment (Minga Peru, n.d.).

Umurage Urukwiye (Rwanda's Brighter Future), which was first broadcast in April 2007, included a radio drama designed to raise awareness and discussion about issues such as reproductive health, HIV/AIDS, wildlife habitat and natural resource preservation, land conservation, and the promotion of civil harmony. The drama role-modeled a community that promoted planting trees to protect the environment and the protection of natural gorilla habitats. The evaluation of the effects of *Umurage Urukwiye* found that listeners were 1.5 times more likely than non-listeners to have talked with their spouse about the connection between family planning and the conservation of natural resources (Barker et al., 2013). Barker et al. concluded that popular entertainment could drive planet-positive behavior change.

Shamba Chef, a reality TV show in Kenya, featured food sources and cooking methods, placing safer cooking methods and environmental issues at the forefront. Apart from cleaner cooking solutions, the show also provided nutritious recipes and expert advice on the best foods to grow and eat (Evans et al., 2020).

Two specific EE and climate change examples from HH&S include: Season 5, Episode 16, "The New Normal" (2019) from *Madam Secretary*, a popular drama on CBS which focused on the global impact of climate change, as illustrated by changing weather patterns and extreme weather events. The third episode of season 18 of *Grey's Anatomy* was titled "Hotter than Hell," and it took inspiration from a real-life heat wave, with the titular character Meredith Grey explaining the impact of heat exhaustion on the human body (Gammon, 2022).

Tom Perrotta's (2011) novel, *The Leftovers*, constitutes one pertinent example of accidental EE on climate change. According to Perrotta, this novel was not meant to be an allegory for climate change, but, when HBO converted the book into a TV show, some critics connected it to climate change, a view he then endorsed (North, 2014). While limited evidence can be found of this type of inclusion in the academic literature, journalists and media bloggers commenting on popular TV have noted that streaming shows such as *Black Mirror* have incorporated specific episodes that deal with climate change as part of interesting narratives, such as the first and last episodes of Season 3. The first episode of the season, "Nosedive," juxtaposed the widespread availability of clean energy with inequality in a totalitarian society. The last episode, "Hated in the Nation," imagined a world where bees went extinct, bringing the U.K. to the brink of an ecological and food crisis (Deep Green Philly, 2016).

What Makes EE Unique

As a part of popular culture, EE holds several advantages when it comes to its feasibility for health education and promotion, engendering behavior and social change. EE extends from theory and evidence, harnesses the power of storytelling, offers flexibility vis-à-vis channel selection and audiences, addresses social and behavioral change across the SEM, and tackles multiple health issues and their determinants simultaneously.

Theory-Driven

Most of the literature traces the roots of modern EE to Miguel Sabido, who famously developed the Sabido methodology of entertainment-education (Frank & Falzone, 2021). Extensive literature exists on the various theoretical traditions from public health and communication sciences upon which EE programs have been developed (Sood et al., 2004). While originally relying heavily on principles of Albert Bandura's (2003) Social Learning Theory, EE scholars and researchers have been applying more innovative and diverse theoretical frameworks to understand why and how EE works (Oliver et al., 2018; Tamborini et al., 2010; Vorderer & Halfmann, 2019). For example, more recent theorizing in EE has incorporated a positive deviance (PD) approach. PD constitutes a community-based approach that attempts to find people with uncommon solutions to problems and diffuse those solutions among the community (Gesser-Edelsburg et al., 2021). Research among the Bedouin population living in the Southern District of Israel employed the PD and Community Based Participatory Research (CBPR) approaches while utilizing theatrical traditions from EE to narratively engage and persuade the Bedouins regarding unintentional injury prevention (Gesser-Edelsburg et al., 2021).

Evidence-Based

The evidence base for EE interventions includes different evaluation methods. On the one hand, scholars have used experimental and quasi-experimental studies to measure various facets of EE programs, for example, the role of engagement, spillover effects, and impact on social and behavior change (Asbeek-Brusse et al., 2015; van Leeuwen, 2015; Wilke et al., 2020). On the other hand, population-based surveys evaluate the effects of large-scale full-coverage programs (W. J. Brown, 2012). Evaluation of EE effects originally focused on how these effects related to social and behavior change. Over time, scholars from multiple disciplines have sought to understand "how" and "why" EE works (Riley, Sangalang, et al., 2021). This focus on the process has encouraged research on multidisciplinary efforts on both cognitive and affective pathways to encourage change.

Along with broadening the theoretical bases to examine EE, the evidence for measuring the effects of EE has also increasingly used participatory research methods and community engagement to foster social change (Garney et al., 2015; Gesser-Edelsburg et al., 2021; Singhal & Rogers, 2004). Storey and Sood (2013) highlighted three themes that have contributed to the increase in the use of participatory research in EE, namely the emphasis on increasing equity, affirming the power of those whose story is told, and expanding opportunities for dialogue and participation. Participatory approaches draw insights and ideas from the population (Singhal & Rattine-Flaherty, 2006), and the more engaged an audience, the higher the likelihood of the EE messages proving to be effective. A review of the EE literature by Riley et al. (2017) identified four categories of participatory methods – visual (photography, video, and drawings), oral (stories, theater, and phone calls), written (diaries and letters), and listening (formal listening groups) – which spanned formative, process, and impact research around EE interventions, therefore providing evidence on the effects and effectiveness of EE interventions using mixed methods approaches (Riley et al., 2017). Another systematic review, summarizing evidence from 22 studies on the effectiveness of EE in communicating health information across various topics, concluded that EE has small but significant effects on health outcomes (Shen & Han, 2018).

Harnesses the Power of Storytelling

By employing the power of storytelling through fictional narratives that reflect real life or serve as aspirational for audiences, EE more likely results in narrative engagement, which, in turn, contributes to changing attitudes and norms. Allowing audiences to situate themselves within a narrative enables them to empathize with and/or relate to characters or situations in their own lives or people that they know; EE caters to both the heart and the head (emotions and cognition). First, the narrative appeal of EE fosters the formation of emotional bonds with characters over time (Wang & Singhal, 2016). Audience members begin to identify with the character and their actions and, eventually, feel that they, too, can perform the health-promoting actions (Sood, 2004). A growing body of evidence attests that people are more likely remember and apply health information when they learn it in a narrative versus a non-narrative format and when narratives and characters are designed to be liked and trusted by the audience (Frank et al., 2015; Huang & Green, 2023; Wang & Singhal, 2021b). Narrative persuasion, a term that comes from the field of Communication, broadly explains how storytelling (or narrative) brings about change. Some of the constructs that explain change include narrative transportation (M. C. Green & Brock, 2000), narrative engagement (Busselle & Bilandzic, 2009), and identification with characters (J. Cohen, 2001). In short, these ideas explain how storytelling brings about individual and social change stemming from exposure to EE programs.

Employs Multiple Channels to Reach Audiences

The use of social media has risen by 3% from January 2022 to January 2023, with 4.8 billion social media user identities as of April 2023 (Smart Insights, 2023). Increasing focus on transmedia EE, which engages with audiences using many different formats, allows EE to be nimble in utilizing different channels in increasingly creative ways (Dudacek, 2015; Pratten, 2011; Schiller, 2018). The idea of transmedia, which refers to utilizing multiple and various platforms to disseminate content, has commonly been used in popular media (Schiller, 2018). For example, the *Star Wars* franchise encompasses one transmedia initiative with global reach. *Star Wars* has utilized a variety of different modalities (a combination of films, screenplays, radio dramas, and novels, as well as immersive experiences at Disney's Hollywood Studios) to reach its audience and create a story world for their consumers to explore (Guynes & Hassler-Forest, 2017).

Furthermore, global programs have also adopted transmedia strategies. One global example of a national transmedia EE initiative took place in Bangladesh from 2018–2019. Practitioners implemented *Icchedana* (On the Wings of Wishes), an EE program, along with social mobilization and community engagement components in three regions with a high prevalence of child marriage. *Icchedana* resulted from collaborations among various partners including government agencies, non-governmental organizations (NGOs), universities, global experts, and funders. Stakeholders launched the transmedia campaign in two phases. The first phase included the use of narratives reinforced across several television advertisements, posters, and billboards. Building on this work, they introduced the 26-episode television series named *Icchedana*. The show portrayed the lives of four girls as they navigated the challenges and risks (including child marriage) of being adolescent girls (Sengupta et al., 2020). The episodes aired for 26 consecutive weeks on four television channels in Bangladesh, with episodes also uploaded on YouTube and UNICEF Bangladesh's website and Facebook pages. The evaluation of the effects of *Icchedana* showed that shifts in social norms around child marriage can be measured over a relatively short period of time and that SBCC exposure relates to shifts in descriptive (what people think other people do) and injunctive norms (what people think others approve and disapprove of) in different ways (Hauer & Sood, 2021).

The series *East Los High*, a teen drama that revolved around the lives of a group of teens navigating their final years at a fictional high school in East LA, on Hulu, comprised a U.S.-based example of a transmedia initiative. Primarily filmed in East Los Angeles, the show included an all-Latino cast and crew. Starting as a 24-episode original drama series, *East Los High* expanded its scope by nudging viewers to visit an *East Los High* website (eastloshigh.com), where they could access nine transmedia narrative extensions. These transmedia elements included extended scenes, news articles, vlogs, recipes, dance tutorials, comic strips, and PSAs. *East Los High* also had a comprehensive resources page with embedded health service widgets. The evaluation of *East Los High* concluded that culturally sensitive transmedia edutainment programs constituted a promising health promotion strategy for minority populations and warrant further investigation (Wang & Singhal, 2016).

Works Across the Social Ecological Model

Academic research has contributed to increasing utilization of EE as a public health communication strategy through extensive monitoring and evaluation of EE programs. This scholarship focuses specifically on what works in EE, with examples of programs that have proven effective across the different levels of the SEM (Riley et al., 2023) to simultaneously change both individual behavior and societies by creating an enabling environment where individual behavior change is possible, accepted, and supported. One example of individual-level effects is the #ISurvivedEbola multimedia campaign, which amplified stories of Ebola survival to decrease stigma during the 2014 outbreak in Liberia, Sierra Leone, and Guinea. The EE radio drama provided life-saving prevention information alongside compelling storytelling and call-in segments where listeners could ask questions and learn how to keep themselves safe (PCI Media, n.d.). The evaluation showed that the campaign not only "worked" but was also nominated for an Emmy award (Riley, Sangalang, et al., 2021).

At the interpersonal level, EE messages can be conversation starters for subjects that may otherwise be taboo or hard to talk about. For example, it might be awkward to discuss condom use with a partner, but by discussing an EE program and its characters' experiences, the subject may be easier to broach. At the community level, researchers hypothesized that EE works by increasing collective efficacy and empowering communities to tackle public health topics and change related social norms (Sood et al., 2017; Williams & Swierad, 2019). The Indian television program *Kyunki ... Jeena Issi Ka Naam Hai* (Because ... That's What Life Is), which aired from 2008-2011, exemplified EE targeting social norms. This program, funded in part by UNICEF, aimed to shift norms on maternal and child health topics, such as breastfeeding and spacing out births to lower the impact on the mother's health and family resources. A large evaluation of 27,000 audience respondents at three different times found that the social norms on many of the topics shifted from the first to the final measurement (Sood et al., 2015).

Evidence also exists in the EE literature on how EE can and has promoted policy-level changes. For example, *Soul City*, a longstanding EE program in South Africa, addressed the topic of domestic violence in Season 4. While domestic violence has often been thought of as a private behavior, *Soul City* illustrated collective action from community members who came out of their homes hitting pots and pans to draw attention to the story of a man physically assaulting his wife. The evaluation of *Soul City* demonstrated that the EE program helped to significantly increase a sense of collective efficacy in addressing domestic violence across the country and contributed directly and indirectly to the passage of the Domestic Violence Act in South Africa (Usdin et al., 2005). In the Dominican Republic, *La Peor Novela*, a soap opera, told the stories of two girls living in rural and urban areas who were forced to marry older men based on their settings. These characters imitated the experiences of thousands of Dominican adolescent girls. *La Peor Novela* reached 24 million people and contributed to making child marriage illegal in the country (Giraldo et al., 2022).

Tackles Multiple Issues Simultaneously

Importantly, EE addresses complex issues well because it allows for a layered treatment of related or multiple themes and stories simultaneously (Singhal et al., 2003). For example, the U.S. television show *East Los High* covered a variety of salient public health topics, including teen pregnancy, sexually transmitted infections, HIV/AIDS, drug use, and violence. Furthermore, in Jordan, the 1001 Nights Civic and Peace Education Program consisted of comic books, an animated TV series, and a curriculum centered on the importance of education, life skills and civic values, human rights, and gender equality for children at Syrian refugee camps and learning centers. This initiative led to a 30% decrease in negative attitudes, especially among at-risk children (Giraldo et al., 2022).

Challenges in EE

Despite EE's unique features, EE practitioners face many challenges associated with its design, implementation, and evaluation. The rapidly expanding reach and exposure to multiple forms of social media and the recent inclusion of AI, machine-based learning, and virtual reality require constant innovation. Another key challenge relates to measurement issues. As EE programs become more imaginative and innovative, theories and research methods must keep pace with them. Some recent critiques of EE programs, for example, assert that much of our evaluation methods lag behind theoretical advances (D. P. Green, 2021). Therefore, EE programs should divert from tried and tested methods borrowed from the natural sciences that may or may not apply to real-life scenarios. For example, although some consider randomized controlled trials (RCTs) to be the gold standard in public health, EE strives to create a full-coverage intervention that reaches the maximum number of people – contrary to the basic principles of conducting RCTs (Grossman & Mackenzie, 2005; Oakley et al., 2006). Although numerous examples of RCTs have been associated with EE programs, scale and sustainability remain problematic (Agide et al., 2018; Orozco-Olvera et al., 2019).

Another challenge faced by EE programs pertains to cost and time. The cost-effectiveness of EE programs has been assessed to ensure that cost needs to be balanced with the cost-effectiveness of other forms of health education and health promotion (Jah et al., 2018; Orozco-Olvera et al., 2019). Research has also shown that EE can be relatively cost-effective, considering the cost per person (De Fossard et al., 2008). For example, the Indian EE TV program *Jasoos Vijay* (*Detective Vijay*) costs just $2.49 per person who changes their behavior (starts using condoms) because of exposure (Sood

& Nambiar, 2006). On the other hand, EE programs can incur high upfront costs, requiring that program developers and funders attain strong buy-in.

Another potential drawback to EE programs in certain settings entails demand for health behaviors, services, and products that may not be available (Grady et al., 2021). Although EE does not constitute a magic bullet, it can encourage change but cannot change the immediate contexts and social determinants that impact behavior and social change in the first place. Thus, a major challenge with EE involves creating programs in partnership with government agencies, NGOs, private companies, and others to ensure that the behaviors and actions promoted through EE programs are supported via an enabling and supportive environment.

Some have also critiqued the ethics involved in trying to influence individuals through subliminal messaging (Gratz, 1984; Valenti, 2018). Scholars have questioned the ethics of using entertainment to mask some of the educational content. Dutta (2017) suggested the use of "culture-centered communication" to ensure ethical planning and implementation of EE. This approach focuses on listening to the voices of those who have been expunged by the dominant narratives, with the conviction of reversing the structures that produce global inequities (Dutta, 2018). Therefore, EE messages should reflect and be based on the realities of the communities rather than blatantly attempting to impose external values and beliefs. Despite these challenges, EE strives to take audiences on a journey of self-reflection and critical thinking that prompts change both among individuals and their social and cultural environments.

Conclusion

Entertainment as a tool for education goes back centuries, and popular culture is instrumental in communicating knowledge and values across diverse societies. Although ample evidence exists regarding the influence of all forms of popular communication, entertainment education generally refers to planned efforts to harness multiple communication channels for promoting social and behavioral change. This strategic use of entertainment to encourage prosocial change has unique strengths and faces multiple challenges. Despite many valid critiques, the literature has demonstrated that entertainment has been and should be used to engender social and behavior change.

References

Asbeek Brusse, E. D., Fransen, M. L., & Smit, E. G. (2015). The more you say, the less they hear: The effect of disclosures in entertainment-education. *Journal of Media Psychology: Theories, Methods, and Applications, 27*(4), 159–169.

Agide, F. D., Garmaroudi, G., Sadeghi, R., Shakibazadeh, E., Yaseri, M., Koricha, Z. B., & Tigabu, B. M. (2018). A systematic review of the effectiveness of health education interventions to increase cervical cancer screening uptake. *European Journal of Public Health, 28*(6), 1156–1162.

Bandura, A. (2003). Social cognitive theory for personal and social change by enabling media. In Singhal, A., Cody, M. J., Rogers, E. M., & Sabido, M. (Eds.). *Entertainment-education and social change: History, research, and practice.* (pp. 97–118). Routledge.

Barker, K., Connolly, S., & Angelone, C. (2013). Creating a brighter future in Rwanda through entertainment education. *Critical Arts, 27*(1), 75–90.

Bauck, W. (2023). 'The visuals of today help create the reality of tomorrow:' Why Hollywood is finally tackling climate change onscreen. https://www.fastcompany.com/90856208/the-visuals-of-today-help-create-the-reality-of-tomorrow-why-hollywood-is-finally-tackling-climate-change-onscreen

BBC. (n.d.). Resilience and climate. https://www.bbc.co.uk/mediaaction/our-work/climate-change-resilience/

Bierman, E. (2015, May 6). Play the award-winning video game preserving Alaska native folklore. *Vice*. https://www.vice.com/en/article/jpvde7/play-the-award-winning-video-game-preserving-alaska-native-folklore

Brown, J. D., & Witherspoon, E. M. (2002). The mass media and American adolescents' health. *Journal of Adolescent Health, 31*(6), 153–170.

Brown, W. J. (2012). Promoting health through entertainment-education media: Theory and practice. In R. Obregon & S. Waisbord (Eds.), *The handbook of global health communication* (pp. 121–143). John Wiley and Sons.

Busselle, R., & Bilandzic, H. (2009). Measuring narrative engagement. *Media Psychology*, *12*(4), 321–347.

CDC. (2023). Gateway to health communication. https://www.cdc.gov/healthcommunication/index.html

Cheung, L., Riley, A. H., Brown, A., & Schmid, C. (2018). Not enough fish in the sea: Community-based entertainment-education to promote sustainable fishing in Belize. *The Journal of Development Communication*, *29*(1), 52–60.

Cohen, B. C. (1963). *The press and foreign policy*. Princeton University Press.

Cohen, J. (2001). Defining identification: A theoretical look at the identification of audiences with media characters. *Mass Communication and Society*, *4*(3), 245–264.

Cooper, C. P., Roter, D. L., & Langlieb, A. M. (2000). Using entertainment television to build a context for prevention news stories. *Preventive Medicine*, *31*(3), 225–231.

Das, E., Nobbe, T., & Oliver, M. B. (2017). Moved to act. Examining the role of mixed affect and cognitive elaboration in "accidental" narrative persuasion. *International Journal of Communication*, *11*, 4907–4923.

Deep Green Philly. (2016, October 26). Climate change makes a subtle yet powerful cameo in Season 3 of Black Mirror. https://deepgreenphilly.medium.com/climate-change-makes-a-subtle-yet-powerful-cameo-in-season-3-of-black-mirror-a009df48720a#:~:text=Green%20Philly%20%7C%20Medium-,Climate%20Change-%20Makes%20a%20Subtle%20Yet%20Powerful,Season%203%20of%20Black%20Mirror&text=The%20possibilities%20are%20endless%20for,tapping%20into%20this%20dramatic%20potential

De Fossard, E., Lande, R., Bernstein, J., Cho, N., & Short, M. (2008). Entertainment-education for better health. *INFO Reports*, *17*(2). https://www.media-diversity.org/additional-files/documents/b-studies-reports/Entertainment-Education%20for%20Better%20Health%20[EN].pdf

Deml, T., & Rippberger, R. (2014). Cinema of change – *Magazine & Film Movement*. https://www.cinemaofchange.com/about-the-magazine/mission-statement/

Dhumal, N. (2023, May 8). The impact of AI on the media and entertainment industry. LinkedIn. https://www.linkedin.com/pulse/impact-ai-media-entertainment-industry-nisha-dhumal

Dudacek, O. (2015). Transmedia storytelling in education. *Procedia-Social and Behavioral Sciences*, *197*, 694–696.

Durá, L., Singhal, A., & Elías, E. (2013). Minga Perú's strategy for social change in the Peruvian Amazon: A rhetorical model for participatory, intercultural practice to advance human rights. *Journal of Rhetoric, Professional Communication, and Globalization*, *4*(1), 33–54.

Dutta, M. J. (2017). Culture-centered communication and social change: Listening and participation to transform communication inequalities. *Intercultural Communication*, *9*, 309–327.

Dutta, M. J. (2018). Culture-centered approach in addressing health disparities: Communication infrastructures for subaltern voices. *Communication Methods and Measures*, *12*(4), 239–259.

Endavo. (n.d.). What is OTT? https://www.endavomedia.com/what-is-ott/

Evans, W. D., Young, B. N., Johnson, M. A., Jagoe, K. A., Charron, D., Rossanese, M., Lloyd Morgan, K., Gichinga, P., & Ipe, J. (2020). The *Shamba Chef* educational entertainment program to promote modern cookstoves in Kenya: Outcomes and dose-response analysis. *International Journal of Environmental Research and Public Health*, *17*, 162–176.

Fisher, W. R. (1984). Narration as a human communication paradigm: The case of public moral argument. *Communications Monographs*, *51*(1), 1–22.

Frank, L. B., & Falzone, P. (2021). Introduction: Entertainment-education behind the scenes. In L. B. Frank & P. Falzone (Eds.), *Entertainment-education behind the scenes: Case studies for theory and practice* (pp. 3–14). Springer Nature.

Frank, L. B., Murphy, S. T., Chatterjee, J. S., Moran, M. B., & Baezconde-Garbanati, L. (2015). Telling stories, saving lives: Creating narrative health messages. *Health Communication*, *30*(2), 154–163.

Gammon, K. (2022, October 7). From 'Grey's Anatomy' to 'Abbott Elementary,' pop culture is finally waking up to the climate crisis. https://www.fastcompany.com/90793460/from-greys-anatomy-to-abbott-elementary-pop-culture-is-finally-waking-up-to-the-climate-crisis

Garney, W. R., Beaudoin, C. E., Clark, H. R., Drake, K. N., Wendel, M. L., McLeroy, K. R., ... & Shaw, R. L. (2015). Using community-based participatory research to disseminate a mass media campaign into rural communities. *Journal of Health Communication*, *20*(7), 799–806.

Gerbner, G. (1972). Violence in television drama: Trends and symbolic functions. In G. A. Comstock & E. Rubinstein (Eds.), *Television and social behavior, Vol. 1, content, and control* (pp. 28–187). U.S. Government Printing Office.

Gerbner, G., & Gross, L. (1976). Living with television: The violence profile. *Journal of Communication*, *26*, 172–199.

Gesser-Edelsburg, A., Alamour, Y., Cohen, R., Abed Elhadi Shahbari, N., Hijazi, R., Orr, D., ... & Singhal, A. (2021). Creating safe spaces to prevent unintentional childhood injuries among the Bedouins in southern Israel: A hybrid model comprising positive deviance, community-based participatory research, and entertainment-education. *PLoS One*, *16*(9), e0257696.

Giraldo, J-P., Jenkins, R., & Tungatarova, A. (2022). The case for edutainment. https://www.unicef.org/blog/edutainment-multiple-pathways-learning

Global Population Speak Out. (n.d.). Entertainment-education. https://populationspeakout.org/solutions/entertainment-education-2/

Grady, C., Iannantuoni, A., & Winters, M. S. (2021). Influencing the means but not the ends: The role of entertainment-education interventions in development. *World Development*, *138*, 105200.

Gratz, J. E. (1984). The ethics of subliminal communication. *Journal of Business Ethics*, *3*, 181–184.

Green, D. P. (2021). In search of entertainment-education's effects on attitudes and behaviors. In L. B. Frank & P. Falzone (Eds.), *Entertainment-education behind the scenes: Case studies for theory and practice* (pp 195–210). Springer Nature.

Green, M. C., & Brock, T. C. (2000). The role of transportation in the persuasiveness of public narratives. *Journal of Personality and Social Psychology*, *79*(5), 701–721.

Grossman, J., & Mackenzie, F. J. (2005). The randomized controlled trial: Gold standard, or merely standard? *Perspectives in Biology and Medicine*, 48(4), 516–534. Project MUSE, https://doi.org/10.1353/pbm.2005.0092

Guynes, S. A., & Hassler-Forest, D. (2017). *Star Wars and the history of transmedia storytelling*. Amsterdam University Press.

Hauer, M. K., & Sood, S. (2021). Exploring knowledge, attitudes, and beliefs about child marriage in Bangladesh through a transmedia entertainment-education initative. *The Journal of Development Communication*, *32*(1), 68–79.

Hollywood, Health, & Society. (2023). Sentinel awards. https://hollywoodhealthandsociety.org/sentinel-awards

Huang, Y., & Green, M. C. (2023). Reducing COVID-19 vaccine hesitancy among African Americans: The effects of narratives, character's self-persuasion, and trust in science. *Journal of Behavioral Medicine*, *46*(1–2), 290–302.

Jah, F., Connolly, S., & Ryerson, W. (2018). Comparing the cost-effectiveness of mass media long-running entertainment-education (EE) for social and behaviour change in Africa. *The Journal of Development Communication*, *29*(1), 61–72.

John Hopkins Center for Communication Programs. (2020). About CCP. https://ccp.jhu.edu/about-ccp/

John Hopkins Center for Communication Programs. (n.d.). Climate Action. https://ccp.jhu.edu/what-we-do/priorities/climate-action/

Kaiser Family Foundation. (1997). Telephone survey of 700 regular ER viewers: Summary of results. http://www.kff. 2org/content/archive/1358ers.html

Kaiser Family Foundation. (2004). Entertainment education and health in the United States. https://www.kff.org/wp-content/uploads/2013/01/entertainment-education-and-health-in-the-united-states-issue-brief.pdf

Kemp, A. (2022, August 2). How 'Reservation Dogs' became a breakthrough hit for Indigenous representation. *PBS*. https://www.pbs.org/newshour/arts/how-reservation-dogs-became-a-breakthrough-hit-for-indigenous-representation

Logan, R. K. (2011). McLuhan misunderstood: Setting the record straight. Reason and Word (76) https://mcluhangalaxy.wordpress.com/2011/06/17/mcluhan-misunderstood-setting-the-record-straight-by-robert-k-logan/

Maher, R. (2009, August 3). Netflix cuts deal with ABC to stream 'Lost', 'Grey's Anatomy'. *Business Insider*. https://www.businessinsider.com/netflix-inks-deal-with-disney-abc-to-stream-popular-tv-shows-2009-8

Mares, M. L., & Pan, Z. (2013). Effects of Sesame Street: A meta-analysis of children's learning in 15 countries. *Journal of Applied Developmental Psychology*, *34*(3), 140–151.

Means Coleman, R. R., & Yochim, E. C. (2008). Symbolic annihilation. In W. Donsbach (Ed.), *The international encyclopedia of communication*. Wiley Publishing.

Minga Peru. (n.d.). A conservation path: Training artisans in the Peruvian Amazon. https://mingaperu.org/en/a-conservation-path-training-artisans-in-the-peruvian-amazon/

Mojang AB. (n.d.). Minecraft education. https://education.minecraft.net/en-us

Nader, K., Toprac, P., Scott, S., & Baker, S. (2022). Public understanding of artificial intelligence through entertainment media. *AI & Society*, 1–14. https://doi.org/10.1007/s00146-022-01427-w

North, A. (2014, July 27). What 'The Leftovers' says about climate change. *The New York Times*. https://archive.nytimes.com/op-talk.blogs.nytimes.com/2014/07/27/what-the-leftovers-says-about-climate-change/

Oakley, A., Strange, V., Bonell, C., Allen, E., & Stephenson, J. (2006). Process evaluation in randomised controlled trials of complex interventions. *British Medical Journal*, *332*(7538), 413–416.

Oliver, M. B., Raney, A. A., Slater, M. D., Appel, M., Hartmann, T., Bartsch, A., ... & Das, E. (2018). Self-transcendent media experiences: Taking meaningful media to a higher level. *Journal of Communication, 68*(2), 380–389.

Orozco-Olvera, V., Shen, F., & Cluver, L. (2019). The effectiveness of using entertainment education narratives to promote safer sexual behaviors of youth: A meta-analysis, 1985–2017. *PLoS One*, *14*(2), e0209969 https://doi.org/10.1371/journal.pone.0209969

PCI Media. (2020). Support media that makes change. https://www.pcimedia.org/category/environment/

PCI Media. (n.d.). Evaluation of PCI media impact's #IsurvivedEbola campaign in Liberia, Guinea, and Sierra Leone. *PCI Media*. https://teamsurvive.org/about-ts/

Perrotta, T. (2011). *The leftovers*. St. Martin's Press.

Petrozzello, D. (1999, June 1). 'ER' is the season's no. 1 med drama leads NBC to five top-10 1998-99 finishes. *New York Daily News*. https://www.nydailynews.com/1999/06/01/er-is-the-seasons-no-1-med-drama-leads-nbc-to-five-top-10-1998-99-finishes/

Population Media Center. (2020). A dedication to diverse stories: Population Media Center presents "Vencer el Miedo" and Virtual Event "Latinas Unidas: Rising Together". https://www.globenewswire.com/news-release/2020/08/27/2085141/0/en/A-Dedication-to-Diverse-Stories-Population-Media-Center-Presents-Vencer-el-Miedo-and-Virtual-Event-Latinas-Unidas-Rising-Together.html#.X0kYNR9uY84.facebook

Pratten, R. (2011). *Getting started with transmedia storytelling*. CreateSpace.

Producers Guild of America. (n.d.). Bringing together the producing team in film, TV, and new media. https://producersguild.org

Rideout, V. (2008). *Television as a health educator: A case study of Grey's Anatomy*. Kaiser

Riley, A. H., & Chattoo, C. B. (2019). Developing multimedia social impact entertainment programming for Hispanics in the United States. *The Journal of Development Communication*, *30*(2), 16–29.

Riley, A. H., Rodrigues, F., & Sood, S. (2021). Social norms theory and measurement in entertainment-education: Insights from case studies in four countries. In L. B. Frank & P. Falzone (Eds), Entertainment-education behind the scenes (pp 175–193). Palgrave Macmillan. https://doi.org/10.1007/978-3-030-63614-2_11

Riley, A. H., Sangalang, A., Critchlow, E., Brown, N., Mitra, R., & Campos Nesme, B. (2021). Entertainment-education campaigns and COVID-19: How three global organizations adapted the health communication strategy for pandemic response and takeaways for the future. *Health Communication*, *36*(1), 42–49. https://doi.org/10.1080/10410236.2020.184751

Riley, A. H., Sood, S., & Robichaud, M. (2017). Participatory methods for entertainment–education: Analysis of best practices. *Journal of Creative Communications*, *12*(1), 62–76.

Riley, A. H., Sood, S., & Wang, H. (2023). Entertainment-education (Effects). *The International Encyclopedia of Health Communication*, 1–7.

Schiller, M. (2018). Transmedia storytelling: New practices and audiences. In I. Christie and A. van der Oever (Eds.) *Stories: Screen narrative in the digital age* (pp. 97–108). Amsterdam University Press.

Sengupta, A., Sood, S., Kapil, N., & Sultana, T. (2020). Enabling gender norm change through communication. *The Journal of Development Communication*, *31*(2), 34–45.

Shaw, D. L., & Martin, S. E. (1992). The function of mass media agenda setting. *Journalism Quarterly*, *69*(4), 902–920.

Shefner-Rogers, C. L., & Rogers, E. M. (1998). Parasocial interaction with the television soap operas "Simplemente Maria" and" Oshin." *Keio Communication Review*, *20*, 3–18.

Shen, F., & Han, J. A. (2018). Effectiveness of entertainment education in communicating health information: A systematic review. In R. Wei (Ed.), *The state of Asian communication research and directions for the 21st century* (pp. 605–616). Routledge.

Singhal, A., Cody, M. J., Rogers, E. M., & Sabido, M. (Eds.). (2003). *Entertainment-education and social change: History, research, and practice*. Routledge.

Singhal, A., Obregon, R., & Rogers, E. M. (1995). Reconstructing the story of Simplemente Maria, the most popular telenovela in Latin America of all time. *Gazette (Leiden, Netherlands)*, *54*(1), 1–15.

Singhal, A., & Rattine-Flaherty, E. (2006). Pencils and photos as tools of communicative research and praxis: Analyzing Minga Perú's quest for social justice in the Amazon. *International Communication Gazette*, *68*(4), 313–330.

Singhal, A., & Rogers, E. M. (1988). Television soap operas for development in India1. *Gazette (Leiden, Netherlands)*, *41*(2), 109–126.

Singhal, A., & Rogers, E. (1989). *Entertainment-education: A communication strategy for social change*. Routledge.

Singhal, A., & Rogers, E. (2004). The status of entertainment-education worldwide. In A. Singhal, M. J. Cody, E. M. Rogers, & M. Sabido (Eds.), *Entertainment-education and social change* (pp. 3–20). Erlbaum.

Singhal, A., Usdin, S., Scheepers, E., Goldstein, S., & Japhet, G. (2004). Entertainment-education strategy in development communication. In C. Okigbo & F. Eribo (Eds.), *Development and communication in Africa* (pp. 141–156). Rowman & Littlefield.

Smart Insights. (2023). Global social media statistics research summary 2023. https://www.smartinsights.com/social-media-marketing/social-media-strategy/new-global-social-media-research/#:~:text=The%20number%20of%20social%20media,the%20rest%20of%20the%20yea

Social Impact Entertainment [SIE] Society. (n.d.). About us. https://siesociety.org/who-we-are/Sood, S. (2002). Audience involvement and entertainment—education. *Communication Theory*, *12*(2), 153–172.

Sood, S., Menard, T., & Witte, K. (2004). The theory behind entertainment-education. In A. Singhal, M. J. Cody, E. M. Rogers, & M. Sabido (Eds.). *Entertainment-education and social change: History, research, and practice* (pp. 117–145). Routledge

Sood, S., & Nambiar, D. (2006). Comparative cost-effectiveness of the components of a behavior change communication campaign on HIV/AIDS in North India. *Journal of Health Communication*, *11*(S2), 143–162.

Sood, S., Riley, A. H., & Alarcon, K. C. (2017). Entertainment-education and health and risk messaging. In M. C. Green & K. Fitzgerald (Eds.), *Oxford research encyclopedia of communication*. Oxford University Press.

Sood, S., Riley, A. H., & Birkenstock, L. (in press). Entertainment-education and climate change: Program examples, evidence, and best practices from around the world. In E. Coren & H. Wang (Eds), *Storytelling to accelerate climate solutions*. Springer Nature.

Sood, S., Riley, A. H., Mazumdar, P. D., Choudary, N., Malhotra, A., & Sahba, N. (2015). From awareness-generation to changing norms: Implications for entertainment-education. *Cases in Public Health Communication & Marketing*, *8*, 3–26.

Storey, D., & Sood, S. (2013). Increasing equity, affirming the power of narrative, and expanding dialogue: The evolution of entertainment education over two decades. *Critical Arts*, *27*(1), 9–35.

Sukkersudha, R. (2023). Gaming for good: Investing in the social impact of video games. LinkedIn. https://www.linkedin.com/pulse/gaming-good-investing-social-impact-video-games-raj-sukkersudha

Takyar, A. (n.d.). Role of AI in the entertainment industry: Real-world use cases & examples. https://www.leewayhertz.com/ai-use-cases-in-entertainment/

Tamborini, R., Bowman, N. D., Eden, A., Grizzard, M., & Organ, A. (2010). Defining media enjoyment as the satisfaction of intrinsic needs. *Journal of Communication*, *60*(4), 758–777.

Tikhonova, S. V. (2022). How cinema changes social reality: The social impact entertainment.

United Nations. (n.d.). SDG Media Compact. https://www.un.org/sustainabledevelopment/sdg-media-compact-about

UN SDG Action Campaign. (2015). UN virtual reality. https://unvr.sdgactioncampaign.org/home/about/#:~:text=The%20UN%20Virtual%20Reality%20Series,danger%20of%20being%20left%20behind

Usdin, S., Scheepers, E., Goldstein, S., & Japhet, G. (2005). Achieving social change on gender-based violence: A report on the impact evaluation of Soul City's fourth series. *Social Science & Medicine*, *61*(11), 2434–2445.

Valenti, M. (2018). *More than a movie: Ethics in entertainment*. Routledge.

van Leeuwen, L. (2015*). I was totally there!: Understanding engagement in entertainment-education narratives* (Doctoral dissertation, Wageningen University and Research).

Vorderer, P., & Halfmann, A. (2019). Why do we entertain ourselves with media narratives? A theory of resonance perspective on entertainment experiences. *Annals of the International Communication Association*, *43*(2), 79–96.

Wang, H., & Singhal, A. (2016). East Los High: Transmedia edutainment to promote the sexual and reproductive health of young Latina/o Americans. *American Journal of Public Health*, *106*(6), 1002–1010. https://doi.org/10.2105/AJPH.2016.303072

Wang, H., Singhal, A. (2021a). Mind the gap! Confronting the challenges of translational communication research in entertainment-education. In L. B. Frank & P. Falzon (Eds.) *Entertainment-education behind the scenes* (pp. 223–241). Palgrave Macmillan. https://doi.org/10.1007/978-3-030-63614-2_14

Wang, H., & Singhal, A. (2021b). Theorizing entertainment-education: A complementary perspective to the development of entertainment theory. In P. Vorderer & C. Klimmt (Eds.) *The Oxford handbook of entertainment theory* (pp. 819–838). Oxford University Press.

Wang, H., Singhal, A., Quist, C., Sachdev, A., & Liu, S. (2019). Aligning the stars in East Los High: How authentic characters and storylines can translate into real-life changes through transmedia edutainment. *Journal of Media and Communication Research, 11(3),* 1–22

Whitehead, S. (2017). Building resilience: How research has been used to develop and evaluate a media and communication approach. *BBC Media Action*. https://dataportal.bbcmediaaction.org/site/assets/uploads/2016/07/Building-Resilience-research-report.pdf

Wilke, A. M., Green, D. P., & Cooper, J. (2020). A placebo design to detect spillovers from an education–entertainment experiment in Uganda. *Journal of the Royal Statistical Society Series A: Statistics in Society, 183*(3), 1075–1096.

Williams, O., & Swierad, E. M. (2019). A multisensory multilevel health education model for diverse communities. *International Journal of Environmental Research and Public Health, 16*(5), 872–879.

Wodzak, S. (2023, March 30). 3 ways Duolingo improves education using AI. Duolingo Blog. https://blog.duolingo.com/ai-improves-education/

Yount, A. (2020). Virtual reality trains public to reverse opioid overdoses. https://www.asc.upenn.edu/news-events/news/virtual-reality-trains-public-reverse-opioid-overdoses

18

SOAP OPERAS RAISING AWARENESS OF PHYSICAL AND MENTAL WELLNESS

Jennifer L. Walton

Soap Operas and Health Awareness

In this chapter, I primarily focus on *General Hospital*, which has been a part of the daytime lineup on the ABC (American Broadcasting Company) in the United States for 60 years. The other soap operas that made up the ABC lineup were canceled many years ago, with two of the three remaining shows on that network (*All My Children* and *One Life to Live*) canceled in 2011 to make way for less expensive lifestyle shows. Both soaps averaged 2.5 million viewers daily which ranked them 5th and 4th, respectively, out of 6 daytime dramas on the air at the time (Rice, 2011). *General Hospital* was not affected by the cuts and continued on the air as of 2024, attracting 2.2 million viewers daily (Lewis, 2024). In all, three daytime dramas remain in production in the United States – *General Hospital* as well as *The Young and the Restless* and *The Bold and the Beautiful*, with the latter two airing on CBS.

To provide background, as a genre, soap operas began on the radio in the 1930s and then successfully transitioned to television. These continuing dramas are characterized by large ensemble casts and often melodramatic plot lines. While these serials were on the radio in the United States, their biggest sponsor was Procter and Gamble, a soap manufacturing company, and those laundry commercials resulted in the genre's nickname of "soap opera" (Ashby, 2006).

Forms of the genre have aired around the world – including long-running shows in the United Kingdom (e.g., *Coronation Street*, *Emmerdale Farm*, and *EastEnders*) and Australia (*Home and Away* and *Neighbors* (see, e.g., IMDB, n.d.; Knox, 2023) – as well as shorter-run telenovelas (see R. Allen, 1995b; Rios & Castaneda, 2011). Soaps in the U.S. have aired for decades like *General Hospital*, making them multigenerational (see R. Allen, 1995b; Ford et al., 2010; Levine, 2020). (*Young and the Restless* has aired for 50 years, with The *Bold and the Beautiful* in its 35th year of production.) It is commonplace to hear people talk about watching soap operas with their mothers, grandmothers, and aunts (Ford et al., 2010). According to Ford et al., the multigenerational, longitudinal nature of soaps creates an intense connection for viewers, given that viewers tune in 5 days a week, 52 weeks a year, unlike the weekly and seasonal nature of primetime television programming (see also related argument by Beck, 2012).

 DOI: 10.4324/9781003436409-21

Positive Effect or Bad Influence?

Soap operas feature powerful positive and negative messages embedded within them. Story arcs in soap operas can be fun and carefree, romance-driven plotlines, but they can also include stark overtones and undertones, while still maintaining an entertainment value. Some critics consider soap operas to be low-quality, low-budget smut that keeps housewives entertained while their children go to school or nap (see R. Allen, 1995a). This contention implies that soap operas hold no redeeming qualities and, certainly, little social value. As such, those critics overlook the values that these dramas depict, never mind their rhetorical potential.

However, I disagree. As I argue in this chapter, soap operas should be explored for their rhetorical effects that potentially impact the attitudes and actions of the viewers. This chapter examines how soap operas can have a positive impact by educating the audience about important mental and physical health issues.

Mental and Emotional Heath

Mental health constitutes a prevailing theme in soap operas, and soap operas have addressed this issue since the beginning (Ford et al., 2010). Psychiatric disorders have been the most frequently visited ailments over the decades, and soap operas have historically not portrayed these conditions in a realistic manner. In recent years, though, soap operas have depicted both men and women suffering from mental illness, which marks a significant change from the early days of soaps when they predominantly treated mental illness as a "female" issue (Ford et al., 2010). In this section, I focus on bipolar disorder and autism spectrum disorder (which comprises a developmental disorder and is not categorized as a mental health issue but can impact emotional health). I argue that, although soap opera storylines tend to include melodramatic circumstances that the characters create as a result of being unwell, positive messages can still be gleaned from the storylines.

Bipolar Disorder

How are issues identified? Residents of *General Hospital*'s fictional town, Port Charles, New York, have come to know mobster Sonny Corinthos as a tough, no-nonsense crime lord who can be deadly if crossed. This reputation has comprised Sonny's outer persona; however, once his loved ones (and the audience) got to know him, he could be kind, sensitive, and perhaps a little moody. After many years, Sonny's moodiness started to take a toll on his personal and professional life. When something did not go his way, he destroyed his home and made other destructive decisions. Eventually, after much encouragement, Sonny sought help, and doctors diagnosed him with bipolar disorder.

According to the National Institute for Mental Health (2023), bipolar disorder constitutes a mood disorder signified by unusual shifts in mood and energy levels. Historically, practitioners referred to the disorder as manic depression, and many considered it to be just simple mood swings. However, the U.S. Department of Health and Human Services (2023a) noted that bipolar is a very serious disorder that can damage relationships, cause poor job performance, and even result in suicide.

To date, Sonny Corinthos has been presented as a volatile character, quick to react and suffer the consequences later. His temper has resulted in divorces, the conception of children, the breakup of friendships, and estrangement from family. Sonny's mood swings started to become severe and threaten his family and business when he went through a particularly traumatic period in his life. Sonny learned that his estranged brother (Ric) planned to marry his ex-girlfriend (Alexis), which would make Ric the stepfather to Sonny's daughter, Kristina. Unfortunately, Ric was waging a personal and professional war against Sonny. Ric and Sonny shared the same mother, and Ric always blamed his mother's death on Sonny, swearing vengeance. Furthermore, Ric worked for the District

Attorney's office in Port Charles. Ric decided that if he could not bring Sonny down personally, he would have him arrested and tried on racketeering charges.

For many years, other characters just envisioned Sonny as unpredictable and dangerous and considered those attributes a part of Sonny's personality that could not be changed – until Emily Quartermaine stepped into the picture. Emily was the younger sister of Sonny's best friend and business partner, Jason Morgan. While Sonny's ex-wife and the mother of his children (Carly) was institutionalized after having a mental breakdown, Emily moved into Sonny's house to help him take care of his children. This move seemed a bit odd because Sonny and Emily had little onscreen presence together up to that point. Thus, the show left viewers to assume that she was doing her brother a favor by helping his best friend and business partner. It did not take long for Sonny and Emily to connect emotionally, romantically, and physically.

Emily began to care about Sonny, and she wanted to take care of him. She could see that he was dealing with a lot of stress and was not handling it well. Sonny was drinking too much and having emotional outbursts that caused him to throw glasses, pitchers, vases, and anything else that could break and cause a scene. Instead of walking out on Sonny, Emily wanted to help him understand his issues and deal with them in a healthier manner.

After many discussions, arguments, and fights, Emily finally got through to him. She helped him realize that his behavior was not normal or healthy, and, as time went on, the situation grew worse. Emily convinced him to stop drinking and seek help for his mood swings. Sonny sought professional assistance from a psychiatrist, and, through therapy and medication, he was able to manage his bipolar disorder.

How are issues used to promote awareness in the audience? This bipolar story arc involved more than another plotline conjured up in the writer's room to boost ratings during sweeps week. The show carefully constructed and placed this story upon the soap opera canvas, not coincidentally featuring Sonny as the character afflicted with this illness. Maurice Benard, the actor who has played Sonny for 30 years, suffers from bipolar disorder, and, since his diagnosis, he has become a face and voice for the illness. In fact, he recently released an autobiography, entitled *Nothing General About It: How Love and Lithium Saved Me On and Off General Hospital* (2020), where he detailed his struggles with mental illness and the challenges that he faced as a young man before his diagnosis. According to ABC News (2008), doctors diagnosed Benard with manic-depressive disorder (as it was known at the time) when he was 21 years old. Benard encountered unbelievable highs and unbearable lows. As Benard wrote in his book, after diagnosis and treatment, he has been managing the illness in a healthy manner for 39 years.

In 2022, Bernard decided that he wanted to continue the conversation that he initiated with his autobiography, and he started hosting a podcast, *State of Mind.* This podcast features his family members and co-stars discussing their mental health challenges. Through his podcast and advocacy work with *General Hospital*, he seeks to erase the stigma that continues to surround discussions about mental health and mental illness.

In 2006, *General Hospital's* head writer (Robert Guza) approached Benard and asked him if he would be interested in Sonny's character having a "breakdown" storyline. Benard responded with a resounding yes, but with one caveat. The breakdown had to be a result of bipolar disorder, and the storyline had to be portrayed in a responsible manner and used to educate the public on bipolar disorder, its symptoms and treatment (ABC News, 2008; Benard, 2020).

Guza granted Benard's request. The show portrayed Sonny's bipolar breakdown realistically and with an educational element. The character of Sonny was compelled to examine his behavior patterns over the years. After much denial and resentment, Sonny finally accepted his diagnosis and started a treatment plan that included therapy and medication. Per Benard's wishes, at the conclusion of each episode featuring the bipolar storyline, a public service announcement aired with Maurice Benard discussing his personal experience. Benard encouraged viewers to consult a physician, call a hotline, or visit a website if they experienced any of Sonny's symptoms.

In the ensuing years, bipolar disorder has been written onto the *General Hospital* canvas occasionally. Morgan Corinthos was Sonny's youngest son, and he was always a good kid—studious and well behaved. When Morgan became a teenager between 2013 and 2016, his behavior changed, and he became unpredictable and reckless. Sonny began to recognize the signs and understood that one can have a genetic predisposition to the illness if a close relative has been diagnosed (U.S. National Library of Medicine, 2021). After a great deal of struggle and strife, the family got Morgan into treatment, but, in true soap fashion, he did not simply live happily ever after. While in one of his manic phases, he fell in love with a much older woman who was rather villainous, Ava Jerome. In a jealous rage, she switched out his lithium with placebos, and Morgan died while making reckless and dangerous decisions. (Morgan died in a car bomb meant for his father.) This storyline gave Maurice Benard another opportunity to raise awareness about bipolar disorder, alerting viewers that the average age of onset is 25 years old but often occurs much earlier (NAMI, 2023).

Over the past 18 years, on occasion, Sonny's life has spun out of control, and he has occasionally decided to stop taking his medication, exacerbating the chaos. Those incidents have put Sonny's bipolar disorder back on the canvas and given Maurice Benard another opportunity to use the storyline to educate the audience about his illness and how it can be managed. *General Hospital* has always handled these storylines responsibly, even if the circumstances surrounding the illness are dramatic and unrealistic.

Autism Spectrum Disorder

How are issues identified? Over the last 46 years of *General Hospital*, the audience has been introduced to multiple generations of the Quartermaine family, including fourth-generation family member, Leo Falconeri Quartermaine. Leo is the son of Olivia Falconeri and Julian Jerome, head of the Jerome Crime family, who is presumed dead. Olivia married Ned Quartermaine, who adopted Leo.

The show introduced Leo as unique and not sharing many of the same interests as his cousins. He tended to spend time alone focusing on books about animals and talking at length about the facts that he learned in those books. When he was seven years old in 2023, Leo visited a local hotel pool and cut his finger. His mother took him to the hospital to get stitches, and a new doctor, Austin Gatlin-Holt (an illegitimate cousin of the Quartermaine clan), treated Leo's finger. While at the appointment, Dr. Gatlin-Holt noticed behaviors that he found curious. Leo didn't make eye contact, showed no interest in holding conversations but, at other times, seemed a bit obsessive about some topics. He also did not listen when people spoke to him and tended to wander off. The National Institute of Mental Health (2023) listed all these behaviors as symptoms of autism spectrum disorder. Since Dr. Gatlin-Holt suspected this diagnosis but was not an expert, he mentioned to Ned and Olivia that Leo might benefit from visiting a specialist and may need to find new ways to learn. He never said autism, but the implication that something might be amiss with Leo outraged Olivia. She emphasized that nothing was wrong with her son and that Dr. Gatlin-Holt needed to stay in his lane.

Ned, however, expressed concern about Leo. He had noticed unusual behaviors and worried about him wandering away. Olivia refused to entertain any possibility of a problem. As an illegitimate cousin of the Quartermaines, Olivia suspected that the doctor sought to exact revenge for being cut out of his grandfather's will and losing out on a sizeable inheritance.

How are issues used to promote awareness? Olivia experienced a very common reaction. Denial of even the hint of autism is usually the first stage of the diagnosis for families (Barbera, 2023). Although common and understandable, denial does not help the autistic child. According to Barbera, the sooner the family starts interventions, the better for the child. Fortunately for Leo, Olivia came around and finally took him to a specialist, but that decision only came as a response to a dangerous situation.

A short time after Dr. Gatlin-Holt suggested a specialist for Leo, the Jerome Gallery held a National Geographic gala. Since the gala featured many photographs of various animals, Olivia and Ned took Leo. Leo wandered out of the gallery onto the docks, where he lay down on the pier next to the water. Leo's disappearance terrified his family, and once they found him and reflected on the potential danger he faced when he wandered off, Olivia agreed to take Leo to a specialist.

General Hospital raised awareness of autism spectrum disorder in an unusual fashion, not typical of the soap's standard playbook. The actor who plays Leo, Easton Rocket Sweda, has autism. He took to Instagram:

> "Hi, I'm Easton Rocket Sweda," he said in a video shared on Instagram, "and I'm Leo from GENERAL HOSPITAL, the famous soap opera. Yesterday, he got diagnosed with autism, but you know what's cool? I have autism, too! I was diagnosed when I was very young," Sweda continued. "And I couldn't speak until I was four. And now look at me. I have a cool life and kids with autism are cool. You have a good life too with autism. Bye." He waved and blew a kiss, then quickly added, "Happy new year!"
>
> *(Sweda, 2022)*

General Hospital presented autism as just an alternate approach to learning and being in the world. The show did not take a negative tone when discussing it. Furthermore, using an actor who has autism was noteworthy because he understood how to play the part. This choice illustrated that children with the diagnosis can lead a happy, fulfilling life, much like Maurice Benard playing a character with bipolar disorder. These storylines on *General Hospital* spotlighted that, with proper intervention and treatment, people who experience these conditions can live normal lives.

Physical Heath

Soap operas specifically avoided physical illness and disease in the earliest days of the genre. They tended not to connect illness and death, and characters typically died of fictitious ailments or external factors such as car accidents, plane crashes, or murder (Ford et al., 2010). This trend continued into the 1960s, with a couple of noteworthy exceptions on *All My Children* and *The Guiding Light*, but, in recent decades, health issues have become more prevalent and realistically portrayed. Health issues such as HIV/AIDS, cancer, and Alzheimer's Disease have been prominently painted onto the soap opera canvas. In this section, I will discuss a few of the physical health issues that have been featured on *General Hospital.*

Cancer

How are issues identified? Several instances of cancer have occurred on *General Hospital* over the years. One of the more powerful cancer storylines focused on Alexis Davis. The character of Alexis has had a sordid history on the show, starting from her arrival in the mid-1990s. Her identity as a Cassadine heir placed her in the midst of the Spencer/Cassadine feud, and that feud made the wedding of Luke and Laura infamous. Luke also saved the world from the Cassadine weather machine back in the early 1980s (with a brief comeback for the weather machine in 2022). Clearly, this rivalry has proven deadly. After the weather machine failed, Port Charles remained free of Cassadines for many years, but writers brought the family back onto the canvas shortly after Luke and Laura returned to Port Charles in the early 1990s.

Beyond the Cassadine drama, Alexis held positions that were at odds with each other over the years. She served as a mob lawyer for Sonny Corinthos and his organization, leading to an affair that resulted in the birth of her daughter Kristina. After it became clear to Alexis that her mob connection ran too deep, she ended both her personal and professional relationships with Sonny and became the District Attorney for the City of Port Charles. This new career path created obvious conflicts of interest because of her former mob connections.

While in the D.A.'s office, Alexis started to have terrible bouts of coughing. After several friends and family members conveyed their concern, she finally went to the hospital, getting confirmation of her biggest fear – she had stage two lung cancer. This diagnosis was quite a shock to everyone because Alexis had never smoked nor had much contact with other carcinogens known to cause lung cancer. After being diagnosed with lung cancer, she left the D.A.'s office and went into private practice, eventually forming a partnership with her dear friend, Diane Miller.

How are issues used to promote awareness in the audience? This storyline promoted awareness in a few different ways. Alexis' diagnosis came just five months after Dana Reeve died from lung cancer. Dana Reeve, who was best known as the widow of Christopher Reeve, died of lung cancer after being a nonsmoker her entire life (ABC News, 2006). This real-life story received a lot of media attention because health care professionals and public opinion alike inevitably linked lung cancer to smoking. According to the ABC News report, Reeve worked as a lounge singer in smoky conditions for most of her life, and doctors attributed her diagnosis to second-hand smoke.

This storyline took an unexpected turn while Alexis received chemotherapy. Damien Spinelli arrived in Port Charles shortly after Alexis' diagnosis. At the time of his arrival, the audience knew very little about Spinelli, other than that he was a college student and computer genius. Alexis' eldest daughter, Samantha, also suspected that he could be an avid marijuana user. Alexis' chemotherapy treatment left her weak and nauseous with no appetite. After researching chemotherapy and possible ways to relieve side effects, Samantha solicited help from Spinelli, assuming, at the very least, his access to a supplier if not an impressive stash of marijuana. At first, Spinelli feigned offense but finally conceded that he could help her mother get relief from the chemotherapy side effects.

After procuring a reasonable dosage, Samantha tried to convince her mother that marijuana would help her nausea and appetite. Convincing Alexis proved quite a task since she was recently an officer of the law. However, after much encouragement from both Samantha and Spinelli and in desperate need of relief, Alexis gave in and tried the herbal remedy. Much to her delight, the marijuana proved to be the magic treatment that cured her weakness, increased her appetite, and gave her the strength to continue the chemotherapy, which eventually cured her cancer. In recent years, marijuana has been regarded as an effective treatment for many of the side effects associated with chemotherapy (Centers for Disease Control, 2020).

General Hospital did not take a stand on medical marijuana on screen or in post-episode PSAs. The show addressed it only as an entertaining storyline with an ironic twist since Alexis had served as the former District Attorney. However, the storyline brought attention to lung cancer, second-hand smoke, and the importance of getting screened for those at risk or experiencing symptoms. Portrayer Nancy Lee Grahn (Alexis) starred in the public service announcements after the episodes that featured her cancer storyline. Grahn stated in the PSAs that her father died of emphysema, and she wanted to honor her father by encouraging others to become healthy by becoming ex-smokers.

HIV/AIDS

How are issues identified? The Robin Scorpio/Stone Cates HIV/AIDS storyline constituted one of the most daring and educational storylines launched by *General Hospital* (ABC7, 2010). In the 1990s, several misconceptions still existed about HIV and AIDS, and *General Hospital* chose to explore the issue in great depth through this impactful storyline.

Viewers watched Robin Scorpio grow up over the years. She started out as a precocious seven-year-old and grew into a beautiful, intelligent young woman. Robin was always the picture of perfection, getting perfect grades, never staying out past curfew, and certainly never getting involved with the wrong boys. All of that remained the same except for the latter when Robin met Stone Cates, changing her life forever.

Stone was a homeless street thug who had recently obtained work with Sonny Corinthos and his organized crime outfit. Sonny took Stone under his wing and became an older brother figure to him. Life took a very positive turn for Stone then, much better than his previous situation on the streets. Sonny was dating Brenda Barrett, a close friend of Robin Scorpio. Through Sonny and Brenda, Robin met Stone. They fell hard and fast for each other and eventually made love. Shortly after consummating their relationship, Stone tested positive for HIV and panicked. He feared that he had infected the woman he loved and that he was going to die, and Robin would die. Robin tested immediately, with an HIV-negative result. Stone felt relieved that Robin had not contracted the disease, but it was too late for Stone. Stone slowly wasted away and died in Robin's arms. After Stone died, Robin tested again and received an HIV-positive result. The first test had been administered too soon after the initial infection.

How are issues used to promote awareness in the audience? This storyline took place in the 1994/1995 seasons of *General Hospital*. The disease was still in its infancy at that point, and the public had several misconceptions about both the facts and myths concerning the illness. Many still believed that only gay men could contract the disease (McCarthy, 2019) and that it could never happen to anyone they knew, including Robin Scorpio. Even though a fictional character, viewers watched Robin grow up from a young child into adulthood, and we felt connected to her through parasocial bonding (see, for example, Forster, 2023; Giles, 2002). Brooks (2023) explained that parasocial bonding comprises the tendency to create a relationship between a viewer and a fictional character. Since so many fans (me included) grew up right alongside Robin, we felt that we knew her, and she was our friend (see related work by Searle & Shea, 2017). This storyline shook us – if Robin can get HIV, anyone can get HIV.

General Hospital posted public service announcements about HIV and AIDS while in the depths of Stone's battle with the disease, providing information about the illness and educational opportunities for the audience at home. Those messages urged audience members to have safe sex, get tested often, and not ignore potential symptoms. The public service announcements did stop after some time had passed, but, close to two decades after the first AIDS-related episode aired, the education and awareness have continued.

General Hospital's awareness campaign did not end with the initial arc. To date, the AIDS and HIV storylines have continued since Robin has remained a prominent character in the history of the show, even though she is not always on the canvas. Kimberly McCullough (who portrayed Robin) eventually left the show but has reprised the role for certain storylines. In the ensuing years, Robin earned her medical degree, studied drug protocols that can be used as less invasive options to surgery, and experienced personal success using HIV drug protocols. The character has treated HIV-positive patients and educated medical staff who were prejudiced against patients who are HIV-positive. She also traveled to Africa to lend her medical skills and research background in combating the disease in one of the most HIV/AIDS-ravaged continents.

The mid-1990s marked a turning point in HIV treatment, and Robin contracted the disease after the medical community had developed a drug therapy that made it possible to live with HIV rather than die from AIDS. In 1991, we learned that Magic Johnson had contracted HIV, and, 30 years later, he is not only surviving but thriving and using a devastating diagnosis to educate the public about the disease (NPR, 2022; Uenuma, 2021; see also Chapter 15, this volume). Robin's storyline parallels this real-life health narrative.

Finally, for years following Stone's death, *General Hospital* held an annual event called the Nurses' Ball. The event constituted a fundraiser to raise money and awareness for HIV/AIDS. From 1994 to 2001 and again from 2013 to the present every spring, *General Hospital* dedicated several weeks to the planning and execution of the Nurses' Ball. The Nurses' Ball, and the ball was not only a fictional fundraiser, but it also actually helped to raise money from viewers. Viewers could buy Nurses' Ball tee shirts and donate money to HIV/AIDS charities. Viewers and characters alike looked forward to the ball each year. One of the most popular characters on the show, Lucy Coe, always served as the emcee, and the ball featured musical numbers performed by popular characters on the show. According to ABC7 News (2023), Lynn Herring (who has portrayed Lucy Coe) stated that "the ball represents everything good that we do in daytime and we have reality for a cause in AIDS/HIV." In that same news report, actress Finola Hughes (who has portrayed Anna Devane, Robin Scorpio's mother) stated that "I think we bring home the conversation about HIV/AIDS and I think it's done in a very elegant and very kind way. We have fun, but we're also reminding people that we have to take responsibility for each other." *Port Charles* – a short-lived spin-off from *General Hospital* that focused on medical school students, interns, residents, and nurses – provided many cross-over opportunities for the Nurses' Ball, increasing the audience and fundraising opportunities.

Robin's character has kept all the HIV storylines educational and true to life. Through it all, *General Hospital* and the character of Robin have increased awareness and, in the process, raised money for HIV/AIDS research.

Alzheimer's Disease

How are issues identified? In my perspective, the Alzheimer's disease storyline on *General Hospital* marked the crowning achievement of the *GH* writers in terms of raising awareness of all aspects of this devastating illness. Not surprisingly, the show featured Maurice Benard (Sonny Corinthos) at the center of this storyline since he drives many of the socially responsible and realistic portrayals of both physical and mental health illnesses. In this story arc, the show reintroduced Sonny's father Mike Corbin. Mike was a major character in the *General Hospital* universe (including the *GH* spin-off *Port Charles*) in the early 2000s, portrayed at the time by Ron Hale. The first several story arcs involved considerable conflict over Sonny's toxic childhood caused by Mike. Mike was an absentee father who had a gambling addiction, causing Sonny's parents to divorce. Sonny's mother remarried, and his stepfather was abusive and cruel. Sonny never really forgave his father, but, over the years, they tried to reconcile with limited success. Mike Corbin left Port Charles in 2010 but reentered the landscape in 2017. Much to the delight of television fans, actor Max Gail from *Barney Miller* fame took over the role.

Sonny and Mike attempted to forge a new relationship after years of estrangement, but doing so proved difficult. Mike began to experience memory lapses occasionally. Although it was initially easy to attribute the memory issues to aging, the problems escalated. Mike was living in Brooklyn at this time, and after Sonny observed Mike and his troubling behavior, Sonny moved Mike to his home in Port Charles.

As a wealthy mobster, Sonny sought the best doctors to help Mike. After many tests and hospital stays, doctors diagnosed Mike with Alzheimer's Disease. According to the Alzheimer's Foundation of America (2022), Alzheimer's Disease comprises a form of dementia. Dementia is a general category that results in a decline in memory, impaired judgment, and complex motor skills. Many different types of dementia-related illnesses exist, but Alzheimer's Disease is the most common in persons aged 65 and older, accounting for 60 to 80% of cases. According to the Centers for Disease Control (CDC, 2023), Alzheimer's Disease and other types of dementia are not a normal part of the aging process.

Alzheimer's Disease is a multifaceted and multistage illness, and *General Hospital* viewers witnessed Mike and Sonny as they navigated each of the stages in a true-to-life and responsible manner. According to the Mayo Clinic (2024), several different stages and behaviors accompany a diagnosis. The patient and families must first accept the reality of the diagnosis—a process requiring time to absorb the information. Following acceptance, patients and their families experience the early, middle, and late stages of the illness and caregiving.

No two patients always exhibit the same symptoms and behaviors, but researchers have identified commonalities. Alzheimer's patients can experience aggression, anxiety, depression, and confusion – all common and understandable symptoms. Some troubling behaviors include delusions and hallucinations (Alzheimer's Foundation of America, 2022). *General Hospital* portrayed a realistic decline for Mike, given his Alzheimer's diagnosis. The show also represented the trauma and impact that the diagnosis has on the Alzheimer's patient's loved ones.

How are issues used to promote awareness in the audience? Alzheimer's Disease is a brutal illness, and it takes some time for the patient and loved ones to come to terms with it. As with other illnesses and issues, *General Hospital* bookended each episode that featured the Alzheimer's storyline with a public service announcement about the disease, symptoms, and a hotline or website where a viewer could learn more about the illness. The show remained consistent in its responsible messaging. However, the show took the message a step further and created a social media campaign to raise awareness and offer fans an outlet to post about their experiences. Maurice Benard (Sonny Corinthos) posted on Facebook: "Our Alzheimer's storyline has shown me how important it is to raise awareness. This disease affects us all" (Alzheimer's Association, 2019). This quote prompted viewers to share their experiences and their opinions on how *General Hospital* portrayed the disease. Comments posted in response to Maurice Benard's post included:

> My sister has Alzheimer's. I thought the show did a good job of showing what it is like living with a person in the early stages. I'm hoping it will continue with the story line. Alzheimer's get much worse. Alzheimer's gets ugly. You have to remember your family member is still in there. They change but they are in there.
>
> *(Alzheimer's Association, 2019)*

> This is such a compelling storyline. Max Gail does a terrific job of Mike, who is afflicted with Alzheimer's. The look of confusion on his face is heartbreaking. Sonny does his best to keep it all together.
>
> *(Alzheimer's Association, 2019)*

> My dad had it as well as a couple brothers and sister and aunt. Now lucky me, I have it. I worry about my son, daughter and granddaughter. It's being studied to death with no cure in sight.
>
> *(Alzheimer's Association, 2019)*

The comments continued for many pages, with nothing but praise for how the show handled the storyline, as well as their own experiences, fears, and hopes for a cure.

Throughout the Alzheimer's story arc (which lasted four years), viewers witnessed all of the common stages of the disease. When Mike appeared back on the *GH* canvas, he had mild symptoms, which included short-term memory loss. That memory loss became apparent when Sonny visited Mike in Brooklyn and prompted the move back to Port Charles. Next, the show depicted difficulty in solving problems, and Mike exhibited frustration when everyday issues became difficult to navigate, leading to changes in his personality (another symptom of mild illness). As more things began to challenge him, he started to exude anger and hostility toward all of his loved ones who were trying to help him. Mike also struggled to organize and express thoughts, which also triggered anger and frustration. Finally, he got lost frequently and misplaced things. On more than one occasion, Mike got lost and couldn't explain who he was or where he was going. For example, very early in his illness, he took his granddaughter

Avery out for ice cream, and he began to think that she was his deceased daughter, Courtney. These events caused great concern to Sonny and his family. The family hired full-time in-home care for Mike, so he didn't wander off or put anyone else in danger. Mayo Clinic (2024) discussed the importance of taking advantage of services like in-home care and memory care facilities when symptoms worsen.

As the disease progressed, Mike entered the moderate phase of Alzheimer's Disease, characterized by greater memory loss. Mike no longer always recognized Sonny and other family members. He needed more assistance with daily tasks and activities. The home health workers helped in this regard since their original role was to keep an eye on him. When his daily routine became a challenge, they stepped in and assisted him when he needed a hand. Finally, he exhibited significant personality changes. Most often, those changes involved anger, hostility, and violent outbursts. The violence became common, and a social worker suggested Sonny place Mike in a care facility that specialized in Alzheimer's Disease and memory care. Sonny felt like he would be giving up on Mike, and he couldn't agree to moving him into a facility full time, but he did compromise and use the care center's adult day care service, benefiting Mike and his family. The facility provided activities and socialization that kept Mike stimulated and less hostile.

The final stage of Alzheimer's Disease is the most traumatic for the patients and their loved ones. In this stage, the patient loses the ability to communicate, requiring constant care. Patients also lose their motor skills, and their muscles become rigid and reflexes abnormal (Mayo Clinic, 2024). When Mike started to suffer from these issues, Sonny moved him into the care facility full-time, and he was confined to his bed 24 hours a day. Once Mike reached this stage, the family realized the end was near. Sonny did arrange some outings to try to jog some of Mike's memories, and, in some cases, it did work. He took him to the stables at the racetrack. As a gambling addict and fan of the racetrack, it proved beneficial for Mike to interact with the horses.

Regrettably, Sonny didn't think of this possibility sooner. According to K. Allen (2021), interacting with animals can benefit Alzheimer's patients by helping with problem behavior, increasing nutritional intake which can result in fewer supplements, thereby lowering the cost of care. Interacting with animals can also reduce anxiety, increase socialization, and motivate patients to exercise, staying active longer. While pets can create a danger for some patients by creating a tripping hazard, and Alzheimer's patients can forget to feed their pets, some programs certify dogs and other pets to visit care facilities and homebound patients. While the interaction isn't as prolonged, patients still benefit. Wherever the setting and whatever kind of animal, the benefits remain. According to Edwards and Beck (2002), pets can make a big difference in the daily life of an Alzheimer's patient, and they provided a positive force in the final weeks of Mike's life. When he visited the horses, he recognized Sonny and his family members.

When a patient enters the end stage of Alzheimer's, they lose the ability to swallow and they lack an appetite (Mayo Clinic, 2024). Mike's condition at the end of his life reflected these symptoms. Sonny seriously considered granting permission for a feeding tube to provide nutrition to his father, but some hospital staff members and family talked him out of it. Sonny came to realize that a feeding tube wasn't going to improve Mike's quality of life. The feeding tube would have been more for Sonny than Mike in the end.

The impact on family and caregivers constitutes one of the most significant concerns in Alzheimer's Disease. According to the Alzheimer's Association (2023), caregiver stress constitutes a serious issue and one that needs attention. Caregiver stress can manifest in many ways – denial, anger, anxiety, and sleeplessness, etc. The stress associated with being a caregiver can cause physical and mental health problems for the caregiver. In *General Hospital*, Sonny and his family struggled with the diagnosis, treatment, and Mike's eventual death. At the behest of Sonny's family, Sonny sought support. Although not the type of person to typically feel comfortable in a support group setting, he and his family found comfort in a social worker.

Stella Henry (played by Vernie Watson-Johnson) proved to be a boon to the Corinthos family. According to London (2023), denial, fear, grief, and a general lack of understanding of the disease can impede a family member's ability to ask the right questions and communicate about the situation at all. Social workers can assist a family in a variety of ways. London argued that social workers can be trained in Alzheimer care and can assist families when they are feeling overwhelmed and helpless. A good social worker can become a messenger, a skilled listener, and an advocate. They can help families make difficult decisions and mediate disputes between stressed-out family members who may have differing opinions on the best way to move forward. Stella became an asset to the family and to Mike, and the family included her in family gatherings. Mike even started thinking of her as his girlfriend and looked forward to seeing her. Stella helped the family understand that they had to take one day at a time and meet Mike where he was. She helped them to see that they were not going to be able to convince him that he was confused and that they should not try to chastise him for not knowing someone or remembering an event.

Conclusion

In this chapter, I addressed the ways in which soap operas educate audiences about serious mental and physical health issues, such as promoting awareness of Alzheimer's Disease, helping viewers learn how to deal with the heartbreak of a cancer diagnosis, or understanding the signs and symptoms of bipolar or autism spectrum disorder. Soaps do not seem to lose any of their entertainment value in the process of promoting wellness, and that means that more and more viewers will continue to benefit from the service soap operas provide (see also related work on entertainment-education in Chapter 17, this volume).

In addition to depicting serious mental and physical health issues in an appropriate manner, soap operas also provide public service announcements with important information for the viewers and create entire social media campaigns to accompany the storyline. These messages contain hotlines and websites, along with the actors from the storylines emphasizing the importance of cancer screenings or getting tested for HIV. I argue that all this information holds value for the audience, especially those devoted viewers who tune in on a daily basis and identify greatly with the characters and their journeys.

Further Reading

Beck, C. S. (2012). Intersecting narratives: Enjoying daytime drama as viewers (and actors) experience the days of their lives. *Communication Studies, 63*(2), 152–171.

This article discusses the importance of soap operas to the viewership because of the multigenerational audiences and the viewers' relationships to both the storylines and the characters in the show.

Brunsdon, C. (2000). *The feminist housewife, and the soap opera*. Clarendon Press.

This book is an interesting piece that establishes soap opera research as a serious topic in scholarship.

Frentz, S. (1992). *Staying tuned: Contemporary soap opera criticism*. Bowling Green State University Press.

This book examines soap operas and discusses why they have continued to interest audiences for decades.

Scodari, C. (2004). *Serial monogamy: Soap Opera, lifespan, and the gendered politics of fantasy*. Hampton Press.

This book is a virtual ethnography that studies email groups, discussion boards, and other online soap opera fan groups.

References

ABC News. (2006, March 7). Friend: Dana Reeve died in peace. https://abcnews.go.com/GMA/story?id=1695995

ABC News. (2008, March 21). The cost of creativity: Bipolar disorder and the stars. https://abcnews.go.com/Health/MindMoodNews/story?id=4439015&page=1

ABC 7 News. (2010, September 28). General Hospital's super couple: Robin and Stone. *ABC 7 News Chicago*. https://abc7chicago.com/archive/7687374/

ABC 7 News. (2023). Music, dance, philanthropy filled nurses ball part of 'General Hospital' 60 year celebration. *ABC7 San Francisco*. https://abc7news.com/general-hospital-nurses-ball-60-anniversary-60th/13052457/

Allen, K. (2021, July 9). Alzheimer's disease: The magic of pets. *BrightFocus*. https://www.brightfocus.org/alzheimers/article/alzheimers-disease-magic-pets

Allen, R. (1995a). Introduction. In R. Allen (Ed.), *to be continued... Soap operas around the world* (pp. 1–26). Routledge.

Allen, R. (Ed.). (1995b). *to be continued... Soap operas around the world*. Routledge.

Alzheimer's Association. (2019). *Home* [Facebook page]. *Facebook*. ttps://m.facebook.com/actionalz/photos/a.10150446402959447/10158477736149447/?type=3&#_=_

Alzheimer's Association. (2023). *Caregiver stress*. Alzheimer's disease and dementia. https://www.alz.org/help-support/caregiving/caregiver-health/caregiver-stress

Alzheimer's Foundation of America. (2022, April 14). About Alzheimer's disease and dementia. https://alzfdn.org/caregiving-resources/about-alzheimers-disease-and-dementia/

Ashby, L. (2006). *With amusement for all*. University of Kentucky Press.

Barbera, M. (2023, April 25). How to get a parent out of autism denial. https://marybarbera.com/autism-denial/

Beck, C. S. (2012). Intersecting narratives: Enjoying daytime drama as viewers (and actors) experience the days of their lives. *Communication Studies*, *63*, 152–171.

Benard, M. (2020). *Nothing general about it: How love and lithium saved me on and off General Hospital*. Harper Collins.

Brooks, A. C. (2023, April 6). Parasocial relationships are just imaginary friends for adults. *The Atlantic*. https://www.theatlantic.com/family/archive/2023/04/parasocial-relationships-imaginary-connections-fans-celebrities/673645/

Centers for Disease Control and Prevention. (2020, October 19). Cancer. https://www.cdc.gov/marijuana/health-effects/cancer.html

Centers for Disease Control and Prevention. (2023, June 29). Recognizing symptoms of dementia and seeking help. *Alzheimer's Disease and Healthy Aging*. https://www.cdc.gov/aging/publications/features/dementia-not-normal-aging.html

Edwards, N. E., & Beck, A. M. (2002). Animal-assisted therapy and nutrition in Alzheimer's Disease. *Western Journal of Nursing Research, 24,* 697–712.

Ford, S., DeKosnik, A., & Harrington, C. L. (2010). Introduction: The crisis of daytime drama and what it means for the future of television. In S. Ford, A. DeKosnik, & C. L. Harrington (Eds.), *The survival of soap opera: Transformations for a new media era* (pp. 3–21). University of Mississippi Press.

Forster, R. T. (Ed.). (2023). *The Oxford Handbook of parasocial experiences*. Oxford University Press.

Giles, D. C. (2002). Parasocial interaction: A review of the literature and model for future research. *Media Psychology*, *4*, 279–305.

IMBD. (n.d.). Long running British and Australian TV soap operas and dramas. https://www.imdb.com/list/ls062058058/

Knox, D. (2023, April 27). Australia's longest running TV shows: Part 1. *TV Tonight*. https://tvtonight.com.au/2023/04/australias-longest-running-tv-shows-pt-i.html

Levine, E. (2020). *Her stories: Daytime soap opera and US television history*. Duke University Press.

Lewis, E. (2024, January 9). Daytime broadcast ratings for the week of January 1-5, 2024. *Soap Opera Network*. https://www.soapoperanetwork.com/2024/01/daytime-broadcast-ratings-for-the-week-of-january-1-5-2024

Mayo Clinic. (2024, February 13). Alzheimer's disease. Mayo Foundation for Medical Education and Research. https://www.mayoclinic.org/diseases-conditions/alzheimers-disease/symptoms-causes/syc-20350447

McCarthy, J. (2019, June 28). *Gallup vault: Fear and anxiety during the 1980s AIDS crisis*. https://news.gallup.com/vault/259643/gallup-vault-fear-anxiety-during-1980s-aids-crisis.aspx

NAMI: National Alliance on Mental Illness. (2023). Bipolar disorder. https://www.nami.org/About-Mental-Illness/Mental-Health-Conditions/Bipolar-Disorder

National Institute of Mental Health. (2023, February). Bipolar disorder. https://www.nimh.nih.gov/health/topics/bipolar-disorder

NPR. (2022, October 4). Magic Johnson on basketball, business, and being the face of HIV: The limits with Jay Williams. https://www.npr.org/2022/10/04/1126788790/magic-johnson-on-basketball-business-and-being-the-face-of-hiv

Rice, L. (2011, April 14). Do canceled soap stars have another life to live. *Entertainment Weekly*. https://ew.com/article/2011/04/14/do-canceled-soap-stars-have-another-life-to-live/

Rios, D. I., & Castañeda, M. (Eds.). (2011). *Soap operas and telenovelas in the digital age*. Peter Lang.

Searle, E., & Shea, S. S. (Eds.). (2017). *Soap opera confidential: Writers and soap insiders on why we'll tune in tomorrow as the world turns restlessly by the guiding light of our lives*. McFarland.

Sweda, E. R. [@easton.rocket.sweda] (2022, February 1). I'm so excited to be on GH today! Thank you so much for all your support! [Video] Instagram. https://www.instagram.com/p/CZceFhdPOM7/?utm_source=ig_embed&utm_campaign=loading

Uenuma, F. (2021, November 4). Magic Johnson's HIV disclosure helped to shatter stigmas. But 30 years later, disparities in treatment remain. *Time*. https://time.com/6113046/magic-johnson-hiv-aids-impact/

U.S. National Library of Medicine. (2021). Bipolar disorder: Medlineplus genetics. https://medlineplus.gov/genetics/condition/bipolar-disorder/

U.S. Department of Health and Human Services. (2023a, February). *Autism spectrum disorder*. National Institute of Mental Health. https://www.nimh.nih.gov/health/topics/autism-spectrum-disorders-asd

19

"DIDN'T RING TRUE FOR ME"

Queering Breast Cancer, Graphic Medicine, and *Kimiko Does Cancer: A Graphic Memoir*

Sathyaraj Venkatesan

Introduction

Is medicine and healthcare accommodative and respectful of queer individuals? Whose stories/narratives receive attention and whose voices are ignored? Whose bodies are legible and whose are not? Is the medical system shaped by the norms and practices of heterosexuality and cisgender standards? Is there an influence of a prevailing heteronormativity on the experiences of queers within a clinic? What are the broader (health) implications of queer negligence and discriminatory practices? How does the genre of graphic medicine address such pressing concerns? This chapter investigates these questions through the close reading of some sections of *Kimiko Does Cancer: A Graphic Memoir* (hereafter *Kimiko*). In this essay, the name "Tobimatsu" will be used to refer to the author/narrator, while *Kimiko* will denote the graphic text co-authored by Kimiko Tobimatsu and illustrated by Keet Geniza. *Kimiko* offers a vital and unique perspective on the intersections of contemporary cancer and queer cultures. Most importantly, the graphic narrative sheds light on the challenges faced by marginalized individuals within healthcare systems and how they often encounter exclusion from cancer support groups that predominantly adhere to a heteronormative framework, emphasizing cure and unwavering optimism. Before I offer such a critical reading of *Kimiko*, it would be instructive to understand the historical emergence and evolution of graphic medicine, queer comics, and the general implications of heteronormativity among others.

Overview of Graphic Medicine

Various forms of media – including films, literature, dance, paintings, and songs – have depicted medical conditions over the years. In recent times, appreciation has grown for the potential of comics, graphic novels, and other forms of visual storytelling to explore a range of critical issues in healthcare. Labeled as graphic medicine in 2007 by a British physician and comics artist, Ian Williams (2015), graphic medicine refers to the intersection of comics and healthcare. Later, Green and Myers (2010) popularized the term in their article, "Graphic Medicine: Use of Comics in Medical Education and Patient Care." Emphasizing the uniqueness of these narratives, Venkatesan defined graphic medicine as "comics' distinctive engagement with and performance of illness experience (2016, p. 93). While graphic medicine has primarily focused on autobiographical and memoir-style narratives, it also encompasses a range of visual media such as graphic non-fiction (*Introducing Psychology*

DOI: 10.4324/9781003436409-22

(2014) by Nigel C. Benson), educational comics (*Rock Steady* (2018) by Ellen Forney), graphic novels (*Black Hole* (2005) by Charles Burns), among others. The critical high point in the evolution of graphic medicine is the publication of Czerwiec et al.'s *Graphic Medicine Manifesto* by Penn State University Press in 2015. This groundbreaking compendium of scholarly essays serves as the inaugural volume in a series devoted to graphic medicine, thus laying a theoretical foundation for this field. In recent years, graphic medicine has expanded its scope, as noted by Czerwiec et al., to include "more work about the environmental contexts in which we all live ... health and social activism, about how our political and financial environments impact our health" (p. 105).

Underground/alternative comics (aka. "comix") of the 1960s and the narrative medicine movement of the 1990s influenced graphic medicine as a field. While narrative medicine emphasized a patient-centered approach, underground comics boldly addressed taboo themes such as masturbation, incest, female sexuality, drugs, affective disorders among others. The roots of narrative medicine lie in the work of Rita Charon (2008), who emphasized the importance of understanding and interpreting patients' stories as a means of improving healthcare outcomes. In the "Introduction" to the *Graphic Medicine Manifesto*, Williams (2015) enunciated the correlation of graphic medicine with the aims of narrative medicine thus: "graphic medicine combines the principles of narrative medicine with an exploration of the visual systems of comic art, interrogating the representation of physical and emotional signs and symptoms within the medium" (p. 1). By harnessing the creative freedom of the comix movement while expanding the fundamental principles of narrative medicine, graphic medicine enables a rich exploration of the diverse interpretations of illness, disease, sickness, and the practice of medicine.

Though several comics, cartoons, comic series, and newspaper strips addressed health and medical issues in the first half of the 20th century (for example, *True Comics, Real Heroes,* etc.), Justin Green's *Binky Brown Meets the Holy Virgin Mary* (1972) inaugurated graphic medicine. As the first confessional autobiographical comics, *Binky Brown Meets the Holy Virgin Mary** is a meditation on sexuality, OCD (Obsessive-Compulsive Disorder), and guilt. Other major graphic medical texts include Al Davison's (1990) *The Spiral Cage*, Harvey Pekar and Joyce Brabner's (1994) *Our Cancer Year*, Marisa Acocella Marchetto's (2006) *Cancer Vixen* (breast cancer), Brian Fies's (2006) *Mom's Cancer* (lung cancer), MK Czerwiec's (2017) *Taking Turns* (HIV/AIDS), Sarah Leavitt's (2010) *Tangles* (Alzheimer's), Stan Mack's (2004) *Janet and Me* (cancer), David B's *Epileptic* (Beauchard, 1996) (seizure disorder), Ken Dahl's *Monsters* (2009) (herpes), Joyce Farmer's (2010) *Special Exits* (aging and dying), Tucky Fussell's *Mammoir* (2005) (breast cancer), Ellen Forney's (2012) *Marbles* (bipolar disorder), and Ian Williams' (2014) *The Bad Doctor* (on doctors). These narratives, often autobiographical in nature, delve into important themes such as medical negligence, the complex doctor–patient relationship, the commercialization of healthcare, patient identity, the role of insurance providers, the challenges of caretaking, medical ethics, and the demands of being a doctor, among others. Together, challenging the authority of medical knowledge and practice through utilizing the subversive potential of comics, graphic medicine articulates several "aspects of social experience that escape both the normal realms of medicine and the comforts of canonical literature" (Squier, 2008, p. 130). As Holmes (2013) reminded us, the word "Graphic" also connotes "the scandalous and subversive potential that is part of the shared histories of comics and representations of the body" (p. 148). Given such strengths, it is not surprisingly, graphic medicine has a wide array of potential readers, ranging from healthcare providers and medical students to patients, caretakers, and anyone interested in gaining insights into the human experience of illness and healing through the medium of comics (Couser, 1997; Williams, 2015b)

Queer Comics and Graphic Medicine

Queer represents a range of identities and orientations that fall outside of the traditional heterosexual and cisgender norms, including, but not limited to, lesbian, gay, bisexual, transgender, and non-binary individuals. In an abstract sense, queerness is an "open mesh of possibilities, gaps, overlaps, dissonances and resonances, lapses and excesses of meaning" (Sedgwick, 1993, p. 8). Graphic narratives, to paraphrase Gardner (2012), have long been known for providing a platform for marginalized voices, offering a unique opportunity for underrepresented groups to tell their respective stories and be heard.

As with graphic medicine, underground comics in the mid-1960s influenced LGBTQ+ comics, and that genre witnessed a phenomenal rise during and after countercultural (1960s) and post-Stonewall (1970s) movements in the U.S. During the 1980s, LGBTQ+ artists revolutionized the portrayal of queer lives in comics as a means of survival in the face of anti-LGBTQ+ prejudice and the HIV/AIDS crisis. Significant ones include *Strip AIDS* (Melia, 1987) and *Strip AIDS U.S.A.: A Collection of Cartoon Art to Benefit People with AIDS* (Robbins et al.,1988) and *Hothead Paisan* (DiMassa, 1993). While many underground and HIV/AIDS comics artists featured queer desire and sexuality, it was Alison Bechdel's (2008) *Dykes to Watch Out For* (1983–2008) and her memoir, *Fun Home: A Family Tragicomic* (2006), which positively consolidated the queer comics genre itself. Further, the mainstream publishers of comics, such as Marvel and DC Comics, also introduced queer characters, thus legitimizing LGBTQ+ lives. To quote Hillary Chute, "[q]ueer comics are one of the most vibrant areas of contemporary comics" (Chute, 2017, p. 349).

Recently (2015–2023), several graphic narratives have specifically explored the queer experiences in the context of healthcare. Representing a diverse range of voices and perspectives, Zena Sharman's (2016b) "*The Remedy: Queer and Trans Voices on Health and Health Care*," for instance, examined the often insensitive medical-industrial complex and the challenges faced by queer and transgender communities within healthcare systems (for related work, see Chapter 9, this volume). Other such graphic narratives that amplify queer experiences of healthcare include A. K. Summers' (2014) *Pregnant Butch*, Meg-John Barker's (2019) *Gender: A Graphic Guide*, Sabrina Symington's (2017) *First Year Out: A Transition Story* among others. These graphic narratives convey complex medical experiences, including harassment, marginalization, discrimination, and stigma undergone by queers. While these narratives predominantly critique the medical system for its queer incompetency, by combining visual storytelling with personal narratives to foster empathy, they also educate healthcare providers and empower patients to advocate for intersectional equity. More importantly, in many ways, these narratives highlight a lack of representation of queer experiences within the medical system. In the "Introduction" to *Pregnant Butch,* Summers, for instance, underscored the absence of stories about queers and emphasized the importance of writing these narratives not only to "broaden the scope of representation" but also to show who gets to tell these stories (p. 160). These narratives, in effect, make "the unseen visible" (n.p.), without which such experiences may be forgotten or ignored ("If you don't get it down, it didn't exist") (n.p.).

Queering Medicine

The medical establishment's historical distrust of queer bodies is an indisputable legacy, and several chapters in this section delve into its examination. For instance, the American Psychiatric Association's Diagnostic and Statistical Manual of Mental Disorders (DSM) removed homosexuality as a disease in its second edition in 1973 (Drescher 2015, p. 565). Worse still, transgender individuals were treated for "gender identity disorder" and subjected to corresponding treatment (e.g., ECT, conversion therapy, etc.). The AIDS crisis further "complicated and exacerbated what had already been a tense relationship between LGBTQ persons and biomedical practice" (Wahlert & Fiester, 2013, p. 86). Put differently, these characterizations medicalize queer bodies and their relational choices and deem them as pathological and unnatural. According to Wahlert and Fiester, "sexuality and gender identity retained a permutation of shame, having now migrated into a discourse of pathology" (p. 87).

In fact, the entire medical system is premised on a "persistent, negative culture … toward sexual and gender minority populations" (Mansh et al., 2015, p. 574). Lee (2018, p. 20) noted:

> Many governments still regard sexual and gender minorities as 'irresponsible' in terms of the global burden of both the HIV epidemic and mental disorders, and such a bias, without reasonable grounds, is one of the greatest impediments that prevents LGBT health from being considered on the global social health agenda.

Despite advancements in queer inclusivity, thanks to the LGBTQ+, feminist, and disability movements, medicine still overlooks queer bodies and renders them unintelligible and invisible in terms of care and treatment. More importantly, queer experiences are either erased or made hyper-visible, leading to undesirable health outcomes. Because sexual orientation and gender identity-related health concerns are "often not recognised, some health systems do not provide treatment guidelines or resources, or specific treatments or interventions may not be covered by health insurance" (Müller, 2022, p.165). Put together, "medical education, training, practice, and knowledge remains largely heteronormative, homophobic, and transphobic" (Robertson, 2019, p. 107). Citing Zeeman et al. (2019) and Mongelli et al. (2019), Pillay (2022) observed that "[t]hese omissions are glaring given the well-established, disproportionate burden of physical and psychosocial health disparities experienced by LGBT+ people, who have higher rates of both communicable and noncommunicable diseases than cisgender, heterosexual people" (p. 574).

Queer insensitivity manifests in various ways in a clinic, which may include one or a combination of the following: "being refused needed care; health care providers refusing to touch them or using excessive precautions; providers using harsh or abusive language; being blamed for their health status; providers being physically rough or abusive" (Sharman, 2016a, p. 13). Denying access to treatments can have serious consequences for queer individuals' mental and physical health, leading to increased rates of depression, anxiety, and suicide. In a book chapter titled "Challenging Heteronormativity in Medicine," Robertson (2019) listed the problems of practicing heteronormativity in medicine. According to Robertson, heteronormativity not only reproduces the extant health inequalities among the LGBTQ+ community but also causes minority stress. Additionally, as Robertson asserted, heteronormativity reduces "all LGBTQ health problems to sexual health" and treats "LGBTQ people as *inherently* more 'at risk' than straight or cisgender people" (p. 109).

A significant obstacle affecting the provision of adequate care to queers constitutes the lack of queer competency among healthcare providers (physicians and formal/paid caregivers). This problem can be attributed, at least in part, to the absence of queer perspectives in medical education and literature. Medical texts, for instance, predominantly adopt a cisgender and heterosexual viewpoint, resulting in a limited understanding of the unique healthcare needs and aspirations of queers. Such a limited perspective perpetuates a pathologizing, constrained, and underdeveloped approach toward queer bodies. This issue must be considered not only within medical and physician education but also among other healthcare professionals, including nurses and pharmacists, who play pivotal roles in providing care. Additionally, the social stigma associated with queerness further compounds the challenges faced by queer individuals in accessing appropriate healthcare. Although the acknowledgment and understanding of multiple intersectional identities has evolved, misogyny, homophobia, and transphobia across clinical contexts remain (Kelly & Rodriguez, 2022). In effect, medicine and healthcare, as Robertson (2019) observed, "absorbs, reflects, and institutionalizes all kinds of sociocultural norms and prejudices, including those concerning gender and sexuality" (p. 105). Tobimatsu's *Kimiko* illustrates how the medical system deals with queer individuals, addressing many of the concerns mentioned in this section. Paradoxically, even within ostensibly progressive environments, instances of heteronormative and ableist marginalization of queer aspirations endure, thus contributing to the marginalization of queers. More importantly, *Kimko* offers a distinctive and experientially rich personal viewpoint on these issues.

Text and Contexts of *Kimiko*

Published in 2020 and set in Toronto, *Kimiko* is a graphic memoir written by Kimiko Tobimatsu (2020a) and illustrated by Keet Geniza.[1] Identified as a cancer patient at the young age of 25, Tobimatsu is an employment and human-rights lawyer. Dedicated to "fellow sick queers," *Kimiko* told the life story of Tobimatsu's (a dyke) tryst with estrogen-positive breast cancer as a young, queer, and mixed-race woman. Reminiscent of the art style of Alison Bechdel in many ways, *Kimiko* exposed the inherent and unconscious biases of the (Canadian) healthcare system, portraying it as deeply entrenched in hetero-cis norms. In so doing, Tobimatsu offered the much-needed "dyke-insight" that Lorde (1980) asserted lacks in breast cancer narratives. Artistically speaking, the drawings in *Kimiko* are simple, direct, and realistic, offering the reader an intimate insight into the complexity of Tobimatsu's arduous cancer journey. Most importantly, *Kimiko* not only brought forth Tobimatsu's life stories that illuminate the unique experiences and challenges faced by queer individuals within the realm of medical care but also filled the gap in representation of queer experiences. To quote Tobimatsu in a related article, "I really came into this story thinking that there are not enough stories out there right now that are talking about queerness and the medical system and how that affects our care" (Käll, 2021, p. 160).

Influenced by Lorde as well as the comedy of Tig Notaro and the writings of Ericka Hart, Tobimatsu worked through various registers of subversion, commentary, and exposition to launch a multi-pronged critique of mainstream cancer culture, highlighting the commodification of cancer, queer negligence despite the promise of inclusivity and diversity, and the impact of cancer treatments (Tobimatsu, n.d., para. 2). In fact, *Kimiko* employed breast cancer as a lens to expose the extant queer denial, heteronormative assumptions of the health care system, and inadequate representation of queers. Summing up, *Kimiko* is, to borrow Sedgwick's (1993) phrase an "adventure in applied deconstruction" (p. 12).

Tracing the Trails: Queer Exclusions

Kimiko was not the first text to discuss the many intersectionalities of breast cancer. Black, lesbian, mother, warrior, poet Audre Lorde, for instance, set the tone when she railed against the imposed silence of breast cancer/mastectomy while challenging breastlessness as "a sign of shame, a token of lost sexuality, and therefore an indicator of cultural worthlessness" (Jain, 2013, pp. 69–70). In fact, in the "Acknowledgments" of *Kimiko*, Tobimatsu admitted the influence of Lorde thus: "Audre Lorde, who wrote a version of this book long before us" (n.p.). Other important voices include Sedgwick (1992, 1993) and Jain (2013, a queer theorist and a cancer butch) among others. In spite of the temporal and generic differences, what binds these authors is the way that they challenged various aspects of heteronormative cancer culture and treatment procedures. In doing so, they ultimately shed light on the particular ways in which their queerness intersected with their experiences as patients.

Importantly, *Kimiko* visualized several concerns already addressed by Ehrenreich (2001) in her provocative essay, "Welcome to Cancerland," that critiqued "the pink sticky sentiment" (p. 44) and what she called the "breast cancer cult," which "serves as an accomplice in global poisoning – normalizing cancer, prettying it up, even presenting it, perversely, as a positive and enviable experience" (p. 53). In her essay, Ehrenreich argued that this cult not only normalizes cancer but also contributes to the commodification and ultra-feminization of the disease. Moreover, she emphasized the significance of feminism in challenging the deeply ingrained gender biases within the medical system, as it exposes the underlying assumptions about gender. Tobimatsu explored similar concerns and challenges the relentless romanticization and reimagination of cancer as an ostensibly positive and enviable experience but also delved into her experiences as a queer individual within healthcare.

Kimiko, for instance, opened with a jolting moment when Tobimatsu shockingly realized that she had "some sort of lump" on her chest (2020a, p. 7). Filled with uncertainty about the lump's nature and fearing it could be cancer, she resolved to sort it out with her mother. Various cancer-related thoughts crisscrossed her as she imagined how she would look "without boobs" and "without hair" (p. 9). She even imagined her death ("What would people say at my funeral?") and the prospects of her job ("Would I keep working?") (p. 9). A series of questions plagued her, all revolving around the ominous presence of the lump in her breast. The dark gray tone of the opening pages further reinforced the broodiness and reflective quality of the panels. Additionally, an apparent lack of connection between words and images further deepened the eerie and suspenseful atmosphere, ultimately enhancing the overall resonance of the scene.

In the next chapter titled "The Diagnosis," Tobimatsu met her gynecologist and a family doctor to assess the lump in her breast. Later, a specialist ran a battery of tests to determine the nature of the lump. The biopsy results confirmed that Tobimatsu had cancer, specifically a rare and non-aggressive cancer with high survival rates (2020a, p. 16). To prevent the recurrence of the cancer, her doctor recommended particular treatment procedures. However, she felt confused by a lack of consensus among the doctors regarding the treatment procedure and pressure to make "snap decisions" (p. 17) regarding her treatment. One such decision involved freezing her eggs as her gynecologist told her that "[y]ou need to decide **today** if you want to freeze your eggs" (p. 18). Interestingly, Tobimatsu remained uncertain about her desire to have children, given the growing emotional distance between her and Ayaan, her lesbian partner, and her inclination toward solitude, along with concerns about climate change. Nevertheless, she ultimately decided to freeze her eggs (p. 229).

Tobimatsu found it disconcerting that her doctor later suggested family planning due to the potential effects of cancer treatment on fertility. What particularly troubled her was the pressure to make a decision hastily as opposed to her usual practice of consulting her parents for significant choices. In fact, with a focus on restoring the appearance of conventional femininity, doctors gave her heteronormative advice on fertility and appearance. As Amy L. Brandzel (2016) asserted, "Throughout mainstream breast cancer, survival has been routed into a white, normative, heterogendered, ableist subjectivity" (p. 129). Put differently, even without conversing with Tobimatsu, the doctor "read" her as a heterosexual adult and decided that Tobimatsu might be interested in becoming a parent and in reconstructive breast surgery – a classic case of what Jain (2007, p. 506) described as the "relentless hyper- and heterosexualization of the disease."

Importantly, Tobimatsu felt alienated from the heterosexual couples around her at the infertility clinic. The page-length panel showed an uneasy-looking Tobimatsu seated between two happy heterosexual couples who were desperate to be parents. Discussing her experience in an interview, Tobimatsu admitted:

> My fertility doctor wasn't talking about why I might not want to have kids at all and why that was just as legitimate a choice. She wasn't talking about how support networks for queer families can look different, that donor parents might be involved in care. Adoption wasn't raised either.
>
> *(Tobimatsu, 2021, p. 162)*

Tobimatsu underscored the lack of discussion on certain important topics related to family planning, especially given that support structures and family dynamics might differ for queer families (families with same-sex parents) compared to traditional heterosexual families. Further, doctors did not mention the involvement of donor parents in the care of the child, which is relevant for families who have used donor assistance in conception. Overall, Tobimatsu expressed disappointment with her fertility doctor's limited perspective on family planning options which are premised on heterosexuality.

In yet another medical consultation regarding the future course of action, a female physician counseled Tobimatsu to consider a mastectomy (removal of the entire breast or a portion of the breast as a treatment for breast cancer) and immediate reconstructive surgery. That interaction irked Tobimatsu because the female physician communicated ignorance of her queer identity and treated her as a heterosexual woman. Ideally, the doctor should have inquired about and responded professionally to Tobimatsu's queer identity and needs. Instead, the doctor seemed to base recommendations on a predetermined image of a breast cancer patient and constructed a normative reference point – white, heterosexual, and able-bodied woman. Intentionally or not, the doctor upheld an epistemic standpoint rooted in hetero-cis-normativity and thus became yet another example of a provider who regularly made "heteronormative assumptions about patients in clinical environments" (Robertson, 2019, p. 109).

After all, as Tobimatsu (2020a) observed in an aside, "Losing my breasts wouldn't be the worst thing in the world" (p. 25) for it allowed her to "play with gender a bit more" (p. 25). With this observation, Tobimatsu implied that breast cancer introduced newer opportunities to explore gender presentation and multiple intersectionalities of her lived experiences. Put boldly, Tobimatsu (2020b) had a loose affiliation with her breasts, and she even felt confident in her appearance: "I already felt cute looking like a teenage boy with my typically hidden breasts" (para. 6). Clarifying her position in her essay, Kimiko (2020b) stated, "To be clear, breast reconstruction and enlargement are totally valid routes for patients. The problem is that it's a foregone conclusion that all patients would want either or both despite there being a whole host of reasons people choose to stay flat" (para. 6).

Elsewhere in an interview, Tobimatsu stated, "[t]hat was just so outside of my norm or my life circle" (Tobimatsu, 2021, p. 161). Despite Kimiko self-identifying as a masculine lesbian or a dyke who considered a "mastectomy" as having "certain appeal" (along with the fear of side effects), doctors recommended that breast reconstruction. In fact, in one of the interviews, Tobimatsu characterized her interaction with the plastic surgeon as "bizarre" (p. 161). While Tobimatsu harbored a desire to "play with gender" (p. 161) that her new look would guarantee after mastectomy, the surgeon insisted on breast reconstruction. In many ways, it echoed Lorde's (1980) *The Cancer Journals,* which revealed the medical staff's insistence on her use of a prosthetic after her mastectomy, underscoring the patriarchal and gendered expectations imposed on women's bodies. Challenging such reductionist gender identity, in an interview, Tobimatsu observed:

> There was one more reason that I sort of liked the idea of a mastectomy – I could mess with people's assumptions. I could turn the typical pity associated with a mastectomy on its head. Or push back on the other likely assumption – that I must be trans. A reminder that gender expression can look all sorts of ways, even within the context of a cis gender identity.
>
> *(p. 169)*

Like Sedgwick (1993), Tobimatsu insisted that breasts are "relatively peripheral to the complex places where sexuality and gender identity really happen" (p. 256). In some ways, Tobimatsu's stance also echoed Jain's (2013) observations about breastlessness when she stated thus: "even breastlessness is a completely conceivable choice for a person like me (queer, out, athletic, relatively confident)" (p. 219). Both authors considered breastlessness and baldness, among other medical side effects of cancer, as "expression[s]" of "specific selfhood" (see Jain, p. 219), as amplifiers of their queer identity, and finally as embodied modes of resistance. Put together, as Judge (2021) asserted, "heterosexuality continues to operate as the privileged, universal and unmarked sexuality, whilst queerness remains minoritised, particularised and othered" (p. 126).

Finally, Tobimatsu (2020a) candidly expressed how she felt about the entire healthcare system: "As a queer woman, I went into this whole experience with some mistrust towards doctors, particularly around sexual and physical health" (p. 26). Collectively, Tobimatsu experienced a deep "mistrust" (p. 26) in her doctors, prompting her to seek answers from her scientist friends and through her own research, implying that her doctors were not very helpful. This perspective also highlighted the limited assistance provided by her medical professionals and emphasized the need to resort to alternative means to comprehend her experience. To exacerbate matters, Tobimatsu found herself contending with a team of doctors who demonstrated varying degrees of insensitivity and helpfulness, underscoring a systemic issue. The magnitude of these challenges became overwhelming for Tobimatsu, as she openly acknowledged, "[i]t was a lot to deal with" (p. 30).

Pinktober to Pinkbashing

Kimiko tackled not only the issue of queer negligence but also posed a strident critique of the prevailing mainstream cancer culture. In the chapter titled "The Others," for instance, Tobimatsu shed light on the excessively optimistic breast cancer discourses and the resultant toxicity that influences the public conversation surrounding cancer. However, what is "mainstream cancer culture"? Mainstream cancer culture hinges on the language of survivorship as well as "corporate complicity, pink iconography, upbeat rhetoric, and privileging of philanthropy over activism" (DeShazer, 2013, p. 1). Elsewhere, Ehrenreich (2001, p. 48) sarcastically described this culture: "one finds very little anger, no mention of possible environmental causes, few complaints about the fact that, in all but the more advanced, metastasized cases, it is the 'treatments,' not the disease, that cause illness and pain."

Additionally, the mainstream culture overlooks the intersectionalities (such as sex, gender, class, and race, etc.) in the context of cancer culture, resulting in their underrepresentation and exacerbation of the social, economic, and emotional repercussions faced by these individuals. To quote Tobimatsu (2020a, p. 39), the cancer community is predominantly "white, feminized, and apolitical," highlighting how the community/narratives surrounding cancer gloss over the unique needs and perspectives of intersectional identities. The lack of inclusivity and sensitivity perpetuates a disservice to those who face this illness from varying backgrounds and sexual orientations. Read this way, *Kimiko* stands out as a disruptive graphic medical narrative in that it defies conventional cancer practices/narratives and challenges cis-heteronormative gender expectations, thus presenting cancer as a distressing and intricate disease condition.

While community-based organizations play a vital role in supporting the health and well-being of individuals with cancer, Tobimatsu's experience in connecting with one such community proved to be unique. She encountered a group that exuded a hyper-feminine appearance, speech, and confidence. Tobimatsu (2020a) introduced readers to three such animated and exuberant cancer survivors – Macy, Stacy, and Lacy – and depicted them as superhuman fairies. These characters symbolized Ehrenreich's (2001) "survivors" who embraced "brightsiding" (p. 49) and the "pumped up optimism of breast-cancer culture" (p. 50). Put differently, they exemplified the normalization of cancer as an enviable experience, embodying the unapologetically positive aspects of cancer culture. As such, Tobimatsu criticized the notion that illness brings about newer opportunities or "enlightenment" for understanding life. That is, Tobimatsu expressed skepticism of such arguments and firmly asserted that illness should not be romanticized or celebrated as a transformative experience. She further emphasized that such narratives can foster unrealistic expectations and impose undue pressure on individuals confronting serious health challenges. Instead, Tobimatsu advocated for a more realistic and compassionate approach to support those dealing with illnesses. Disappointed, Tobimatsu later joined a queer cancer support group which was also riven by "differences" (p. 41).

In yet another instance, a researcher invited Tobimatsu to participate in a research study but, in doing so, revealed that she was being included merely to fulfill the role of the "token diverse participant" (2020a, p. 40). As Tobimatsu stated, "I was only being called on to fill a role" (p. 40).

Tobimatsu's (2020a) critique in *Kimiko* went beyond the focus on cancer, as she also drew attention to the disproportionality in resource allocation, with a heavy emphasis on treatment and cure rather than investing in prevention efforts. The penultimate chapter titled "New Normal" deliberated this aspect and depicted the demands placed on cure (as opposed to care and preventive measures). In drawing readers' attention to the big banners and towering buildings where such captions appear (e.g., "Yes. We will do everything for the cure," p. 60), Tobimatsu attended to the politics of cure and the false promises of the medicine/health systems. These statements constitute ambitious declarations, displaying an optimistic belief in medical advancements and reflecting a collective determination to eradicate cancer. However, as Jain (2013) and other cancer theorists reminded us, many of the available cancer treatments are as old as the Second World War, which is ironic. Again, the excessive emphasis on "cure" (Cole et al., 2015; Venkat, 2021) and "conquer cancer" puts undue pressure on cancer patients and portrays them as defeated individuals.

Elsewhere, Tobimatsu highlighted a lack of corporate support for vital causes like immigration. In a striking set of panels, Tobimatsu symbolically transferred a cancer donation box to a migrant workers fund, effectively challenging the imbalanced distribution of funds and advocating for a more equitable approach to supporting marginalized groups. The passage also spotlighted the stark contrast between the attention given to cancer patients and the overlooked issues faced by migrants. The graphic narrative boldly critiqued various aspects, including the toxic fandom surrounding cancer, the corporatization of the cancer experience, the over-sentimentalization of it, ageism, and the commercialization of the cancer journey through products like cancer cards, specialized food, and care, among others. Overall, *Kimiko* transcended the boundaries of traditional narratives and illuminated the urgent need for society to address these disparities and embrace a more inclusive and compassionate approach to supporting vulnerable and marginalized communities.

Overcoming Adversity or Masking Pain?

Mainstream cancer culture often overlooks the adverse impact of cancer treatments on the suffering individual. Worse still, it discourages sufferers from openly expressing their pain and misery, promoting a stoic attitude instead. In fact, according to Tobimatsu (2020a), "the ingrained [cultural] pattern" (p. 94) is to suffer silently or endorse a narrative of "overcoming adversity" (p. 92) to present an optimistic version of cancer treatments. As Ehrenreich (2001, p. 48) observed, "so pervasive is the perkiness of the breast-cancer world that unhappiness requires a kind of apology." Unlike the mainstream cancer culture, *Kimiko* courageously delved into the negative impact of breast cancer treatment on her personal and professional life. Particularly, Tobimatsu challenged these normative cultural responses to cancer and courageously presents multiple realities and "new limitations" (p. 93) brought forth by the disease and treatments. Through her candid storytelling, she exposed her vulnerable self, shedding light on the struggles that many others face in silence.

Titled "The Impact," Chapter three, for instance, documented the adverse impact of breast cancer treatment and cancer-preventing medications (such as scarring, induced menopause, insomnia, and fatigue) on Tobimatsu's personal and professional life. While menopause slowed her sexual interest with Ayaan, hot flashes disrupted her professional life and even made "her bedtime treacherous" (Tobimatsu, 2020a, p. 50). In essence, as Tobimatsu later admitted, "I hate how they intrude on my life – not only are they uncomfortable, they also remind me that I had cancer" (p. 52). The chapter also revealed the ways in which Tobimatsu was compelled to reshape her lifestyle to mitigate the disruptive nature of hot flashes. Furthermore, the panels also captured how her existence was reduced to a process of trial and error, characterized by the formidable challenge of selecting the most suitable course of medication and action.

The emotional vulnerability and anxieties stemming from her battle with cancer were effectively conveyed to the readers through the poignant use of a mirror. Mirrors play a crucial role as tropes and sites in health humanities and in graphic medical narratives. For example, both Ellen Forney's *Marbles* (2012) and Georgia Webber's *Dumb* (2018) employed mirror scenes to effectively convey inner conflicts, self-doubts, and embodiment. In the final page of "The Impact" chapter, Tobimatsu (2020a) encountered a mirror and contemplated whether the cancer had metastasized. Here the mirror became a site of

> repeated stand-offs between hope and disappointment, confidence and frank incredulity, between yesterday when things were looking up and the cold light of today. This unsteadiness is not just a function of the mirror, of course, for it occurs within ourselves.
>
> *(Cumming, 2009, p. 148)*

Put differently, the mirror served as a symbolic gateway, allowing Tobimatsu to confront her inner struggles, doubts, and physical realities as she navigated the delicate balance between optimism and skepticism, and ultimately, gained a deeper understanding of herself.

Significantly, the "Epilogue" chapter functioned as a visual representation of Ehrenreich's (2001) insight that "it is the 'treatments,' not the disease, that cause illness and pain" (p. 48). Within this chapter, Tobimatsu (2020a) meticulously documented the aftermath of her cancer treatment, revealing its profound influence on her life and sense of self. She contemplated whether cancer should be classified as an "ongoing disability" (p. 92) due to the persistent side effects of treatment, even during periods of remission. By characterizing cancer as a form of "disability" and reflecting on her ambivalent medical identity (chronic illness or disability?), Tobimatsu addressed how the illness typically impairs a person's ability to engage in major life activities, thus shedding light on cancer's enduring impact on physical, emotional, and social well-being. Ironically, the discussion surrounding cancer as a disability is often absent ("not a lot of writing out there on cancer and disability") (p. 92), leading to a lack of validation for those enduring such hardships. Though the memoir concluded with Tobimatsu acknowledging her emotional vulnerability and embracing her past, present, and future, she eloquently challenged the overly optimistic and one-sided approach taken toward embracing cancer, thereby failing to capture the profound hardship that cancer brings.

Coda

To conclude, *Kimiko* not only exposed how queer bodies are excluded from the medical system but also questioned the hegemonic and mainstream breast cancer discourses, which is premised on heterosexual/cisgender norms. Through meticulously recounting her experiences of breast cancer, Tobimatsu articulated how medical and healthcare systems transmit cultural meanings of the human body. That is, *Kimiko* uncovered the gendered assumptions, predominantly masculinist ones, and the heterosexual orthodoxy of medicine undergirding medical practice. In bold terms, medicine operates on normative principles that often lead to the neglect and concealment of queer experiences.

At one level, *Kimiko* is an expose of the underlying biases and assumptions of the healthcare system and the way cancer is culturally mainstreamed, heterosexualized, and ultra-feminized. At another level, this graphic medical narrative, through realistic illustrations and vivid storytelling, persuades the readers to embrace a more inclusive and equitable society wherein stakeholders acknowledge and respect individual experiences. Within healthcare, this approach translates into a consideration of perspectives, agencies, and voice of queers. In so doing, *Kimiko* not only emphasized the need for queer competency and pedagogical repair but also persuasively implied how such inclusions are necessary for creating responsible healthcare cultures in medicine.

Finally, *Kimiko* comprised a much-desired alternative text in that it boldly challenges the triumphalist discourses surrounding cancer. Characterizing triumph as only a half-story of cancer, Tobimatsu (2020a) presented her pain, fear of death, emotional vulnerabilities and disruptions occasioned by cancer. Taking cues, as it were from Conway's question, "[w]hat harm can there be in a story of triumph?" (Conway, 2013, p. 17), Tobimatsu dismantled trite tropes and stereotypical responses to cancer. In the process, Tobimatsu insisted that any illness is a "soul-wrenching encounter with loss, limitation, and the reality of death" (Conway, 2013, p. 2), thus refraining from a "cancer made me a better person" narrative. *Kimiko* is an important work in that the queer comic offers a unique perspective on the intersection of queerness and healthcare while exposing the inequities within healthcare settings and the underlying structures of the cancer-industrial complex.

Collectively, *Kimiko* emerges as a significant text in health communication by shedding light on the ongoing exclusion of queer individuals from (cancer) healthcare narratives and environments. This thought-provoking work underscores the critical need to address these systemic omissions, providing a perspective on the intersection of queerness and health. More importantly, as an alternative narrative, *Kimiko* lays bare prevailing norms within the broader cancer culture, exposing heteronormative aspects of medicine and highlighting the marginalized experiences of non-binary individuals facing breast cancer. As a health communication text, *Kimiko* advocates for the integration of diverse voices and narratives in medical practices to promote inclusivity and empathy within the healthcare environment.

Further Reading

Visit the Graphic Medicine website at https://www.graphicmedicine.org. *PathoGraphics: Narrative, Aesthetics, Contention, Community*, edited by Susan Merrill Squier and Irmela Marei Krüger-Fürhoff; *The Undying: A Meditation on Modern Illness* by Anne Boyer is an unsentimental account of cancer; *Flat: Reclaiming My Body from Breast Cancer* by Catherine Guthrie; see themed special issues on graphic medicine: *Configurations* (Volume 22, Number 2, Spring 2014), *AMA* (Volume 20, Number 2, 2019), *Biography: An Interdisciplinary Quarterly* (Volume 44, Number 2 & 3, 2021), and *Journal of Literary and Cultural Disability Studies* (Volume 17, Issue 3, 2023).

Note

1 Keet Geniza is a queer Filipinx-Canadian illustrator and comic artist. Geniza's debut book is *Kimiko Does Cancer*. Drawing inspiration from her intimate experience with cancer as she witnessed her father's battle with the disease, Geniza presents a compassionate perspective on the hardships of dealing with cancer.

References

Barker, M.-J. (2019). *Gender: A graphic guide*. Icon Books, Limited.
Beauchard, D. (1996). *Epileptic*. Fantagraphics.
Bechdel, A. (2006). *Fun home: A family tragicomic*. Jonathan Cape.
Bechdel, A. (2008). *The essentials dykes to watch out for*. Jonathan Cape.
Benson, N. C. (2014). *Introducing psychology: A graphic guide*. Icon Books Ltd.
Brandzel, A. L. (2016). The subjects of survival: The anti-intersectional routes of breast cancer, *Women's Studies Quarterly*, *44*(1/2), 128–151.
Burns, C. (2005). *Black hole*. Pantheon.
Charon, R. (2008). *Narrative medicine: Honoring the stories of illness*. Oxford University Press.
Chute, H. (2017). *Why comics? From underground to everywhere*. HarperCollins.

Cole, T. R., Carlin. N. S., & Carson, R. A. (2015). *Medical humanities: An Introduction*. Cambridge University Press.
Conway, K. (2013). *Beyond words: Illness and the limits of expression*. University of New Mexico Press.
Couser, G. T. (1997). *Recovering bodies: Illness, disability, and life writing*. University of Wisconsin Press.
Cumming, L. (2009). *A face to the world: On self-portraits*. Harper Press.
Czerwiec, M. K. (2017). *Taking turns: Stories from HIV/AIDS care unit 371*. Penn State University Press.
Czerwiec, M. K., Williams, I., Squier, S., Green, M. J., Myers, K. R., & Smith, S. T. (2015). *Graphic medicine manifesto*. Penn State University Press.
Dahl, K. (2009). *Monsters*. Secret Acres.
Davison, A. (1990). *The spiral cage: An autobiography*. Active Images.
DeShazer M. K. (2013). *Mammographies: The cultural discourses of breast cancer narratives*. University of Michigan Pres.
DiMassa, D. (1993). *Hothead Paisan: Homicidal lesbian terrorist*. Giant Ass Pub.
Drescher, J. (2015). Out of DSM: Depathologizing homosexuality. *Behavioral Sciences*, *5*(4), 565–575. https://doi.org/10.3390/bs5040565
Ehrenreich, B. (2001, November). Welcome to cancerland. *Harper's Magazine*, 43–53.
Farmer, J. (2010). *Special exits*. Fantagraphics Books.
Fies, B. (2006). *Mom's cancer*. Abrams.
Forney, E. (2012). *Marbles: Mania, depression, Michelangelo, and me: A graphic memoir*. Penguin.
Forney, E. (2018). *Rock steady: Brilliant advice from my bipolar life*. Fantagraphics Books.
Fussell, T. (2005). *Mammoir: A pictorial odyssey of the adventures of a fourth grade teacher with breast cancer*. AuthorHouse.
Gardner, J. (2012). *Projections comics and the history of twenty First-century storytelling*. Stanford University Press.
Green, J. (1972). *Binky brown meets the holy virgin Mary*. McSweeney's Books.
Green, M. J., & Myers, K. R. (2010). Graphic medicine: Use of comics in medical education and patient care. *BMJ*, *340*.
Holmes, M. S. (2013). Cancer comics: Narrating cancer through sequential art. *Tulsa Studies in Women's Literature*, *33*(1), 147–162.
Jain, S. L. (2007). Cancer butch. *Cultural Anthropology*, *22* (4), 501–538. https://doi.org/10.1525/can.2007.22.4.501
Jain, S. L. (2013). *Malignant: How cancer becomes Us*. University of California Press.
Judge M. (2021). Queer at 25: A critical perspective on queerness, politics and futures. *Journal of Asian and African Studies, 56*, 120–134.
Käll, F. (2021). Kimiko does cancer. *Lambda Nordica*, *27*(2–3), 158–173, https://doi.org/10.34041/ln.v27.745
Kelly, T., & Rodriguez, S. B. (2022). Expanding underrepresented in medicine to include lesbian, gay, bisexual, transgender, and queer individuals. *Academic Medicine*, *97*(11), 1605–1609.
Leavitt, S. (2010). *Tangles: A story about Alzheimer's, my mother and me*. Jonathan Cape.
Lee, P. (2018). The demagogies of 'Lack': The WHO's ambivalence to the right to health of LGBT people. *Global Health Governance*, *12*(1), 17–21.
Lorde, A. (1980). *The cancer journals*. Penguin Random House.
Mack, S. (2004). *Janet & me: An illustrated story of love and loss*. Simon & Schuster.
Mansh, M., Garcia, G., & Lunn, M. R. (2015). From patients to providers: Changing the culture in medicine toward sexual and gender minorities. *Academic Medicine*, *90*(5), 574–580.
Marchetto, M. A. (2006). *Cancer vixen: A true story*. Knopf.
Melia, D. (Ed.). (1987). *Strip AIDS*. Willyprods/Small Time Ink
Mongelli, F., Perrone, D., Balducci, J., Sacchetti, A. F., Mattei, S., & Galeazzi, G., et al. (2019). Minority stress and mental health among LGBT populations: An update on the evidence. *Minerva Psichiatrica*, *60*(1), 27–50.
Müller, A. (2022). Sexual orientation and gender identity as determinants of health and illness. In K. Chamberlain & A. Lyons (Eds.), *Routledge international handbook of critical issues in health and illness* (pp. 155–168). Routledge.
Pekar, H., & Joyce, B. (1994). *Our cancer year*. Frank Stack.
Pillay, S. R., Ntetmen, J. M., & Nel, J. A. (2022). Queering global health: An urgent call for LGBT+ affirmative practices. *The Lancet Global Health*, *10*(4), e574–e578.
Robertson, W. J. (2019). Challenging heteronormativity in medicine. In A. Bleakley (Ed.) *Routledge handbook of the medical humanities* (pp. 105–113). Routledge.
Robbins, T., Sienkiewicz, B., & Triptow, R. (Eds.). (1988). *Strip AIDS U.S.A.: A collection of cartoon art to benefit people with AIDS.* Last Gasp.

Sedgwick, E. K. (1992). White glasses. *The Yale Journal of Criticism*, *5*(3), 193–208.
Sedgwick, E. K. (1993). *Tendencies*. Duke University Press.
Sharman, Z. (2016a). Introduction: Why queer and trans health stories matter. In Z. Sharman (Ed.), *The remedy: Queer and trans voices on health and health care* (pp. 9–23). Arsenal Pulp Press.
Sharman, Z. (Ed.). (2016b). *The remedy: Queer and trans voices on health and health care*. Arsenal Pulp Press.
Squier, S. M. (2008). Literature and medicine, future tense, making it graphic. *Literature and Medicine, 27*(2), 124–152.
Summers, A. K. (2014). *Pregnant butch: Nine long months spent in drag*. Soft Skull Press.
Symington, S. (2017). *First year out: A transition story*. Jessica Kingsley Publishers.
Tobimatsu, K. (2020a). *Kimiko does cancer: A graphic memoir.* Arsenal Pulp Press.
Tobimatsu, K. (2020b). What breast cancer awareness month & the pink ribbon get wrong. *Refinery29*. https://www.refinery29.com/en-us/2020/10/10101858/breast-cancer-awareness-month-racism-women-of-color
Tobimatsu, K. (2021). *Kimiko does cancer* [Interview]. *Lambda Nordica*, *2*(3), 159–173.
Tobimatsu, K. (n.d.). Navigating breast cancer as a young, queer, mixed-race woman. *Rethink Bread Cancer*. https://rethinkbreastcancer.com/navigating-breast-cancer-as-a-young-queer-mixed-race-woman/
Venkat, B. J. (2021). *At the limits of cure*. Duke University Press.
Venkatesan, S. (2016). Graphic medicine manifesto, by M. K. Czerwiec, Ian Williams, Susan Merrill Squier, Michael J. Green, Kimberly R. Myers, and Scott T. Smith. *Journal of Graphic Novels Comics, 7*(1), 93–94.
Wahlert, L., & Fiester, A. (2013). Queer in the clinic. *Journal of Medical Humanities*, *34*(2), 85–91.
Webber, G. (2018). *Dumb: Living without a voice*. Fantagraphics Books
Williams, I. (2014). *The bad doctor: The troubled life and times of Dr Iwan James.* Myriad Edition.
Williams, I. (2015). Introduction. In M. K. Czerwiec, I. Williams, S. M. Squier, M. J. Green, K. R. Myers, & S. T. Smith, S. (Eds.) *Graphic medicine manifesto* (pp. 1–20). Penn State University Press.
Zeeman, L., Sherriff, N., Browne, K., McGlynn, N., Mirandola, M., Gios, L., et al. (2019). A review of lesbian, gay, bisexual, trans and intersex (LGBTI) health and healthcare inequalities. *European Journal of Public Health*, 29(5), 974–980.

20

WHAT DID I JUST WATCH? MEDIA LITERACY'S RELATIONSHIP WITH HEALTH COMMUNICATION AND POP CULTURE

Andrew D. Sutherland and Erica Weintraub Austin

Introduction

It's time to read a chapter.
It's time to pop the culture.
It's time to learn about health communication.
When it comes to Media Literacy tonight.

For some readers, the previous blurb can prompt thoughts of *The Muppets*' opening theme song. The iconic history of *The Muppets* and *Sesame Street*, programs both created by puppeteer Jim Henson, has helped to shape popular culture (Garlan & Graham, 2009) by featuring celebrity guests, parodying current events, and blending comedy with lessons encouraging critical thinking made accessible to people of all ages. The use of nonsensical goofy humor and fundamental human connectedness earned mainstream popularity amongst adults and children alike (Abate, 2009). *The Muppets* and *Sesame Street* also have raised awareness of healthy foods and behaviors (Kotler et al., 2016), emotional health related to children and families dealing with military deployment (Desens & Hughes, 2013), and navigating complicated health topics such as COVID-19 (Riley et al., 2020) and H.I.V. and AIDS (Arak, 2002).

In such ways, popular culture often presents valuable information and spreads innovative ideas through platforms such as television, music, comics, and the internet. Media and pop culture also can influence people's purchase decisions and shape their identities (Boden, 2006), affirming the views and values of the dominant culture (Giroux, 2002), and reinforcing ideas and perceptions around race, class, gender, and sexual orientation (Browne, 2005; Tisdell & Thompson, 2007). Whether applied to the use of pop culture for marketing, health campaigns, or the framing of information to educate their audience, media literacy serves as a vital skill for individuals to evaluate the intent and content of persuasive messages over media. This chapter, therefore, explores media literacy and its relationship with Health Communication and pop culture.

The Muppets and other entertainment programming have successfully introduced unfamiliar and controversial topics to young and older audiences through entertainment education (see also Chapters 17 and 23 [Lifespan and Entertainment Education], this volume). *Sesame Street* demon-

DOI: 10.4324/9781003436409-23

strated how effectively pop culture can educate even the youngest viewers, and it also helped to demonstrate that these youngest participants comprise active information processors, not passive sponges soaking up every media effect in the same way as every other child does. Individuals can learn vicariously through media but are not necessarily able or motivated to reproduce what they observe, as famously demonstrated by social cognitive theorist Albert Bandura (1986, 2001). However, passive acceptance of promoted messages without critical thinking about sources and content can risk acquiring dangerous misinformation, unhealthy behaviors, and can create a marketer's bonanza (see also Chapter 11 [Misinformation], this volume). Media literacy, therefore, can equip media consumers to obtain the most value from pop culture, particularly when the often-blurred separation between fiction and nonfiction holds implications for real-life decision-making and health outcomes.

Media Literacy: An Overview

Educators commonly use media and pop culture to encourage their students to engage in critical thinking around media and representation (Tisdell, 2008; Tisdell & Thompson, 2007). The use of popular culture to teach and apply media literacy makes the material relevant, unique, and entertaining. Pop culture entertainment's association with pleasure and emotional engagement, however, can also can lead people to refrain from logically analyzing the message. Buckingham (2003) noted that movies and television often constitute a source of pleasure, leading individuals to focus on emotional connections rather than evaluation of content. When pop culture, such as film and television, combines entertainment with information and persuasion, perhaps intended for the message designer's benefit or for what the message designer thinks is for the message recipient's benefit, the lessons learned will depend on how the content is interpreted. These many variables of intent, skill, emotional response, and message interpretation all make it important for individuals to understand how to critically evaluate pop culture through media literacy.

A great need exists for media users to realize the need to think more critically about the information with which they engage through media and online. Various personal factors like socio-demographics and individual literacy skills, current health situation, social and media environment, and access to information can significantly influence how an individual approaches health media literacy behavior (Levin-Zamir & Bertschi, 2018). Lyons et al. (2021) found that three in four American Facebook users surveyed drastically overestimated their own abilities to distinguish between legitimate and false news, which leads to more sharing of misinformation. While individuals believe that they can distinguish between accurate and inaccurate information, a difference can exist between one's beliefs about what they can do and what they actually know how to do or have practiced doing. However, as people experience and critically engage with media, they start to develop those skills. For example, as children get older, they develop the abilities to figure out the persuasive intentions of advertisers (Grohs et al., 2012). Much like learning to perform gymnastics, media literacy requires skills and benefits from practice.

As media literacy has gained stronger support in the public eye, scholars have developed different and more expansive definitions (Potter, 2010). The National Association of Media Literacy Education (N.A.M.L.E., 2023) built upon prior definitions and research on media literacy and its elements as the active measures to "access, analyze, evaluate, create, and act" (p. 1) when engaging with communication actions. By recognizing people as consumers and creators of media, media literacy promotes a mindful and empowering relationship with media by encouraging individuals to develop media literacy skills for civic life (N.A.M.L.E., 2023). The ability to access, analyze, comprehend, and critically assess media and media material remains at the center of media literacy, with many advocates also encouraging media users to produce media and use it in a variety of contexts by applying their knowledge of how to effectively develop media-based messages (Aufderheide, 1993; Hobbs, 1998).

Although sometimes framed as competing perspectives, two approaches known as protectionist and empowerment allow users to engage thoughtfully with potential adverse effects of mass media and find practical means to engage with media outside of the classroom or laboratory. The protectionist perspective has argued for the use of media literacy as a defensive skill to enable users to identify and critically analyze information to determine its accuracy; whereas, the empowerment perspective emphasizes that critical thinking skills, paired with skills for media creation, expand intercultural understanding, help individuals to form their identities, and can facilitate positive change (Cole et al., 2007; Hobbs, 1998). In the protectionist perspective, individuals should respond with skepticism when they encounter pop culture figures to question their message intent and content. Empowerment perspectives would encourage individuals to also create their own media messages and consider using pop culture figures or images to do so.

As both perspectives demonstrate, successful engagement with media requires a combination of abilities, competencies, and skills, some of which develop with age and maturity, some of which can be taught, and all of which benefit from practice (Austin, 2014; Potter, 2004). Social media and smartphone apps powered by Artificial Intelligence (AI) algorithms increasingly require users to possess an understanding of media construction skills.

Primary caregivers can help youth through intervention techniques that include media choice, parents' social co-viewing, their own example and discussion styles, and active discussion with their youth that encourage inquiry and critical thinking, all of which have implications for health outcomes (Chen & Austin, 2012; Collier et al., 2016; Valkenburg et al., 1999). Adolescents need this support because they often opt to "follow" marketers that they may consider to be entertaining and important for staying up-to-date on how to maintain their popularity, with less healthy brands having the most followers (Rummo et al., 2020; Wong et al., 2023). Even young children demonstrate an affinity for marketing messages that affect family purchases, increase obesity risk, and impact body image (Smith et al., 2019). Media literacy interventions and pop culture can blunt this influence and help children begin to develop lifelong media literacy skills even from a young age (Kaiser et al., 2024; Rasmussen et al., 2016).

The American Academy of Pediatrics (2023) recommended combining media literacy instruction with media use management, especially limits on screen use for youth, but they acknowledge that a realistic approach must emphasize effective media use over preventing media use. Currently, formal media literacy instruction exists in some K–12 classrooms, and states and countries have begun to develop standards for media literacy curricula. Unfortunately, many programs lack assessments and accountability and offer uneven access. Further, adults need real-time media literacy skills training too (van der Linden et al., 2023). This lack of media literacy education access can lead to uncritical engagement with social media content, such as TikTok, which promotes 'infotainment' that blurs the lines of facts, fiction, sales, and politics.

Entertainment – and influencer-focused social media, including Facebook, Instagram, and TikTok, now represent leading sources of news, especially for Americans under 30 (Liedke & Wang, 2023), encouraging sharing without fact-checking (Lyons et al., 2021), the glorification of appearance (Kaiser et al., 2024) and the engagement with outrage and emotionally driven content (Rathje et al., 2021).

Some online resources exist through games that focus on the correction of misinformation (see University of Cambridge, 2021) along with organizations that promote media literacy outside of the classroom, such as in libraries and other public places (see C.O.R., n.d.; News Literacy Project, 2023). Yet again, access remains uneven, and these organizations often focus on correcting misinformation rather than dealing with media literacy in other forms such as marketing and entertainment, including songs, games, and other forms of popular culture.

In particular, media literacy education tends to focus on improving people's abilities to identify trustworthy sources, websites, and content (N.A.M.L.E., 2023). For example, a popular curriculum, the S.I.F.T. method, developed by Caulfield (2021), takes a step-by-step approach for individuals to quickly evaluate online content to determine its accuracy by:

1. **Stop** and reflect on how they feel about the content.
2. **Investigate** the source of the claim,
3. **Find** better coverage
4. **Trace** claims, quotes, and media to understand the original context.

These various media literacy skills hold relevance beyond the classroom. For example, the Stanford Civic Online Reasoning (C.O.R., n.d.) provides a free curriculum to help people evaluate online information through video lessons. In addition to teaching media literacy skills, these resources and strategies introduce the idea of "prebunking" based on inoculation theory.

Inoculation theory, a social psychological framework that takes a preemptive resistance to persuasive messaging, similar to medical inoculation, aims to protect a person from a threat preemptively (Compton, 2013; McGuire & Papageorgis, 1961). Similar to getting a flu shot to prevent disease, "prebunking" teaches people how to identify misinformation and manipulative strategies before their intended miscommunicators strike (Roozenbeek & van der Linden, 2019a, 2019b; Roozenbeek et al., 2020). This type of media literacy strategy has been shown to reduce the effects of health misinformation (Compton et al., 2016) and to reduce the appealing effects of conspiracy theories and propaganda (Banas & Miller, 2013). These types of approaches can help prime people to think critically of persuasive information and to consider the accuracy of information.

Some scholars have even played to the theme of pop culture by developing free online video games such as those developed by Cambridge Social Decision-Making Lab Inoculation Science. Games like "GoViral!" are designed to help protect against COVID-19 misinformation, and "Bad News" teaches people various ways to identify manipulated content (Roozenbeek et al., 2023; University of Cambridge, 2021). The "Go Viral!" online game reduces manipulative messages' effects, improves the ability to spot misinformation, and minimizes the willingness to share misinformation (Basol et al., 2021). According to Basol et al., this type of media literacy strategy can reduce the effects of misinformation around vaccines and COVID-19 misinformation.

Roll to Investigate: Drawbacks of the Cognitive Approach

Yet, this practice requires people to "stop and think" and to engage in critical analysis that involves checking multiple sources, such as pausing before sharing an entertaining social media post or clicking on an enticing purchase that might sell out before ensuring its promised benefits. It requires intent and motivation in addition to skills. The reality, according to the Limited Capacity Model of Motivated, Mediated Message Processing (LC4MP), is that the human cognitive system has a limited capacity to process information and cannot process everything contained in a message all at once as we encode, store, or retrieve information (Lang, 2009). The LC4MP holds that people allocate cognitive resources in two forms: 1) Controlled processing, or the conscious and voluntary allocation of attention to media, and 2) the automatic processing, or unconscious processing of information (Lang, 2009; Potter & Bolls, 2012). At the same time, more approachable information, such as humorous or engaging content, can capture an audience's attention and enhance creative thinking (Clore et al., 2001; Lang, 2006). From a media literacy perspective, educators who expect individual media users to engage more actively with media through controlled processing on a sustained level, unfortunately, expect them to engage in an unsustainable level of cognitive activity.

If people possess the skills to engage skeptically with messages more heuristically, they can assess whether and when they need to invest more cognitive energy in critical analysis. Media literacy, therefore, can aim to teach both necessary skills and an awareness of how emotions can inform the critical processing of messages. Austin (2014) suggested that people apply media literacy much as they ride a bicycle, by developing the equivalent of muscle memory through practice and consistency. Individuals need enough training to practice media literacy behaviors just as they would practice riding bicycles on easy and progressively more challenging trails. As with riding a bicycle, people can put less cognitive effort into thinking about riding the "easy trails," can ask friends and experts about unfamiliar ones, and can "stop and think" about dangerous spots. So, just like the Muppets in *The Muppets Great Caper*, let us jump on a bike and "just a push and we are on our way. Yes, could we ride, side by side. Couldn't we ride" (Hensen, 1981).

Media Literacy Stages: A Bicycle Built for You

Media literacy crosses platforms and disciplines, enabling individuals to engage with media critically and develop their own media. The media literacy theory of change, as shown in Figure 20.1, explains how people interact with media and make decisions from that interaction. The skill-building process of media literacy includes critical thinking about sources and content, helps individuals assess forewarning clues about sources' credibility, and then can motivate people to consider the accuracy, representativeness, and currency of message content. Media literacy skills take time to develop, like riding a bicycle, whereby individuals develop appropriate techniques and practice, some of which can become as automatic as muscle memory (Austin, 2023; Austin et al., 2023). Media literacy interventions for health topics, particularly those based on inoculation and forewarning, have shown effectiveness across topics and age groups as individuals are motivated to avoid letting themselves or others fall for manipulation and misinformation (Bergsma & Carney, 2008; Kaiser et al., 2024; Vahedi et al., 2018; Xie et al., 2019).

The motivation to think more critically about the source and the message content facilitates outcome beliefs and expectations of possible conclusions while building evidence-based confidence in a media consumer's abilities (efficacy) toward certain actions and possible outcomes. For example, media literacy interventions have been shown to help with health decisions to reduce risky behaviors, such as decrease alcohol consumption among youths (Austin et al., 2016). These logic-based

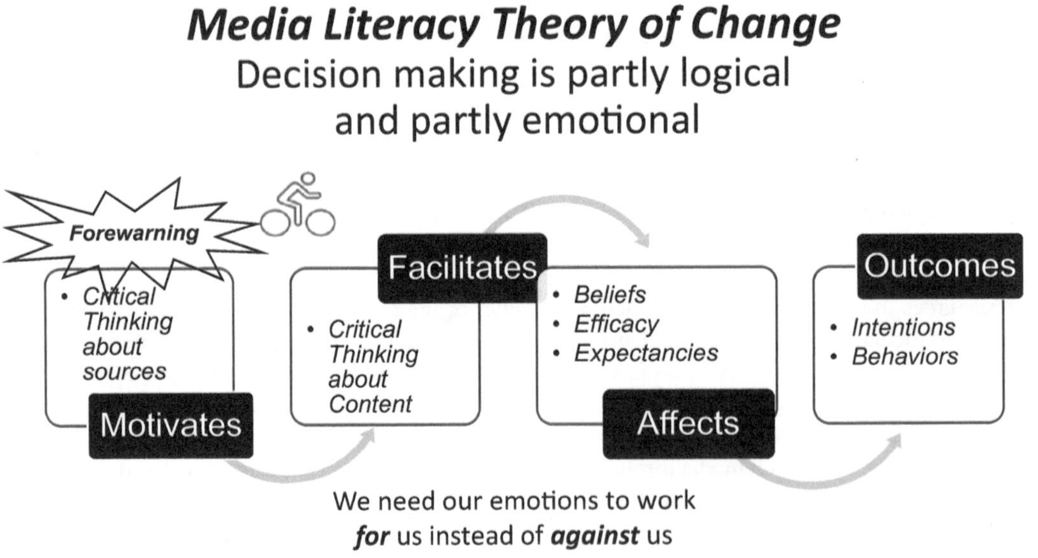

Figure 20.1 The Media Literacy Theory of Change (Austin, 2023)

outcomes can lead to specific intentions or behaviors, but importantly, the media literacy theory of change considers emotions in addition to logical processing.

Emotions can provide useful insight for media users in relation to various situations and topics (Clore et al., 2001). Emotions can provide valuable clues to make sense of information, experiences, and the world (Oatley, 1992; Opdahl, 2002). An awareness of emotions and biases can open the opportunity to dive deeper into a topic to understand why a message makes someone feel or respond a certain way to a specific message. Emotions, therefore, can act as a kind of forewarning radar to help people prevent bad-faith actors from taking advantage of these emotions. Grey Imm, a high school student, noticed how he'd been drawn in by the humor of Zyn appeals on TikTok: "He [Max VanderAarde] would create all these funny phrases or things that would make it funny and joke about it and make it relevant to us" (Dreyfuss, 2024; para. 29). He fought back against the nicotine purveyors with a poll and column in his high school newspaper.

Jenkins (1997) proposed that media literacy education should take this type of approach, teaching people to actively participate when they critically reflect on the media with which they engage and the pop culture they embrace, rather than accept passive consumption of content. To empower media users, rather than protect consumers, media literacy interventions must partner with people in ways that reflect how their brains function. To do so, the Message Interpretation Process (MIP) model has provided a successful approach for media literacy interventions (Vahedi et al., 2018; Xie et al., 2019).

The MIP model acknowledges that, as individuals engage with information, they evaluate messages by applying a combination of logical analyses of the messages, reflections based on their personal experiences and perceptions, and affective reactions, which together determine the extent to which the individual accepts or rejects the presented message content (Austin, 2007). The MIP model draws from Social Cognitive Theory (Bandura, 1997, 2001), expectancy theory (Goldman et al., 1987), and theories of heuristic and systematic message processing (Chen & Chaiken, 1999). Scholars often use this model to test the outcomes of media literacy interventions. For example, Social Cognitive Theory explains that people make decisions through a process of experiencing the world actively and vicariously, with their observations influencing their decisions through a process that requires attention, representation, translation, and knowledge gain, as well as motivation and skill to reproduce behaviors observed (Bandura, 1986).

The MIP model has been tested with youth as young as third grade to demonstrate that individuals will interpret a media message by reflecting on their experiences, testing media portrayals on logic-based beliefs such as perceived realism, and reflecting on affect-oriented beliefs such as how desirable portrayals seem (Vahedi et al., 2018; Xie et al., 2019). A particularly influential belief associated with the MIP model is wishful identification with a media character or influencer. Wishful identification describes the belief held by consumers who idealize media personalities. The desire to "be like" or "do things that" people in media are doing can influence intentions of behaviors (Feilitzen & Linné, 1975). For example, Bond and Drogos (2014) found that when people experienced wishful identification with the personalities of the MTV pop culture reality show, *The Jersey Shore*, young adults tended to hold positive attitudes and perceptions toward sexual behaviors. Desirable messages tend to predict wishful identification, and wishful identification tends to predict positive expectancies, the belief that performing a behavior will produce beneficial results.

People tend to combine their logic-based reasoning and affective processing, and the media literacy theory of change suggests that improved skills for noticing characteristics of media sources and for critical thinking about content can reduce the influence of emotion on decision-making. Prior research that used the MIP model found that media literacy interventions can enable people to recognize the inaccurate and glamorized depictions of sexual portrayals in media, for example, and equip them to think more critically about those portrayals (Pinkleton et al., 2012). These interventions strengthen an individual's logic-based processing networks so that they can continue to enjoy media messages without the desirability of messages exerting as much strength over decision-making (e.g., Kaiser & Austin, 2020).

In this way, the LC4MP and the MIP Model together show that "gut feelings" inform decision-making about media because logic and emotion both influence it, and people's skills and motivations affect the level of cognition applied to message processing. Thus, a person's cognitive effort will vary depending on whether information seems approachable and if they think they need to put up their defenses against it (Lang, 2006). For example, the show *Reservation Dogs,* a coming-of-age FX series on Hulu created by Sterlin Harjo and Taika Waititi about young Indigenous youth and their life on an Oklahoma reservation, has incorporated deeper meaning and social commentary through humor (Harjo et al., 2021-Present). In the episode "*What About Your Dad*" from Season 1 Episode 4, the cast prepared for the local Indian Health Service diabetes outreach event (Freeland et al., 2021). The episode focused on the lack of access to healthy food options and exemplified how product labeling can create misperceptions. It combines characters' efficacy and (lack of) knowledge toward choosing healthy options with the topic of diabetes within a cultural context, using irony and humor to provide supportive and culturally specific health information to create a less threatening message through entertainment. The show engaged an active audience to think more critically to understand the jokes and learn lessons about both health and culture.

This example leads to an important feature of the Message Interpretation Process Model: that critical thinking about media does not result in disliking the media. Although media literacy education teaches that marketers routinely cultivate undue desirability of products and personalities, often without realism, this model also acknowledges that people can enjoy likable messages without necessarily believing them. Tests of this principle have been called "The double-edge desirability effect" and have indicated that increasing awareness of the techniques used by marketers and disinformation purveyors can decrease the persuasive effectiveness of these techniques (Austin et al., 2007, 2015, 2018). Similarly, games based on inoculation theory also have shown some effectiveness by revealing the techniques used in misinformation messages (Roozenbeek & van der Linden, 2022). In other words, individuals motivated to evaluate a message analytically tend to process the desirability of a message with more skepticism, which can make a message less persuasive through an increased understanding of media literacy techniques (Kaiser & Austin, 2020). This description explains why the Message Interpretation Process Model describes the decision-making process as both logic- and affect-oriented.

Media Literacy, Pop Culture Content, and Health Communication

Media literacy principles make a difference when viewing pop culture messages in relation to Health Communication. Advertising and pop culture can promote both healthy and problematic content, encouraging individuals to think more critically about messages as the producers of *Reservation Dogs* have done (Harjo et al., 2021-Present). People who critically consider the sources and content of media messages tend to engage in a more thoughtful process of information seeking (Bergsma & Carney, 2008). Health communicators, however, need to avoid promoting an automatic distrust among media users that can deter more in-depth information seeking. Whereas cynicism shuts down further consideration of critical thinking, healthy skepticism encourages inquiry about specific characteristics that should affect the presentation of a message, raising the bar for quality control.

Opportunities and risks both exist in the unique relationship that celebrities and pop culture icons have with the public based on their relatability, reach, and storytelling abilities. They can engage successfully with audiences to address health-related topics on an emotion-oriented, heuristic level (Myrick, 2017; see also Chapter 16, this volume). According to Myrick et al., celebrities' disclosure of their health issues can lead to increases in health awareness and information seeking (Myrick et al., 2013). Their disclosures also can reduce stigmatization and seeking of treatment, such as when Tom

Hanks's disclosure of testing positive for COVID-19 increased perceptions among the public of their own susceptibility to the virus (Cohen, 2020). Unfortunately, however, celebrities and pop culture figures also can spread misinformation. Celebrities hold a certain trust with the public, and people may become disarmed to persuasive messages and less skeptical of misinformation, including about health (Hoffman et al., 2017; White et al., 2023; for related information, see Chapters 11 and 15 [11 Misinformation and 15 Celebrities], this volume). For example, celebrities and pop culture figures who promoted dangerous dietary advice and misinformation have influenced audiences to emulate their behavior due to individuals' trust and identification with the celebrities and their perceptions of social norms (Myrick & Erlichman, 2020). Nevertheless, celebrities and pop culture can promote a product, inform the public on certain topics due to their ability to attract attention, or even discuss their personal struggle with health issues (Myrick, 2017).

Body image represents an especially important example of health-related messaging in pop culture (see Chapters 5 [Body Image] and 15 [Celebrities], this volume). For example, Levine and Harrison (2009) argued that professional wrestling portrayed exceptionally muscular wrestlers such as Hulk Hogan and Dwayne "The Rock" Johnson through television, video games, and toys, shaping expectations of body image through an economic presence. With these portrayals exhibited in pop culture and the underlying meaning associated with body image, professional wrestling presents these body images as desirable and realistic, even if not achievable healthily (Soulliere & Blaire, 2004). Media literacy interventions can build skepticism about the realism portrayed in depictions of beauty and improve perceptions of one's own body image (McLean et al., 2016). Such interventions can lead to increased self-esteem and body satisfaction, critical thinking about food advertisements, and reflection on food intake and nutrition outcomes (Kaiser et al., 2024, see also Chapter 4 [Food and Nutrition], this volume). Meanwhile, people can continue to enjoy some of the content, although they also may decide that they like some of it less upon critical reflection.

Pop culture memes have been used as a tool to promote health education, while also helping individuals develop media literacy skills. Tsene (2022) noted that comic books comprise an engaging learning tool that serves as a "superpower" that can promote skills like critical thinking, creativity, understanding reality, and the promotion of empathy with characters. Graphic novels and comic books can serve as a more engaging medium than textbooks as they use both text and pictures, which allows readers to critically evaluate multimodal media (Jacobs, 2007; Schwarz, 2007; see also Chapter 19 [Queering - Graphic Memoir], this volume). For example, manga or Japanese comics have been used as an intervention medium for readers to consider the nutrition quality of snacks, resulting in an increase in the self-efficacy of teenagers (Leung et al., 2014). In this case, comics and pop culture can serve as an empowerment intervention that helps individuals to think more critically about their health needs.

The use of media literacy in relation to Health Communication and pop culture can vary. Individuals, organizations, and even governments might use pop culture figures such as celebrities or fictional characters to promote a public health message or affect a desired outcome (see also Chapter 24 [Looking to the Future], this volume). In these cases, they seek to persuade an audience to take a certain action in relation to a specific health behavior. For example, memes during the 2020 Covid-19 pandemic became a powerful form of coping and efficacy-building strategies during a time of social isolation. They fostered the expression of stress, the ability to find humor in the world, and a concise means of information sharing (Myrick et al., 2022).

As with other types of media, however, memes do not necessarily provide correct information and require skeptical analysis. Bad-faith actions, conspiracy theories, and political actors can use memes to promote their messages. For example, DiRusson and Stansberry (2021) explored anti-vaccination advocates' use of social media and their spread of vaccine misinformation. These individuals presented themselves as critics and experts of health information while reframing health information in a way that reinforces their previous beliefs and shared values. In one specific post, they pointed to a meme of Beaker, a Muppet scientist, with the text, "That awkward moment when you realize you are the smartest person in the room … and you are in the doctor's office" (p. 323). This meme positions the targets as informed experts while framing official sources of information as untrustworthy (DiRusson & Stansberry, 2021). This example reminds readers that they should consider the motives of the source and the implications of the content.

Resources to Learn More About Media Literacy

As awareness and research about media literacy have increased, resources have continued to develop both inside and outside of the classroom. These organizations and the people who have developed these resources have dedicated themselves to educating others about practical approaches to media literacy. For example, as mentioned earlier, N.A.M.L.E. offers various resources such as a parents' guide to media literacy and safe online behaviors. N.A.M.L.E. offers a wide range of resources to fight misinformation and promote social justice using media literacy as a civic engagement skill. "The News Literacy Project" provides resources for educators and the general public, including their SIFT newsletter about misinformation trends, journalism, and press freedom. Their Checkology e-learning program also provides lessons on media bias, misinformation, and fact-checking strategies (News Literacy Project, 2023). Finally, the American Academy of Pediatrics (AAP, 2021, 2023) provides evidence-based resources to help health professionals and families use media in a healthy manner.

More topic-specific resources exist from the Center for Disease Control and Prevention (2021), which developed steps to address misinformation focused on COVID-19 but which still have relevance beyond the single topic. In addition, organizations such as FirstDraft combat online dis/misinformation and provide research, tools, and resources to help people develop "prebunking" skills (Garcia, 2022). Many local schools, universities, and public libraries also have sections dedicated to digital or media literacy.

Future Directions

This chapter demonstrates that pop culture can entertain, educate, and empower for health while also achieving commercial success. Because media literacy skills apply across topics and media platforms, these skills can strengthen pop culture's ability to communicate health information. They also can help consumers avoid accepting misinformation into their decision-making when it arrives in the form of entertainment.

Researchers, producers, and practitioners all benefit from taking further action to extend and refine their knowledge, collaborate, and make efforts at outreach and empowerment in this complex and multidisciplinary field. Future success can build on research that continues to pursue how media literacy processes correspond to how the brain functions, through cognitive and affective processing and throughout the lifespan. Media literacy interventions also need to further explore how opportunities can harness pop culture and can do so across communities and situations. Additionally, health communicators can partner more with pop culture producers, including members of their target audiences, to connect more effectively with their patients and communities. In doing so, Health Communicators can cultivate media literate audiences and simultaneously ensure they can achieve media literacy assessments of source and content credibility with each subculture they intend to embrace. Including members of the community in Health Communication research and content creation can help build trust and lead to healthy success.

But now it's the end of the chapter,
Why don't you reflect on this,
It's time to get empowered,

On the most accessible, analytical, comprehendible, critical,
This is what we call Media Literacy!

References

Abate, M. A. (2009). Taking silliness seriously: Jim Henson's *the Muppet Show*, the Anglo-American tradition of nonsense, and cultural critique. *The Journal of Popular Culture*, *42*(4), 589–613. https://doi.org/10.1111/j.1540-5931.2009.00698.x

American Academy of Pediatrics. (2021, June 4). Media and Children. *Home*. https://www.aap.org/en/patient-care/media-and-children/

American Academy of Pediatrics. (2023, May 21). Screen time guidelines. *Home*. https://www.aap.org/en/patient-care/media-and-children/center-of-excellence-on-social-media-and-youth-mental-health/social-media-and-youth-mental-health-q-and-a-portal/middle-childhood/middle-childhood-questions/screen-time-guidelines/

Arak, J. (2002, July 12). Muppet with HIV joining "sesame" cast. *CBS News*. https://www.cbsnews.com/news/muppet-with-hiv-joining-sesame-cast/

Aufderheide, P. (1993). *Media literacy: A report of the national leadership conference on media literacy*. Aspen Institute.

Austin, E. W. (2007). The message interpretation process model. In J. J. Arnett (Ed.), *Encyclopedia of children, adolescents, and the media* (pp. 535–536). SAGE.

Austin, E. W. (2014). A bicycle riding theory of media literacy. In A. Silverblatt (Ed.), *The Praeger handbook of media literacy* (pp. 538–543). Praeger.

Austin, E. W., Austin, B. W., French, B. F., & Cohen, M. A. (2018). The effects of a nutrition media literacy intervention on parents' and youths' communication about food. *Journal of Health Communication, 23*(2), 190–199. https://doi.org/10.1080/10810730.2018.1423649

Austin, E. W. (2023). The media literacy theory of change model. In E. W. Austin., P. Bolls, N. H. O'Donnell, Z. Edwards, S. Domgaard, D. Mu, B. W. Austin,P. Rose, A. Sheftel, C. Payne, & L. Fox. (2023, Alphabetical listing after PI). *Getting to the heart and mind of the matter: A toolkit to build confidence as a trusted messenger of health information* (3rd ed., pp. 70). EXCITE (Extension Collaborative on Immunization Teaching and Engagement), Extension Foundation.

Austin, E. W., Austin, B. W. Power, T. G, Parker, L., Kaiser, C. K., & Edwards, Z. (2023). Youth perspectives on the effects of a family-centered media literacy intervention to encourage healthier eating. *Health Communication, 39*, 122–135. https://doi.org/10.1080/10410236.2022.2160078

Austin, E. W., Muldrow, A., & Austin, B. W. (2016). Examining how media literacy and personality factors predict skepticism towards alcohol advertising. *Journal of Health Communication, 21*, 600–609. https://doi.org/10.1080/1081730.2016.1153761

Austin, E. W., Pinkleton, B. E., Chen, Y., & Austin, B. W. (2015). Processing of sexual media messages improves due to media literacy effects on perceived message desirability. *Mass Communication and Society, 18*, 399–421. https://doi.org/10.1080/15205436.2014.1001909

Austin, E. W., Pinkleton, B. E., & Funabiki, R. P. (2007). The desirability paradox in the effects of media literacy training. *Communication Research, 34*, 483–506. https://doi.org/10.1177/0093650207305233

Banas, J. A., & Miller, G. (2013). Inducing resistance to conspiracy theory propaganda: Testing inoculation and metainoculation strategies. *Human Communication Research, 39*(2), 184–207.

Bandura, A. (1986). *Social foundations of thought and action: A social cognition theory*. Prentice-Hall.

Bandura, A. (1997). *Self-efficacy: The exercise of control*. Freeman and Company. W. H. Freeman/Times Books/Henry Holt & Co. https://doi.org/10.4135/9780857025753.n178

Bandura, A. (2001). Social cognitive theory of mass communication. *Media Psychology*, *3*(3), 265–299. https://doi.org/10.1207/S1532785XMEP0303_03

Basol, M., Roozenbeek, J., Berriche, M., Uenal, F., McClanahan, W. P., & Linden, S. van. (2021). Towards psychological herd immunity: Cross-cultural evidence for two prebunking interventions against COVID-19 misinformation. *Big Data & Society*, *8*, 1–18. https://doi.org/10.1177/20539517211013868

Bergsma, L. J., & Carney, M. E. (2008). Effectiveness of health-promoting media literacy education: A systematic review. *Health Education Research, 23*(3), 522–542. https://doi.org/10.1093/her/cym084

Boden, S. (2006). Dedicated followers of fashion? The influence of popular culture on children's social identities. *Media, Culture & Society*, *28*(2), 289–298. https://doi.org/10.1177/0163443706061690

Bond, B. J., & Drogos, K. L. (2014). Sex on the shore: Wishful identification and parasocial relationships as mediators in the relationship between jersey shore exposure and emerging adults' sexual attitudes and behaviors. *Media Psychology, 17(1)*, 102–126. https://doi.org/10.1080/15213269.2013.8720

Browne, R. B. (2005). *Popular culture studies across the curriculum: Essays for educators*. McFarland.

Buckingham, D. (2003). *Media education: Literacy, learning, and contemporary culture*. Polity Press.

Caulfield, M. (2021, February 15). *SIFT (the four moves)*. Hapgood. https://hapgood.us/2019/06/19/sift-the-four-moves/

Center for Disease Control and Prevention. (2021, November 3). *How to address COVID-19 vaccine misinformation*. Center for Disease Control and Prevention. https://www.cdc.gov/vaccines/covid-19/health-departments/addressing-vaccine-misinformation.html

Chen, Y., & Austin, E. W. (2012). The role of parental mediation in the development of Media Literacy and the prevention of substance use. In E. Scharrer (Ed.), *Media effects/media psychology* (pp. 1–19). Blackwell-Wiley Publishing. doi:10.1002/9781444361506.wbiems1.

Chen, S., & Chaiken, S. (1999). The heuristic-systematic model in its broader context. In S. Chaiken & Y. Trope (Eds.), *Dual-process theories in social psychology* (pp. 73–96). Guilford.

Clore, G. L., Wyer, R. S. Jr., Dienes, B., Gasper, K., Gohm, C., & Isbell, L. (2001). Affective feelings, as feedback: Some cognitive consequences. In L. L. Martin, & G. L. Clore (Eds), *Theories of mood and cognition: A user's guide* (pp. 27–62). Erlbaum.

Cohen, E. L. (2020). Stars—They're sick like us! The effects of a celebrity exemplar on COVID-19-related risk cognitions, emotions, and preventative behavioral intentions. *Science Communication, 42*(5), 724–741. https://doi.org/10.1177/1075547020960465

Cole, C., Biel, L., Pai, S., & Chand, A. (2007). Projecting youth voices: Sisimpur rural filmmak- ers' project in Bangladesh. *Journal of Children and Media, 1*(1), 88–92.

Collier, K. M., Coyne, S. M., Rasmussen, E. E., Hawkins, A. J., Padilla-Walker, L. M., Erickson, S. E., & Memmott-Elison, M. K. (2016). Does parental mediation of media influence child outcomes? A meta-analysis on media time, aggression, substance use, and sexual behavior. *Developmental Psychology, 52*(5), 798–812. https://doi.org/10.1037/dev0000108

Compton, J. (2013). Inoculation theory. In J. P. Dillard & L. Shen (Eds.). *The SAGE handbook of persuasion: Developments in theory and practice* (2nd ed., pp. 220–236). SAGE. https://doi.org/10.4135/9781452218410

Compton, J., Jackson, B., & Dimmock, J. A. (2016). Persuading others to avoid persuasion: Inoculation theory and resistant health attitudes. *Frontiers in Psychology, 7,* 1–16. https://doi.org/10.3389/fpsyg.2016.00122

Cor. (n.d.). *Civic online reasoning*. Home. https://cor.stanford.edu/

Desens, L. C., & Hughes, L. (2013). Entertainment-education and strategic communication: A case study of Sesame Workshop's "talk, listen, connect" initiative for military families. *International Journal of Strategic Communication, 7,* 292–309. https://doi.org/10.1080/1553118x.2013.7779

DiRusson, C., & Stansberry, K. (2021). Unvaxxed: A cultural study of the online anti-vaccination movement. *Qualitative Health Research, 32*, 317–329. https://doi.org/10.1177/10497323211056050

Dreyfuss, E. (2024, January 12). Our kids are living in a different Digital World. *The New York Times*. https://www.nytimes.com/2024/01/12/opinion/children-nicotine-zyn-social-media.html

Feilitzen, C., & Linné, O. (1975). The effects of television on children and adolescents: Identifying with television characters. *Journal of Communication, 25*(4), 51–55.

Freeland, S. (Director), Wilson, B. (Writer), Pico, T. (Writer), & Harjo, S. (Writer). (2021, August 23). What about your dad (Season 1, Epsiode 4) [TV series episode]. In S. Harjo, T. Waititi, & G. Basch (Executive Producers), *Reservation dogs.* FX Productions.

Garcia, L. (2022, September 2). *A guide to prebunking: A promising way to inoculate against Misinformation*. First Draft. https://firstdraftnews.org/articles/a-guide-to-prebunking-a-promising-way-to-inoculate-against-misinformation/

Garlen, J. C., & Graham, A. M. (2009). *Kermit culture: Critical perspectives on Jim Henson's muppets*. McFarland.

Giroux, H. (2002). *Breaking into the movies: Film and the culture of politics*. Blackwell.

Goldman, M. S., Brown, S. A., & Christiansen, B. A. (1987). Expectancy theory: Thinking about drinking. In H. T. Blane & K. E. Leonard (Eds.), *Psychological theories of drinking and alcoholism* (pp. 181–226). Guilford Press.

Grohs, R., Wagner, U., & Steiner, R. (2012). An investigation of children's ability to identify sponsors and understand sponsorship intentions. *Psychology & Marketing, 29*(11), 907–917. https://doi.org/10.1002/mar.20573

Harjo, S. (Executive Producer), Waititi, T. (Executive Producer), & Basch, G. (Executive Producers). (2021-Present). *Reservation dogs.* FX Productions.

Henson, J. (Director). (1981). *The Muppets great caper.* [Film]. The Jim Henson Company.

Hobbs, R. (1998). The seven great debates in the media literacy movement. *Journal of Communication, 48*(1), 16–32.

Hoffman, S. J., Mansoor, Y., Natt, N., Sritharan, L., Belluz, J., Caulfield, T., Freedhoff, Y., Lavis, J. N., & Sharma, A. M. (2017). Celebrities' impact on health-related knowledge, attitudes, behaviors, and status outcomes: Protocol for a systematic review, meta-analysis, and meta-regression analysis. *Systematic Reviews, 6*, 1–13. https://doi.org/10.1186/s13643-016-0395-1

Jacobs, D. (2007). More than words: Comics as a means of teaching multiple literacies. *English Journal, 96*, 19–25.

Jenkins, H. (1997). Empowering children in the digital age: Towards a radical media pedagogy. *Radical Teacher*, 50, 30–35.

Kaiser, C. K., & Austin, E. W. (2020). Media Literacy and advertising. In J. van den Bulck & D. R. Ewoldsen (Eds.), *The International Encyclopedia of Media Psychology* (pp. 984–991). Wiley Blackwell. https://doi.org/10.1002/9781119011071.iemp0230

Kaiser, C. K., Edwards, Z., & Austin, E. W. (2024). Media literacy practices to prevent obesity and eating disorders in Youth. *Current Obesity Reports, 13*, 1–9. https://doi.org/10.1007/s13679-023-00547-8

Kotler, J. A., Truglio, R. T., & Betancourt, J. (2016). R is for responsive: How Sesame Street meets the changing needs of children in the United States. In C. Cole & J. Lee (Eds), *The sesame effect: The global impact of the longest street in the world* (pp. 71–91). Routledge.

Lang, A. (2006). Using the limited capacity model of motivated mediated message processing (LC4MP) to design effective cancer communication messages. *Journal of Communication, 56*, 1–24.

Lang, A. (2009). The limited capacity model of motivated mediated message processing. In R. L. Nabi & M. B. Oliver (Eds.), *The SAGE handbook of media processes and effects* (193–204). SAGE.

Levine, M. P., & Harrison, K. (2009). Effects of media on eating disorders and body image. In J. Bryant & M. B. Oliver (Eds.), *Media effects: Advances in theory and research* (pp. 490–516). Routledge.

Levin-Zamir, D., & Bertschi, I. (2018). Media health literacy, eHealth literacy, and the role of the social environment in context. *International Journal of Environmental Research and Public Health, 15*, 1–12. https://doi.org/10.20944/preprints201805.0478.v1

Leung, M. M., Tripicchio, G., Agaronov, A., & Hou, N. (2014). Manga comic influences snack selection in black and Hispanic New York City youth. *Journal of Nutrition Education and Behavior, 46*(2), 142–147. https://doi.org/10.1016/j.jneb.2013.11.004

Liedke, J., & Wang, L. (2023, November 15). Social media and news fact sheet. Pew Research Center's Journalism Project. https://www.pewresearch.org/journalism/fact-sheet/social-media-and-news-fact-sheet/

Lyons, B. A., Montgomery, J. M., Guess, A. M., Nyhan, B., & Reifler, J. (2021). Overconfidence in news judgments is associated with false news susceptibility. *Proceedings of the National Academy of Sciences, 118*, 1–10. https://doi.org/10.1073/pnas.2019527118

McGuire, W. J., & Papageorgis, D. (1961). The relative efficacy of various types of prior belief-defense in producing immunity against persuasion. *Journal of Abnormal and Social Psychology, 62*(2), 327–337.

McLean, S. A., Paxton, S. J., & Wertheim, E. H. (2016). The role of media literacy in body dissatisfaction and disordered eating: A systematic review. *Body Image, 19*, 9–23. https://doi.org/10.1016/j.bodyim.2016.08.0

Myrick J. G. (2017). Celebrity-based appeals in health and risk messaging. In R. Parrott (Ed.), *Oxford research encyclopedia of health and risk message design and processing*. Oxford University Press.

Myrick, J. G., & Erlichman, S. (2020). How audience involvement and social norms foster vulnerability to celebrity-based dietary misinformation. *Psychology of Popular Media, 9*, 367–379. https://doi.org/10.1037/ppm0000229

Myrick, J., Willoughby, J., Noar S., & Brown, J. (2013). Reactions of young adults to the death of Apple CEO Steve Jobs: Implications for cancer communication. *Communication Research Reports, 30*(2), 115–126. https://doi.org/10.1080/08824096.2012.762906

Myrick, J. G., Nabi, R. L., & Eng, N. J. (2022). Consuming memes during the COVID pandemic: Effects of memes and meme type on Covid-related stress and coping efficacy. *Psychology of Popular Media, 11*, 316–323. https://doi.org/10.1037/ppm0000371

NAMLE. (2023, May 27). *Core principles*. https://namle.net/resources/core-principles/

News Literacy Project. (2023, July 12). News literacy project. *News Literacy Project*. https://newslit.org/

Oatley, K. (1992). *Best laid schemes: The psychology of the emotions.* Cambridge University Press.

Opdahl, K. M. (2002). *Emotion as meaning: The literary case for how we imagine.* The Rosen Publishing Group.

Pinkleton, B. E., Austin, E. W., Chen, Y. C. Y., & Cohen, M. (2012). The role of media literacy in shaping adolescents' understanding of and responses to sexual portrayals in mass media. *Journal of Health Communication, 17*(4), 460–476. https://doi.org/10.1080/10810730.2011.635770

Potter, W. J. (2004). *Theory of media literacy: A cognitive approach.* SAGE.

Potter, W. J. (2010). The state of media literacy. *Journal of Broadcasting & Electronic Media, 54*, 675–696.

Potter, R., & Bolls, P. D. (2012). *Psychophysiological measurement and meaning: Cognitive and emotional processing of media*. Routledge.

Rathje, S., Van Bavel, J. J., & Van Der Linden, S. (2021). Out-group animosity drives engagement on social media. *Proceedings of the National Academy of Sciences, 118*(26), e2024292118.

Rasmussen, E. E., Shafer, A., Colwell, M. J., White, S., Punyanunt-Carter, N., Densley, R. L., & Wright, H. (2016). Relation between active mediation, exposure to *Daniel Tiger's neighborhood*, and US preschoolers' social and emotional development. *Journal of Children and Media, 10*(4), 443–461. https://doi.org/10.1080/17482798.2016.1203806

Riley, A. H., Sangalang, A., Critchlow, E., Brown, N., Mitra, R., & Campos Nesme, B. (2020). Entertainment-education campaigns and COVID-19: How three global organizations adapted the health communication strategy for pandemic response and takeaways for the future. *Health Communication, 36*(1), 42–49. https://doi.org/10.1080/10410236.2020.1847

Roozenbeek, J., Basol, M., & van der Linden, S. (2023, January 17). A new way to inoculate people against misinformation - by Jon Roozenbeek, Melisa Basol, and Sander van der Linden. *Behavioral Scientist*. https://behavioralscientist.org/a-new-way-to-inoculate-people-against-misinformation/

Roozenbeek, J., & van der Linden, S. (2019a). Fake news game confers psychological resistance against online misinformation. *Palgrave Communications, 5*, 1–10. https://doi.org/10.1057/s41599-019-0279-9

Roozenbeek, J., & van der Linden, S. (2019b). The fake news game: Actively inoculating against the risk of misinformation. *Journal of Risk Research, 22*, 570–580. https://doi.org/10.1080/13669877.2018.1443491

Roozenbeek, J., & van der Linden, S. (2022). How to combat health misinformation: A psychological approach. *American Journal of Health Promotion, 36*(3), 569–575. https://doi.org/10.1177/08901171211070958

Roozenbeek, J., van der Linden, S., & Nygren, T. (2020). Prebunking interventions based on "inoculation" theory can reduce susceptibility to misinformation across cultures. *Harvard Kennedy School (HKS) Misinformation Review, 1*, 1–23. https://doi.org/10.37016//mr-2020-008

Rummo, P. E., Cassidy, O., Wells, I., Coffino, J. A., & Bragg, M. A. (2020). Examining the relationship between youth-targeted food marketing expenditures and the demographics of social media followers. *International Journal of Environmental Research and Public Health, 17*(5), 1–12. https://doi.org/10.3390/ijerph17051631

Schwarz, G. (2007). Media literacy, graphic novels, and social issues. *Simile, 7*, 1–18. https://doi.org/10.3138/sim.7.4.002

Smith, R., Kelly, B., Yeatman, H., & Boyland, E. (2019). Food marketing influences children's attitudes, preferences and consumption: A systematic critical review. *Nutrients, 11*, 1–14. https://doi.org/10.3390/nu11040875

Soulliere, D., & Blair, J. (2004). Muscle-mania: The male body ideal in professional wrestling. *International Journal of Men's Health, 5*, 268–286. https://doi.org/10.3149/jmh.0503.268.

Tisdell, E. J. (2008). Critical media literacy and transformative learning. *Journal of Transformative Education, 6*, 48–67. https://doi.org/10.1177/1541344608318970

Tisdell, E. J., & Thompson, P. M. (2007). 'Seeing from a different angle': The role of pop culture in teaching for diversity and critical media literacy in adult education. *International Journal of Lifelong Education, 26*(6), 651–673. https://doi.org/10.1080/02601370701711349

Tsene, L. (2022). Using comics as a media literacy tool for marginalized groups: The case of Athens comics library. *Media and Communication, 10*, 289–293. https://doi.org/10.17645/mac.v10i4.5716

University of Cambridge. (2021). Interactive games. *Social Decision-Making Lab: Inoculation Science*. https://inoculation.science/inoculation-games/

Vahedi, Z., Sibalis, A., & Sutherland, J. E. (2018). Are media literacy interventions effective at changing attitudes and intentions towards risky health behaviors in adolescents? A meta-analytic review. *Journal of Adolescence, 67*(1), 140–152. https://doi.org/10.1016/j.adolescence.2018.06.007

Valkenburg, P. M., Krcmar, M., Peeters, A. L., & Marseille, N. M. (1999). "Instructive mediation,' "restrictive mediation," and "social coviewing." *Journal of Broadcasting & Electronic Media, 43*, 52–66.

van der Linden, S., Albarracín, D., Fazio, L., Freelon, D., Roozenbeek, J., Swire-Thompson, B., & Van Bavel, J. (2023). Using psychological science to understand and fight health misinformation: An APA consensus statement. *PsycEXTRA Dataset*, 1–43. https://doi.org/10.1037/e506432023-001

White, B. M., Melton, C., Zareie, P., Davis, R. L., Bednarczyk, R. A., & Shaban-Nejad, A. (2023). Exploring celebrity influence on public attitude towards the COVID-19 pandemic: Social media shared sentiment analysis. *BMJ Health & Care Informatics Online, 30*, 1–7. https://doi.org/10.1136/bmjhci-2022-100665

Wong, I. H., Fan, C. M., Chiu, D. K. W., & Ho, K. K. W. (2024). Social media celebrities' influence on youths' diet behaviors: A gender study based on the Aida Marketing Communication Model. *Aslib Journal of Information Management*, *75*(5), 778–799. https://doi.org/10.1108/ajim-11-2022-0495

Xie, X., Gai, X., & Zhou, Y. (2019). A meta-analysis of media literacy interventions for deviant behaviors. *Computers & Education*, *139*, 146–156. https://doi.org/10.1016/j.compedu.2019.05.008

21

MEDICAL ETHICS, HEALTH COMMUNICATION, AND POPULAR CULTURE

Evie Kendal

Introduction

The relationship between health and media consumption is complex. Using the COVID-19 pandemic as an example, Cascini et al.'s (2022) systematic review of the influence of social media on vaccine uptake found online communities sharing misinformation impacted vaccination rates and promoted behaviors "not in line with public health recommendations globally" (p. 38). Cascini et al. suggested that pro-vaccination campaigns should, therefore, seek to harness the power of social media to get their message out as well. The pandemic also dominated news media, including numerous articles focused on inequitable distribution of limited medical supplies, including vaccines (Naftulin & Akhtar, 2021; Ovalle, 2023). Political leanings also influenced both the types and sources of news media consumed and the adoption of health protective behaviors, with the former further entrenching the latter through reinforcement and confirmation bias (Ansell et al., 2021; Barbieri & Bonini, 2021; Modgil et al., 2021; Nguyen & Catalan-Matamoros, 2022; Ovalle, 2023). As Ovalle asserted, in the context of COVID-19, political ideologies and influences led to a disparity in excess deaths caused by the virus across political affiliations.

While predominantly aimed at entertainment, popular media also contributes to the public's knowledge of health and healthcare systems, with Cambra-Badii et al. (2021) noting "[s]everal authors have suggested that medical dramas are a potential tool for teaching students in health science disciplines" (p. 509). However, it is not just programs explicitly focused on medicine that have this potential, but any popular media considering the kinds of social issues that face healthcare providers and consumers.

In this chapter, I will consider a particularly challenging example from both a medical ethics and health communication standpoint: The issue of healthcare resource rationing. Using two episodes of popular television from outside the medical drama genre, I will demonstrate how the abstract rationing methods discussed in bioethics scholarship can come alive in fictional narratives, providing an accessible mode for public discussion. The two episodes have been specifically chosen as rare examples where healthcare resource rationing is explicitly discussed in shows not set within the familiar hospital setting. Further, various bioethical frameworks are either directly referenced or indirectly described throughout, making these episodes well-suited to stimulate ethical discussion. First, I explore the *Star Trek: Voyager* episode "Critical Care" (Kahn & Windell, 2000), which dramatized elements from several competing healthcare rationing models, including utilitarianism and broad

 DOI: 10.4324/9781003436409-24

social utility versus egalitarianism and human rights theory. Second, I examine the *Law & Order: Organized Crime* episode "Not Your Father's Organized Crime," which explicitly tackled COVID-19 vaccine distribution and fairness (Chaiken & Girotti, 2021). Considered "free advertising" for law enforcement agencies, the latter comprised one of many police and legal procedurals to incorporate a COVID-19 storyline during the pandemic (Yu, 2022, p. 582). Time will tell whether such attempts at real-world relevance have influenced recruitment; however, previous research suggests that it likely enhanced viewers' knowledge and awareness of health ethics, including the rationale behind limited vaccine allocation decisions (see, e.g., related work by Pew Research Center, 2014).

I begin this chapter by briefly outlining some of the key healthcare rationing methods from the bioethics literature before exploring their depiction in "Critical Care" and "Not Your Father's Organized Crime." In so doing, I highlight the important role of popular culture in mediating health communication and discussions of the ethics of healthcare rationing in society. This treatment includes both standard and disaster triage protocols, including various examples employed during the COVID-19 pandemic.

Healthcare Resource Allocation Methods: Just Health vs. Libertarian Approaches

In his book, *Just Health: Meeting Health Needs Fairly*, Daniels (2008) argued that a just state must provide healthcare and health promotion services to protect each citizen's share of the "normal opportunity range" for someone at their stage of life (p. 175). Wilson (2009) noted that, while Daniels supported his argument by appealing to the idea that health is a "necessary condition" for access to various other opportunities – such as education and employment – he also advocated for limitations to be set on state-subsidized healthcare. Daniels claimed that the just state has a responsibility only to subsidize care that can be said to promote, restore, or maintain "normal species functioning," as a method of protecting the ideal of equal opportunity in society (p. 29). Where normal functioning cannot be attained, as in the case of chronic illness or long-term disability, the role of healthcare entails bringing people *as close as possible* to that ideal and preventing further deviation from it.

A major strength of Daniels' (2008) theory involved its focus on establishing minimum standards for state-subsidized healthcare, allowing private health insurers and clients to opt for "luxury" services without compromising the basic standard of care for all citizens. It also imposes maximum standards. For example, when rejecting the use of public funds for cosmetic surgeries, Daniels did not rely on resource scarcity as a defense but rather made the justice claim that, regardless of a country's level of wealth, limitations should be set on publicly funded healthcare entitlements. However, this perspective exposed a weakness regarding citizens with incurable diseases or permanent disabilities, as Daniels focused almost entirely on providing long-term care and ensuring equal opportunity in the workplace, rather than pursuing research and experimental treatments which could, in the future serve a curative function. Schmidt (2009) also criticized this theory for attributing little to no responsibility for personal lifestyle choices that may have contributed to a person's poor health when attempting to determine a reasonable healthcare resource allocation.

An alternative allocation method can be found in Nozick's influential 1974 text, *Anarchy, State, and Utopia*, where he outlined a libertarian approach to the allocation of healthcare, dictating that justice requires only that health resources be traded according to free-market values in the absence of coercion. This reliance on procedural justice for healthcare resource allocation directly conflicts with Daniels' (2008) argument in *Just Health*, where he characterizes healthcare as a "special" good that should not be reserved solely for those able to afford it. According to Nozick, however, healthcare resources – like any other resources – should be distributed according to ability to pay, keeping taxation to a minimum and protecting citizens from subsidizing the healthcare of others. In Nozick's view, ill-health is "unfortunate but not unfair," and, thus, no special claim exists for healthcare resources to be allocated any differently from other goods or services, for which exchange is dictated by market values rather than according to need (p. 32). For Nozick, as long as assets are fairly exchanged, no ethical problem emerges with allowing those in possession of more to use these to access better healthcare.

Nozick's (1974) theory fails to account for the kinds of injustices that may lead to wealth concentration among some members of a society at the expense of others. Reinhardt (1987) further noted that the libertarian goal of promoting free-market healthcare is not shared by "the world at large," claiming, "literally no country seems prepared to surrender the delivery of personal health services and products completely to arbitration by unfettered market forces" (p. 168). He further pointed to a shared instinct to impose certain ethical restraints on the free-market trade of healthcare services, which transcends physical and political borders. However, a common argument in favor of Nozick's user-pay system of healthcare is that it would increase individual responsibility for health, even if failing to recognize the complex socio-economic factors influencing health behaviors (Marchand et al., 1998).

Healthcare Resource Allocation Methods: Human Rights and Universal Healthcare vs. Pure Utilitarianism and Cost-Benefit Analysis

Another common way of discussing healthcare resource allocation relates to health as a human right. Article 12(1) of the United Nations' International Covenant on Economic, Social and Cultural Rights discusses this right, which requires that the State recognize "the right of everyone to the enjoyment of the highest attainable standard of physical and mental health" (United Nations, 1960). Noting that this right cannot feasibly entail a duty to guarantee "a healthy state for each person," Susser (1993) claimed that the societal obligation instead necessitates "equity between groups as a fundamental principle" (p. 419). For Susser, the steps toward discharging the State's obligation here include providing equal access to "curative, preventive and promotive" health services, making "good faith" attempts to promote health among citizens suffering disadvantage, engaging in effective evaluation of health services, and ensuring "equitable sociopolitical arrangements that give a voice to all groups" regarding matters of health (p. 420). Clearly, the libertarian perspective that would allow wealthier citizens to purchase better healthcare runs afoul of this equity principle.

A strength of the health as a human right argument is that it promotes respect for every individual as an equal, without demanding equality of outcomes regarding health status. It also forms the basis of the World Health Organization's (WHO, 2023) definition of universal health coverage, which demands that "all people have access to the full range of quality health services they need, when and where they need them, without financial hardship" (para. 1). However, even if one accepts health as a human right, the issue of resource allocation remains, as the need for health resources always outstrips supply on the local, national, and international levels. The utilitarian response involves using all resources to maximum benefit, even if doing so means tolerating significant inequalities between individuals in the relevant community.

Classical utilitarianism dictates that an act can only be considered right if it can reasonably be expected to produce the greatest utility for the greatest number of people affected by the act. According to Mill (1906), *greatest utility* can be conceived of in practical terms as the *greatest happiness*, with each individual's happiness counting equally. When used in healthcare resource allocation, "utility" typically refers to health. As various states of health cannot be directly compared, public health officials often employ metrics like cost-benefit analysis, quality-adjusted life years (QALYs), and disability-adjusted life years (DALYs) as proxies to calculate which interventions should be prioritized for which patients to achieve the "biggest bang for the buck" (Prieto & Sacristán, 2003). Daniels (2008) alluded to this principle in *Just Health* when advocating for "aggregate welfare" (p. 49). As I discuss later in this chapter, utilitarianism also constitutes a major influence in triage situations.

COVID-19 has exposed various inequalities within and between nations that have significantly influenced population health. In the United States, despite higher rates of infection and severe illness,

African American, Latinx, and people of lower socio-economic status lacked vaccination coverage compared to wealthier communities and Caucasian citizens (Naftulin & Akhtar, 2021). Bollyky et al. (2023) also noted COVID deaths "disproportionately clustered in US states with lower mean years of education, higher poverty rates, [and] limited access to quality health care" (p. 1352). Bollyky et al. partially attributed these disproportionate deaths to the fact that essential workers and those who could not work remotely were more likely to belong to disadvantaged communities, and, thus, were more likely to be exposed to the virus due to an inability to socially distance.

The disparities in both vaccination rates and disease outcomes are even more stark when viewed from an international perspective, with Jecker et al. (2021) reminding us that "[b]ioethical debates over allocating scarce healthcare resources often take for granted that distribution will occur at a local level" (p. 308). When the disease of interest encompasses a global pandemic, however, allowing wealthier nations to hoard limited vaccines is both ethically and practically problematic. Jecker et al. noted that, without a focus on equitable global vaccine distribution, "country of residence will likely become the single most important factor" in who gets access (p. 308). They observed that tragic implication conflicts with various resource allocation methods and philosophies, including moral cosmopolitanism, which argues that we owe the same consideration to everyone regardless of their "place of origin," and both sufficitarian and prioritarian justice principles (p. 309). The former holds that everyone has the right to "have enough opportunity and capability to lead a minimally decent life," while the latter suggests fair distribution of goods requires that we "place more weight on improving the situation of those who are worse off" (p. 309). Bayati et al. (2022) also argued that the injustice attached to inequitable vaccine distribution is not just limited to health disparities, but also the rate of economic recovery that vaccination promotes. While less obvious than the wealthy individual using their personal wealth to skip the queue, inequities on the nation-state level can affect large numbers of people and violate the principles underpinning the human rights approach to health.

In response to concerns about global inequity, the COVID-19 Vaccines Global Access (COVAX) initiative aimed to close the gap in vaccine coverage between high- and low-income countries by incentivizing collaborative vaccine research and purchasing agreements over competitive ones. Nevertheless, writing in February 2021, Yamey reported that more than 75% of the vaccines administered at the time had gone to people in just 10 countries, with the 2.5 billion citizens of some 130 other countries having received none (p. 529). Quite apart from the ethical obligation to provide for disadvantaged communities, Yamey referenced the utilitarian argument in favor of sharing vaccine supply, as it is "in everyone's interests … to boost vaccinations" to control the virus globally (p. 529).

Healthcare Resource Allocation in Popular Culture: *Star Trek: Voyager* "Critical Care" s7e5

One of the major contributions that popular culture makes to the field of bioethics involves providing compelling narratives that dramatize ethical dilemmas and bring them out of the abstract (Hughes & Lantos, 2001). For resource allocation decisions, such narratives put a face to an otherwise anonymous category of persons who are to be provided or denied healthcare resources under the system being debated. *Star Trek: Voyager*'s episode "Critical Care" represents a particularly potent example, illustrating several of the methods discussed above and how they yield conflicting priorities.

"Critical Care" opened with the starship's Emergency Medical Hologram, or EMH, having been kidnapped and sold to an alien hospital. Known only as "The Doctor," this artificial intelligence initially declared that he would not "perform medical services for a pair of common thieves," but, when faced with the victims of a mining accident, he stated that he could not withhold his services as he was "programmed with the Hippocratic Oath." Nevertheless, The Doctor was horrified to discover that the ward, Level Red, lacked even basic medical supplies and personnel. There, he met a young patient, Tebbis, who was dying of a "chromo-viral infection" that could be easily cured with the right medication, but none had been administered. Before he could get to the bottom of this situation, the director of the facility, Chellick, informed The Doctor that he was being transferred to Level Blue. "Level Blue is your critical care area, I presume," The Doctor said, to which Chellick responded: "Level Blue is the area where it's most critical that we provide excellent care."

On arrival, the Doctor observed that Level Blue comprised a luxurious facility replete with modern technology and high-quality treatments, including access to the medication that Tebbis needed to survive. The Doctor demanded an explanation, and Chellick responded that the Allocator assigned a treatment coefficient (T.C.) to each patient that determined the level of care that they would receive, based on a calculation of their social utility.

> The Doctor: "How is this coefficient derived?"
> Chellick: "Through a complex formula that involves professions, skills, accomplishments … "
> The Doctor: "How is any of that relevant to medical treatment?"
> Chellick: "An agricultural engineer is obviously more important than a waste processor."
> The Doctor: "Important to whom?"
> Chellick: "Society. When your resources are limited, you have to prioritize."
> The Doctor: "So you base treatment on whether patients have particular abilities?"
> Chellick: "It's much more complicated than that. The Allocator assesses the entire individual."
> The Doctor: "And reduces his life to a number."
>
> *(11:04–11:38)*

The Doctor was further distressed to learn the injections that Tebbis needed were routinely allocated to Level Blue patients to prevent "arterial aging," with the justification that it would enhance life expectancy for this cohort. That disadvantaged Level Red patients were being de-prioritized for life-saving treatment so elite members of society could use these resources for non-urgent reasons violates various justice principles; however, Chellick defended this practice on purely utilitarian grounds. Chellick admitted that the system may seem "impersonal," but he argued that it served the greater good as it lifted society out of chaos and promoted overall survival.

While the scenes in "Critical Care" were deliberately provocative, the idea of a resource allocation system that allows social utility to influence treatment priority is not far-fetched. In fact, many used some variant of this argument to support the prioritization of frontline workers for early COVID-19 vaccination, on the grounds that the special circumstance of the pandemic justified preferential treatment (Bhatia, 2020). The rationale again appealed to the greater good, as Bhatia affirmed that "[b]y prioritising their healthcare needs, we can benefit others" since frontline workers contribute to the provision of essential services, including healthcare (p. 733). Bhatia reminded us that healthcare rationing is not limited to crises like the pandemic, though, with emergency room triage and pharmaceutical government subsidies routinely prioritizing services for some patients and not others, often on economic grounds (p. 733). However, she also noted that law courts have been reluctant to weigh in on matters of healthcare rationing, "presumably because notions of placing a monetary value on life are ethically and morally repugnant" (p. 734). In this regard, an artificial intelligence like The Allocator might alleviate some of the guilt arising from making allocation decisions that will have profound effects on people's lives.

Cheung and Parent's (2021) account of "narrow social utility" in COVID-19 vaccine distribution models also matched Chellick's position in the previous quote, noting "judgements about the instrumental value of certain jobs or positions" often underlie the intuition that healthcare workers should be prioritized for vaccination if supplies are limited (p. 76). These authors rejected the other major argument in favor of healthcare worker prioritization – namely, the claim of reciprocity – but also argued that narrow social utility is "a procedurally fickle principle to operationalize and therefore prone to inconsistencies" (p. 76). Interestingly, "Critical Care" portrayed The Allocator's judgements as unfair and discriminatory, but not procedurally unsound. At least according to its own programming, the system seems robust; for example, it resisted tampering after The Doctor tried to trick it into authorizing treatment for Tebbis by manipulating his T.C. through listing additional in-need skills against his profile. The fact that The Allocator prioritized Level Blue patients due to their overall calculated value to society, rather than their contribution to a specific project, indicated that it employed a broad, rather than narrow, social utility metric. However, in so doing, it violated the rights of less advantaged citizens who may have had more pressing health needs, like Tebbis.

The Doctor's claim that Tebbis had "as much right to treatment as anyone" aligned with the health as a human right perspective, as did his focus on distributing resources according to medical need, without reference to social status, wealth, education, or other factors. Furthermore, prioritizing the young person whose opportunities had been limited due to poor health also fulfilled Daniels' (2008) requirement for the state to protect each citizen's "normal opportunity range" (p. 175). In his Prudential Lifespan Account of resource rationing, Daniels advocated for the reasonable budgeting of limited healthcare resources over the lifespan, allowing the use of age-based rationing as a last resort when dealing with extreme resource scarcity. According to this aspect of the *Just Health* argument, prioritizing injections for Tebbis would support "age-relative" normal functioning, while using the same medication to prevent the naturally occurring "arterial aging" would not. Chellick's arguments about saving society, rather than any given individual, would resonate with utilitarians. Meanwhile, the libertarian perspective would uphold a right for the more elite members of society to use their advantages to procure better healthcare services; however, it would be less in favor of the state provided treatment facility making allocation decisions.

Ford and Pretorius (2017) claimed that "Critical Care" should be incorporated into medical ethics curricula due to its exploration of justice and beneficence and the need to balance patient needs against available resources. Ford and Pretorius noted that ethics education allows students to be "professionally socialised and gain an understanding of appropriate ethical behaviour in their discipline," with the framing of this narrative supporting the dominant Western model of biomedical ethics (p. 133). However, while the writing primed the audience to accept The Doctor's egalitarian perspective on resource allocation and assume that he was more moral than Chellick, The Doctor engaged in many behaviors throughout the episode that violated basic ethical precepts. He lied to a patient about their medication, allowed an untrained person to administer injections without supervision, stole medical supplies from one ward to use in another, falsified medical records, indirectly caused discomfort and death for various Level Red patients by exceeding their annual medication allowances leading to The Allocator discharging them prematurely, and eventually kidnapped and poisoned Chellick to force him to release more resources to Level Red. Only the latter gave him pause, though, with The Doctor requesting a diagnostic of his "ethical subroutines" when the Voyager crew eventually rescued him. The diagnostic is run by Seven of Nine, a former member of the Borg Collective, a machine intelligence that represented one of the greatest evils in the show due to their extreme utilitarianism and abandonment of individuality. When The Doctor received a "clean bill of health," he admitted that he had hoped that his behavior in torturing Chellick to save his other patients could be explained by a malfunction. Seven responded: "You were prepared to sacrifice an individual to benefit a collective," to which The Doctor answered: "No offense, Seven, but I don't exactly aspire to Borg ideals."

Resource Rationing: Standard and Disaster Triage

A more extreme version of healthcare resource rationing occurs in standard and disaster triage scenarios, which forms the basis for discussion of the second text to be considered in this chapter. According to Ghanbari et al. (2021, n.p.), triage protocols are subject to criticism by the "competing philosophies of utilitarianism and egalitarianism," with the first focused on benefiting the most people and the second on treating everyone as fairly as possible. Bhatia (2020) also added prioritarianism, where doctors give preference to the most disadvantaged, and social utility models, focused on preserving useful roles in society. She claimed that COVID-19 brought healthcare rationing conversations to the fore, with substantial public attention paid to ventilator allocation decisions, but that emergency triage probably represents the most highly recognizable form of rationing as medical professionals devote resources according to the "severity of need and/or likelihood of recovery" (pp. 731–732). Childress (2004) claimed that all systems of triage have an "implicit or explicit utilitarian rationale," while also aiming to meet the justice requirement of treating like cases alike (p. 207). He further noted that it is generally appropriate for healthcare workers to treat the most severely injured or unwell patients first, "in the confidence that others can wait their turn without undue burden or risk" (p. 207). Okorie (2019) asserted that doctors employ triage to ensure that they do not waste limited resources on patients who will survive without them or on patients who will likely die regardless. However, Okorie criticized this focus on "survivability" as the very elements that contribute to it are likely to "mirror the socioeconomic vulnerabilities of patients" (p. 77). For example, systemic racism may be the reason that a patient with particular characteristics may have historically suffered worse outcomes than another patient, so selecting for predicted survival does not compare these patients fairly. Far from being neutral, such supposedly value-free judgments based on survivability data might simply replicate other social biases.

Repine et al. (2005) claimed that triage is necessary as a conflict exists between citizens who believe healthcare is an entitlement, rather than a privilege, and thus will settle for nothing less than "maximal care," and the providers "who must determine who can realistically receive care" in resource-constrained settings (p. 505). Previous methods for making such determinations have suffered fierce criticism on the grounds of discrimination, but Orfali (2021) asserted that alternatives like "first-come, first-served" or lottery-based methods are not considered viable options (p. 16). Practitioners generally understand that urgent, life-threatening cases will take priority, but studies show the application of triage protocols across providers is inconsistent (Sevimli et al., 2015). Srinivas et al. (2021) suggested that such differences of opinion could be overcome using normative economics, where priorities can be assigned values according to the benefits accruing to the relevant population – not dissimilar to the T.C. algorithm featured in "Critical Care."

While most people have experienced standard triage, disaster triage operates under a different principle where the most severe cases may be deprioritized for care due to the low likelihood of meaningful recovery or the resource-intensive process required to attempt treatment in a situation of scarcity. According to Ghanbari et al. (2021), it is unacceptable for healthcare providers to make ad hoc decisions in a mass casualty event regarding who will be treated and who will not, advocating instead for "robust policies and procedures" that can be followed in an emergency. Inconsistent policies for the allocation of ventilators during the first waves of COVID-19, or evacuation resources during Hurricane Katrina, indicate that many places lack such protocols, feeding into public distrust that scarce resources will be managed fairly and effectively in a crisis (Cheung & Parent, 2021; Chuang et al., 2022). Childress (2004) agreed that, without firm protocols, "confusion and even chaos will reign" during a disaster. However, he also noted the moral distress attending resource allocation decisions by individual healthcare professionals, particularly when shifting from a standard to disaster triage policy (p. 206). In such instances, a healthcare worker's instinct to prioritize the patient most at risk may conflict with the new directive to concentrate resources where they likely make the most impact, even if this choice means sacrificing the worst off. As Wagner and Dahnke (2015) asserted, in disaster triage, health professionals face the reality where "[t]he decision to advocate for the sickest patient is overruled by the utilitarian principle of doing the greatest good for the greatest number" (p. 303). When the resource being decided is a ventilator, Truog et al. (2021) reminded us that the likely outcome for the patient denied access will be death, a confronting situation for decision-makers.

Farrell et al. (2020) also claimed that various age cut-offs for accessing resources during COVID were ethically problematic from an ageism perspective and would have switched the usual priority system where the elderly are seen more rapidly, due to greater frailty. Some people tried to justify age limits either by appealing to the higher likelihood of survival for younger and fitter people or to principles resembling Daniels' Prudential Lifespan Account, the so-called "fair innings" framework, or other life cycle models that posit the young should be prioritized as they've had the least opportunities to progress through life's stages (2008, p. 1145; White, 2020, p. 1773). Whether life expectancy or quality of life estimations should form part of the allocation process constitutes the subject of much debate in bioethics scholarship (Joebges & Biller-Adorno, 2020). As with vaccine prioritization, ethicists hotly debate whether healthcare professionals should be given preferential access to ventilators and other life-saving interventions during a public health emergency (Cheung & Parent, 2021).

Case Study: COVID-19 Vaccine Rollout in the News

The need to have procedures for resource allocation in place before emergencies occur has been illustrated well, both in the news media from the original COVID-19 vaccine rollout and in the episode, "Not Your Father's Organized Crime." Writing for *Business Insider*, Naftulin and Akhtar (2021, n.p.) noted that the public's hope with the announcement of the vaccine "soon curdled when Americans discovered congressional lawmakers, billionaire nursing-home benefactors, and hospital executives were getting the vaccine more quickly than the average person," observing that these individuals took advantage of "loopholes, using money and connections to jump the line." Such behavior would be well-tolerated within a Nozickian world where the free-market reigns; however, Naftulin and Akhtar argued that the wealthy purchasing a "first-class ticket" for a health resource billions of people were in desperate need of did not sit well with the majority of citizens. This reaction was particularly the case, given the wealthy were already better protected than most, given the higher likelihood they could self-isolate and work remotely (Thomson & Sprague, 2020). Bengali et al. (2020) also reported in the *Los Angeles Times* that the COVID-19 pandemic was unusual, in that it was carried across countries by the wealthy. According to Bengali et al., "Pandemics throughout history have been associated with the underprivileged, but in many developing countries the coronavirus was a high-class import – carried in by travelers returning from business trips in China, studies in Europe, ski vacations in the Rockies" (para. 3). These authors also recounted various instances where entitled rich citizens knowingly broke quarantine rules, leading to disease spread. Writing for *The Australian Financial Review Magazine,* Thomson and Sprague (2020) also highlighted that billionaires often dodged state quarantine rules by flying privately and isolating in their own mansions.

Healthcare Rationing in Popular Culture: *Law & Order – Organized Crime* "Not Your Father's Organized Crime" s1e2.

The numerous news media items following rich people behaving badly during lockdown likely influenced the decision to have a vaccine rorting storyline feature in the newest installment of the *Law & Order* franchise. In the episode, "Not Your Father's Organized Crime," the local gang hijacked a vaccine delivery truck with the intent to sell the medicines to doctors treating wealthy clients. When Detective Elliott Stabler questioned the mob boss, Richard Wheatley, he mentioned that the stolen vaccines were intended for the Harlem hospital, for "people who need 'em. The elderly, frontline workers, folks who can't afford to have a private doctor show up at their house with a vaccine shot and a glass of Chardonnay." Later, when Stabler tried to convince one of the women set to receive a vaccination from a stolen vial to tell him where the clinic providing the illegal doses was, he told her: "It's stolen vaccines. They were meant to go to other people. Vulnerable people, the elderly, your parents, kids." The show positioned the queue-jumping as immoral and unfair and did not provide any reason for the audience to excuse any of the wealthy vaccine recipients.

The clock ticked as the police struggled to recover the vaccines before they spoiled. Meanwhile, wealthy people hosted vaccination parties at their homes and injected their friends. When authorities made an arrest, they captured one of the "Park Avenue doctors" who bought some of the stolen vaccine supply, and a number of his wealthy clients in the clinic waiting room then faced the music. It may be cathartic for audiences to witness these entitled people taken down a notch, but the true villains (the mob thieves) were not punished in this episode, and the misappropriation of limited resources continued apace.

In an educational moment, Stabler asked his Sergeant, "Didn't the governor make it illegal to jump the line?" – in addition to providing details for the vaccine allocation triage. The show reminded viewers that the immunocompromised and healthcare workers remained at higher risk of exposure and should be prioritized, and that others would have to wait their turn to receive a vaccine, much like having to wait in the emergency room when a more severe case presents itself.

Throughout COVID-19, an individual's adherence to public health advice – including social distancing, testing, using personal protective equipment, and getting vaccinated when able – depended heavily on their political views and media consumption (Ansell et al., 2021; Barbieri & Bonini, 2021; Wallace et al., 2023). However, Bayati et al. (2022) pointed to socio-economic status as the greatest predictor for vaccine availability in an area, indicating inequitable distribution of preventive health measures among those most at risk, including poorer citizens and those experiencing homelessness. The righteous anger brought on by the misuse of COVID-19 vaccines in "Not Your Father's Organized Crime" reinforced the justification for triage and reminded individuals where they were in the queue. This episode represented just one of countless COVID story arcs in television series since the pandemic started, but it provided a rare example discussing the mechanics of healthcare rationing in action.

Conclusion

Healthcare rationing comprises a politically and ethically fraught issue, and health professionals have proposed various methods for managing the use of scarce healthcare resources in bioethics literature. *Star Trek: Voyager*'s "Critical Care" and *Law & Order: Organized Crime*'s "Not Your Father's Organized Crime" depicted several key issues: the struggle to balance egalitarianism and utilitarianism, moral distress in triage, and the need to establish trust with the public to promote adherence to public health guidelines. Research has shown that using television dramas, particularly watching whole episodes in the classroom, can help make ethical issues more real for students considering these issues, while also providing an outlet for health communication with the wider public (Spike, 2008). When it comes to medical education in particular, fictional representations of real-life dilemmas provide a source for future healthcare providers to draw on when forming their own professional identities and deciding what kind of practitioner they want to be (Weaver et al., 2014).

For the general public, studies have demonstrated that popular television can serve a public health communication role in countries at every economic development level (Elkamel, 1995; Haq et al., 2010; Kato et al., 2017). In the cases referenced in this chapter, future nurses, doctors, and administrators may find role models to emulate or villains to shun in characters like The Doctor or Chellick. Meanwhile, current and future patients may gain a deeper awareness and understanding of standards of triage or healthcare rationing decisions from watching Detective Stabler enforce resource allocation policies. For all viewers, *Star Trek: Voyager*'s "Critical Care" and *Law & Order: Organized Crime*'s "Not Your Father's Organized Crime" provide engaging content to fuel ethical debates, humanizing otherwise abstract concepts of distributive and procedural justice as they apply to health as a human right.

References

Ansell, B., Cansunar, A., & Elkjaer, M. A. (2021). Social distancing, politics and wealth, *West European Politics, 44*(5–6), 1283–1313. https://doi.org/10.1080/01402382.2021.1917154

Barbieri, P. N., & Bonini, B. (2021). Political orientation and adherence to social distancing during the COVID-19 pandemic in Italy. *Economia Politica, 38*, 483–504. https://doi.org/10.1007/s40888-021-00224-w

Bayati, M., Noroozi, R., Ghanbari-Jahromi, M., & Jalali, F. S. (2022). Inequality in the distribution of Covid-19 vaccine: A systematic review. *International Journal for Equity in Health, 21*, 122. https://doi.org/10.1186/s12939-022-01729-x

Bengali, S., Linthicum K., & Kim, V. (2020, May 8). How coronavirus – a 'rich man's disease' – infected the poor. *Los Angeles Times.* https://www.latimes.com/world-nation/story/2020-05-08/how-the-coronavirus-began-as-a-disease-of-the-rich

Bhatia, N. (2020). We need to talk about rationing: The need to normalize discussion about healthcare rationing in a post COVID-19 era. *Journal of Bioethical Inquiry, 17*, 731–735. https://doi.org/10.1007/s11673-020-10051-6

Bollyky, T. J., Castro, E., Aravkin, A. Y., Bhangdia, K., Dalos, J., Hulland, E. N., et al. (2023). Assessing COVID-19 pandemic policies and behaviours and their economic and educational trade-offs across US states from Jan 1, 2020, to July 31, 2022: An observational analysis. *Lancet, 401,* 1341–1360. https://doi.org/10.1016/S0140-6736(23)00461-0

Cambra-Badii, I., Moyana, E., Ortega, I., Baños, J-E., & Sentí, M. (2021). TV medical dramas: Health sciences students' viewing habits and potential for teaching issues related to bioethics and professionalism. *BMC Medical Education, 21*, 509–519.

Cascini, F., Pantovic, A., Al-Ajlouni, Y. A., Failla, G., Puleo, V., Melnyk, A., et al. (2022). Social media and attitudes towards a COVID-19 vaccination: A systematic review of the literature. *Lancet, 48,* 1–44.

Chaiken, I. (Writer), & Girotti, K. (Director). (2021, April 8). Not Your Father's Organized Crime (Season 1, Episode 2). In Wolf, D. et al. (Executive producers), *Law & Order: Organized Crime*, Universal Television.

Cheung, A. T. M., & Parent, B. (2021). Mistrust and inconsistency during COVID-19: considerations for resource allocation guidelines that prioritise healthcare workers. *Journal of Medical Ethics, 47,* 73–77.

Childress, J. F. (2004). Disaster triage: Triage duties in the event of a medical disaster have different ethical rules than normal situations. *Virtual Mentor*, *6*(5), 206–208.

Chuang, E., Grand-Clement, J., Chen, J-T, Chan, C. W., Goyal, V., & Ng Gong, M. (2022). Quantifying utilitarian Outcomes to inform triage ethics: Simulated performance of a ventilator triage protocol under Sars-CoV-2 pandemic surge conditions. *AJOB Empirical Bioethics*, *13*(3), 196–204.

Daniels, N. (2008). *Just health: Meeting health needs fairly*. Cambridge University Press.

Elkamel, F. (1995). The use of television series in health education. *Health Education Research, 10*(2), 225–232.

Farrell, T. W., Francis, L., Brown, T., Ferrante, L. E., Widera, E., Rhodes, R., et al. (2020). Rationing healthcare resources in the COVID-19 era and beyond: Ethical considerations regarding older adults. *Journal of the American Geriatrics Society, 68*, 1143–1149.

Ford, A., & Pretorius, L. (2017). Balancing the needs of the many against the needs of the few: Aliens, holograms and discussions of medical ethics. In E. Kendal & B. Diug (Eds.), *Teaching medicine and medical ethics using popular culture* (pp. 133–147). Palgrave.

Ghanbari, V., Ardalan, A., Zareiyan, A., Nejati, A., Hanfling, D., Bagheri, A., et al. (2021). Perceptions on principle of priority setting in disaster triage: A Q-method study. *International Emergency Nursing, 59*, 101064. https://doi.org/10.1016/j.ienj.2021.101064

Haq, Z. U., Sood, S., Yansen, S., Javeed, S, & Ali, N. (2010). Using TV talk show for public health media advocacy: A case study. *JPMA: The Journal of the Pakistan Medical Association, 60*(6), 460–464.

Hughes, J. J, & Lantos, J. (2001). Medical ethics through the Star Trek lens. *Literature and Medicine, 20*(1), 26–38.

Jecker, N. S., Wightman, A. G., & Diekema, D. S. (2021). Vaccine ethics: An ethical framework for global distribution of COVID-19 vaccines. *Journal of Medical Ethics, 47,* 308–317.

Joebges, S., & Biller-Adorno, N. (2020). Ethics guidelines on COVID-19 triage—an emerging international consensus. *Critical Care, 24,* 201–205.

Kahn, J. (Writer), & Windell, T. (Director). (2000, November 1). Critical Care (Season 7, Episode 5). In Berman, R. (Executive producer), *Star Trek: Voyager*. Paramount.

Kato, M., Ishikawa, H., Okuhara, T., Okada, M., & Kiuchi, T. (2017). Mapping research on health topics presented in prime-time TV dramas in "developed" countries: A literature review. *Cogent Social Sciences, 3*(1), 1318477.

Marchand, S., Wikler, D., & Landesman, B. (1998). Class, health and justice. *The Milbank Quarterly, 76*(3), 449–467.

Mill, J. S. (1906. *Utilitarianism.* Longman's, Green and Company.
Modgil, S., Singh, R. K., Gupta, S., & Dennehy, D. (2021). A confirmation bias view on social media induced polarisation during Covid-19. *Information Systems Frontiers*, 26, 417–441. https://doi.org/10.1007/s10796-021-10222-9
Naftulin, J., & Akhtar, A. (2021, February 5). Some rich people are gaming the system to get COVID-19 vaccines using hefty donations and cozy relationships with CEOs. *Business Insider*. https://www.businessinsider.com/rich-poor-covid-vaccine-disparity-2021-2
Nguyen, A., & Catalan-Matamoros. (2022). Anti-vaccine discourse on social media: An exploratory audit of negative tweets about vaccines and their posters. *Vaccines, 10*(12), 2067.
Nozick, R. (1974). *Anarchy, state, and utopia.* Basic Books.
Okorie, N. (2019). Partiality, impartiality and the ethics of triage. *Developing World Bioethics, 19,* 76–85.
Orfali, K. (2021). Getting to the truth: Ethics, trust, and triage in the United States versus Europe during the Covid-19 Pandemic. *Hastings Center Report, 51*(1), 16–22.
Ovalle, D. (2023, July 24). Vaccine politics may be to blame for GOP excess deaths, study finds. *The Washington Post.* https://www.washingtonpost.com/health/2023/07/24/covid-vaccines-republicans-deaths/
Pew Research Center. (2014, March 7). Millennials in adulthood: Detached from institutions, networked with friends. http://www.pewsocialtrends.org/2014/03/07/millennials-in-adulthood/
Prieto, L., & Sacristán, J. A. (2003). Problems and solutions in calculating quality-adjusted life years (QALYs). *Health and Quality of Life Outcomes, 1,* 80.
Reinhardt, U. (1987). Resource allocation in health care: The allocation of lifestyles to providers. *The Milbank Quarterly, 65*(2), 153–176.
Repine, T. B., Lisagor, P., & Cohen, D. J. (2005). The dynamics and ethics of triage: Rationing care in hard times. *Military Medicine, 170*(6), 505–509.
Schmidt, H. (2009). Just health responsibility. *Journal of Medical Ethics 35*, 21–26.
Sevimli, Ş., Dursan, R., & Karadaş, S. (2015). Health professionals of emergency service: Evaluation of triage and ethical values in disaster medicine. *Eurasian Journal of Emergency Medicine, 14,* 107–112.
Spike, J. (2008). Television viewing habits and ethical reasoning: Why watching *Scrubs* does a better job than most bioethics classes. *The American Journal of Bioethics, 8*(12), 11–13.
Srinivas, G., Maanasa, R., Meenakshi, M., Adaikalam, J. M., Seshayyan, S., & Muthuvel, T. (2021). Ethical rationing of healthcare resources during COVID-19 outbreak: Review. *Ethics, Medicine and Public Health, 16,* 100633. https://doi.org/10.1016/j.jemep.2021.100633
Susser, M. (1993). Health as a human right: An epidemiologist's perspective on public health. *American Journal of Public Health, 83*(3), 418–426.
Thomson, J., & Sprague, J. (2020, October 26). How COVID-19 rocked the rich in Australia this year. *The Australian Financial Review Magazine*. https://www.afr.com/rich-list/how-covid-19-rocked-the-rich-in-australia-this-year-20200917-p55wlu
Truog, R. D., Mitchell, C., & Daley, G. Q. (2021). The toughest triage: Allocating ventilators in a pandemic. *New England Journal of Medicine, 382*(21), 1973–1975.
United Nations International Covenant of Economic, Social and Cultural Rights (1960). https://www.ohchr.org/en/instruments-mechanisms/instruments/international-covenant-economic-social-and-cultural-rights
Wagner, J. M., & Dahnke, M. D. (2015). Nursing ethics and disaster triage: Applying utilitarian ethical theory. *Journal of Emergency Nursing, 41*(4), 300–306.
Wallace, J., Goldsmith-Pinkham, P., & Schwartz J. L. (2023). Excess death rates for Republican and Democratic registered voters in Florida and Ohio during the COVID-19 pandemic. *JAMA Internal Medicine, 183*(19), 916–923.
Weaver, R., Wilson, I., & Langendyk, V. (2014). Medical professionalism on television: Student perceptions and pedagogical implications. *Health, 18*(6), 597–612.
White, D. B. (2020). A framework for rationing ventilators and critical care beds during the COVID-19 pandemic. *The Journal of the American Medical Association, 323*(18), 1773–1774.
Wilson, J. (2009). Not so special after all? Daniels and the social determinants of health. *Journal of Medical Ethics, 35*, 3–6.
World Health Organization (WHO). 2023. Universal health coverage. https://www.who.int/health-topics/universal-health-coverage#tab=tab_1
Yamey, G. (2021). Rich countries should tithe their vaccines. *Nature, 590*, 529.
Yu, H. H. (2022). An examination of Asian American officers in State and Federal law enforcement. *Public Integrity*, *24*(6), 573–585.

PART IV

Understanding Health Issues in Popular Culture from Diverse Perspectives

22

RACE, ETHNICITY, POPULAR CULTURE, AND HEALTH COMMUNICATION

Amanda R. Martinez

Introduction

Popular culture encompasses many types of content, channels of communication, and interests of lay people. Audience size and reach, in addition to reasons people choose to engage to varying extents of intensity, dictate what becomes popular (Dunn & Young, 2017). Mass media dominates due to its mainstay as a fixture spanning decades and generations. Popular culture within mass media helps to construct shared narratives surrounding health topics, and some argue that "global popular culture is often drawn on by families and health professionals to develop a shared story of hope" (Mattingly, 2006, p. 497). I challenge readers to consider how health issues and messages are racially framed and how those messages influence the masses (Grossberg et al., 2006). Popular culture promotes, produces, and often reflects "deeper structural conditions—such as poverty, racism, sexism, and homophobia—and economic disparities woven into major social institutions" (Sternheimer, 2013, p. ix). What do these messages communicate about health along racial and ethnic lines, to whom, why, and how?

Many people turn to social media sites for their news and seek information through other, more traditional channels of transmission too (Social Media and News Fact Sheet, 2023). Within diverse societies, "it is inevitable that the cultural mindset of various racial and ethnic groups will reflect differences resulting from their unique social, subcultural, political, and economic experiences" (Oliver, 2000, p. 538). Social media provides an important counterspace to the top-down mass media by functioning as a bottom-up or horizontal form of communication driven by a wide audience scope and, in fact, "new media like the Internet have *increased* public discourse" (Sternheimer, 2013, p. 73). We must be health and mass/social media literate to navigate the information landscape (see also Chapter 20, this volume). I focus on popular mass and social media contexts because they are widely available and draw attention to issues about or of concern to a given population's racial and ethnic identity groups in health contexts. Whether messages resonate with audiences opens ways to engage with racialized health communication as "the limited effects model reminds us of the web of influences, including personality factors, social situations, climates of opinion and culture" (Grossberg et al., 2006, p. 293). I explore recent popular culture health communication topics with high-profile racialization relevance gauged by public attention.

DOI: 10.4324/9781003436409-26

Key Concepts Defined: Race, Ethnicity, Culture, and Racialization

I first explore the definitions and connotative tensions surrounding this chapter's key concepts. Race commonly refers to "grouped physical human differences such as skin, hair, and eye color, and genetic differences among people originating from different areas of the planet" (Hesmondhalgh & Saha, 2013, p. 180). Race does not hold scientific, biological meaning as it was once believed several decades ago, and those views have been thoroughly debunked and discredited (Bradby, 1995). Concerning health, scientific racism dates back at least to the 1600s and still permeates our healthcare structures with the most impact upon society's most vulnerable groups (for a review of the history of medicinal racism, see Byrd & Clayton, 2001). The enduring legacy and intertwinement of psychiatry, Eurocentrism, and colonial technologies permeates mental health realms too (Joseph, 2015).

The term "race" has a long, essentialist history rooted in oppression and a stubbornly dichotomous Black and white binary wherein Black connotes deficit and white connotes privilege. The racial binary shortchanges the myriad other racialized ethnic groups that do not succinctly fit, such that Asian, Hispanic/Latinx, Native/Indigenous, and multiracial and multiethnic people might be arbitrarily categorized or made to choose a category, rendering the categorization insufficient and limited in its explanatory power. Colorism (i.e., preferential treatment among similarly racialized people for whiteness or lighter complexion) complicates the racial grouping system because one's skin complexion can prompt essentialist ponderings about whether one truly belongs; the example of a white-passing person of color illustrates this point, which is rooted in white supremacist hierarchical thinking (Similly, 2023). As many scholars assert, the explicitly held belief in racial categories as meaningfully distinctive and deterministic is rare now; however, a stubborn system of evaluation persists that includes discourse about negative characteristics and features attributed to some groups, which upholds a racist ideological structure (Bradby, 1995; Miles, 1989). It becomes glaringly apparent that "cultural production in the modern world cannot be adequately understood without taking account of race and ethnicity, and their relation to oppression" (Hesmondhalgh & Saha, 2013, p. 180).

As Collins and Solomos (2010, p. 3) reminded us, though race signifies social groups with different physical attributes laden with socially constructed importance, and ethnicity denotes "language, culture, place of origin or common membership of a descent group without distinguishing physical characteristics," scholars often use the terms together. The danger in our socialization to assume that racial groupings carry some universally shared commonality lies in the fact that racial groupings are overly simplistic social constructions that fail to account for intragroup diversity, including ethnic and cultural distinctions that matter greatly to the racialization experience. Fenton (1999) poignantly asserted that the process of racialization fundamentally describes the realities of discourse and practices that surround race, racism, and now also include ethnicity, such as the long-standing historical realities of "modern racialized slavery, colonial domination, and political and economic oppression" (p. 61). The concept of racialization is, itself, historically flexible and imprecise. Multiculturalism and neoliberalism scholars argue that the antagonisms resulting from public discourse that invoke migration patterns, religious diversity, and national citizenry further agitate the entwinement of race with racism (Hesmondhalgh & Saha, 2013; Lentin & Titley, 2011).

Importantly, though no similarly parallel concept for ethnicity exists as racism is to race (Collins & Solomos, 2010), ethnicity demonstrates its dynamism in its characterization "by its relationship to forms of heritage (national, linguistic, culture), notions of belonging and external recognition of such claims, but also by its malleability, flexibility and situationality," including as "a marker of identity, a vehicle for community mobilization and a possible indicator of disadvantage, discrimination or privilege" (Ahmad & Bradby, 2007, p. 796). Furthermore, the slippage between the interchangeable use of race and ethnicity, a long-standing practice in health contexts, functions as deterministic when considering ethnicity and health (Bradby, 1995). Singer et al. (2016) documented the history of failed progress in the health sciences to adequately articulate population group differences so that researchers might more effectively study cultural processes that influence health and behaviors. Singer et al. asserted that concerted efforts to reach consensus on race and ethnicity as variables used in health research have progressed in over 15 years, but the use of culture as a factor remains muddled in both definition and usage.

Though not limited to Health Communication, those who argue in favor of a postracial society may prefer "culture" as a sweeping term that encompasses race and ethnicity to soften discussion about racialization and diminish potential accusations of racism. This pattern, however, invokes problematic tendencies for an interpersonal and large-scale reliance on stereotypes, which can lead to inequality in healthcare system experiences, the institutionalization of racist practices and policies, and the perpetuation of ignorance related to ethnic group differences in health-related outlooks and remedies (Bradby, 1995). The "danger exists in looking at how illness (but not good health) might be patterned by ethnicity, whereby ethnicity is transformed into a risk factor for ill-health" (Bradby, 1995, p. 412). Racialization discourse that relies on postracialism as a form of colorblindness creates an environment in which whiteness as the racial majority remains unquestionably in the backdrop as the comparison point and, concerning health, "conditions thus become racialized, with ethnic or cultural features over-emphasized to the extent that commonly understood aetiological or prognostic factors are ignored and new solutions invented, aimed at changing the presumed deficient culture of the communities concerned" (Ahmad & Bradby, 2007, p. 802). Perhaps among the most extreme outcomes in this type of racialized health communication climate, the afflicted might be blamed for their own ills.

Furthermore, a culture of prioritizing and prizing the biomedical healthcare model maintains its mainstream status while simultaneously de-emphasizing complementary healing systems that may hold culture-specific foundations (Dutta & Zoller, 2009). In a medical editorial that cites several health outcomes studies, Egede (2006) stated that "the current definition of ethnicity is arbitrary and ill-defined. For example, the term "Hispanic" includes over 400 million people from many different ethnic groups and subgroups, in more than 20 different countries" (p. 667). According to Egede, the persistence of using race as a variable should be approached critically because, even when medical researchers use self-reported racial identity, its meaningfulness reaches quick limits because more genetic variation exists within races than between them, rendering race a much more social rather than biological construct. Beyond the details of study designs, structural issues abound in racialized ethnic and cultural terms including stereotypical behavior of health professionals as well as conscious and unconscious biases and prejudices, and a shortage of minorities in health professions from recruitment, retention, nurturing interest, and then networking and mentoring them towards belonging in the professional community (López, 2003; Manson, 2003).

Critical Issues and Topics: Current Contributions and Research

The Medical Establishment and People of Color

The medical field in the U.S. has become less explicitly racist, xenophobic, and sexist, considering malicious atrocities inflicted upon people of color and the poor since well before the days of informed consent and more rigorous scientific research standards for the ethical treatment of patients. Scientific racism spans the entirety of civilization as we know it, with roots going back about 2,500 years (Byrd & Clayton, 2001). A pattern of hesitation and distrust commonly imbues communities of color due to the history of abuse at the hands of medical professionals spanning both physical and mental health. Among the best-known examples, news media have highlighted the Tuskegee experiments, the horrific research that began in 1932 on Black men with syphilis, who were misled about the study's purposes, and once penicillin was developed in the 1940s to treat it, were purposefully untreated and, in some cases, not made aware of their diagnosis. The Center for Disease Control's (2022) website features a timeline about this racist medical history entitled, "The Untreated Syphilis Study at

Tuskegee Timeline." Beyond this infamously explicit lack of concern for Black men's health, public discourse that links negative features or characteristics to people of color (Bradby, 1995; Miles, 1989) historically fuels a racist attitudinal assumption that people of color can endure more pain or that they should be approached with infantile communication about health.

In April 2022, tennis superstar Serena Williams penned an essay published in *Elle* magazine describing her harrowing near-death experience giving birth to her daughter in 2017, which described how she required several surgical medical interventions. The headline gripped readers' attention: "How Serena Williams Saved Her Own Life," followed by the subheading: "Black women are nearly three times more likely to die after childbirth than white women. Serena Williams was almost one of them" (Williams, 2022). *Good Morning America* (GMA) republished Williams' essay online, emphasizing this stunning quote from Williams: "No one was really listening to what I was saying" (Kindelan, 2022, para. 6). GMA online cited many health research statistics that corroborate Williams' experience, such as "Black women are more likely than white, Asian or Latina women to die from pregnancy-related complications regardless of their education level or their income" (Kindelan, 2022, para. 14). In remarks by Vice President Harris in a conversation on reproductive rights with Lieutenant Governor Tisch Sussman, Harris referred to Williams' birth experience as "a well-known story" about how racial bias leads to Black and Native women not being taken seriously in medical contexts (The White House, Speeches and Remarks, 2022, para. 58). Harris highlighted the importance of racial bias training for medical professionals to help remedy discriminatory patterns in medical treatment. Thanks to Williams using her celebrity platform to tell her story, other powerful sources with mass media access helped further expand its reach (see also Chapter 15, this volume).

Another example that haunts our public imagination and has received widespread public and media attention is the history of forced sterilization practices that largely targeted women of color, immigrants, and the poor for several decades and was often justified with racism-fueled laws under the guise of mental health and fitness (Shoichet, 2020). Villarosa (2022) authored a report in *The New York Times Magazine*, The Long Shadow of Eugenics in America, and chronicled recent acknowledgments, apologies, and long overdue compensation for sterilization survivors, but this sequence of remedies has taken years. In 2003, the North Carolina Senate overturned a sterilization law in place since 1919, presumably after pressure from the public in the aftermath of *The Winston-Salem Journal*'s publication of "Against Their Will," which comprised a multi-part series on the state's eugenics program (Villarosa, 2022). The state of North Carolina named a historical commemoration in Raleigh, North Carolina for the thousands of victims, developed a foundation to find survivors to share stories and compensate them, and finally in 2013, dedicated $10 million as a compensation package for survivors of the eugenics program. In 1907, Indiana passed the first state eugenics sterilization law, followed shortly by another 31 states, resulting in an estimated 60,000 forced sterilizations, with most laws not being repealed until the 1970s; most sterilizations were conducted on women of color with variation by state reflecting population (i.e., women of Mexican descent in California, Black women in North Carolina) (Shoichet, 2020, para. 9). According to Shoichet, eugenics laws amplified racism and sexism because the justification was driven by mindsets that deemed some people "unfit" to reproduce because of their "feeble-minded" or "mentally defective" status, a racist judgment by medical personnel given that women of color have been disproportionately forcibly sterilized (para. 10). In 2020, amidst ongoing political tensions surrounding immigration along the U.S.–Mexico border, allegations arose about poor ICE custody conditions after a nurse "reported concerns about a high rate of hysterectomies and alleged medical neglect" (para. 5).

Oftentimes, history's past horrors reappear in modern day, and, though they have gained traction in respected mass media outlets that have then prompted public outrage, accountability, and action from institutions and governing bodies, it may be hard for racist health topics to become widespread knowledge because of the fragility and discomfort they invoke. Disparities in healthcare delivery, access, care, and subsequent treatment are thoroughly documented, and the intersections of socio-economic class status overlaid with racialized ethnicity groupings have long captured the attention of the medical establishment (Cogburn, 2019; Egede, 2006; Johnson & Smith, 2002; López, 2003).

Mass Media, Health, and Racialized Ethnic Representation

Media representations, in both sheer volume in comparison to population proportions and the nature of those representations, are important. Across genres and types of programming, decades' worth of content analyses show that U.S. racial and ethnic minority group members have long been underrepresented in comparison to population proportions (Dixon & Linz, 2000; Mastro, 2009; Yamamoto, 2000). Black, Latinx, Asian, Indigenous, and multiracial people are far underrepresented, if not completely invisible (Behm-Morawitz & Ortiz, 2013; Bogle, 2016). This staggering reality results from the "overwhelming evidence of the dominance of white people over Black and ethnic minority populations when it comes to working in media organizations" (Hesmondhalgh & Saha, 2013, p. 183). Representational politics matter because they communicate whose stories and perspectives are valued and told. Absence speaks volumes in the same vein that proportional overrepresentation does and racist media messages further communicate a devaluation to people of color in society (Dogan et al., 2022).

Content analyses demonstrate that white people are overrepresented across media and are typically complex in character and storyline development; whereas for minoritized racial and ethnic groups, representations are typically negative, unidimensional, and stereotypical (Dixon, 2019; Dixon & Linz, 2000; Mastro, 2009). This long-term rampant marginalization shows the starkly skewed reality that we live in with major impact "on the range of perspectives that are heard in the media, and the most interesting research from that perspective tackles more concertedly the issue of what the lack of participation *off-screen* means for the representation of minorities *onscreen*" (Hesmondhalgh & Saha, 2013, p. 183). Of course, studies demonstrate the positive effects of media representation for the minoritized, as research has shown increases in self-esteem and empowerment of Black people (Dogan et al., 2022) and stronger identification with Black characters (Dixon et al., 2009), and even a resistance to media that does not affirm racial identity positively (Hoplamazian & Knobloch-Westerwick, 2014).

To date, the popular TV show "*Grey's Anatomy*" (created, written, and produced by Shonda Rhimes) comprises primetime's longest-running medical drama series (see Dugan Ramirez, 2022). The show has included lead people of color characters in the fictitious hospital, including Chandra Wilson, James Pickens Jr., Sandra Oh, and Sara Ramirez. Warner (2015) defined the practice of blindcasting as show writers' choice to not write race into scripts, which intends to function as a progressive step in the equitable treatment of actors. Long (2011) argued that Rhimes' blindcasting furthers colorblindness, obscures racial differences, and ultimately erases the stubbornly pervasive reality of structural, intersecting barriers to racial equality specifically. Instead, it emphasizes similarities such as "gender, location of origin, and individual merit or personality traits" (p. 1069). Warner asserted that Shonda Rhimes neutralizes race as an implied solution to racial inequality by intentionally including "racialized bodies as signifiers of historical progress in the struggle of televisual racial representation" while "undermining the diversity of those bodies through a laundering, or whitewashing, of social and cultural specificity" (p. 633), which makes racial diversity "more gimmick than innovation" (p. 635). As Long argued, even though blindcasting seems progressive, "it functions more accurately as a discursive band-aid for a political bullet hole" (p. 1079), effectively ignoring and maintaining intersectional oppression and systemic power differentials.

Eguchi and Ding (2017) analyzed another of ABC's comedy-drama medical-focused TV shows, *Dr. Ken*, which aired from 2015-2016 and featured Asian American medical doctor-turned-comedian Ken Jeong's life experiences. In contrast to Warner's (2015) critique of Rhimes' blindcasting, Jeong stated in an interview that Dr. Ken is "refreshingly uncultural," and he framed this unculturalism positively "because a white writer would tend to overtly introduce Asian jokes into the sitcom" (Eguchi & Ding, 2017, pp. 296–297). Eguchi and Ding contended that Jeong's unculturalism masked the cultural as it "operat[ed] as a rhetorical method of postracialism, that is, colorblinding the historical and contemporary realities of racism to secure the territory of whiteness as the center" (p. 297). Within a white supremacist society, the pervasive model minority stereotype describes Asian Americans when they are doing better in life than other racialized ethnic minorities, and the yellow peril stereotype resonates when Asian Americans do better than white people. So, according to Eguchi and Ding, "they coexist and are inseparable to redefine invisible territory of whiteness as the center" (p. 299). *Dr. Ken*'s uncultural appeal downplays racialized cultural otherness to appeal as simply U.S. Americans.

Edutainment or infotainment media messages serve as a prime example of how existing channels of communication can reach target populations with health-tailored information (see also Chapter 17, this volume). For example, Oliver (2000) discussed how culture-specific radio campaigns leveraged gospel music to reach African Americans with pertinent information about domestic violence prevention and interventions to promote health within the community. In an interdisciplinary study that attended to the types and frequency of health risk behaviors enacted by white and Black main characters in popular films, results revealed that, across a sample of 63 films, Black characters were more likely to be portrayed engaging in sex, tobacco, and alcohol use, and white characters were more likely to engage in violence and alcohol use (Ellithorpe et al., 2017; for related work, see also Chapter 10, this volume). When AIDS dominated the news headlines in the 1980s, media framing created an association in audiences' minds of the disease linked to homosexuality while simultaneously "concealing other equally pertinent facts: for example, that the majority of AIDS cases in NYC are among people of color, with a rising percentage among women" (Grossberg et al., 2006, p. 241). According to Reitmanova et al. (2015), Canadian media misrepresented HIV/AIDS "as an imported problem that could be addressed only by excluding suspect immigrant groups, rather than by sound and multifaceted disease prevention strategies" (p. 476; for related work, see also Chapter 11, this volume). Victim blaming, accusations of poor personal responsibility, and social ostracism often unfold in the wake of widespread racialized illness to quell paranoia (Weinstock, 1997).

Herd's (2008) research on drug use prevalence in rap music and how social attitudes shifted over two decades showed a noteworthy increase in drug use presence in popular rap and a widespread liberal attitude about drugs. Importantly, given rap's African American roots, Herd observed that the disproportionate actual drug use patterns were similar between African American and white people, with use of most drugs being less among African American youth compared to other groups; however, Black people are much more likely to be arrested for drug possession, convicted, and imprisoned for it compared to white people. Conversely, Peterson et al. (2018) analyzed newspaper reports on meth use to compare the social constructions underlying a meth epidemic hotspot through racialized lenses of whiteness, especially because recent years' framing around national drug use crises has focused on poor white drug users from rural areas. They argued that the media pseudo-racializes white people as "white trash" meth users, and news accounts often pit rural and urban white people against each other to cope with how this "White drug scare" threatens perceptions of White cultural superiority" (p. 4). Furthermore, pop culture sensationally frames meth as uniquely composed of highly addictive chemicals rendering white meth users powerless against addiction and, by focusing on backstories to highlight redemption journeys, this colorblind excuse-making for whiteness scapegoats non-white drug addicts as the true drains on social systems.

Mental health and learning difference diagnoses provide an interesting example as a newer form of racialized health communication portrayed through popular culture. Matthews (2019) reminded us of the powerful impact of the scarce popular culture portrayals of autism in his analysis of Sheldon Cooper in the CBS sitcom, *The Big Bang Theory*. Cooper, a white male genius scientist with obvious social awkwardness tendencies, occupied an important role for his mainstay popularity on a long-running TV show that became a common referent for the autism community in assessing spectrum placement and mannerisms. Matthews ultimately concluded that the show embodied a "visual rhetoric conflation of autism and whiteness" that "fuels a racial narrative that equates ethnic whiteness with intellectual superiority" (p. 57), though the assumption that autism constitutes a white male-specific condition is common but rarely questioned. According to Matthews, Cooper comprised one of many examples in popular media that "serve the rhetorical function of converting stigma and marginalization, in gendered and ethnic terms, into glorification and intellectual giftedness" (p. 62). Ratto et al. (2016) argued that cultural factors impact rates of diagnoses for autism spectrum disorders, and they found that ethnic minority children, namely, Latinos, tend to receive diagnoses much later than their white peers on average. The implications for media to repeatedly provide frames of incomplete health complexities hold potential for informing attitudes and consequences in already deeply established structural inequalities in health contexts (Grossberg et al., 2006).

Bodily Transformations: Whiteness, Thinness, and Constant Changes

Focus on bodies remains a highly racialized site for health and physical desirability measured by socially constructed narrow standards (see also Chapter 5, this volume). Body transformations usually emphasize thinness as ideal, and the danger lies in the reality that "because emaciated celebrities often parade before us … American girls have been monitoring their body size and comparing themselves unfavorably to others for at least a century" (Sternheimer, 2013, p. 211). The news media perpetuate negative, stereotypical images of obese people and can create social distance, anti-fat attitudes, and sentiments of laziness and dislike, all strong indicators of weight stigmatization reinforcement, with higher ratings of social distance and dislike for African American women compared to white people in Puhl et al.'s (2013) study.

The aesthetic, cosmetic bodily changes showcased in popular culture often display extremes for their sensationalistic qualities, such as surgical procedures and weight loss competitions. An overall tone of striving for perfection and achieving Western standards of beauty invoke thinness and colorism when people of color are present that rewards lightness (Covino, 2001; Similly, 2023). For example, skin lightening procedures and practices persist among people of color (Regencia et al., 2023), and double eyelid surgery (which is sometimes aesthetic and other times due to medical needs) to create a larger crease and wider eyelid space remains popular, particularly among Asian women (Chow, 2014). These practices, though adherent to the dominant narrow standards, may improve the mental health and self-esteem of those who elect to engage in these procedures, a reality that complicates temptations to judge others for upholding rigid standards by conforming to them. Popular culture representations have undoubtedly influenced the public's acceptance of the aesthetic surgery industry as American household surveys from the 1990s through the early 2000s show that the majority of women and men approve of cosmetic surgery, and, as Covino stated, "we see that aesthetic surgery is for everybody: the well-adjusted, the maladjusted, and the over-achievers are all motivated to a lesser or greater extent toward body improvement" (p. 99). According to Covino, the industry is racialized such that everyone receives the specific message to strive for racialized white "Caucasian features (through rhinoplasty and skin bleaching)" (p. 100).

Ritter (2023) analyzed the plight to achieve thinness for women of color in the reality TV show, *Fat Chance*, in which "fatness and singlehood are constructed as undesirable temporary states, with the diet being presented as the rite of passage toward the acceptable states of thinness and being coupled" (p. 1). Makeover shows pedestalize the thin body type as desirable and other body shapes as deviant and in need of change through diets and makeovers. Ritter argued that universality emanates through achieving thinness to become worthy of love, as men and women, heterosexual and homosexual people, and people of color, regardless of sociocultural background, are featured in the show. The personal responsibility theme frames the only two women of color in need of weight loss to become better people and to love and accept themselves, shortchanging the impact of possible socioeconomic and structural barriers.

In the last decade, "popular culture has seen a shift in what constitutes an attractive, desirable body. Beyoncé and other entertainers, actresses, and athletes such as Sofia Vergara, Serena Williams, and Jennifer Lopez have helped normalize curvy figures" (Similly, 2023, p. 4). The following phenomenon takes shape: Though many curvaceous women of color have achieved success in the entertainment industry, even as curvy bodies have largely been perceived as "overweight and undesirable," white women appropriate curvy women of color aesthetics as evidenced by the growing trend of buttock augmentation procedures (Similly, 2023, p. 4). Recent research shows that eating disordered behavior and body image issues constitute a pattern among upper-class white women, women of color, men, and those from low-income households; however, the underrepresented and marginalized have historically been underdiagnosed and undertreated due to different ways racialized minorities display symptoms and discuss body image issues (Ciciurkaite & Perry, 2017).

Though mass media stubbornly pedestal thinness achievements, social media spaces offer counter brand messaging, such as Dove's Campaign for Real Beauty, which celebrates a variety of body shapes, sizes, and different racialized ethnic women. The fat positive movement and the simple mantra "all bodies are good bodies" fill internet spaces to counter thinness and whiteness idealism. Social media influencers and celebrities contribute to diversifying body messages, too, as the fitspiration content positively emphasizes health and fitness through exercise and clean eating compared to the thinspiration content that motivates people to strive towards thinness regardless of whether the means are healthy (see also Chapter 16, this volume). Cooking shows have also diversified to debunk the cost and access barriers for healthy eating with shows like *Struggle Meals*, led with a comedic tone by Chef Frankie Celenza on YouTube, who teaches audiences how to eat well inexpensively (see also Chapter 4, this volume). Next, I detail the race-norming controversy and lawsuit concerning professional football players' concussion assessments as a high-profile case study.

The NFL as Modern-Day Plantation: Football, Concussions, and Racialized Outcomes

Professional sports require elite athleticism, and for high-contact, violent, male-dominated sports like football, players may feel pressure to play through pain in an imminent culture of hegemonic masculinity wherein admitting pain equals weakness (see also Chapter 14, this volume). Similar prized values span Western cultures and sports: success, progress, achievement, patriotism, individualism, and recognition (Volkwein-Caplan, 2013). Bell et al. (2019) made the metaphorical connection between football and war rhetoric with sacrificing to win as priority; masculine social organizations like sports and military abide by the pain principle, the attitude that pain inevitably occurs and strengthens character. An unfortunate reality persists: "injuries often overlooked due to desire for acceptance in the hegemonic masculine space have long-term effects, sometimes without revealing significant impact for years or even decades after an initial injury" (Bell et al., 2019, p. 34). Only recently has the culture shifted, and players increasingly self-report long-term impact from game injuries.

Consider football's racialized organizational structure: the NFL represents a "modern-day plantation system" (Benson, 2017, p. 320) where Black players constitute the racial majority at about 68%, with an overwhelmingly white spectator fanbase at about 83% white and 64% male, and a vast majority of white men occupy leadership as league executives, team owners, front-office personnel, and coaches. Furthermore, Black men are estimated to be in the single-digit proportion of college undergraduates but comprise over half of college football players, with only about 1% of college football players drafted into the NFL (for an in-depth analysis on the NFL as plantation, see Prior, 2006; Sailors, 2015). Fletcher and Hylton (2016) observed a "clustering of black bodies in lower positions of administration and leadership, or even the highest levels of performance, without being able to consistently break through glass ceilings" (p. 94). Beyond the racialized skews, Ferriter (2016) recalled that, "in sport, biological distinctions are consistently reinforced through racialized discourse regarding sporting performances" (p. 24).

For example, studies document that "white people assume that Black people feel less pain" (Benson, 2017, p. 322). Fletcher and Hylton (2016) argued:

> Assumptions of natural ability in football, athletics ... were flattering facilitators of insiderness and hegemonic masculinity. Yet, at the same time, those assumptions based upon racial stereotypes also inferred other things about intellectual capacity and propensities for success in academic as well as sporting domains. We should not be surprised that these subtle patterns retain a certain resilience today, given racism's ability to adapt and be reinvented over time.
>
> *(p. 88)*

Benson (2017) drew attention to the language used in mainstream news reports that referred to football players as "modern day gladiators," including NFL running back Marshawn Lynch, aka "Beast Mode," and NFL receiver Calvin Johnson, aka "Megatron" (named after a Transformer action figure); both players' nicknames were meant as compliments about their size and strength (p. 321). Similarly, NFL linebacker James Harrison earned his nickname, "The Hitman," as a combination of his "violent celebrity" and "voice of contestation" against the "unfair levying of fines from new rules, especially those fines against Black players" (Bell et al., 2019, p. 37). Older former NFL players Mike Webster and Jim Otto each garnered nicknames as "ironmen" because they played hard and paid for it later (Bell et al., 2019). No matter how tough football players are, they experience pain and may struggle to recover from sports injuries because they are human beings with bodies that require recovery when injured.

In 2013, thousands of former NFL football players and their families filed a class action lawsuit against the NFL on the grounds that it concealed the dangers of concussions. The NFL settled the lawsuit and allocated $765 million for medical exam expenses to compensate players for health issues related to a history of sustained concussions (Alsup & Sutton, 2021). In 2020, Najeh Davenport and Kevin Henry, two retired Black NFL players, sued the NFL for racial discrimination in the cognitive assessment baseline measurement referred to as "race-norming" that resulted in their denied claims. As part of the required diagnostic criteria in a claim, doctors must process a "premorbid intellectual ability" which assesses cognitive functioning preceding football-related head trauma (Balsam, 2021). The two models used to make this assessment include: 1) demographic data (race, ethnicity, sex, and education) and 2) race-norming, a practice that "assume[s] that black players start at a lower level of cognitive functioning than white players," which renders the model to "effectively require black players to show larger cognitive declines to qualify for compensation" (Balsam, 2021, p. 6; for a thorough review of the lawsuit, see Balsam, 2021). Using race to "norm" cognitive ability not only assumes that Black players have lower cognition before they are tested for evidence of brain damage (Walton et al, 2022) but fails to consider complex factors like "health, level of education, or economic background" (Brett et al., 2023, p. 3095).

Employing race essentially as a proxy for multiple complex factors communicates that race itself is a meaningful variable and begs the question: what about multiracial people who do not fit into the oversimplified racial categories? Ironically, the rationale for creating lower scores for Black people when race-norming was introduced was to prevent them from being subject to overdiagnosis of cognitive impairment, which means race-norming attempts to adjust for racial biases in cognitive tests. However, instead of eliminating these biases, the practice essentializes Black people and, in the context of the class action lawsuit, adds a racist hurdle that makes it harder for Black applicants to prove they have suffered cognitive impairment (Ventresca & Henne, 2020).

Race-norming is an old, racially discriminatory neuropsychology practice, much like using racial differences in IQ, that attempts to account for historical trends by using race to represent life-long social experiences meaningfully. These discriminatory practices are thoroughly debunked such that "both public and medical opinion has evolved to discredit the methodology," and "as a result, in June 2021, the NFL renounced the use of race-norming" (Balsam, 2021, p. 7). In 2022, a federal judge modified the NFL's settlement to end the use of race norms, and Black players who were previously denied can have their tests rescored or file new claims (Almasy, 2022). As Ventresca and Henne (2020) asserted, "Davenport and Henry's complaint, however, highlights inequalities beyond workplace compensation. It is an example of how racial science continues to harm Black people by upholding racist beliefs about white superiority" (para. 3). As Goldberg (2013) stated, "given its overwhelming power, capital, and influence in shaping sport culture at all levels, the NFL is a crucial player" in taking head injuries seriously, recognizing their long-term impact, and treating players humanely with appropriate recovery regimens without pressure to play through pain (p. 190).

In an episode of *The Takeaway* (2021) radio program, Ken Jenkins, a former NFL running back, pointed out that it took public outcry and players' families loudly complaining to draw attention to race-norming, even though attorneys had already been working on the issue for over three years. Thanks to journalists, football players themselves, and popular documentaries such as *Head Games* (2012), *League of Denial* (2013) and *Concussion* (2015) – starring Will Smith as Dr. Bennet Omalu, the forensic pathologist who discovered CTE among football players showing neurological deterioration similar to that found in Alzheimer's patients – the severity and prevalence of CTE among football players pushed the topic into mainstream public discourse (Bell et al., 2019). According to Bell et al.'s analysis, these films emphasize themes that humanize NFL players beyond the field and portray the long-term tragic and uncomfortable impact on them and their families by showcasing the connection between science and football and the role of whistleblowers and media. Together, according to Bell et al., they reveal "a sad truth of sport: the better an athlete performed usually equaled a longer-than-likely playing career and a greater risk for long-term brain injuries" (p. 114). The lawsuit revealed racism in medical practices that created a tangible disproportionate discriminatory impact on Black former NFL players. The power of the people – including those afflicted and with platforms to amplify the stories – cannot be underestimated, even against massively powerful institutions like the NFL. Now, I explore the disproportionate health impact on Asian people because of racialized popular discourse surrounding the COVID-19 pandemic.

Spreading Sicknesses: Anti-Asian Violence Amidst a Pandemic

The year 2020 will forever jog our collective memory as the onset of the COVID-19 pandemic that drastically disrupted life routines worldwide. For most of the global population, enduring their first pandemic experience already presented challenges to our healthcare systems and personal health and well-being, and soon popular discourse took a sinister turn once the media identified Wuhan, China as the virus's origin (Schumaker, 2020). Mass panic and fear swept across nations as people felt urgently vulnerable, which soon fueled xenophobic outcries and outright blame of Chinese people for spreading the disease – and in many cases, anyone who physically appeared or was assumed to be of Asian descent.

For example, in Japan, the hashtag #ChineseDon'tCometoJapan trended on Twitter, thousands of Singapore's residents signed a petition to ban Chinese nationals from the country, and businesses in Hong Kong, South Korea, and Vietnam posted unwelcome signs aimed at Chinese customers (Rich, 2020). In India, Sri Lanka, and Myanmar, reports of attacks and discrimination against Muslims in relation to pandemic threats and hate speech have been documented, as well as similar physical and verbal (including slurs, jokes, and other racist or racially insensitive expressions) attacks against Asian people in the U.S., United Kingdom, Russia, and Australia ("Covid-19 fueling anti-Asian racism," 2020). The governor of Veneto, Italy, told journalists that Italians would better handle the virus than the Chinese because they have a "culturally strong attention to hygiene ... whereas we have all seen the Chinese eating mice alive," a statement for which he later apologized ("Covid-19 fueling anti-Asian racism," 2020, para. 6). Brazil's education minister tweeted that the pandemic was part of the Chinese government's "plan for world domination" ("Covid-19 fueling anti-Asian racism," 2020, para. 6). Former U.S. President Donald Trump used shorthand descriptors referring to the pandemic as "Kung Flu" and the "Chinese Virus," and they quickly gained traction as social media hashtags. U.S. Secretary of State Mike Pompeo used "Wuhan virus" to refer to COVID-19 ("Covid-19 fueling anti-Asian racism," 2020). As Ng (2021) explained, "the adjective 'Chinese' in 'Chinese virus' is particularly problematic as it metaphorizes the devastation of the pandemic with an ethnicity," (para. 22) which functions to marginalize all members from the group identity.

In Hswen et al.'s (2021) analysis of anti-Asian hashtags from March 9–23, 2020, which was the week before and after Trump's "Chinese Virus" tweeting, they urged all people to "use neutral, non-judgmental language to avoid stigmatizing communities and perpetuating discrimination" because they found that "Chinese virus" was related to more than twice as many hate expressions across many states in the U.S. compared with the referent "COVID-19" and even the latter neutral descriptor was associated with anti-Asian sentiment in social media hashtags. An aggregated report by Stop AAPI Hate found that verbal harassment, shunning, and physical assault incidents increased from one year to the next during the pandemic, with most incidents reported by women and taking place in public spaces like streets and businesses ("More than 9,000 anti-Asian incidents," 2021). Beyond the bodily harm ever present in pandemics and the resultant hate crimes tied to panic and racist discourse, discrimination in the form of social exclusion and adverse economic impact proliferated too. In Huang et al.'s (2023) examination of Asian-owned restaurants, an important market sector to gauge impact due to their ubiquity as small businesses that sell varieties of ethnically-entwined goods, they found that "Asian restaurants experienced an 18.4% decrease in traffic (estimated US $7.42 billion lost revenue in 2020) relative to comparable non-Asian restaurants, with greater decreases in areas with higher levels of support for Donald Trump" (p. 682).

Some public health experts have stated that, during a new widespread illness, the public panics and people want to distance themselves from any possibility of contracting the virus. So, their fear prompts the targeting of others, and, in this case, Asian people writ large, given reports about COVID originating in Wuhan (Rich, 2020). Discriminatory actions and sentiments toward an "other" in times of public health panic constitute a pattern documented throughout history, and xenophobic foreign "othering" quickly gained traction (Ng, 2021). In Reitmanova et al.'s (2015) critical discourse analysis of Canadian daily news reports over the course of a decade racialized immigrants' bodies as disease breeders and irresponsible health fraudsters, essentially blaming them for threatening the health of the host population and burdening healthcare systems economically by taking up too much space. Health threats may directly inform policies and be fueled by racist scapegoating because "the press ran stories calling for tightened borders and immigration policies and improving medical screening and surveillance of immigrants to protect the health of Canadian-born citizens" (p. 482). Indeed, the discourses of collective blame, and ethnically homogenizing and misidentifying others explain the power that anti-China rhetoric held in harming Asian Americans in general in the U.S. (Huang et al., 2023). These modern examples of panic amidst widespread health threats exemplify "the establishment of human hierarchies to rationalize violence through the implementation of racial and eugenic rationale" (Joseph, 2015, p. 1022).

Weinstock (1997) aptly described virus omnipresence as the cause of generalized anxiety and infection paranoia that, quite harshly, re-stigmatizes those already afflicted with oftentimes life-threatening ailments in many cases. This rings true for the COVID-19 pandemic. Adding insult to injury, the anti-Asian racism in the U.S. contributed to many members of Asian American households, particularly seniors, being fearful to venture outside their homes, which caused health-related problems such as food insecurity, avoidance of doctor's appointments, and abandonment of outdoor exercise routines.

Recommendations for Practice

In today's world, our limited attention economies require that information engage us meaningfully, as we have seemingly limitless access to digital devices and vast quantities of information at the touch of a button. This media saturation means that we must continually refine our mass media, social media, and health literacies and see them as intertwined and mutually reinforcing rather than siloed realms that simply co-exist. Understanding the messages that we receive and the channels through which they greet us requires a personal ethic of ongoing vigilance to dig beyond the surface into the deeper implications of what might otherwise seem like simply neutral and general health information. We hone our empowerment and agency by also using the many channels of communication to reach potentially mass audiences and networks and talk back to these top-down messages while simultaneously parsing the legitimate from the sensationalized clickbait health information, recognizing perspective slants all the while.

Diversifying our thinking about research designs, intended purposes, and potential impact must assume a central position in the work of scholars and practitioners going forward. As the world becomes increasingly diverse – multicultural, multiracial, and multiethnic – achieving a thorough understanding of intersectionality and the historical and long-standing impact of racism as a global form of domination and oppression helps us address health-focused research and practice in more heterogeneous, better representative ways. We must internalize a reflex to always ask questions and wonder: *Who or what is missing from consideration here? What are the potential monoliths we take for granted? What do we mean by "culture" and why are "race" or "ethnicity" designations appropriate to inform our research focus? What are the consequences of our chosen focus? Who is not being represented and why?*

At a very basic minimum, we benefit by collectively rejecting colorblindness and instead filling our educational gaps around the very real, consequential, historical, and modern-day realities of scientific and medicinal racism, health disparities, cultural competencies, and a wide array of ways of knowing that transcend the biomedical model of healthcare. These considerations include cultural knowledge and preferences that inform health experiences. By identifying our individual ignorance and embracing it instead as a collaborative opportunity to expand our knowledge locus, we inherently keep asking tough questions, compartmentalize our fragilities, and strive to do better for everyone by fully seeing everyone in heterogeneous identity-intersecting ways. Though public figures (like celebrities and politicians) and widespread shared experiences (like global pandemics and Sunday night football) more readily amplify health issues, we, too, have a responsibility to use any platform where we have even a small amount of power to contribute to discourse and help amplify a richer range of messages. We hold knowledge and learn from each other, our communities, the experts, history, and popular culture. Undoing racism in health contexts by recognizing and dissecting racialized ethnic cultural nuances is our perpetual shared responsibility.

References

Ahmad, W. I., & Bradby, H. (2007). Locating ethnicity and health: Exploring concepts and contexts. *Sociology of Health & Illness*, *29*(6), 795–810.

Almasy, S. (2022, March 4). Judge approves changes to NFL concussion settlement that ends use of race norms. *CNN*. https://www.cnn.com/2022/03/04/sport/nfl-concussion-settlement-black-players-spt/index.html

Alsup, D., & Sutton, J. (2021, October 21*)*. NYT: Agreement reached to scrap race as a factor in NFL concussion settlements. *CNN*. https://www.cnn.com/2021/10/21/us/nfl-concussion-settlement-race-spt/index.html

Balsam, J. S. (2021). Fraud, race norming, and delays: How the NFL's concussion settlement fund is faring five years later. *Law In Sport*. https://www.lawinsport. com/topics/item/fraud-race-norming-delays-how-the-nfl-s-concussion-litigation-fund-is-faring-five-years-on
Behm-Morawitz, E., & Ortiz, M. (2013). Race, ethnicity, and the media. In K. E. Dill (Ed.), *The oxford handbook of media psychology* (pp. 252–262). Oxford University Press.
Bell, T. R., Applequist, J., & Dotson-Pierson, C. (2019). *CTE, media, and the NFL: Framing a public health crisis as a football epidemic*. Rowman & Littlefield.
Benson, P. (2017). Big football: Corporate social responsibility and the culture and color of injury in America's most popular sport. *Journal of Sport and Social Issues*, *41*(4), 307–334.
Bogle, D. (2016*). Toms, coons, mulattoes, mammies, and bucks: An interpretive history of Blacks in American films*. Bloomsbury Publishing Inc.
Bradby, H. (1995). Ethnicity: Not a black and white issue. A research note. *Sociology of Health & Illness*, *17*(3), 405–417.
Brett, B. L., Aggarwal, N. T., Chandran, A., Kerr, Z. Y., Walton, S. R., DeFreese, J. D., ... & Mannix, R. (2023). Incorporation of concussion history as part of the LIfestyle for BRAin Health (LIBRA) modifiable factors risk score and associations with cognition in older former National Football League players. *Alzheimer's & Dementia, 19*, 3087–3097.
Byrd, W. M., & Clayton, L. A. (2001). Race, medicine, and health care in the United States: A historical survey. *Journal of the National Medical Association*, *93*(3 Suppl), 11S.
Chow, K. (2014, November 18). The many stories behind double-eyelid surgery. *Code Switch*. https://www.npr.org/sections/codeswitch/2014/11/18/364670361/the-many-stories-behind-the-double-eyelid-surgery
Ciciurkaite, G., & Perry, B. L. (2017). Body weight, perceived weight stigma and mental health among women at the intersection of race/ethnicity and socioeconomic status: Insights from the modified labelling approach. *Sociology of Health & Illness*, *40*(1), 18–37.
Cogburn, C. D. (2019). Culture, race, and health: Implications for racial inequities and population health. *The Milbank Quarterly*, *97*(3), 736–761.
Collins, P., & Solomos, J. (2010). Introduction: Situating race and ethnic studies. In P. H. Collins & J. Solomos (Eds.), *The SAGE handbook of race and ethnic studies* (pp. 1–16). SAGE. https://doi.org/10.4135/9781446200902
Covid-19 fueling anti-Asian racism and xenophobia worldwide: National action plans needed to counter intolerance. (2020, May 12). *Human Rights Watch*. https://www.hrw.org/news/2020/05/12/covid-19-fueling-anti-asian-racism-and-xenophobia-worldwide
Covino, D. C. (2001). Outside-in: Body, mind, and self in the advertisement of aesthetic surgery. *Journal of Popular Culture*, *35*(3), 91–102.
Dixon, T. L. (2019). Media stereotypes: Content, effects, and theory. In M. B. Oliver, A. A. Raney, & J. Bryant (Eds.) *Media effects: Advances in theory and research* (4th ed. pp. 243–257). Routledge.
Dixon, T. L., & Linz, D. (2000). Overrepresentation and underrepresentation of African Americans and Latinos as lawbreakers on television news. *Journal of Communication,* 50(2), 131–154.
Dixon, T. L., Zhang, Y., & Conrad, K. (2009). Self-esteem, misogyny and Afrocentricity: An examination of the relationship between rap music consumption and African American perceptions. *Group Processes and Intergroup Relations*, *12*(3), 345–360. https://doi.org/10.1177/1368430209102847
Dogan, J. N., Rosenkrantz, D., Wheeler, P. B., & Hargons, C. N. (2022). Exploring identity and coping among Black viewers of Marvel's *Black Panther*. *Psychology of Popular Media*, *11*(2), 183.
Dugan Ramirez, C. (2022, January 10). Ellen Pompeo will return for 19th season of 'Grey's Anatomy.' *People*. https://people.com/tv/greys-anatomy-renewed-for-19th-season/
Dunn, J. C., & Young, S. L. (2017). *Pursuing popular culture: Methods for researching the everyday*. Kendall Hunt.
Dutta, M. J., & Zoller, H. M. (2009). Theoretical foundations: Interpretive, critical, and cultural approaches to health communication. In H. Zoller & M. J. Dutta (Eds.) *Emerging perspectives in health communication* (pp. 11–38). Routledge.
Egede, L. E. (2006). Race, ethnicity, culture, and disparities in health care. *Journal of General Internal Medicine*, *21*(6), 667–669.
Eguchi, S., & Ding, Z. (2017). "Uncultural" Asian Americans in ABC's Dr. Ken. *Popular Communication*, *15*(4), 296–310.
Ellithorpe, M. E., Bleakley, A., Hennessy, M., Weitz, I., Jamieson, P., & Khurana, A. (2017). Differences in the portrayal of health risk behaviors by black and white characters in popular films. *Journal of Health Communication*, *22*(6), 451–458.
Fenton, S. (1999). *Ethnicity: Racism, class and culture*. Rowman & Littlefield.

Ferriter, M. (2016). The anthropology of race and ethnicity in sport: Unfolding the map. In J. Nauright & D. K. Wiggins (Eds.) *Routledge handbook of sport, race and ethnicity* (pp. 21–34). Routledge.

Fletcher, T., & Hylton, K. (2016). 'Race', whiteness and sport. In J. Nauright & D. K. Wiggins (Eds.) *Routledge handbook of sport, race and ethnicity* (pp. 87–106). Routledge.

Goldberg, D. S. (2013). Mild traumatic brain injury, the National Football League, and the manufacture of doubt: An ethical, legal, and historical analysis. *Journal of Legal Medicine*, *34*(2), 157–191.

Grossberg, L., Wartella, E., Whitney, D. C., & Wise, J. M. (2006). *Mediamaking: Mass media in a popular culture* (2nd ed.). SAGE.

Herd, D. (2008). Changes in drug use prevalence in rap music songs, 1979–1997. *Addiction Research & Theory*, *16*(2), 167–180.

Hesmondhalgh, D., & Saha, A. (2013). Race, ethnicity, and cultural production. *Popular Communication: The International Journal of Media and Culture*, *11*(3), 179–195.

Hoplamazian, G. J., & Knobloch-Westerwick, S. (2014). The color of their collar: Effects of social status portrayal in advertising on self-esteem. *Howard Journal of Communications*, 25(4), 378–398. https://doi.org/10.1080/10646175.2014.955930

Hswen, Y., Xu, X., Hing, A., Hawkins, J. B., Brownstein, J. S., & Gee, G. C. (2021). Association of "#covid19" versus "#chinesevirus" with anti-Asian sentiments on Twitter: March 9–23, 2020. *American Journal of Public Health*, *111*(5), 956–964.

Huang, J. T., Krupenkin, M., Rothschild, D., & Lee Cunningham, J. (2023). The cost of anti-Asian racism during the COVID-19 pandemic. *Nature Human Behaviour*, *7*, 1–14.

Johnson, J. C., & Smith, N. H. (2002). Health and social issues associated with racial, ethnic, and cultural disparities. *Generations: Journal of the American Society on Aging*, *26*(3), 25–32.

Joseph, A. J. (2015). The necessity of an attention to Eurocentrism and colonial technologies: An addition to critical mental health literature. *Disability & Society*, *30*(7), 1021–1041.

Kindelan, K. (2022, April 6). Serena Williams says she had to advocate to save her life after giving birth. *Good Morning America*. https://www.goodmorningamerica.com/wellness/story/serena-williams-advocate-save-life-giving-birth-83893049

Lentin, A., & Titley, G. (2011). *The crises of multiculturalism: Racism in a neoliberal age*. Bloomsbury Publishing.

Long, A. (2011). Diagnosing drama: Grey's anatomy, blind casting, and the politics of representation. *Journal of Popular Culture*, *44*(5), 1067–1084.

López, S. R. (2003). Reflections on the Surgeon General's report on mental health, culture, race, and ethnicity. *Culture, Medicine and Psychiatry*, *27*, 419–434.

Manson, S. M. (2003). Extending the boundaries, bridging the gaps: Crafting mental health: Culture, race, and ethnicity, a supplement to the Surgeon General's Report on Mental Health. *Culture, Medicine and Psychiatry*, *27*, 395–408.

Mastro, D. E. (2009). Effects of racial and ethnic stereotyping. In J. Bryant & M. B. Oliver (Eds.), *Media effects: Advances in theory and research* (pp. 325–341). Routledge.

Matthews, M. (2019). Why Sheldon Cooper can't be black: The visual rhetoric of autism and ethnicity. *Journal of Literary & Cultural Disability Studies*, *13*(1), 57–74.

Mattingly, C. (2006). Pocahontas goes to the clinic: Popular culture as lingua franca in a cultural borderland. *American Anthropologist*, *108*(3), 494–501.

Miles, R. (1989). *Racism*. Routledge.

More than 9,000 anti-Asian incidents have been reported since the pandemic began. (2021, August 12). *The Associated Press*. https://www.npr.org/2021/08/12/1027236499/anti-asian-hate-crimes-assaults-pandemic-incidents-aapi

Ng, R. (2021). Anti-Asian sentiments during the COVID-19 pandemic across 20 countries: Analysis of a 12-billion-word news media database. *Journal of Medical Internet Research*, *23*(12), e28305.

Oliver, W. (2000). Preventing domestic violence in the African American community: The rationale for popular culture interventions. *Violence Against Women*, *6*(5), 533–549.

Peterson, J. C., Gubrium, A., & Fiddian-Green, A. (2018). Meth mouth, white trash, and the pseudo-racialization of methamphetamine use in the US. *Health Communication*, *34*(10), 1–10.

Prior, A. E. (2006). *The slave side of Sunday*. Stone Hold Books. com.

Puhl, R. M., Luedicke, J., & Heuer, C. A. (2013). The stigmatizing effect of visual media portrayals of obese persons on public attitudes: Does race or gender matter? *Journal of Health Communication*, *18*(7), 805–826.

Ratto, A. B., Reznick, J. S., & Turner-Brown, L. (2016). Cultural effects on the diagnosis of autism spectrum disorder among Latinos. *Focus on Autism and Other Developmental Disabilities*, *31*(4), 275–283.

Regencia, Z. J. G., Gouin, J. P., Ladia, M. A. J., Montoya, J. C., & Baja, E. S. (2023). Effect of body image perception and skin-lightening practices on mental health of Filipino emerging adults: A mixed-methods approach protocol. *BMJ [British Medical Journal] Open*, *13*(5), 1–12.

Reitmanova, S., Gustafson, D. L., & Ahmed, R. (2015). “Immigrants can be deadly”: Critical discourse analysis of racialization of immigrant health in the Canadian press and public health policies. *Canadian Journal of Communication*, *40*(3), 471–487.

Rich, M. (2020, February 13). As coronavirus spreads, so does anti-Chinese sentiment. *The New York Times*. https://www.nytimes.com/2020/01/30/world/asia/coronavirus-chinese-racism.html

Ritter, S. (2023). ‘When I lose the weight, we’ll go on a date’–fatness, singleness and liminality in Fat Chance. *Popular Communication*, *21*, 1–13.

Sailors, P. R. (2015). Personal foul: An evaluation of the moral status of football. *Journal of the Philosophy of Sport*, *42*(2), 269–286.

Schumaker, E. (2020, September 22). Timeline: How coronavirus got started. *ABC News*. https://abcnews.go.com/Health/timeline-coronavirus-started/story?id=69435165

Shoichet, C. E. (2020, September 16). In a horrifying history of forced sterilizations, some fear the US is beginning a new chapter. *CNN*. https://www.cnn.com/2020/09/16/us/ice-hysterectomy-forced-sterilization-history/index.html

Similly, L. (2023). Bootylicious yellow bone: Beyoncé's physicality as a site of racialized, socio-political angst concerning beauty, class, and essentialized Blackness. *The Journal of Popular Culture*, *56*(3–4), 1–21.

Singer, M. K., Dressler, W., George, S., Baquet, C. R., Bell, R. A., Burhansstipanov, L., ... & Williams, D. (2016). Culture: The missing link in health research. *Social Science & Medicine*, *170*, 237–246.

Social Media and News Fact Sheet. (2023, November 15). Pew Research Center. https://www.pewresearch.org/journalism/fact-sheet/social-media-and-news-fact-sheet/

Sternheimer, K., (2013). *Connecting social problems and popular culture: Why media is not the answer* (2nd ed.). Routledge. https://doi.org/10.4324/9780429495342

The Takeaway (2021, June 9). After practice or “race-norming” is exposed, Black former players remain skeptical of NFL. [Radio broadcast transcript]. *New York Public Radio*. https://www.wnycstudios.org/podcasts/takeaway/segments/after-practice-race-norming-exposed-black-former-players-remain-skeptical-nfl

The Untreated Syphilis Study at Tuskegee Timeline. (2022, December 5). Centers for Disease Control and Prevention. https://www.cdc.gov/tuskegee/timeline.htm

The White House, Speeches and Remarks. (2022, October 22). Remarks by Vice President Harris in a conversation on reproductive rights. https://www.whitehouse.gov/briefing-room/speeches-remarks/2022/10/22/remarks-by-vice-president-harris-in-a-conversation-on-reproductive-rights-3/

Ventresca, M., & Henne, K. (2020, September 17). NFL concussion lawsuit payouts reveal how racial bias in science continues. *The Conversation*. https://theconversation.com/nfl-concussion-lawsuit-payouts-reveal-how-racial-bias-in-science-continues-145987

Villarosa, L. (2022, June 8). The long shadow of eugenics in America. *The New York Times Magazine*. https://www.nytimes.com/2022/06/08/magazine/eugenics-movement-america.html

Volkwein-Caplan, K. (2013). *Sport fitness culture* (Vol. 12). Meyer & Meyer Verlag.

Walton, S. R., Kerr, Z. Y., Mannix, R., Brett, B. L., Chandran, A., DeFreese, J. D., ... & Echemendia, R. J. (2022). Subjective concerns regarding the effects of sport-related concussion on long-term brain health among former NFL players: An NFL-LONG study. *Sports Medicine*, *52*, 1–15.

Warner, K. J. (2015). The racial logic of Grey’s Anatomy: Shonda Rhimes and her “post-civil rights, post-feminist” series. *Television & New Media*, *16*(7), 631–647.

Weinstock, J. A. (1997). Virus culture. *Studies in Popular Culture*, *20*(1), 83–97.

Williams, S. (2022, April 5). How Serena Williams saved her own life. *Elle*. https://www.elle.com/life-love/a39586444/how-serena-williams-saved-her-own-life/

Yamamoto, T. (2000). In/visible difference: Asian American women and the politics of spectacle. *Race, Gender & Class*, *7*(1), 43–55.

23

POPULAR CULTURE AND HEALTH COMMUNICATION ACROSS THE LIFESPAN

Jennifer Stevens Aubrey, Heather Gahler, and Jiaqi Zeng

Just as health concerns will inevitably change over people's lifespans, so too will their attention and sensitivity to health topics that are covered in popular culture. In this vein, a guiding assumption of the present chapter is that health communication practitioners (e.g., writers/producers, campaign directors) who are correspondingly sensitive to the developmental tasks and milestones of the age groups they are targeting will have better success at connecting with audiences in ways that will lead to their intended outcomes. Given our focus on the developmental tasks of people as they move through the lifespan, Erik Erikson's (1959, 1968) theory of psychosocial development guides our perspective. Erikson contended that an individual's personality develops through eight stages of the lifespan, and living a healthy, well-adjusted life depends on the successful completion of the core developmental task of each stage. Thus, in this chapter, we strive to explore the health messaging that connects with these developmental tasks throughout the lifespan.

To this end, we will, first, review Erikson's theory of psychosocial development, using a popular television sitcom, *Modern Family*, as an illustrative text. We then examine the messaging, impact, and notable examples of health topics addressed in popular culture that either focus on issues especially relevant to certain developmental stages (e.g., unplanned pregnancy in adolescence, death/dying in older adulthood), or were specifically created for and/or tested on audiences of certain developmental stages.

Psychosocial Development and the Major Stages of Life through *Modern Family*

In his model of psychosocial development, Erikson (1959, 1968) asserted that identity emerges in stages, and this development requires restructuring over time. Although the theory has been criticized for focusing too much on the notion of discrete stages and for assuming that the completion of one stage is a prerequisite for the next stage of development (Maree, 2021), we argue that the theory holds utility if we focus on the developmental tasks in each stage without assuming that they are discretely completed before the next stage begins. In this vein, Erikson articulated eight sequential stages of individual human development that are influenced by biological, psychological, and social factors throughout the lifespan (Orenstein & Lewis, 2022).

In each stage, individuals face a core tension or crisis, consisting of opposing psychological tendencies – one developmentally positive, resulting in an identity strength (i.e., an "ego virtue"), and

DOI: 10.4324/9781003436409-27

the other developmentally negative, leading to an identity weakness (Erikson, 1959). The resolution of the core crisis in each stage fosters change within the individual, expanding connections between the self and the environment (Kropf & Greene, 2017). If an individual resolves the core crisis in favor of an ego virtue, that person gains skills to complete subsequent stages of development and adds to a stable foundation for core belief systems (Orenstein & Lewis, 2022). If the individual resolves the core crisis in favor of the identity weakness, the result will be maldevelopment, and subsequent stages may be delayed and/or increasingly difficult to navigate.

Modern Family, a sitcom that was on ABC for 11 seasons (2009-2020), captured both critical and popular success. The show told the stories of three related families, who were united by their relationship to Jay Pritchett. At the beginning of the show, Jay had recently married a younger woman, Gloria, and cohabitated with Gloria and her son, Manny, who was 11. Jay also had two adult children, Claire and Mitchell, who had their own families. The show centered on the relationships and situations of these three families, and notably, the audience saw these experiences through the lenses of characters at various developmental stages (Caballero & Richardson, 2023). Jay was 61 when the show started, and the next generation of characters (Gloria, Claire, Claire's husband Phil, Mitchell, Mitchell's husband Cameron) were in middle adulthood. Claire and Phil had three kids (ranging in age from 11-16) at the show's start, and Mitchell and Cameron had recently adopted a baby. During the series run, the characters (and the actors who played them) age in real time. Thus, *Modern Family* provides useful examples of the stages of psychosocial development. In the following, we will describe each stage and a relevant character from *Modern Family*, whose storyline illustrates each stage. See Figure 23.1 for a partial family tree of *Modern Family* and the associated stage of psychosocial development.

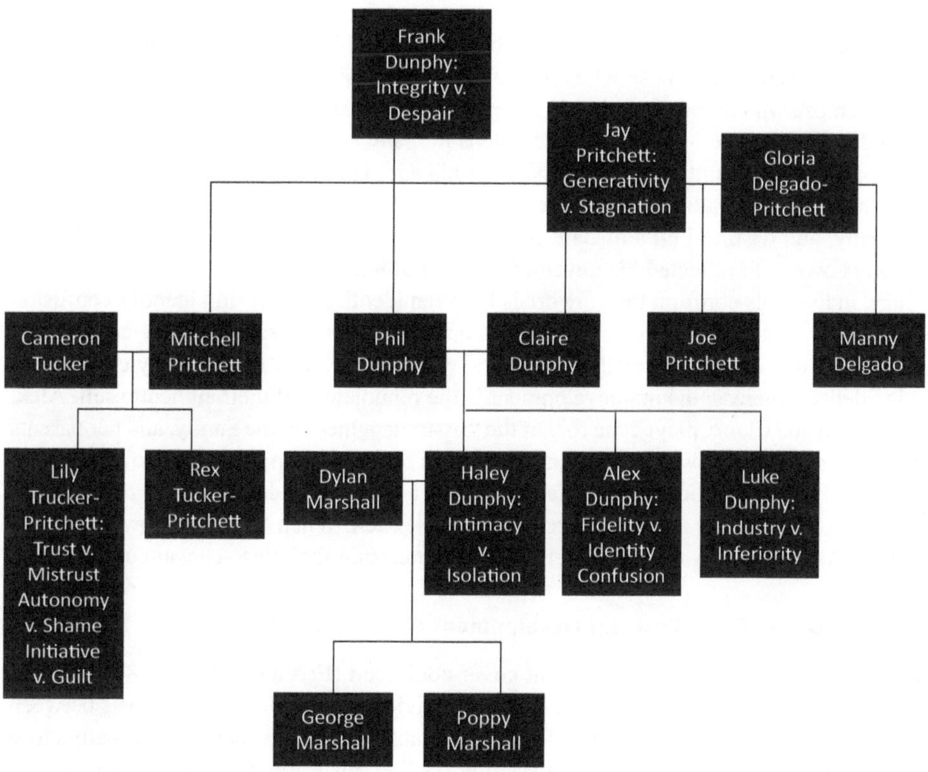

Figure 23.1 Partial Family Tree of Modern Family and Associated Stages of Psychosocial Development.

The Stages of Psychosocial Development during Childhood and Adolescence

The first four stages of psychosocial development cover childhood (Erikson 1959, 1968). Infancy, the first stage of development, reflects a struggle between trust and mistrust. Infants must learn to trust that their caregivers are going to adequately respond to their needs. If they do, the ego virtue is hope, but if they do not, the maldevelopment is withdrawal. *Modern Family*'s Lily, who was raised in a Vietnamese orphanage before being adopted by Mitchell and Cameron, had questions about her origins, indicating that she was grappling with issues related to trust. Mitchell and Cameron fretted when Lily bonded with an Asian female doctor and called her "mommy," likely because Lily was reminded of her caretakers in Vietnam.

The next stage occurs during early childhood (i.e., toddlerhood), and the core crisis is between autonomy and shame. If the toddler learns to take care of their basic needs and develops confidence in their own physical competencies, the ego virtue is will. However, if others discourage them from doing so or force them before they are ready, the maldevelopment is compulsion. On *Modern Family*, Cameron was extremely attentive to toddler Lily, hovering over her basic needs, such as dressing herself. However, after Lily became overly attached to Cameron while rejecting Mitchell, her other dad, Cameron realized that allowing Lily to dress herself would increase her confidence and autonomy.

Occurring during the preschool age, the next stage involves the core crisis between initiative and guilt. If the child learns to assert themselves in their environment, the ego virtue is purpose, but if they do not, they will have inhibitions about taking initiatives. For example, in *Modern Family*, Cameron and Mitchell rushed to intervene when Lily experienced bullying at kindergarten, but after they arranged a playdate for Lily and the boy who bullied her, the pair became fast friends. Thus, Mitchell and Cameron learned that trusting Lily to solve her own conflicts likely allowed her to develop the agency to do so in the future.

The next stage of childhood covers school age, and the core crisis covers industry and inferiority. Children in this stage explore their interests and competencies, while reflecting on other people's evaluations of these competencies. Those who resolve this crisis positively experience the ego virtue of competence, and those who do not experience a prevailing sense of inferiority. Luke, the youngest child of Claire and Phil, followed in his father's footsteps in many ways, but he struggled to develop interests and hobbies that were authentic to him because his dad insisted that Luke participate in his hobbies, such as magic, cheerleading, and dance. However, Luke did not take an interest in these activities. Eventually, and despite Phil's disdain for it, Luke wrestled for his school's team. Luke's decision to forge his own path reflected his developing sense of industry.

In adolescence, individuals confront the core crisis between identity fidelity and identity confusion (Erikson, 1959, 1968). Adolescents need to develop an adequate sense of self that they can express authentically and know that others, especially their peers, will validate them for it. If they can do that, the ego virtue is fidelity; whereas, the maldevelopment is the repudiation of their authentic self. Alex, the middle child of Phil and Claire, played the role of the "smart daughter" in the family, and her parents tended to neglect her because she was self-reliant and driven to succeed on her own. However, after suffering a panic attack in front of her extended family during her 16th birthday party, her parents realized that they never considered the amount of pressure that Alex felt. When Claire acknowledged this perspective to Alex, Alex gratefully embraced her, feeling appreciated for being seen and understood.

Stages of Psychosocial Development during Adulthood

The last three stages of psychosocial development cover adulthood (Erikson 1959, 1968). In young adulthood (typically called "emerging adulthood" today), individuals confront the core crisis between intimacy versus isolation. With the developmental task of establishing an intimate, emotionally close relationship with another person, those who successfully resolve this stage develop the capacity for love, and those who do not develop a tendency to distance themselves from intimate relationships. On *Modern Family*, this stage was well-illustrated by the relationship between Haley, Phil and Claire's oldest daughter, and her on-again, off-again boyfriend, Dylan. After falling in love during high school, Haley broke up with Dylan when she went to college because she wanted to be free from commitment. Although Haley and Dylan broke up and got back together many times, mostly due to Haley's fear of commitment, the two ended up together, married, and became parents of twins by the end of the series.

In the next stage, covering mid-adulthood, the core crisis addresses generativity versus stagnation. In this stage, individuals will face the task of taking care of others and not only themselves. If they can create a healthy and supportive environment for the next generation, they will experience the ego virtue of care, but if they reject future generations, they will develop rejectivity. On *Modern Family*, Jay, the patriarch, reflected on his own parenting when he found himself on the brink of becoming a great-grandfather. In a speech to the entire extended family, he reminded them that "you never know the last time you're going to pick up your kids," as he fought back tears. In this way, he expressed to his family that generativity is the ultimate pursuit of adulthood.

The final stage, occurring during old age, reflects the core crisis between integrity and despair. This stage often involves taking stock of one's life. If individuals feel generally satisfied with their lives, they will experience wisdom, but if they do not, they will experience despair. On *Modern Family*, Phil and his father, Frank, who suffered from dementia, had a meaningful conversation about the end of life. When Phil asked Frank whether he wished that he had another child to carry on the family business, Frank replied that he never wished for that, and he assured Phil that he had, in fact, carried on the family business of keeping life fun and light. Shortly after, Frank died. Thus, in this last conversation, Frank demonstrated that he achieved wisdom by appreciating his loved ones and feeling satisfaction about the course that his life had taken.

Mediated Health Messaging and Effects across the Lifespan

In the following sections, the stages of psychosocial development guide our understanding of how health messaging connects to major developmental tasks. We highlight two or three topics especially relevant to illustrating each developmental stage in light of messaging in popular culture.

Health Messaging in Childhood

It is developmentally normal for children to be unaware of their health. "Even under the most dire circumstances, it is children's nature to be energetic, engaged, and happy. Children expect physical, mental, and social well-being – they focus on exploring life, expanding their worlds, and they are often oblivious to risk" (Borzekowski & Rich, 2012, p. 1). Thus, when we consider the potential health effects of media on children's health, media present both potential risks, in that they might be encouraging unhealthy behaviors without the child's awareness, and potential benefits, in that the media can encourage children to develop healthy habits that will sustain their health throughout their lifespan. In this section, we will focus on narrative health messaging targeting children (ages 0–12), focusing on three domains: nutrition and childhood obesity, mental health, and alcohol use.

Nutrition and Childhood Obesity. In toddlerhood, early childhood, and school age, the developmental tasks for children involve learning to attend to their own needs (Erikson, 1950). Making their own nutritional choices comprises an essential aspect of building this autonomy. However, the World Health Organization recognized childhood obesity as a global epidemic in 1997, and many subsequently identified the media as a negative influence in this domain (Stephenson & Banet-Weiser, 2007). Certainly, media consumption typically constitutes a sedentary activity that displaces active behaviors and lifestyles (e.g., Strasburger et al., 2010). However, we can attribute the responsibility for the epidemic of childhood obesity more directly to food marketing (Harrison et al., 2015). For the most part, food marketing targeting children encourages them to consume high-energy, low-nutrient foods. Children see about 13 food ads on television every day, and 9 out of 10 of these ads promote products high in salt, sugar, and fat (LoDolce, 2015). Randomized, controlled experiments have provided evidence that exposure to fast-food advertising has an impact on children's food beliefs and preferences (e.g., Robinson et al., 2007). For example, Harrison et al. (2012) linked television viewing with increased intake of high-energy, low-nutrient foods and decreased intake of fruits and vegetables among 2–4-year-olds – effects largely resistant to parental mediation. In an earlier study, Harrison (2005) suggested that television viewing results in decrements in nutritional knowledge and reasoning, especially in relation to foods that tend to be marketed for weight loss.

As with many socially relevant issues in childhood, Sesame Workshop, the organization that develops and evaluates *Sesame Street* and associated products, has been at the forefront of using its platform to encourage healthy habits regarding nutrition and exercise. *Sesame Street*'s "Healthy Habits for Life" curriculum features characters who model fun ways to move and play and encourage children to explore and enjoy healthy foods. As an intervention, Sesame Workshop (2013) evaluated the effectiveness of the televised curriculum, in conjunction with a resource kit, in childcare centers, and 98% of childcare providers reported an improvement in children's food choices.

Mental Health. Parents, teachers, and health professionals often overlook the mental health of children, but in 2022, in the wake of the COVID-19 pandemic and associated school closures and lockdowns, the American Academy of Pediatrics declared a mental health emergency in U.S. children (Karpman et al., 2023). School-age children benefit from the opportunity to take on increasingly complex assignments, and their teachers, coaches, and counselors contribute significantly to this part of their development (Maree, 2021). However, during the early stages of the COVID-19 pandemic, children experienced considerable isolation from these significant interactions. At the same time, their media use and exposure increased significantly (Hedderson et al., 2023). Using a longitudinal design, Rosen et al. (2021) found that U.S. children who had less passive screen time were less likely to develop psychopathological symptoms.

Moreover, between the ages of 7–11, children's cognitive ability to conceptualize separation from others makes it possible to develop prejudice toward others, including the stigma of mental illness (Mueller et al., 2016). Czeisler et al. (2020) concluded that stigmatized attitudes about mental illness emerge from ages 7–8 and persist into young adulthood, when individuals encounter the highest risk of developing a mental health disorder of their own. Thus, children should be provided with realistic and humanistic portrayals of mental illness. Unfortunately, content analyses of children's films (Wahl et al., 2003) and television programming (Wahl et al., 2007) have revealed a tendency to identify characters with a psychiatric disorder by the use of words like "crazy," "nuts," and "psycho." Children's films and TV shows largely depicted characters who had a mental illness as aggressive and threatening and were treated by other characters with fear, exclusion, and disrespect. In light of mostly negative depictions of mental illness, Mueller et al. (2016) identified the media as a sociocultural source of mental health stigma.

Although *Sesame Street* has created research-based content to support children's social-emotional wellbeing for the duration of its 50-year-plus run, new offerings directly tackle current issues in children's mental health. In May 2023, Sesame Workshop released *Elmo's Mindfulness Spectacular*, a 45-minute program on YouTube, as well as a PSA campaign, curricular materials, and podcasts. In the YouTube special, the *Sesame Street* Muppets learn how to calm anxiety by learning about mindfulness. According to Sesame Workshop, this new initiative seeks to highlight the importance of parents nurturing their children's emotional well-being and to lessen the stigma associated with seeking help for children's mental health.

Health Messaging in Adolescence

Much of the research on health messaging in adolescence centers on risk-taking. We have two developmental explanations for this focus. First, given adolescents' core crisis of identity cohesion versus confusion (Erikson, 1959, 1968), peers comprise the significant relationships for adolescents, and as such, they are often tempted to engage in risky behaviors to fit in socially (DiClemente et al., 1996). Second, another hallmark of adolescence involves the belief in one's "personal fable," adolescents tend to believe that they are so special and unique that life's risks and difficulties will not affect them (Elkind, 1967). Because of these beliefs, risk-taking behaviors, such as substance use and unsafe sexual behaviors, spike in adolescence. Wide-ranging health risks and problem behaviors occur in adolescence, but in this chapter, we focus on unsafe sexual behaviors and disordered eating (Strasburger et al., 2010).

Unsafe Sexual Behaviors and Teen Pregnancy. Given the importance of sexual development in adolescence, it is not surprising that most research examining media effects on sexual risk-taking utilizes adolescent samples (typically starting around the age of 12–13), when the social forces of peer groups and pubertal development coalesce into an interest in sexual media content. A meta-analysis, reporting results from 59 studies, revealed that exposure to sexual media had a small but significant effect on both sexual attitudes and behaviors, and the effects were strongest for adolescents (Coyne et al., 2019). (For related work on sexual health and popular culture, please see Chapter 6, this volume.)

In general, researchers explain the link between exposure to sexually oriented media and sexual risk-taking through the lens of social cognitive theory (Bandura, 2009). That is, adolescents who consume media that include depictions of attractive characters who enjoy having sexual intercourse and rarely suffer negative consequences from it will be more likely to model the behavior (e.g., Eyal & Kunkel, 2008; Finnerty-Myers, 2011). For example, Bond and Drogos (2014) found that late adolescents who viewed the sex-laden reality show *Jersey Shore* expressed stronger parasocial relationships (i.e., feeling like their favorite *Jersey Shore* character was a friend) and wishful identification (i.e., the desire to be like a favorite *Jersey Shore* character), which both subsequently predicted more positive attitudes toward uncommitted sexual exploration. Indeed, content analytic research has shown that television's portrayals of sex rarely contain safe sex messages, particularly among programs that target teen viewers (see Aubrey & Gamble, 2017, for review). If stakeholders in public health want to prevent or discourage irresponsible sexual behaviors, television characters are unlikely to serve as effective behavioral models, given that they rarely experience negative consequences for their risky behavior.

In examining the link between sexually oriented television exposure and reproductive health outcomes, Chandra et al. (2008) connected frequent exposure to sexual content on television with a significantly greater likelihood of teen pregnancy in the following three years. The authors argued that television does not typically depict the negative consequences of sex, including unplanned pregnancies, and, thus, television fails to send a cautionary message about unprotected sex. MTV's *16 and Pregnant*, a reality show that aired between 2014–2019, and its spinoff series, *Teen Mom*, which remained in production as of late 2023, exemplify television shows addressing teen pregnancy. Each episode of *16 and Pregnant* featured a 16–year-old girl who experienced hardships while going through pregnancy, labor and delivery, and the early postpartum weeks. The producers sought to combat teen pregnancy by serving as a cautionary tale about the realities of teen pregnancy (Dinh, 2010). However, the national attention and quasi-celebrity that the actual teen moms experienced might have undermined the show's intention (Martins & Jensen, 2014). Additionally, some of the consequences portrayed – such as getting engaged to the baby's father and bonding with adorable (albeit demanding) infants – could be interpreted as positive outcomes by some adolescents (Martins et al., 2016). As such, research evaluating the impact of *16 and Pregnant* and *Teen Mom* on adolescent viewers' attitudes and behavioral intentions regarding teen pregnancy demonstrated that the show did *not* deter them from teen pregnancy but encouraged it (Aubrey et al., 2014; Behm-Morawitz et al., 2019; Martins & Jensen, 2014).

On a more positive note, some recent television shows (e.g., *Big Mouth*, *Sex Education*) have arguably filled in the gap that poor sex education curricula in many schools leave for adolescents. Aptly titled *Sex Education*, a British comedy-drama series on Netflix, has been lauded for being *actually* educational on sexual topics (Smythe, 2020). The storylines cover everything from how to prevent transmission of chlamydia to the best types of lubricant to use, and these "lessons" are packaged in empathetic, nuanced, and complex explorations of the teen characters' lives. For example, one of the recurring themes in *Sex Education* is sexual consent. In one episode, teen characters Otis and Ola discussed their feelings, concerns, and levels of comfort not only before getting intimate but also during and after the sexual activity. Episodes like this normalize the conversations around sex necessary for active sexual consent (e.g., Edwards et al., 2022). More broadly, the teen characters educated and gave each other practical, yet responsible advice, resulting in engaging storylines and relatable teenage characters.

Disordered Eating. Eating disorders, such as anorexia nervosa and bulimia nervosa, constitute the extremes of a "disordered eating behavior" spectrum and often encompass negative body image, binge eating, and unhealthy forms of weight and shape management (Levine & Smolak, 2006). (For related research on body image and popular culture, please see Chapter 5, this volume.) The prevalence of unhealthy body image, usually measured as body dissatisfaction, is widespread and normative, especially among adolescents (Dion et al., 2015). Rapid body changes during puberty make adolescents sensitive to understanding the sociocultural appearance ideals for bodies, particularly for the members of their social group. During adolescence, individuals absorb the rules and judgments about what society considers to be attractive and whether their bodies measure up. Also, during adolescence, a major developmental task is the construction of a coherent identity (Erikson, 1968), and certainly, body image comprises an important aspect of that (Markey, 2010). Some adolescents will stake their identity strongly on their physical appearance, and these adolescents will be especially vulnerable to mediated messages and narratives about bodies and weight.

Messages in popular culture about attractiveness, body image norms, self-control, and weight management can be considered part of the broader ecosystem of adolescents' lives (Levine & Harrison, 2009). As such, meta-analyses have demonstrated a modest relationship between media exposure and body image disturbance among adolescents (Grabe et al., 2008; Groesz et al., 2002; Hausenblas et al., 2013; Huang et al., 2021). For example, a meta-analysis demonstrated a small but significant increase in eating disorder symptoms in pretest-posttest experimental designs (Hausenblas et al., 2013).

Alongside mainstream messages and imagery that tell adolescents what ideal bodies look like, a darker sub-universe of pro-eating disorder content exists in online spaces. Pro-anorexia (pro-ana) and pro-bulimia (pro-mia) websites instruct visitors on how to successfully maintain an eating disorder, and they promote eating disorders as a lifestyle rather than serious health conditions (Norris et al., 2006). Pro-ana and pro-mia websites strengthen users' eating disorder identity and worsen their eating pathology (Rodgers et al., 2016). Accordingly, major platforms (such as Facebook, Pinterest, Instagram, Twitter, and Tumblr) have banned pro-ED communities, but they still hide in plain sight. Some are invitation-only, and some use secretive names such as butterfly, angel, and dragonfly (Custers, 2015). Moreover, despite some notable attempts to portray the recovery of adolescent characters dealing with an eating disorder in a nuanced and sensitive way, media portrayals also showcase the "how-tos" of eating disorders, which can trigger those who are recovering from the disease (Gilbert, 2017). For example, the 2017 movie *To the Bone* portrayed Ellen, a young affluent white woman, as anorexic. In the narrative arc of the movie, she became a patient at a treatment center. There she got better, and then she got worse. By the end of the movie, she ultimately decided on recovery, but during the movie, the audience witnessed Ellen engage in all manner of anorexic behaviors, likely planting ideas among those who have considered anorexia and triggering those who already suffer from anorexia (Gilbert, 2017).

Health Messaging in Emerging Adulthood

Spanning late teens to late twenties, characteristics of emerging adulthood include a growing sense of self-reliance and identity exploration (Arnett, 2007). Thus, emerging adulthood may be an important but overlooked, developmental period for establishing long-term health behaviors. During this period, opportunities exist for enhancing emerging adults' health literacy, which will benefit their long-term health behaviors (Vaterlaus et al., 2015).

Mental Health and Substance Use Disorders. Certainly, in childhood and adolescence, mental health is a concern, but during emerging adulthood, temporary bouts of poor mental health can bloom into full-blown disorders. Moreover, emerging adults still feel a sense of invulnerability to injury, harm, and danger; therefore, they are prone to mental health issues and substance use disorders (Sussman & Arnett, 2014). In a 2007 national survey of U.S. respondents aged 18–29, 56% agreed with the statement, "I often feel anxious," and 32% agreed with the statement, "I often feel depressed" (Arnett et al., 2014). Thwarted milestones and increased isolation during the COVID-19 pandemic only made the situation worse for emerging adults. In 2020, 74.9% of emerging adult respondents (ages 18–24) reported having one or more mental health symptom – more than any other age group (Czeisler et al., 2020). In 2020, one in four emerging adults had considered suicide within the past month (25.5%), and about the same percentage (24.7%) reported starting or increasing substance use to cope with pandemic-related emotions (Czeisler et al., 2020).

Much research and policy attention have examined the link between social media use and mental health problems among adolescents and emerging adults (Keles et al., 2020). Indeed, the relationship between social media use and mental well-being strengthens as young people move toward emerging adulthood (Marino et al., 2018). As one plausible explanation, social media can lead to difficulties with emotion regulation because emerging adults utilize social media to negatively cope with difficult emotions (Rasmussen et al., 2020). Poor emotional regulation, in turn, leads to more stress and consequently more mental health problems.

Additionally, emerging adults tackle considerable identity work. A developmental task for emerging adults (that actually starts in adolescence) involves determining how they resemble (and differ from) peers. Thus, one of the key motivations influencing how emerging adults make media choices may be their desire to affiliate with similar people while simultaneously distinguishing themselves from others (Brown, 2006). In this vein, emerging adults can be especially sensitive to the ostensibly positive self-portrayals of others on social media. When they negatively compare themselves to their peers on social media, they lack a sense of belonging and are more likely to engage in suicidal ideation (Spitzer et al., 2023).

This period of increased identity exploration can also contribute to both substance use and the clinical diagnoses of substance dependence/disorders, both of which occur more in emerging adulthood than at any other developmental period (Arnett et al., 2014). First, in their quest for identity exploration, emerging adults might want to try out substances before they accept the responsibilities and commitments of adult life (Arnett, 2005). Thus, emerging adults might consider this time as their chance to "sow their wild oats" in many respects, including substance use. Second, most emerging adults find identity exploration that begins in adolescence to be confusing and difficult (Arnett, 2005). However, unlike during adolescence, emerging adults have increased independence from their parents and other authority figures, so they have expanded opportunities to use substances as a welcome relief from identity confusion.

Because the tobacco and alcohol industries target young, potentially new customers of tobacco and alcohol, these industries have long targeted emerging adults. At the same time, emerging adults spend a great deal of time on screen media. Thus, emerging adults are frequently exposed to digital marketing of substances via brand websites, social media marketing campaigns, and product placements (Jackson et al., 2018), in addition to messages about substance use on social media daily, especially on Snapchat and Instagram.

In one observational study, emerging adults encountered during their regular social media use three posts per day on cigarettes on Snapchat and one per day on Instagram, one post per day on e-cigarettes on both Snapchat and Instagram, two posts per day on cannabis on Snapchat and two on Instagram, and nine posts per day on alcohol on Snapchat and seven per day on Instagram (Burnell et al., 2022). Among the same participants, those who *posted* about e-cigarettes, marijuana, and alcohol (but not cigarettes) used more of each of those substances, and those who viewed other people's posts used more cigarettes and e-cigarettes. Additionally, another study connected greater daily social media use among emerging adults to more alcohol consumption, more problematic alcohol use, and more frequent drug use (the latter for women only; Ohannessian et al., 2017). Beyond social media, those who viewed depictions of people being drunk or high across media types, including advertising, television, and social media, used more alcohol, via perceived alcohol norms (Davis et al., 2019).

HBO's *Girls* (2012–2017) offered a raw and controversial look at the lives of a group of emerging adults navigating their 20s in New York City. The show received both praise and critique for its portrayal of mental health and substance use. For example, it drew praise for its accurate depiction of the main character Hannah's anxiety and obsessive-compulsive disorder (OCD), which the show portrayed as a complex condition triggered by stressful events (Muller, 2017). Another main character, Adam, had a substance use disorder (i.e., alcoholism), but he was in recovery throughout the series and was not defined by his history with substance abuse (Bonner, 2012). On the other hand, the other characters' reliance on drugs (including cocaine, heroin, and oxycontin) to negatively cope with their mental health did not end with serious consequences for the characters.

Health Messaging in Mid-Adulthood

Although research on popular media health messages often includes those in mid-adulthood (Wakefield et al., 2010), few messages specifically target this age group. Perhaps health advocates focus on younger age groups out of greater concern for their future well-being or older adults because of the health concerns that often come with aging. In contrast, those in adulthood possess the efficacy to implement what has been learned from past health messages, yet they do not yet need messages directed at older adults.

Generativity, defined as "a concern for establishing and guiding the next generation" (Erikson, 1959, p. 79), comprises the main developmental task of mid-adulthood, and we propose two major health implications. First, in mid-adulthood, individuals will likely be motivated to maintain and maximize their own health so that they can be around to guide younger generations. Second, adults will likely attempt to model healthy behaviors for their children.

Health Screenings. Preventative health behaviors, such as health as screenings, constitute a way for adults to accomplish the developmental task of generativity. For example, showing women getting papanicolaou (PAP) smears and undergoing screening mammography on popular TV programs has increased uptake in these routine screenings (Wakefield et al., 2010). Social media have been used to promote disease and cancer prevention awareness among adults, and some evidence indicates that social media users do have better awareness of preventative behaviors related to some diseases (e.g., HPV, Hepatitis C) but not others (e.g., colon cancer, breast cancer, prostate cancer; Qin et al., 2021).

In line with an entertainment-education strategy, increasing awareness of health prevention and screenings has been a hallmark of medical dramas on television (Hoffman et al., 2017). (For related information on entertainment-education and health communication, please see Chapter 17, this volume.) Hether et al. (2008) examined the effects of storylines about the BRCA1 breast cancer gene mutation that were aired within approximately three weeks of each other on *ER* and *Grey's Anatomy*. Among those who had watched one of the two storylines, the show had a modest impact on adult women's knowledge, attitudes, and behavioral intentions related to breast cancer; however, those who had viewed both storylines showed more consistent and profound effects on their knowledge, attitudes, behavioral intentions, and even their own behaviors in getting screened for the BRCA1 gene after exposure.

Role Modeling of Healthy Behaviors. In mid-adulthood, messages related to being a healthy role model for the younger generation likely appeal to the developmental task of generativity. Examples of these types of messages include smoking-cessation campaigns (Wakefield et al., 2010) and sunburn reduction efforts (O'Riordhan et al., 2003), while others focus on longevity in one's life for the sake of one's larger community, such as AIDS messaging towards LGBTQ+ adults (Wakefield et al., 2010). Some messages combine these ideas, giving adults the ability to help themselves *and* their children, such as the campaign to increase netting use to combat mosquito-borne illnesses in Cameroon (Bowen, 2013).

For example, one effective interventional strategy in combating childhood obesity has entailed using the media to promote parents' role modeling of behaviors related to nutrition and exercise to their children (Evans et al., 2010). These messages have been particularly effective when the messages aim at not just changing the adults' behaviors for their own health but instead changing the adults' behavior for the sake of their children. For example, one media-based intervention in Chicago, 5-4-3-2-1 Go!, targeted parents as agents of change in childhood obesity (Evans et al., 2007).

Health Messaging in Older Adulthood

The developmental task of older adulthood involves fully accepting one's life and coming to terms with death (Erikson, 1959). In general, the media do not offer many inspiring portrayals to aid in this task. Indeed, one truism of media representation is that older adults tend to be extremely underrepresented, and typical representations put them in ill-health (see Harwood, 2007, for a review). Nevertheless, older adults tend to seek out a great deal of information about their health, which may emerge from older adults' search for integrity and/or an attempt to achieve a good death, which is a death that comes with dignity (van Wijingaarden & Sanders, 2022).

Health Information Seeking. Older adults use the internet and social media to obtain health information. Tennant et al. (2015) concluded that older adults experience confidence in their ability to find health information online but uncertainty about how to evaluate it and that women utilize social media almost three times more for health information than men. Potentially, women serve as not only the primary health information seekers for themselves but also for loved ones, therefore increasing their motivation to find health information on the Internet.

Older adults in China benefited from the use of WeChat, a Chinese social media website similar to Facebook, for sharing health information (Shang et al., 2021) as well as for bettering their health (Wei et al., 2022). Wei and colleagues found that the use of WeChat improved older adults' subjective well-being as well as their self-rated health and their mental health status, with women's mental health benefiting more. The health benefits may be due to the social connectedness embedded in WeChat, which alleviates the loneliness that many older adults experience (Ang, 2018). For older men, Wei et al. determined that WeChat often provided a method of health information transmission. When deciding what health information to share, older adults prioritize information that offers hope over severe consequences across a diverse range of health information, thus sharing active trends rather than creating social panic (Shang et al., 2021).

During the COVID-19 pandemic, older adults' health information seeking on social media increased, while their mental health declined (Negarestani et al., 2021). Although this trend was not uncommon across other age groups during the COVID-19 pandemic, according to Negarestani et al., older adults experienced more pronounced effects, probably because they were the most vulnerable to the detrimental effects of COVID-19.

Death and Dying. As older adults are developmentally tasked with taking stock of their lives and hopefully judging them as well-lived, it would be appropriate, too, for them to want to face the end of life with dignity. In content analyses of popular films in 2015 and 2016, researchers found that older characters most often died as a result of violence, unlike their actual most common cause of death (i.e., heart disease; Smith et al., 2016, 2018). Such depictions also highlight victimhood in their deaths, and clearly, they do not offer the dignity of a life well-lived. In an analysis of newspaper coverage of death and dying in Dutch newspapers from 2010-2020, the dominant frame centered on choice, positioning older people as active subjects who autonomously determine their own death (van Wijingaarden & Sanders, 2022). However, the two other dominant frames presented death as a risk or as a burden, requiring care from others and society. These latter frames construed older people as passive and acted upon in their dying process, thus denying them discourses that are based on dignity. (For related work on death and popular culture, please see Chapter 9, this volume.)

In this vein, entertainment-education efforts have sought to improve the accuracy and sensitivity of depictions of terminal illness and death in TV and movies, including storylines about end-of-life care, pain management, biomedical ethics, and rights of the terminally ill (Chartrand & Lazaro, 2022; Kaiser Family Foundation, 2004). For example, *A Million Little Things* followed the terminal cancer diagnosis of one of the main characters, and at the end of the series, the patient and his loved ones grapple with his choice to use medical assistance to end his life (Pardo et al., 2023). Despite such efforts, a recent analysis by the Norman Lear Center suggests that television programs, for the most part, do not effectively connect with older adults' developmental task of achieving a sense of control and dignity about their deaths (Pardo et al., 2023). For example, discussions about estate plans, advance directives, end-of-life care, and death planning were mentioned rarely in scripted television shows (e.g., *Chicago Med*, *Grey's Anatomy*, *Criminal Minds*). Moreover, Pardo et al. (2023) found that rather than granting agency and complexity to dying characters, they were often portrayed passively, without discussion of the choices and emotions that come at the end of life. They concluded that such depictions limit the potential for viewers to initiate their own conversations about end of life.

Conclusion

In this chapter, we examined how health topics pertain to developmental tasks throughout the lifespan. In this analysis, we examined both fictional messages with incidental health implications (e.g., *Sex Education*, *Girls*), as well as targeted media-based health strategies (e.g., *Sesame Street*, *16 and Pregnant*). For future health messaging, we recommend a developmentally grounded approach that connects to individuals' ability to resolve their core developmental crises in favor of their ego virtues. We argue that the effectiveness of health messaging will likely be enhanced if audiences connect the messages to their developmental tasks. In order to effectively implement and evaluate these ideas, it would be necessary for health communication practitioners (1) to develop a knowledge of the developmental tasks across the lifespan, (2) to create storylines, imagery, and messages that provide some solutions or relevance to these developmental tasks, and (3) to include assessments that address the successful resolution of these developmental tasks.

Further Reading

Borzekowski, D., & Rich, M. (2012). Children, media, and health. *Journal of Children and Media, 6*(1), 1–4. http://doi.org/ 10.1080/17482798.2011.633394

Brown, J. D. (2006). Emerging adults in a media-saturated world. In J. J. Arnett & J. L. Tanner (Eds.), *Emerging adults in America: Coming of age in the 21st century* (pp. 279–299). American Psychological Association. https://doi.org/10.1037/11381-012

Erikson, E. H. (1959). *Identity and the life cycle.* WW Norton and Co.

Harwood, J. (2007). *Understanding communication and aging: Developing knowledge and awareness*. SAGE. https://doi.org/10.4135/9781452225920.n8

Wakefield, M. A., Loken, B., & Hornik, R. C. (2010). Use of mass media campaigns to change health behavior. *The Lancet, 376*(9748), 1261–1271. https://doi.org/10.1016/S0140-6736(10)60809-4

References

Ang, S. (2018). Social participation and health over the adult life course: Does the association strengthen with age? *Social Science Medicine. 206*, 51–59. https://doi.org/10.1016/j.socscimed.2018.03.042

Arnett, J. J. (2005). The developmental context of substance use in emerging adulthood. *Journal of Drug Issues, 35*(2), 235–254. https://doi.org/10.1177/002204260503500202

Arnett, J. J. (2007). Emerging adulthood: What is it, and what is it good for? *Child Development Perspectives, 1*(2), 68–73. https://doi.org/10.1111/j.1750-8606.2007.00016.x

Arnett, J. J., Žukauskienė, R., & Sugimura, K. (2014). The new life stage of emerging adulthood at ages 18–29 years: Implications for mental health. *The Lancet, 1*(7), 569–576. https://doi.org/10.1016/S2215-0366(14)00080-7

Aubrey, J. S., Behm-Morawitz, E., & Kim, K. (2014). Understanding the effects of MTV's 16 and Pregnant on adolescent girls' beliefs, attitudes, and behavioral intentions toward teen pregnancy. *Journal of Health Communication*, 19, 1145–1160. https://doi.org/10.1080/10810730.2013.872721

Aubrey, J. S., & Gamble, H. (2017). Media influence on sexuality and sexual health. In P. Rössler, C.A. Hoffner & L. Zoonen (Eds.), *International Encyclopedia of Media Effects.* Wiley. https://doi.org/10.1002/9781118783764.wbieme0152

Bandura, A. (2009). Social cognitive theory of mass communication (3rd edition). In J. Bryant & D. Zillmann (Eds.), *Media effects: Advances in theory and research* (pp. 94–124). Erlbaum.

Behm-Morawitz, E., Aubrey, J. S., Pennell, H., & Kim, K. B. (2019). Examining the effects of MTV's *16 and Pregnant* on adolescent girls' sexual health: The implications of character affinity, pregnancy risk factors, and health literacy on message effectiveness. *Health Communication, 34*(2), 180–190. https://doi.org/10.1080/10410236.2017.1399506

Bond, B. J., & Drogos, K. L. (2014). Sex on the shore: Wishful identification and parasocial relationships as mediators in the relationship between *Jersey Shore* exposure and emerging adults' sexual attitudes and behaviors. *Media Psychology, 17*(1), 102–126. https://doi.org/10.1080/15213269.2013.872039

Bonner, K. (2012, June 14). Character studies: Adam Sackler, Girls. *Slate*. https://slate.com/culture/2012/06/adam-sackler-adam-driver-on-hbo-s-girls-provides-a-fascinating-appalling-glimpse-of-young-male-adulthood.html

Borzekowski, D., & Rich, M. (2012). Children, media, and health. *Journal of Children and Media, 6*(1), 1–4. http://doi.org/ 10.1080/17482798.2011.633394

Bowen, H. L. (2013). Impact of a mass media campaign on bed net use in Cameroon. *Malaria Journal, 12*(1), 36–36. https://doi.org/10.1186/1475-2875-12-36

Brown, J. D. (2006). Emerging adults in a media-saturated world. In J. J. Arnett & J. L. Tanner (Eds.), *Emerging adults in America: Coming of age in the 21st century* (pp. 279–299). American Psychological Association. https://doi.org/10.1037/11381-012

Burnell, K., Andrade, F. C., & Hoyle, R. H. (2022). Emerging adults' exposure to and postings about substance use on social media: An observational study. *Emerging Adulthood, 10*(6), 1395–1408. https://doi.org/10.1177/21676968221119947

Caballero, D., & Richardson, M. (2023, December 23). 'Modern Family' character ages vs. their real-life counterparts. *Collider*. https://collider.com/modern-family-character-actor-ages/

Chandra, A., Martino, S. C., Collins, R. L., Elliott, M. N., Berry, S. H., Kanouse, D. E., & Miu, A. (2008). Does watching sex on television predict teen pregnancy? Findings from a national longitudinal survey of youth. *Pediatrics, 122*(5), 1047–1054. https://doi.org/10.1542/peds.2007-3066

Chartrand, L., & Lazaro, J. (2022). Entertainment-education: What are *Grey's Anatomy* and *Saving Hope* teaching us about death? *OMEGA - Journal of Death and Dying.* https://doi.org/10.1177/00302228221146345

Coyne, S. M., Ward, L. M., Kroff, S. L., Davis, E. J., Holmgren, H. G., Jensen, A. C., Erickson, S. E., & Essig, L. W. (2019). Contributions of mainstream sexual media exposure to sexual attitudes, perceived peer norms, and sexual behavior: A meta-analysis. *Journal of Adolescent Health, 64*(4), 430–436. https://doi.org/10.1016/j.jadohealth.2018.11.016

Custers, K. (2015). The urgent matter of online pro-eating disorder content and children: Clinical practice. *European Journal of Pediatrics, 174*, 429–433. https://doi.org/10.1007/s00431-015-2487-7

Czeisler, M. E., Lane, R. I., Petrosky, E., Wiley, J. F., Christensen, A., Njai, R., Weaver, M. D., Robbins, R., Facer-Childs, E. R., Barger, L. K., Czeisler, C. A., Howard, M. E., & Rajaratnam, S. M. W. (2020). Mental health, substance use, and suicidal ideation during the COVID-19 pandemic. *Morbidity and Mortality Weekly Report, 69*(32), 1049–1057. https://doi.org/10.15585/MMWR.MM6932A1

Davis, J. P., Pedersen, E. R., Tucker, J. S., Dunbar, M. S., Seelam, R., Shih, R., & D'Amico, E. J. (2019). Long-term associations between substance use-related media exposure, descriptive norms, and alcohol use from adolescence to young adulthood. *Journal of Youth and Adolescence, 48*(7), 1311–1326. https://doi.org/10.1007/s10964-019-01024-z

DiClemente, R. J., Hansen, W. B., & Ponton, L. E. (1996). Adolescents at risk. In R. J. DiClemente, W. B. Hansen, & L. E. Ponton (Eds.), *Handbook of adolescent health risk* (pp. 1–4). Springer.

Dinh, J. (2010, December 22). MTV's '16 and Pregnant' credited for decline in teen pregnancy rates. *MTV News*. http://www.mtv.com/news/1654818/mtvs-16-and pregnant-credited-for-decline-in-teen-pregnancy-rates

Dion, J., Blackburn, M.E., Auclair, J., Laberge, L., Veillette, S., Gaudreault, M., Vachon, P., Perron, M., & Touchette, E. (2015). Development and aetiology of body dissatisfaction in adolescent boys and girls. *International Journal of Adolescence and Youth, 20*(2), 151–166. https://doi.org/10.1080/02673843.2014.985320

Edwards, J., Rehman, U. S., & Byers, E. S. (2022). Perceived barriers and rewards to sexual consent communication: A qualitative analysis. *Journal of Social and Personal Relationships, 39*(8), 2408–2434. https://doi.org/10.1177/02654075221080744

Elkind, D. (1967). Egocentrism in adolescence. *Child Development, 38*, 1025–1034.

Erikson, E. H. (1950). *Childhood and Society*. W. W. Norton & Company.

Erikson, E. H. (1959). *Identity and the life cycle.* W. W. Norton & Company.

Erikson, E. H. (1968). *Youth and crisis*. W. W. Norton & Company.

Evans, W. D., Christoffel, K. K., Necheles, J. W., & Becker, A. B. (2010). Social marketing as a childhood obesity prevention strategy. *Obesity, 18*(n1s), S23–S26. https://doi.org/10.1038/oby.2009.428

Evans, W. D., Necheles, J., Longjohn, M., & Christoffel, K. K. (2007). The 5-4-3-2-1 Go! intervention: Social marketing strategies for nutrition. *Journal of Nutrition Education and Behavior, 39*(2), S55–S59. https://doi.org/10.1016/j.jneb.2006.08.024

Eyal, K., & Kunkel, D. (2008). The effects of sex in television drama shows on emerging adults' sexual attitudes and moral judgments. *Journal of Broadcasting & Electronic Media, 52*(2), 161–181.

Finnerty-Myers K. (2011). Understanding the dynamics behind the relationship between exposure to negative consequences of risky sex on entertainment television and emerging adults' safe-sex attitudes and intentions. *Mass Communication & Society*, 14(6), 743–764.

Gilbert, S. (2017, July 14). *To the Bone*: The trouble with anorexia on film. *The Atlantic*. https://www.theatlantic.com/entertainment/archive/2017/07/to-the-bone-review-netflix/533517/

Grabe, S., Ward, L. M., & Hyde, J. S. (2008). The role of the media in body image concerns among women. *Psychological Bulletin, 134*(3), 460–476. https://doi.org/10.1037/0033-2909.134.3.460

Groesz, L. M., Levine, M. P., & Murnen, S. K. (2002). The effect of experimental presentation of thin media images on body dissatisfaction: A meta-analytic review. *International Journal of Eating Disorders, 31*, 1–16. https://doi.org/10.1002/eat.10005

Harrison, K. (2005). Is 'fat free' good for me? A panel study of television viewing and children's nutritional knowledge and reasoning. *Health Communication, 17*(2), 117–132. http://dx.doi.org/10.1207/s15327027hc1702_1.

Harrison, K., Liechty, J. M., & STRONG Kids Team (2012). U.S. preschoolers' media exposure and dietary habits: The primacy of television and the limits of parental mediation. *Journal of Children and Media, 6*(1), 18–36. https://doi.org/10.1080/17482798.2011.633402

Harrison, K., Peralta, M., & STRONG Kids Team. (2015). Parent and child media exposure, preschooler dietary intake, and preschooler healthy-meal schemas in the context of food insecurity. *Journal of Communication, 65*(3), 443–464. https://doi.org/10.1111/jcom.12153

Harwood, J. (2007). *Understanding communication and aging: Developing knowledge and awareness.* Sage. https://doi.org/10.4135/9781452225920.n8

Hausenblas, H. A., Campbell, A., Menzel, J. E., Doughty, J., Levine, M., & Thompson, J. K. (2013). Media effects of experimental presentation of the ideal physique on eating disorder symptoms: A meta-analysis of laboratory studies. *Clinical Psychology Review*, *33*(1), 168–181. https://doi.org/10.1016/j.cpr.2012.10.011

Hedderson, M. M., Bekelman, T. A., Li, M., Knapp, E. A., Palmore, M., Dong, Y., Elliott, A. J., Friedman, C., Galarce, M., Gilbert-Diamond, D., Glueck, D., Hockett, C. W., Lucchini, M., McDonald, J., Sauder, K., Zhu, Y., Karagas, M. R., Dabelea, D., & Ferrara, A. (2023). Trends in screen time use among children during the COVID-19 pandemic, July 2019 through August 2021. *Journal of the American Medical Association (JAMA) Network Open*, *6*(2), e2256157. https://doi.org/10.1001/jamanetworkopen.2022.56157

Hether, H. J., Huang, G. C., Beck, V., Murphy, S. T., & Valente, T. W. (2008).

Entertainment-education in a media-saturated environment: Examining the impact of single and multiple exposures to breast cancer storylines on two popular medical dramas. *Journal of Health Communication*, *13*(8), 808–823. https://doi.org/10.1080/10810730802487471

Hoffman, B. L., Shensa, A., Wessel, C., Hoffman, R., & Primack, B. A. (2017). Exposure to fictional medical television and health: A systematic review. *Health Education Research*, *32*(2), 107–123. https://doi.org/10.1093/her/cyx034

Huang, Q., Peng, W., & Ahn, S. (2021). When media become the mirror: A meta-analysis on media and body image. *Media Psychology*, *24*(4), 437–489. https://doi.org/10.1080/15213269.2020.1737545

Jackson, J. M., Janssen, T., & Gabrielli, J. (2018). Media/marketing influences on adolescent and young adult substance abuse. *Current Addiction Reports*, *5*(2), 146–157. https://doi.org/10.1007/s40429-018-0199-6

Kaiser Family Foundation. (2004, Spring). Entertainment education and health in the United States. https://www.kff.org/wp-content/uploads/2013/01/entertainment-education-and-health-in-the-united-states-issue-brief.pdf

Karpman, H. E., Frazier, J. A., & Broder-Fingert, S. (2023). State of emergency: A crisis in children's mental health care. *Pediatrics*, *151*(3), 1–2. https://doi.org/10.1542/peds.2022-058832

Keles, B., McCrae, N., & Grealish, A. (2020). A systematic review: The influence of social media on depression, anxiety and psychological distress in adolescents. *International Journal of Adolescence and Youth*, *25*(1), 79–93. https://doi.org/10.1080/02673843.2019.1590851

Kropf, N. P., & Greene, R. R. (2017). Erikson's eight stages of development: Different lenses. In R. R. Greene (Ed.), *Human behavior theory: A diversity framework* (pp. 75–92). Routledge.

Levine, M. P., & Harrison, K. (2009). Effects of media on eating disorders and body image (3rd edn.). In J. Bryant & D. Zillmann (Eds.), *Media effects: Advances in theory and research* (pp. 490–515). Erlbaum.

Levine, M. P., & Smolak, L. (2006). *The prevention of eating problems and eating disorders: Theory, research, and practice*. Erlbaum.

LoDolce, M. (2015, Summer). *Food marketing to children: A wolf in sheep's clothing*. Obesity Action Coalition. https://www.obesityaction.org/resources/food-marketing-to-children-a-wolf-in-sheeps-clothing/

Maree, J. G. (2021). The psychosocial development theory of Erik Erikson: Critical overview. *Early Child Development and Care*, *191*(7–8), 1107–1121. https://doi.org/10.1080/03004430.2020.1845163

Marino, C., Gini, G., Vieno, A., & Spada, M. M. (2018). The associations between problematic Facebook use, psychological distress and well-being among adolescents and young adults: A systematic review and meta-analysis. *Journal of Affective Disorders*, *226*, 274–281. https://doi.org/10.1016/j.jad.2017.10.007

Markey, C. N. (2010). Invited commentary: Why body image is important to adolescent development. *Journal of Youth and Adolescence*, *39*, 1387–1391. https://doi.org/10.1007/s10964-010-9510-0

Martins, N., & Jensen, R. E. (2014). The relationship between "Teen Mom" reality programming and teenagers' beliefs about teen parenthood. *Mass Communication and Society*, 17, 830–852. https://doi.org/10.1080/15205436.2013.851701

Martins, N., Malacane, M., Lewis, N., & Kraus, A. (2016). A content analysis of teen parenthood in "Teen Mom" reality programming. *Health Communication*, *31*(12), 1548–1556. https://doi.org/10.1080/10410236.2015.1089465

Mueller, J., Callanan, M. M., & Greenwood, K. (2016). Communications to children about mental illness and their role in stigma development: an integrative review. *Journal of Mental Health*, *25*(1), 62–70. http://doi.org/ 10.3109/09638237.2015.1021899

Muller, R. T. (2017). Lena Dunham's representations of mental illness. *Psychology Today*. https://www.psychologytoday.com/us/blog/talking-about-trauma/201703/lena-dunhams-representations-mental-illness

Negarestani, M., Rashedi, V., Mohamadzadeh, M., & Borhaninejad, V. (2021). Psychological effects of media use on mental health of older adults during the COVID-19 pandemic. *Salmand: Iranian Journal of Aging*, *16*(1), 74–85. http://salmandj.uswr.ac.ir/article-1-2094-en.html

Norris, M. L., Boydell, K. M., Pinhas, L., & Katzman, D. K. (2006). Ana and the Internet: A review of pro-anorexia websites. *International Journal of Eating Disorders*, *39*, 443–447. https://doi.org/10.1002/eat.20305

Ohannessian, C. M., Vannucci, A., Flannery, K. M., & Khan, S. (2017). Social media use and substance use during emerging adulthood. *Emerging Adulthood*, *5*(5), 364–370. https://doi.org/10.1177/2167696816685232
Orenstein, G. A., & Lewis L. (2022). *Erikson's stages of psychosocial development.* StatPearls Publishing.
O'Riordan, D. L., Geller, A. C., Brooks, D. R., Zhang, Z., & Miller, D. R. (2003). Sunburn reduction through parental role modeling and sunscreen vigilance. *The Journal of Pediatrics*, *142*(1), 67–72. https://doi.org/10.1067/mpd.2003.mpd039
Pardo, R., Wheeler, T., & Ungerleider, S. (2023). *Death on television: Flipping the script.* The Norman Lear Center. https://drive.google.com/file/d/1FblL61oQlG4-Js_w6wzh4CF0XWY4_US1/view
Qin, L., Zhang, X., Wu, A., Miser, J. S., Liu, Y.-L., Hsu, J. C., Shia, B.-C., & Ye, L. (2021). Association between social media use and cancer screening awareness and behavior for people without a cancer diagnosis: Matched cohort study. *Journal of Medical Internet Research*, *23*(8), e26395. https://doi.org/10.2196/26395
Rasmussen, E. E., Punyanunt-Carter, N., LaFreniere, J. R., Norman, M. S., & Kimball, T. G. (2020). The serially mediated relationship between emerging adults' social media use and mental well-being. *Computers in Human Behavior*, *102*, 206–213. https://doi.org/10.1016/j.chb.2019.08.019
Robinson, T. N., Borzekowski, D. L. G., Matheson, D. M., & Kraemer, H. C. (2007). Effects of fast food branding on young children's taste preferences. *Archives of Pediatrics & Adolescent Medicine*, *161*(8), 792–797. https://doi.org/10.1001/archpedi.161.8.792
Rodgers, R. F., Lowy, A. S., Halperin, D. M., & Franko, D. L. (2016). A meta-analysis examining the influence of pro-eating disorder websites on body image and eating pathology. *European Eating Disorders Review*, *24*(1), 3–8. https://doi.org/10.1002/erv.2390
Rosen, M. L., Rodman, A. M., Kasparek, S. W., Mayes, M., Freeman, M. M., Lengua, L. J., Meltzoff, A. N., & McLaughlin, K. A. (2021). Promoting youth mental health during the COVID-19 pandemic: A longitudinal study. *PloS One*, *16*(8), e0255294. https://doi.org/10.1371/journal.pone.0255294
Sesame Workshop. (2013, July 19). A healthy dose of Sesame for children worldwide. https://downloads.cdn.sesame.org/sw/SWorg/documents/SW_GlobalHeath.pdfe
Sesame Workshop. (2023). Children's mental health in the spotlight. https://sesameworkshop.org/about-us/news/emotional-well-being-launch/
Shang, L., Zhou, J., & Zuo, M. (2021). Understanding older adults' intention to share health information on social media: The role of health belief and information processing. *Internet Research, 31*(1), 100–122. https://doi.org/10.1108/INTR-12-2019-0512
Smith, S. L., Pieper, K., & Choueiti, M. (2016). The rare and ridiculed: Senior citizens in the top 100 films of 2015. Media, Diversity, & Social Change Initiative. https://annenberg.usc.edu/sites/default/files/2023/04/28/MDSCI_Rare%20and%20Ridiculed%20Report%20Final_1.pdf
Smith, S. L., Pieper, K., & Choueiti, M. (2018). Still rare, still ridiculed: Portrayals of senior characters on screen in popular films from 2015 and 2016. Media, Diversity, & Social Change Initiative. https://annenberg.usc.edu/sites/default/files/2023/04/28/Still%20Rare%20Still%20Ridiculed%20Final%20Report%20January%202018.pdf
Smythe, P. (2020, January 22). 'It answered my weird questions': What do teens really think of Netflix's *Sex Education*? *The Guardian*. https://www.theguardian.com/tv-and-radio/2020/jan/22/it-answered-my-weird-sex-questions-what-teens-really-think-of-sex-education-netflix
Spitzer, E. G., Crosby, E. S., & Witte, T. K. (2023). Looking through a filtered lens: Negative social comparison on social media and suicidal ideation among young adults. *Psychology of Popular Media, 12*(1), 69–76. https://doi.org/10.1037/ppm0000380
Stephenson, R. H., & Banet-Weister, S. (2007). Super-sized kids: Obesity, children, moral panic, and the media. In A. J. Bryant (Ed.), *The children's television community* (pp. 272–293). Routledge. https://doi.org/10.4324/9781410614452
Strasburger, V. C., Jordan, A. B., & Donnerstein, E. (2010). Health effects of media on children and adolescents. *Pediatrics*, *125*(4), 756–767. https://doi.org/10.1542/peds.2009-2563
Sussman, D., & Arnett, J. J. (2014). Emerging adulthood: Developmental period facilitative of the addictions. *Evaluation & the Health Professions*, *37*(2), 147–155. https://doi.org/10.1177/0163278714521812
Tennant, B., Stellefon, M., Dodd, V., Chaney, B., Chaney, D., Paige, S., & Alber, J. (2015). eHealth literacy and web 2.0 health information seeking behaviors among baby boomers and older adults. *Journal of Medical Internet Research, 17*(3), e70. https://doi.org/10.2196/jmir.3992
Vaterlaus, J. M., Patten, E. V., Roche, C., & Young, J. A. (2015). #Gettinghealthy: The perceived influence of social media on young adult health behaviors. *Computers in Human Behavior*, 45, 151–157. https://doi.org/10.1016/j.chb.2014.12.013

van Wijngaarden, E., & Sanders, J. (2022). 'I want to die on my own terms': Dominant interpretative repertoires of 'a good death' in old age in Dutch newspapers. *Social Science & Medicine (1982), 311*, 115361. https://doi.org/10.1016/j.socscimed.2022.115361

Wahl, O., Hanrahan, E., Karl, K., Lasher, E., & Swaye, J. (2007). The depiction of mental illnesses in children's television programs. *Journal of Community Psychology, 35*(1), 121–133. https://doi.org/10.1002/jcop.20138

Wahl, O., Wood, A., Zaveri, P., Drapalski, A., & Mann, B. (2003). Mental illness depiction in children's films. *Journal of Community Psychology, 31*(6), 553–560.

Wakefield, M. A., Loken, B., & Hornik, R. C. (2010). Use of mass media campaigns to change health behaviour. *The Lancet, 376*(9748), 1261–1271. https://doi.org/10.1016/S0140-6736(10)60809-4

Wei, N., Sun, D., & Huang, W. (2022). Effects of WeChat use on the subjective health of older adults. *Frontiers in Psychology, 13,* 919889. https://doi.org/10.3389/fpsyg.2022.919889

PART V

Pop Culture and Health Communication

Looks to the Future

24

LOOKING TO THE FUTURE OF POPULAR CULTURE AND THE FUTURE OF PUBLIC HEALTH INTERVENTIONS

Suraj Arshanapally

Introduction

On April 28, 2017, Logic, the popular hip-hop artist, debuted his song titled "1-800-273-8255," the number of the US National Suicide Prevention Lifeline. This track centered around someone calling the Lifeline, expressing mental health struggles and a desire to end their life. Four months later, he released the song's accompanying music video. The video told the story of a young black man grappling with discrimination and bullying due to his sexual orientation. As the video unfolded, he contemplated suicide, but ultimately decided to call the Lifeline, marking a turning point toward his recovery and resolution (Logic, 2017).

Since the release of this song, the mainstream media promoted it by connecting it with messages of hope and healing. In August 2017, Logic performed the song at the MTV Video Music Awards (Moniuszko, 2017), which significantly amplified the message of suicide prevention among viewers. The song quickly moved into the Top 10 of the Billboard Hot 100 music charts within the United States (Rutherford, 2017). To date, the song has amassed over a billion streams on Spotify and the music video has obtained over 440 million views on YouTube.

While the song and music video made a splash in popular culture, they also made a public health impact. The Lifeline received an excess of 9,915 calls after the song's release, the MTV Video Music Awards in 2017, and the Grammy Awards in 2018 (Niederkrotenthaler et al., 2021). Additionally, Niederkrotenthaler et al. observed a reduction of 245 suicides during the periods with the most social media discourse about the song. Another study found that Google searches for the 'Suicide Hotline' increased 49% more than expected the day following the release of Logic's song (Torgerson et al., 2021). Logic's remarkable ability to craft a song that not only resonated widely with the general public but also had a significant influence on public health serves as a case study in harnessing the potential of popular culture for public health interventions.

Imagine a world where all popular culture mediums such as Hollywood films and television shows, social media platforms, and gaming technologies seamlessly spread vital public health information to millions of people. These mediums could captivate audiences while also raise awareness about public health issues and motivating them to take action toward healthier lifestyles. The fusion of popular culture and public health communication can shape the future of public health interventions, blurring

DOI: 10.4324/9781003436409-29

the lines between entertainment and education, and leveraging the power of media for social change. This chapter highlights multiple methods and examples within popular culture, specifically entertainment media, social and digital media, and gaming technologies that continue to pave the way for the future of public health interventions.

Entertainment-Education (Example: East Los High)

East Los High is a television drama series that showcased the lives, struggles, and aspirations of a group of teenagers living in East Los Angeles, a predominantly Latino neighborhood. Centered on the students of East Los High School, the show offered storylines related to their relationships, family dynamics, identity, culture, and personal struggles. Among these storylines, we observe important public health topics such as sexual health, domestic violence, substance abuse, and immigration being portrayed (Population Media Center, n.d.; see also Chapter 17, this volume).

According to Population Media Center (PMC, n.d.), the show garnered significant attention in popular culture, as it became one of the top five shows on Hulu during its first season and received six Emmy nominations. Similar to Logic's song about the U.S. National Suicide Prevention Lifeline, *East Los High* also had a meaningful public health impact.

In a study conducted by Wang and Singhal (2016), the *East Los High* website obtained 215,964 visits from unique visitors during the nine months of tracking, primarily after Season 1. The study also noted that viewers of *East Los High* accounted for 22% of the total 26,414 Planned Parenthood widget web views. The widgets directed viewers to health resources such as local health clinics. Their StayTeen.org partner noted that their website received almost 4,000 web visits during the premiere day, which is more than double the traffic on a typical day. According to Wang and Singhal, for the first month, their website received about 566,000 web visits, which is 11% higher than during a comparable period.

Half of the participants in Wang and Singhal's (2016) study reported learning at least one fact about correct condom use, and 36% reported learning at least one fact about birth control pills and emergency contraception. Eighty-six percent responded that they were likely to adopt emergency contraception. As a result of watching *East Los High*, viewers' willingness to get tested for sexually transmitted infections, HIV, and pregnancy increased.

While this series successfully demonstrated the potential to communicate important health information through an entertainment medium, it did not occur by chance. PMC, the creator of Season 1 of *East Los High*, comprises a prominent non-profit organization leading entertainment-education efforts globally. Entertainment-education (E-E), commonly referred to as edutainment, constitutes a framework that combines entertainment and educational elements to raise awareness about public health issues, disseminate prosocial messages, and promote social and behavior change through storytelling mediums (Singhal & Rogers, 2002; see also Chapter 17, this volume). Edutainment can utilize interesting narratives and relatable characters as a device to influence the attitudes, beliefs, and behaviors of an audience and establish a foundation for the future of public health interventions in entertainment media. Indeed, studies have attested to the success of the E-E framework in communicating a variety of public health topics such as HIV/AIDS in Tanzania (Singhal et al., 2003), maternal and child health in Brazil (Waisbord et al., 2011), and children's nutrition in the United States (Zhou et al., 2019).

In the case of *East Los High,* PMC drew from a variety of social and behavior change theories (Bandura & Walters, 1977; Bandura, 1986; Bentley, 2000; Horton & Wohl, 1956; Jung, 1969; Sood, 2002) and extensive research to train writers on how to develop culturally relevant storylines and relatable characters. They employed a mix of positive, negative, and transitional characters to provide audiences with a nuanced understanding of health behaviors. The positive characters portrayed healthy decision-making. The negative characters displayed unhealthy decision-making. The transitional characters exemplified the journey from unhealthy to healthy decision-making, or the reverse. Similar to real life, decision-making around health can be challenging. Therefore, PMC's use of transitional characters served as a unique tool for showcasing complex and realistic situations.

Additionally, PMC can attribute part of its success in making a public health impact to its partnerships with several non-governmental organizations such as Planned Parenthood Federation of America. Fostering a network of collaborative multilateral partnerships provided it with access to accurate, evidence-based information as well as resources to support viewers (PMC, n.d.).

East Los High provided a prime example of how a public health organization can utilize an entertainment medium to address complex and sensitive health topics in a way that resonates with viewers. The show not only captivated audiences' attention but also imparted valuable insights and directed them to helpful resources. The success of shows like *East Los High* has created a roadmap for more television shows in Hollywood to incorporate public health storylines using the E-E framework. As more creators and producers recognize the potential of this strategy, we can expect to see more television storylines that empower individuals to make healthier choices and contribute to the overall well-being of their communities.

Hollywood and Public Health Partnerships (Example: Royal Pains)

Royal Pains, a comedy and drama television series, centered around Dr. Hank Lawson, a private doctor for the wealthy elite of the Hamptons. Lawson worked with his brother to set up a concierge medical practice, leading them on a journey of dealing with the medical needs of their clients while also navigating the challenges of high-society life. This USA Network show explores unique medical cases and interesting character archetypes.

On June 23, 2015, an episode titled "The Prince of Nucleotides" aired and featured a storyline where Lawson treated Anna, a 15-year-old girl suffering from a blood clot (Internet Movie Database, n.d.). Lawson learned that Anna identified as transgender and had started administering estrogen as part of her transition from male to female. Throughout her journey, Anna experienced health complications due to a genetic disorder, which could increase her risk of clotting. After having multiple conversations with Anna, Lawson ultimately found a dose of estrogen that would allow her to continue her transition, but not put her health at risk.

This episode's storyline was developed as a partnership between the writing team for *Royal Pains* and the public health program, Hollywood, Health & Society (HH&S). HH&S bridges the gap between the entertainment industry and public health. HH&S collaborates with professionals in the entertainment industry to provide them with accurate and up-to-date information, resources, and guidance on incorporating public health and social issues into their storylines (HH&S, n.d.b).

In February 2015, the writing team had questions about hormone replacement therapy for transgender teens, the prevalence of depression among transgender youth, and changing attitudes among medical professionals on the optimal age for transitioning (Gillig et al., 2018). HH&S supported the writing team by directing them to an expert in the field and resources on the topic. They have earned a trustworthy reputation for providing writers and producers with essential resources, including tip sheets, briefings, and consultations, enabling writers to craft narratives in an evidence-based manner (HH&S, n.d.b).

HH&S has actively collaborated with over 1,100 television series and pilots, including *black-ish, The Good Doctor, and Grey's Anatomy* (HH&S, n.d.a). Through these partnerships, they have received over 4,300 inquiries from television writers and conducted 1,587 expert briefings. Their briefings and consultations led to over 2,600 storylines being aired from 2012 to 2020.

Crafting storylines about those who have often been marginalized in mainstream media, such as transgender individuals, requires a social responsibility to handle the portrayal of these characters conscientiously and appropriately (Berry, 2009). In the realm of storytelling, empathy holds immense power (Gupta & Jha, 2022). Viewers immerse themselves in the lives of the characters. The emotional connection evoked by the journeys of these characters attests to the powerful parasocial relationship established between the audience and the character (Scherer et al., 2022). This phenomenon enables viewers to identify with characters as if their experiences were their own (Cohen, 2018). On the other hand, the opposite is also true. A poorly executed portrayal can unintentionally perpetuate stigma and misconceptions, jeopardizing public health efforts (Corrigan & Watson, 2002).

Fortunately, HH&S equipped the writing team behind *Royal Pains* with accurate public health information and invaluable resources, resulting in a transgender storyline that was both culturally sensitive and relevant. As a result, this episode of *Royal Pains* and other storylines portraying transgender individuals were associated with more supportive attitudes toward transgender people and the policies that affect them (Gillig et al., 2018).

The partnership forged between HH&S and the writing team stands as a notable example of effective collaboration between the public health sector and the entertainment industry. As public health topics continue to serve as popular storylines in entertainment media, it presents an opportunity for public health organizations to partner with writers and producers to ensure accurate and evidence-based information is being communicated.

Multimedia Campaigns (Example: MTV Shuga)

MTV Shuga is a multimedia campaign implemented by the MTV Staying Alive Foundation – a foundation established by MTV Networks International in partnership with the Joint United Nations Program on HIV/AIDS. The foundation focuses on raising awareness and addressing the global HIV/AIDS epidemic, particularly among young people. Through popular culture and entertainment media, this partnership leverages MTV's platform to engage young people in conversations about sexual health, safe practices, and HIV prevention (MTV Staying Alive Foundation, n.d.b).

As of 2024, *MTV Shuga* remains a popular television drama in sub-Saharan Africa (MTV Staying Alive Foundation, n.d.a). Accompanied by radio, digital, and social media, *MTV Shuga* has also functioned as a multimedia campaign spreading awareness about sexual and reproductive health and rights. On the website (www.mtvshuga.com), viewers can watch episodes of the show, read and interact with profiles of the characters, get "backstage" video content, find answers to frequently asked questions about sexual and reproductive health and rights, and share content on their social media platforms (MTV Staying Alive Foundation, n.d.a). People became immersed in the fictional world when multiple mediums enabled them to connect with the entertaining drama.

MTV Shuga has reached 96% of sub-Saharan African countries and has been broadcast in 72 countries globally (MTV Staying Alive Foundation, n.d.a). According to a report by the World Bank, people who interacted with *MTV Shuga* content significantly improved their knowledge and attitudes toward HIV and risky sexual behaviors. These people were twice as likely to get tested for HIV eight months after the intervention (Banerjee et al., 2019). In a study conducted among 15- to 24-year-olds in Eastern Cape, South Africa, the participants who were exposed to the *MTV Shuga* campaign increased knowledge about their HIV status as well as elevated awareness of HIV self-testing more than those who did not experience the campaign (Birdthistle et al., 2022).

In addition to the virtual programming, MTV Staying Alive Foundation also organized a Peer Education program to provide viewers with on-the-ground support. Peer educators created safe spaces for young people to share their stories and connect them to resources. This program reached over 215,000 young people and distributed over 120,000 HIV tests (MTV Staying Alive Foundation, n.d.c).

The team behind *MTV Shuga* has demonstrated the power of combining entertainment media – such as television dramas or social and digital channels – and traditional public health interventions, such as peer education programming. In addition, the brand power of MTV has played a significant role in bringing awareness to topics such as sexual health and HIV prevention. Given the success of *MTV Shuga*, global entertainment brands similar to MTV may create foundations and programs dedicated to implementing multimedia public health interventions that educate their massive viewer bases on public health topics and motivate them to adopt healthier lifestyle choices.

Reality Television (Example: Queer Eye)

While scripted television dramas such as *East Los High*, *Royal Pains*, and *MTV Shuga* can be used to communicate nuanced public health topics in entertaining and engaging ways, reality television can be used to touch on social issues that impact real-world communities. *Queer Eye* is a popular reality television series available on Netflix (Netflix, n.d.). It originally aired in 2003 but was rebooted in 2018. The 2018 series featured a team of five queer men, commonly referred to as the "Fab Five," who specialized in areas such as fashion, grooming, culture, design, and food. The team included Jonathan Van Ness, Bobby Berk, Karamo Brown, Antoni Porowski, and Tan France.

In each episode, the Fab Five visited a person, typically referred to as a "hero," who had been nominated by their friends or family for a "makeover." Each hero brought a personal struggle or aspiration that the Fab Five helped them overcome or achieve through guidance, support, and expertise. While the show operated as a "makeover" show, it went beyond the surface. It addressed issues related to self-confidence, self-care, relationship building, mental and physical health, and personal growth.

From a public health standpoint, this reality show provided viewers with examples of how to live healthier lives. According to the social cognitive theory (Bandura, 1986), people learn from observing others, particularly through modeling or imitation. *Queer Eye* equipped viewers with social scripts on how to have difficult conversations, express emotions, and live healthier lives. In the first episode of Season 7 of *Queer Eye*, culture expert Karamo Brown sat with a group of male college students in a fraternity to discuss the importance of expressing emotion. In the heartfelt scene, the fraternity brothers confided their personal challenges with one another, expressing a range of emotions (Rosen, 2023). It served as a prime example of social cognitive theory, as viewers could learn how to share their own personal struggles by modeling their conversations after the conversation that Karamo had with the heroes.

One characteristic of social cognitive theory is self-efficacy (Bandura, 1991), which refers to a person's belief in their own capability to perform a particular behavior or achieve a goal. Throughout the series, each member of the Fab Five supported the heroes in their respective abilities to reach their goals. With a little bit of help, such as Antoni Porowski providing them with tips on how to cook or Bobby Berk redesigning their space, they created an environment where the heroes could thrive.

In addition to supporting viewers in their self-confidence, the show also touched on important social and public health topics relevant to the general public, such as LGBTQ+ health and rights, race, religion, and more (O'Neill, 2018). While reality shows are still entertainment mediums, and many do not truly showcase all aspects of real-world living, *Queer Eye* served as a positive example of utilizing reality television for public health communication. It expanded conversations about important issues and modeled how one can live healthier lives. Given the popularity of reality television, public health organizations may consider partnering with certain shows to incorporate examples and models of healthy living.

Radio Dramas (Example: La Caldera)

La Caldera comprised a 21-episode Bolivian radio drama that followed the stories of three characters, Canela, Simón, and Mr. X. Canela was a courageous teenager who suffered from the hardships of sexual exploitation. An innocent child brought by himself from another country to do domestic chores, Simon lived in a wealthy neighborhood. Mr. X returned from a center where he worked for many years against his will. Human trafficking connected these three characters (UNODC, n.d.).

Designed for low-income children and adolescents in Bolivia, *La Caldera* educated listeners about common tactics used by human trafficking networks, informed the public about supporting victims, and directed listeners to legal services offered by the government and non-profit organizations. By breaking down intense topics such as labor exploitation, sponsorship and/or servitude, and commercial sexual exploitation into easy-to-follow storylines, parents and teachers could openly discuss these topics with their children and students.

In collaboration with partners such as the United Nations Office on Drugs and Crime, the United States Embassy, and the Dutch Inter-Church Organization for Development Cooperation, PCI Media developed this radio program. PCI Media is a non-profit organization focused on entertainment-education to promote positive outcomes in public health, environment, and social justice (PCI Media, n.d.b).

With a listenership of over 1.2 million people, *La Caldera* has engaged over 200 local partners to support the radio program, and over 20,000 people have participated in their community mobilization efforts (PCI Media, 2019). Classrooms in Bolivia have used the radio program to raise awareness and action around human trafficking and forced labor. PCI Media Impact and its partnering agencies also developed discussion guides to support radio station hosts in leading educational conversations with listeners to discuss the topics touched upon in each episode (UNODC, n.d.). The show has reached 6,159 students and collaborated with 1,750 school community members (PCI Media, n.d.a). *La Caldera* exemplifies how radio dramas can be a unique popular culture medium to communicate public health messages and lay the foundation for future public health interventions to utilize radio to educate and mobilize communities.

Medical YouTubers (Example: Doctor Mike)

YouTube is an online video-sharing platform accessed by billions of monthly logged-in users (YouTube, n.d.a). It allows any person to create videos and share them on the platform. While this platform uplifts voices from all communities, it also threatens the credibility of the information that we receive, given that it has contained and disseminated misleading medical information that contradicts credible sources (Madathil et al., 2015; Marwah et al., 2023; Narayanan & Basch, 2023). In spite of governments and public health agencies creating videos with reliable information, viewers still likely experience videos with misleading information (see also Chapter 11, this volume). With YouTube spreading this medical misinformation, more authoritative sources should create YouTube channels and debunk medical myths.

For this reason, medical YouTubers – or medical professionals who create and share videos that inform the public about important health topics – have emerged. Dr. Mikhail Varshavski, commonly known as Doctor Mike, is a board-certified family medicine physician and YouTuber (Atlantic Health System, n.d.). With over 11 million followers on YouTube (Varshavski, n.d.a), Doctor Mike has created and shared videos addressing medical misinformation and promoting healthy lifestyle choices through entertaining methods. In one series, he has referred to inaccuracies present in popular medical television shows, such as *Grey's Anatomy*, to educate his followers about how medical care and procedures actually work (Varshavski, n.d.b). In a separate series, he has used popular medical internet memes as a way to debunk myths and misinformation in medicine (Varshavski, n.d.c).

Additionally, Doctor Mike has created videos to educate his followers on mental health, nutrition, and healthy routines. During the COVID-19 pandemic, Doctor Mike employed his platform to debunk misinformation being spread about the virus, conduct interviews with experts such as Dr. Anthony Fauci, and educate his followers on a variety of topics such as vaccines. As of August 2023, Doctor Mike's YouTube channel has over two billion views.

The company behind YouTube recognized that the platform had become a hub for health-related content, including medical misinformation, especially during the COVID-19 pandemic (YouTube Health, n.d.a). As a response, YouTube amplified authoritative sources of information on the site and implemented fact-check information panels to reduce the spread of misinformation (YouTube, n.d.b). To facilitate more accurate information, YouTube has established public health partnerships with the American Public Health Association, Cleveland Clinic, The Forum at the Harvard School of Public Health, Mayo Clinic, Osmosis, Psych Hub, and the National Academy of Medicine to create high-quality videos on health education and awareness for the general public (American Public Health Association, 2021).

Over 100 countries use YouTube across 80 languages, and YouTube Shorts averages over 70 billion views per day (YouTube, n.d.a), making YouTube a major driver of popular culture around the world. Medical YouTubers like Doctor Mike play a large role in educating the general public about medical information and empowering them to speak with their healthcare providers (Rietchel, 2017). With features such as livestreams, closed captioning, and multi-language audio, YouTube is an ideal tool for medical professionals to provide updates during infectious disease outbreaks or emergency disaster situations. As more people look to YouTube as a search engine for medical and public health information (YouTube Health, n.d.b), we can expect more medical professionals to utilize YouTube as a channel to disseminate public health messages.

Follow-Along Fitness Videos (Example: Yoga With Adriene)

Follow-along fitness videos constitute instructional videos that focus on physical exercise, workout routines, and other fitness-related activities. These videos guide viewers through specific exercises, such as a push-up or crunch, or full workout routines, such as Pilates or yoga (see also Chapter 16, this volume).

Adriene Mishler created and hosts *Yoga with Adriene*, a popular YouTube channel. With over 12 million followers, she shares videos that direct her viewers through a variety of yoga routines and practices. In her videos, she emphasizes self-care and mindfulness, and she reminds viewers that yoga can be practiced by all experience levels, body types, and backgrounds (Mishler, n.d.). Her videos include yoga practices focused on stretching, breathing, and meditation.

While the *Yoga with Adriene* channel provided viewers with a follow-along yoga practice, yoga is not the only form of exercise being promoted on YouTube. With over 8 million followers, the channel *blogilates*, hosted by Cassey Ho, offered entertaining and effective Pilates and cardio workouts (Ho, n.d.). Maddie Lymburner developed the channel, *MadFit*, with high-intensity interval training (HIIT) workout videos – another platform with over eight million followers (Lymburner, n.d.). Matt Steffanina, a popular dancer, choreographer, and YouTuber, produced a dance channel with tutorials for his dance routines and boasts over 13 million followers (Steffanina, n.d.).

Interestingly, studies reveal mixed results for the impact of fitness videos on YouTube on people's intentions to exercise at home. According to Sokolava and Perez (2021), physically active people expressed motivation from fitness videos, while fitness videos did not inspire people who were not already physically active. However, McDonough et al. (2022) implemented a 12-week YouTube video-delivered intervention for 64 young adults. The intervention involved weekly aerobic and muscle-strengthening physical activity YouTube videos. The researchers found that the intervention improved free-living physical activity and removed barriers to exercise.

Some people may not have access to expensive gym memberships or yoga studios, or know how to perform an exercise safely. Creators on YouTube have filled these gaps with accessible, educational videos on physical fitness, virtual workouts, healthy lifestyle messaging, and expert advice. We must also strive for more physical therapists, athletic trainers, and other licensed professionals to create follow-along fitness videos on YouTube that could impact the future of public health interventions around physical exercise.

Short-Form Food Recipe Videos (Example: Tasty)

Short-form food recipe videos have become popular in internet culture. *Tasty* is a food recipe brand developed by the media company Buzzfeed (Buzzfeed, n.d.). The *Tasty* social media channels include short, captivating videos with step-by-step recipes and cooking techniques (see www.facebook.com/buzzfeedtasty for Facebook; see www.youtube.com/buzzfeedtasty for YouTube). They use short-form video and hands-on demonstrations of cooking, making them easy to follow and understand for people with varying levels of cooking skills (see also Chapter 4, this volume).

The *Tasty* channels have obtained a large following on social media (Buzzfeed, n.d.). As of late 2023, the main *Tasty* channel has garnered over 105 million followers on Facebook, 45 million followers on Instagram, and 21 million followers on YouTube. Buzzfeed also manages a portfolio of *Tasty* channels, targeting various audiences based on dietary preferences and geographical areas, including *Tasty Vegetarian* with 11 million followers on Facebook and *Tasty Japan* with 7 million followers on Instagram.

Schlussel and Frosh (2023) determined that part of *Tasty*'s success can be attributed to its heightened multisensory experience. From a visual standpoint, the videos have showcased colorful ingredients presented in an appetizing way. As chefs have prepared the ingredients, the videos have engaged viewers auditorily through sounds such as sizzling or chopping. While viewers could not touch the ingredients in the video, they could see the textures, evoking tactile sensations associated with actual cooking. The video format told a story, taking the viewer on a journey of creating a snack or meal through a series of steps. This multisensory experience helped viewers to develop an emotional connection with the videos.

Potential exists for these videos to communicate information about healthy eating. While not all of the *Tasty* videos have focused on healthy foods (Tasty, 2018), the successful short-form video format could be leveraged for public health interventions. Ngqangashe and De Backer (2021) researched the impact of short-form online culinary videos on adolescents' appetites. The researchers found that these short-form videos influenced food choice behaviors, liking of the foods, and their intentions to prepare and eat the foods. Notably, the short-form videos of sweet snacks reduced the liking of fruits and vegetables, and the short-form videos of fruits and vegetables lessened the liking of sweet snacks. Therefore, public health agencies can take advantage of this format to educate viewers on nutrition-related topics such as healthy ingredients, portion control, healthy lifestyles, and diverse food options.

Social Media Movements (Example: #MeToo)

In 2006, Tarana Burke, a survivor of sexual assault and an activist, wanted to support women and girls of color who had similar experiences. She coined the phrase "Me Too" to help other women stand up for themselves (Ohlheiser, 2017). On October 15, 2017, actress Alyssa Milano tweeted, "If you've been sexually harassed or assaulted, write "me too" as a reply to this tweet," which turned Burke's work into a viral movement ("Me Too: A Timeline of Events," 2021). Twelve million social media posts within the following twenty-four hours showcased the millions of people who stood in solidarity with Tarana Burke, Alyssa Milano, and the many others who have been sexually harassed or assaulted (Burke, 2022).

#MeToo has become an international movement against sexual violence, dedicated to creating opportunities for healing, justice, action, and leadership (Me Too, n.d.). A content analysis of the tweets with #MeToo conducted by Hosterman et al. (2018) revealed that the messages included informational support and directive support, which refer to messages that communicate a call for collective action and address larger social issues that contribute to violence and harassment.

The #MeToo movement initiated a series of events in various industries and sectors. Temin and Company (2018), a crisis and management company, logged 810 high-profile figures accused of sexual harassment. California and 12 other states banned non-disclosure agreements in cases that involved sexual assault, harassment, or sex-based discrimination (National Conference of State Legislatures, n.d.). Governments from around the world gathered at the International Labor Organization Convention on Violence and Harassment at Work and voted to adopt measures to address harassment at work and provide survivors with access to services and protect them from retaliation if they speak up (Human Rights Watch, n.d.).

Social media movements have become integral to popular culture for advocacy and activism (Kidd & McIntosh, 2016). Other movements include the #BlackLivesMatter movement, which focuses on addressing systemic racism against Black individuals (Black Lives Matter, n.d.) and the Movember annual campaign, which challenges men to grow their mustaches during November to raise awareness and funds for men's health issues such as prostate cancer and mental health (Movember, n.d.).

As social media remains a constant in our lives, public health organizations should continue to utilize these platforms to disseminate public health messages. While starting a social media movement may not be an easy endeavor, public health organizations can employ online strategies and partnerships to increase the reach of their messages. If a social media movement arises out of these efforts, then potential exists to create an international and institutional impact for public health, similar to #MeToo.

Celebrity Platforms (Example: Deepika Padukone)

Deepika Padukone is an Indian actress and producer and one of the most prominent celebrities in Bollywood, the film industry in India. Some of her popular Bollywood movies include *Pathaan, Padmaavat, Bajirao Mastani, Chennai Express, and Yeh Jawaani Hai Deewani* (Padukone, n.d.). She has gained international recognition and popularity, earning her awards with *Time 100* (Bruner & Law, 2022) and *Variety Magazine* (Garrett, 2021) as well as over 75 million followers on Instagram.

In 2014, Padukone was diagnosed with clinical depression, drawing public attention toward the topic of mental health and depression (Lang, 2018). As Lerner (2006) observed, increased news media coverage about a health issue tends to occur after celebrities make announcements about their health issues. In the case of Deepika Padukone's announcement, Jain et al. (2017) linked the parasocial relationships that her fans have established with her with fans' intent to obtain mental healthcare (for related work, see Chapters 3 and 15).

Similar to Deepika Padukone, other celebrities have also publicly shared their struggles with a health issue. In 2011, the singer Demi Lovato shared her struggle with bipolar disorder with her followers (Heiser, 2021). Wong et al. (2017) conducted a study on Demi Lovato's announcement and found that people's social distance and negative stereotypes toward people with bipolar disorder were reduced after Lovato's disclosure about her diagnosis.

Celebrity platforms can serve as powerful tools to draw attention toward public health issues such as depression or bipolar disorder. Following her public announcement, Deepika Padukone founded a mental health organization called Live Love Laugh (LLL). According to a press statement, LLL has supported 1,200 people with mental illness and their caregivers who reside in 131 villages within Chhindwara, Madhya Pradesh, India (LLL, 2023). The organization has also educated over 210,000 students, sensitized 21,000 teachers, and trained 2,383 doctors on mental health, according to their website (LLL, n.d.).

As celebrities remain an integral component of popular culture, public health organizations should consider connecting with celebrities who are willing to share more about a mental or physical health challenge. This collaboration could help the celebrity communicate health information in an accurate and evidence-based manner as well as use their platforms for social good, benefiting the public health organization, the celebrity, and their followers.

Augmented Reality Mobile Games (Example: Pokémon Go)

Augmented reality (AR) is a technology that combines digital platforms with the real-world environment. Unlike virtual reality, which immerses users in entirely virtual environments, AR places digital content over real-world content through the use of a mobile device or glasses.

One of the most popular examples of augmented reality is Pokémon Go, a mobile game developed by Niantic, Nintendo, and The Pokémon Company. Launched in 2016, Pokémon Go has been downloaded over 800 million times (Chamary, 2018). The game blends the real world with virtual Pokémon elements in an immersive way. One of the goals in the game is to catch Pokémon. When players hold up their smartphones, they may find a Pokémon character appear based on their location. If they do not see one, they can pull up a game map to find landmarks in the real world where Pokémon may be available. They also have the opportunity to battle their Pokémon with others that they encounter in the real world. Pokémon Go gained popularity for its innovative and interactive nature, but, from a public health standpoint, it successfully encouraged outdoor exploration, social interaction, and exercise.

A systematic review of studies on the impact of Pokémon Go on physical activity found that playing Pokémon Go correlated with an increase in the number of steps per day by 1,446 steps (Khamzina et al., 2020). Wang and Skjervold (2021) conducted a study on how Pokémon Go impacts different groups of people. They found that half of the Pokémon Go players reported positive health benefits, including weight loss, a loss in body fat, and a gain in muscle mass. In addition, they concluded that the game motivated groups who typically struggle to be physically and socially active. Lee et al. (2021) determined that Pokémon Go improved players' social interactions and their moods as well as selective attention and concentration in adolescents, and memory in young adults.

Augmented reality mobile games like Pokémon Go provide an innovative and interactive experience for game-lovers. They blend digital entertainment with real-world physical activity, providing players with an opportunity to live a healthy lifestyle in a fun and engaging way. We can expect more AR mobile games to be developed by technology companies to improve health and social outcomes.

Exergames (Example: Nintendo Wii)

Exergames, also referred to as 'exercise games,' comprise a type of video game that combines physical activity with interactive gameplay. Exergames encourage players to participate in physical activity while also playing a video game. In order to play the game, players must move their bodies to perform physical activities like jumping or walking.

In 2006, Nintendo released Wii Sports alongside its launch of the Nintendo Wii. This system included various sports games, such as tennis, bowling, golf, baseball, and more. In order to play these games, players have to physically move their bodies as if playing these sports in the real world. In 2008, Nintendo released Wii Fit, an exergame that came with a Wii Balance Board, a specialized game controller that players would stand on to measure their balance and weight. Wii Fit offered games and exercises focused on aerobics, strength training, yoga, and more (Nintendo, n.d.).

Studies performed on the impact of exergames demonstrated positive results on physical activity among gamers. For instance, Bock et al. (2019) concluded that people who played exergames such as the Nintendo Wii engaged in more moderate to vigorous physical activity for 30 minutes per week compared to those who followed a standard exercise routine and 85 more minutes per week than people in a control group. Hurkmans et al. (2010) determined that Wii Sports tennis and boxing provided adults with bilateral spastic cerebral palsy with moderate-intensity exercise, suggesting that these exergames can be used to promote healthy lifestyles among these patients. In a study conducted among undergraduate students, Jacobs et al. (2011) found significant improvements in body mass index, weight, and exercise motivation after playing the exergames. These studies suggest that Wii

Sports and Wii Fit can be used as public health interventions among occupational therapists, particularly for weight control and exercise reasons.

Since Wii Sports and Wii Fit were released, other exergames have gained popularity, including the Nintendo Switch console. The Nintendo Switch offers exergames such as Ring Fit Adventure and Fitness Boxing. Ring Fit Adventure is a role-playing game that uses a ring-shaped controller and a leg strap to monitor body movements. The game takes players on fitness-themed adventures and challenges. Fitness Boxing simulates boxing workouts on the Nintendo Switch gaming console. Players can select various workout routines and personal trainers and follow instructions on how to box (Nintendo, n.d.).

In addition, exergames may help individuals create plans to achieve their physical activity goals. For instance, Wii Fit offers individuals the opportunity to select goals for the amount of exercise they want to participate in regularly, weight loss, and more (Nintendo, n.d.). Michalovic et al. (2018) found that physical activity communications that utilize gain frames – messages that focus on positive outcomes – may be more effective at getting individuals to make an action plan when it comes to physical activity than loss frames, messages that focus on negative outcomes (see, e.g., O'Keefe & Jensen, 2007). Public health organizations may consider collaborating with gaming companies to incorporate messaging strategies, such as gain message frames, into exergames to motivate participants to adhere to their physical activity goals.

Innovative Technologies (Example: Virtual Reality)

Virtual reality (VR) constitutes a computer-generated, immersive technology that creates a three-dimensional and interactive environment or experience. People can interact with a computer-generated world, as if they are physically present in that environment. VR has been primarily used in the gaming industry; however, large potential exists for public health impact.

VR can be utilized for public health education, providing educational simulations and training programs. For instance, immersing public health professionals in a virtual emergency risk setting can provide them with a realistic understanding of how to handle emergency situations. VR could also be beneficial for mental health care, such as exposure therapy, where an individual may be exposed to stimuli in a controlled manner virtually. Additionally, immersing people into VR environments around the world can help increase empathy and global awareness. Whether it involves virtually immersing people in refugee camps in other countries or in communities with limited access to healthy food options, it can provide public health professionals and organizations with a better understanding of the living conditions of different groups of people and inform how they implement policies and programs to support them.

Future Directions

The field of public health, with its noble goal of enhancing community well-being, has to navigate a complex landscape of competing messages. In a world flooded with information and media channels, public health agencies must rise to the challenge of reimagining how to convey accurate, timely, and essential messages about health and safety to communities in need. The case studies above demonstrate the power of leveraging popular culture mediums to reimagine public health interventions and health communication efforts.

In particular, popular culture utilizes stories, a powerful tactic for human connection (Yoder-Wise & Kowalski, 2003). The human brain is naturally wired to respond to narratives (Storr, 2020); therefore, we should embed public health messages into popular narratives. According to Storr, whether they are conveyed through entertainment media, social media platforms, or gaming technologies, stories have the potential to educate and inform audiences. Stories can be better positioned to compete for attention in a media-saturated world when an audience-centric approach is utilized (Leow

& Ch'ng, 2021). Public health agencies must work with popular culture outlets to tailor messages to specific audiences based on their needs, preferences, and behaviors, similar to how the MTV Staying Alive Foundation developed the show *MTV Shuga* primarily for audiences in sub-Saharan Africa (MTV Staying Alive Foundation, n.d.b).

As public health professionals seek to refine their communication approaches, it is imperative that the field of public health supports their professional development. Educational programs such as the Master of Science in Media, Medicine, and Health offered by Harvard Medical School comprise a prime example of equipping students with an evidence-based, multidisciplinary storytelling and arts-driven curriculum focused on public health interventions (Harvard Medical School, n.d.). By pairing students with seasoned mentors, students in this program have the opportunity to develop public health communication skills in popular culture mediums such as filmmaking, creative nonfiction, podcasting, and graphic design. Students learn how to build creative public health interventions while also remaining competitive in the media landscape.

Additionally, the field of public health must recognize and celebrate the popular culture mediums created by public health professionals. One prime example is the American Public Health Association's (APHA) Public Health Film Festival (American Public Health Association, n.d.). A part of the APHA Annual Meeting, the APHA Public Health Film Festival raises awareness, improves understanding, and sparks conversations about local, national, and global public health issues through creative films. By featuring short, animated videos to full-length films, this film festival aims to educate, inspire, and encourage a change for a healthier future. Film festivals can be organized on a local scale as well. Students and alumni at the Yale University School of Public Health (YSPH) organized a film festival, modeled after the APHA Public Health Film Festival (Arshanapally et al., 2019). The YSPH Film Festival featured a series of five films with expert panels following each film. The panels were composed of academics, researchers, filmmakers, and members of the community. The goal was to spark conversation among the local community about public health issues covered in the films. When the field of public health prioritizes and applauds Health Communication efforts through popular culture mediums, it can encourage more public health professionals to think creatively when disseminating health information, countering medical misinformation, combating stigma around public health topics, or more.

The fusion of popular culture and public health represents a powerful force for positive social change. It is a space where creativity, storytelling, gaming, and technology come together to reach audiences on a vast array of medical and public health issues. The impact has been evaluated, from increased awareness of public health issues to shifting behaviors and social norms. When we harness the cinematic universe of film and television, the lifestyles of celebrities, the reach of social media, and the technologies of gaming, we open doors to a world where public health communication is not just educational but engaging, relatable, and empowering.

As we move forward into the future, the potential for popular culture to serve as a catalyst for progress in public health is endless. The Hollywood storylines are yet to be written, the YouTube videos yet to be produced, and the virtual gaming worlds yet to be created. With strategic partnerships, multimedia campaigns, augmented reality mobile games, and innovative technologies, we can continue to leverage the allure of popular culture to inspire healthier and safer lives for all.

Disclaimer

This chapter was prepared or accomplished by Suraj Arshanapally in his personal capacity. The opinions expressed in this article are the author's own and do not reflect the views of the Centers for Disease Control and Prevention, the Department of Health and Human Services, or the United States government.

Further Reading

Singhal, A., & Rogers, E. (2012). *Entertainment-education: A communication strategy for social change*. Routledge. (A detailed overview of entertainment-education.)

References

American Public Health Association (APHA). (n.d.). APHA Public Health Film Festival. https://www.apha.org/Events-and-Meetings/Annual/Program/Film-Festival

American Public Health Association (APHA). (2021, January 13). YouTube announces a new team, led by Garth Graham, to bring more authoritative, engaging health content to the platform. https://www.apha.org/news-and-media/news-releases/apha-news-releases/2021/youtube-announces-partnership

Arshanapally, S., Bergonzi-King, L., & Sulentic, R. (2019). The community benefits of organizing a public health film festival at a school of public health. *Perspectives in Public Health, 139*(1), 19–20.

Atlantic Health System. (n.d.). About Mikhail Varshavski. https://findadoctor.atlantichealth.org/provider/Mikhail+Varshavski/639510

Bandura, A. (1986). *Social foundations of thought and action*. Prentice Hall.

Bandura, A. (1991). Social cognitive theory of self-regulation. *Organizational behavior and human decision processes, 50*(2), 248–287.

Bandura, A., & Walters, R. H. (1977). *Social learning theory* (Vol. 1). Prentice Hall.

Banerjee, A., La Ferrara, E., & Orozco-Olvera, V. H. (2019). *The entertaining way to behavioral change: Fighting HIV with MTV* (No. w26096). National Bureau of Economic Research.

Bentley, T. (2000). Drama as a tool for health promotion. *Health Education, 100*(1), 11–20.

Berry, G. L. (2009). Television, social roles, and marginality: Portrayals of the past and images for the future. In N. Pecora, J. P. Murray, & E. A.Wartella (Eds.). *Children and television: Fifty years of practice* (pp. 107–130). Routledge.

Birdthistle, I., Mulwa, S., Sarrassat, S., Baker, V., Khanyile, D., O'Donnell, D., ... & Cousens, S. (2022). Effects of a multimedia campaign on HIV self-testing and PrEP outcomes among young people in South Africa: A mixed-methods impact evaluation of 'MTV Shuga Down South.' *British Medical Journal [BMJ] of Global Health, 7*(4), e007641.

Black Lives Matter. (n.d.). Black lives matter. https://blacklivesmatter.com/

Bock, B. C., Dunsiger, S. I., Ciccolo, J. T., Serber, E. R., Wu, W. C., Tilkemeier, P., ... & Marcus, B. H. (2019). Exercise videogames, physical activity, and health: Wii heart fitness: A randomized clinical trial. *American Journal of Preventive Medicine, 56*(4), 501–511.

Bruner, R., & Law, T. (2022, March 28). Deepika Padukone on living with 'purpose, authenticity, and mindfulness' as she Accepts TIME100 Impact Award. *TIME*. https://time.com/collection/time100-impact-awards/6161152/time100-dubai-deepika-acceptance/

Burke, T. (2022, October 12). Tarana Burke: What 'Me Too' made possible. *TIME*. https://time.com/6221110/tarana-burke-me-too-anniversary/

Buzzfeed. (n.d.). *Tasty*. https://tasty.co

Chamary, J. (2018, February 10). Why 'Pokémon GO' is the world's most important game. *Forbes*. https://www.forbes.com/sites/jvchamary/2018/02/10/pokemon-go-science-health-benefits/?sh=2de7defc3ab0

Cohen, J. (2018). Defining identification: A theoretical look at the identification of audiences with media characters. In R. Wei (Ed.). *Advances in foundational mass communication theories* (pp. 253–272). Routledge.

Corrigan, P. W., & Watson, A. C. (2002). Understanding the impact of stigma on people with mental illness. *World Psychiatry, 1*(1), 16.

Garrett, D., et al. (2021, March 4). From Maria Bakalova to Hikari: Women that have made an impact in global entertainment. *Variety*. https://variety.com/lists/varietys-international-womens-impact-report-2021/

Gillig, T. K., Rosenthal, E. L., Murphy, S. T., & Folb, K. L. (2018). More than a media moment: The influence of televised storylines on viewers' attitudes toward transgender people and policies. *Sex Roles, 78*, 515–527.

Gupta, R., & Jha, M. (2022). The psychological power of storytelling. *The International Journal of Indian Psychology, 10*(3), 606–614.

Harvard Medical School. (n.d.). Master of Science in Media, Medicine, and Health. https://ghsm.hms.harvard.edu/education/master-science-media-medicine-and-health

Heiser, C. (2021, May 20). Demi Lovato speaks up about living with bipolar disorder. *Women's Health*. https://www.womenshealthmag.com/health/a19925262/demi-lovato-be-vocal-campaign/

Ho, C. (n.d.). Blogilates. *YouTube*. https://www.youtube.com/@blogilates

Hollywood, Health & Society (HH&S). (n.d.a). *HH&S by the numbers.* https://hollywoodhealthandsociety.org/about-us/history-hhs-numbers

Hollywood, Health & Society (HH&S). (n.d.b). Hollywood, Health & Society. https://hollywoodhealthandsociety.org

Horton, D., & Richard Wohl, R. (1956). Mass communication and para-social interaction: Observations on intimacy at a distance. *Psychiatry*, *19*(3), 215–229.

Hosterman, A. R., Johnson, N. R., Stouffer, R., & Herring, S. (2018). Twitter, social support messages, and the# MeToo movement. *The Journal of Social Media in Society*, *7*(2), 69–91.

Human Rights Watch. (n.d.). Two years after #MeToo erupts, a new treaty anchors workplace shifts. https://www.hrw.org/world-report/2020/country-chapters/global-1

Hurkmans, H. L., van den Berg-Emons, R. J., & Stam, H. J. (2010). Energy expenditure in adults with cerebral palsy playing Wii Sports. *Archives of Physical Medicine and Rehabilitation*, *91*(10), 1577–1581.

Internet Movie Database. (n.d.) *Royal pains. The Prince of Nucleotides.* https://www.imdb.com/title/tt4703184/?ref_=ttfc_fc_tt

Jacobs, K., Zhu, L., Dawes, M., Franco, J., Huggins, A., Igari, C., ... & Umez-Eronini, A. (2011). Wii health: A preliminary study of the health and wellness benefits of Wii Fit on university students. *British Journal of Occupational Therapy*, *74*(6), 262–268.

Jain, P., Pandey, U. S., & Roy, E. (2017). Perceived efficacy and intentions regarding seeking mental healthcare: Impact of Deepika Padukone, a Bollywood celebrity's public announcement of struggle with depression. *Journal of Health Communication*, *22*(8), 713–720.

Jung, C. G. (1969). *The collected works of CG Jung: The archetypes and the collective unconscious (Volume 9, Part 1)*. Translated by RFC Hull. Princeton University Press.

Khamzina, M., Parab, K. V., An, R., Bullard, T., & Grigsby-Toussaint, D. S. (2020). Impact of Pokémon Go on physical activity: A systematic review and meta-analysis. *American Journal of Preventive Medicine*, *58*(2), 270–282.

Kidd, D., & McIntosh, K. (2016). Social media and social movements. *Sociology Compass*, *10*(9), 785–794.

Lang, C. (2018). Deepika Padukone opens up about struggle with depression and why she's '#NotAshamed' of mental illness. *TIME*. https://time.com/5420395/deepika-padukone-depression-not-ashamed/

Lee, J. E., Zeng, N., Oh, Y., Lee, D., & Gao, Z. (2021). Effects of Pokémon GO on physical activity and psychological and social outcomes: A systematic review. *Journal of Clinical Medicine*, *10*(9), 1860.

Leow, F. T., & Ch'ng, E. (2021). Analysing narrative engagement with immersive environments: Designing audience-centric experiences for cultural heritage learning. *Museum Management and Curatorship*, *36*(4), 342–361.

Lerner, B. H. (2006). *When illness goes public: Celebrity patients and how we look at medicine*. JHU Press.

Live Love Laugh Foundation (LLL). (2023 June 13). LiveLoveLaugh (LLL) expands rural mental health program to Chhindwara, Madhya Pradesh, Impacting 1200 individuals and caregivers across 131 villages. https://cdn.thelivelovelaughfoundation.org/the_live_love_laugh/uploads/media/source/LYZvuW-13-June_LiveLoveLaugh-LLL-Expands-Rural-Mental-Health-Program-to-Chhindwara-Madhya-Pradesh-Impacting-1200-Individuals-and-Caregivers-across-131-Villages.pdf

Live Love Laugh Foundation (LLL). (n.d.). *Live Love Laugh.* https://www.thelivelovelaughfoundation.org/

Logic. (2017, August 17). Logic - 1-800-273-8255 ft. Alessia Cara, Khalid (Official Video). [Video]. *YouTube*. https://www.youtube.com/watch?v=Kb24RrHIbFk

Lymburner, M. (n.d.). *MadFit.* YouTube. https://www.youtube.com/@MadFit

Madathil, K. C., Rivera-Rodriguez, A. J., Greenstein, J. S., & Gramopadhye, A. K. (2015). Healthcare information on YouTube: A systematic review. *Health Informatics Journal*, *21*(3), 173–194.

Marwah, H. K., Carlson, K., Rosseau, N. A., Chretien, K. C., Kind, T., & Jackson, H. T. (2023). Videos, views, and vaccines: Evaluating the quality of COVID-19 communications on YouTube. *Disaster Medicine and Public Health Preparedness*, *17*, e42.

Me Too. (n.d.). *Me Too.* https://metoomvmt.org/

#MeToo: A timeline of events. (2021, February 4). *Chicago Tribune*. https://www.chicagotribune.com/lifestyles/ct-me-too-timeline-20171208-htmlstory.html

McDonough, D. J., Helgeson, M. A., Liu, W., & Gao, Z. (2022). Effects of a remote, YouTube-exercise intervention on young adults' physical activity, sedentary behavior, and sleep during the COVID-19 pandemic: Randomized controlled trial. *Journal of Sport and Health Science*, *11*(2), 145–156.

Michalovic, E:, Hall, S., Duncan, L. R., Bassett-Gunter, R., & Sweet, S. N. (2018). Understanding the effects of message framing on physical activity action planning: The role of risk perception and elaboration. *International Journal of Behavioral Medicine*, *25*, 626–636.

Mishler, A. (n.d.). *Yoga with Adriene.* YouTube. https://www.youtube.com/@yogawithadriene

Moniuszko, S. (2017, August 28). Logic's MTV VMAs performance of '1-800' was an emotional triumph with a powerful message. *USA Today*. https://www.usatoday.com/story/life/entertainthis/2017/08/27/logics-mtv-vmas-performance-1-800-emotional-triumph-powerful-message/606928001/
Movember. (n.d.). Movember. https://us.movember.com/
MTV Staying Alive Foundation (n.d.a). MTV Shuga. https://www.mtvshuga.com/downsouth/
MTV Staying Alive Foundation. (n.d.b). *MTV Staying Alive Foundation*. https://www.mtvstayingalive.org
MTV Staying Alive Foundation (n.d.c). *Peer Education*. https://www.mtvstayingalive.org/peer-education/
Narayanan, S., & Basch, C. H. (2023). YouTube and COVID-19 vaccines: A mini scoping review. *Human Vaccines & Immunotherapeutics*, *19*(1), 2202091.
National Conference of State Legislatures (NCSL). (n.d.). Research & policy. https://www.ncsl.org/research/about-state-legislatures/2018-legislative-sexual-harassment-legislation
Netflix. (n.d.). *Queer Eye*. https://www.netflix.com/title/80160037
Ngqangashe, Y., & De Backer, C. J. (2021). The differential effects of viewing short-form online culinary videos of fruits and vegetables versus sweet snacks on adolescents' appetites. *Appetite*, *166*, 105436.
Niederkrotenthaler, T., Tran, U. S., Gould, M., Sinyor, M., Sumner, S., Strauss, M. J., ... & Draper, J. (2021). Association of Logic's hip hop song "1-800-273-8255" with Lifeline calls and suicides in the United States: Interrupted time series analysis. *BMJ*, *375*, e067726
Nintendo. (n.d.). *Nintendo*. https://www.nintendo.com/
O'Keefe, D., & Jensen, J. (2007). The relative persuasiveness of gain-framed and loss-framed messages for encouraging disease prevention behaviors: A meta-analytic review. *Health Communication*, *12*(7), 623–644.
O'Neill, L. (2018, June 27). 'Queer Eye' will talk about race, religion, and gender – but not about class. *The Washington Post*. https://www.washingtonpost.com/news/posteverything/wp/2018/06/27/queer-eye-will-talk-about-race-religion-and-gender-but-not-about-class/
Ohlheiser, A. (2017, October 19). Meet the woman who coined 'Me Too' 10 years ago — to help women of color. *Chicago Tribune*. https://www.chicagotribune.com/lifestyles/ct-me-too-campaign-origins-20171019-story.html
Padukone, D. (n.d.). Deepika Padukone. https://www.deepikapadukone.com
PCI Media. (2019 October 21). A world in migration. https://www.pcimedia.org/a-world-in-migration/
PCI Media (n.d.a). Empowered people. https://www.pcimedia.org/programs/empowered-people/
PCI Media. (n.d.b). PCI Media. https://www.pcimedia.org
Population Media Center (PMC). (n.d.) *East Los High*. https://www.populationmedia.org/projects/east-los-high
Rietchel, L. (2017). Young physicians on YouTube: Helping patients connect with health care. *Statistics*, 11(2), 38–39.
Rosen, L. (2023 August 15). Three 'Queer Eye' heroes who are forever grateful to the Fab Five. *Los Angeles Times*. https://www.latimes.com/entertainment-arts/awards/story/2023-08-15/queer-eye-fab-five-help-these-heroes
Rutherford, K. (2017 September 14). Logic's '1-800-273-8255' breaks into top 10 on streaming songs chart. *Billboard*. https://www.billboard.com/pro/logic-1-800-273-8255-top-10-streaming-songs-chart/
Scherer, H., Diaz, S., Iannone, N., McCarty, M., Branch, S., & Kelly, J. (2022). "Leave Britney alone!": Parasocial relationships and empathy. *The Journal of Social Psychology*, *162*(1), 128–142.
Schlussel, H., & Frosh, P. (2023). The taste of video: Facebook videos as multi-sensory experiences. *Convergence*, 13548565231179958.
Singhal, A., Cody, M. J., Rogers, E. M., & Sabido, M. (2003). Entertainment-education and HIV/AIDS prevention: A field experiment in Tanzania. *Journal of Health Communication*, *8*(4), 389–433.
Singhal, A., & Rogers, E. M. (2002). A theoretical agenda for entertainment-education. *Communication Theory*, 12(2), 117–135.
Steffanina, M. (n.d.). Dance tutorials [Matt Steffanina]. YouTube. https://www.youtube.com/playlist?list=PLo3hNPeEYeTCMv7CYv7dXwt1sNPzhFEPW
Storr, W. (2020). *The science of storytelling: Why stories make us human and how to tell them better*. Abrams.
Sokolova, K., & Perez, C. (2021). You follow fitness influencers on YouTube. But do you actually exercise? How parasocial relationships, and watching fitness influencers, relate to intentions to exercise. *Journal of Retailing and Consumer Services*, *58*, 102276.
Sood, S. (2002). Audience involvement and entertainment—education. *Communication Theory*, *12*(2), 153–172.
Tasty. (2018, November 19). Mouthwater recipes for junk food lovers. *YouTube*. https://www.youtube.com/watch?v=R5c4anO0m-k
Temin and Company. (2018, October 3). Between Cosby and Kavanaugh – 810 high-profile public figures accused of sexual harassment. *PR Newswire*. https://www.prnewswire.com/news-releases/between-cosby-and-kavanaugh--810-high-profile-public-figures-accused-of-sexual-harassment-300723738.html

Torgerson, T., Swayze, C., Sanghera, S., Cooper, C., Beaman, J., Hartwell, M., & Vassar, M. (2021). Public awareness of the National Suicide Prevention Lifeline following the release of a hip-hop song. *British Medical Journal Evidence-Based Medicine*, *26*(4), 191.

United Nations Office on Drugs and Crime (UNODC). (n.d.). Sale "La Caldera" una radionovela educativa sobre la trata de personas en el país. https://www.unodc.org/bolivia/es/stories/la-caldera.html

Varshavski, M. (n.d.a). *Doctor Mike*. YouTube. https://www.youtube.com/@DoctorMike

Varshavski, M. (n.d.b). *Grey's Anatomy* reviews [Doctor Mike]. YouTube. https://www.youtube.com/playlist?list=PLJRbJuI_csVD4Gv4kMaKQE5BJSwSwT9YF

Varshavski, M. (n.d.c). Medical memes review [Doctor Mike]. YouTube. https://www.youtube.com/playlist?list=PLJRbJuI_csVDOmeEsBumpBhm-hDMCAprj

Wang, H., & Singhal, A. (2016). *East Los High*: Transmedia edutainment to promote the sexual and reproductive health of young Latina/o Americans. *American Journal of Public Health*, *106*(6), 1002–1010.

Waisbord, S., Larson, H. J., Guthmann, J. P., Beaman, V., & Toso, M. (2011). Audience research in support of entertainment-education campaigns: The case of the Brazilian telenovela Salve Jorge. *Journal of Health Communication*, *16*(2), 136–150.

Wang, A. I., & Skjervold, A. (2021). Health and social impacts of playing Pokémon Go on various player groups. *Entertainment Computing*, *39*, 100443.

Wong, N. C., Lookadoo, K. L., & Nisbett, G. S. (2017). "I'm Demi and I have bipolar disorder": Effect of parasocial contact on reducing stigma toward people with bipolar disorder. *Communication Studies*, *68*(3), 314–333.

Yoder-Wise, P. S., & Kowalski, K. (2003). The power of storytelling. *Nursing Outlook*, *51*(1), 37–42.

YouTube. (n.d.a). YouTube for press. https://blog.youtube/press/

YouTube. (n.d.b). Expanding fact checks on YouTube to the United States. YouTube Official Blog. https://blog.youtube/news-and-events/expanding-fact-checks-on-youtube-to-united-states/

YouTube Health. (n.d.). *Learn more about our health mission*. YouTube Health. https://health.youtube/our-mission/

Zhou, Y., Turner, M. M., Litchfield, R. E., Hingle, M., & Sherry, C. L. (2019). Using entertainment-education to promote children's fruit and vegetable consumption: A pilot study. *Journal of Nutrition Education and Behavior*, *51*(9), 1054–1061.

25

LOOKING TO THE FUTURE OF POPULAR CULTURE AND HEALTH COMMUNICATION

Theorizing and Advocacy

Elisia L. Cohen

Introduction

The ways in which popular culture communicates about health hold important implications for theorizing and advocacy. While popular culture may be a source of inaccurate or misleading health information, it also constitutes a source of making complex medical and health problems visible and accessible to publics who lack formal or academic training about media and health topics. To address these concerns, in this chapter, I begin by considering theories of audience to identify the ways that active or more passive understandings of audience relationships with popular media influence sociocultural understandings of media power and effects.

Second, I identify how popular culture influences health behaviors and review how popular entertainment media act as storytellers to shape audience understandings of wellness, safety, addiction, and other health concerns. Third, I explore how technological changes and narratives in popular culture provide resources for contemporary and future visions of health in popular culture. Fourth, I discuss how popular culture provides diverse resources for broadening conceptions of health and medicine, who practices medicine, and representations of illness, disability, and disease. I conclude by examining how future landscapes of popular mediated culture may offer different affordances to audiences and the ways in which they develop understandings of and advocate for health and well-being.

Framing Popular Culture Audiences for Theorizing and Advocacy

The ways that scholars in this and other volumes conceptualize the agency of popular culture audiences matter for theorizing and advocacy. Many theorists of audiences and popular culture focus on the power and effects popular culture and media have on people (Huang et al., 2021; Oliver & Raney, 2023; Rosen, 2022). Whether theorists have been interested in the effects of media on social learning (Bandura, 1977), its uses and gratifications (e.g., Rubin & Windahl, 1986), or the conditions that give rise to media power and constraints on individuals (Ball-Rokeach, 1998), by systematically studying

DOI: 10.4324/9781003436409-30

the effects of mediated popular culture on audiences, researchers examine the interactions between media, audiences, and society.

Researchers explore distinguishing media features of popular mediated culture, for example, embedded commercial images in magazines compared to television, or influences between non-commercial peer or celebrity social comparators on social media to study their power and influence. The omnipresence of media in daily life, ranging from engagement with mobile media through social network platforms (Fardouly & Vartanian, 2015) to videos shared on mobile, television, or other devices, raises concerns about its influence on how individuals view body image (Ferguson et al., 2014). Huang et al.'s (2021) meta analyses of scholarship examining media's effects on body images establish that irrespective of audience gender or national origin, audiences are influenced by thin/athletic-ideal media exposure. Their research found that media with a commercial purpose had the greatest influence on body image concerns and was "most influential in provoking eating disorder and internalization of the thin-ideal" measured (Huang et al., 2021, p. 437; see also related work in Chapter 5, this volume).

How Popular Entertainment Media Help Inform, Frame, and Represent Health

Studies in the first section of this volume consider the ways that popular culture helps inform, frame, or select a representation of reality that may privilege certain representations or problem definitions of health and illness in popular culture to support rendering moral judgments or stigma around health and illness. Whether considering representations of mental illness (Chapter 3, this volume), body image (Chapter 5, this volume), or the LGBTQIA+ community (Chapter 8, this volume), mediated popular culture in its representation of behaviors or beliefs can exert a normalizing influence by making them accessible, seen, and heard by mass audiences and individuals in society. Research shows that people rely on mediated popular culture to learn about others who differ from them, whether a person with disabilities (Darke, 2004), experiencing mental illness (Wahl, 1992), or to reaffirm gender or sexuality-based identities (Robertson, 2018).

Popular entertainment media have also have been studied for their influence on individual cognitions related to infidelity (Alexopoulos et al., 2022), sexual attitudes (Ward, 2003), risky behaviors (Lin et al., 2020), and rape myths (Coyne et al., 2019). For example, Chapter 6 (this volume) examines the framing of sexual health in popular culture. While sexual health can be considered broadly, sexual consent comprises a communicative and physical act, and the #MeToo movement in public culture has galvanized attention to sexual violence and consent. According to Popova (2019), what constitutes consent (or non-consent or lack of consent) expressed and understood in sexual harassment or violating sexual encounters has been contested in recent high-profile court cases, including Harvey Weinstein, Bill Cosby, and others. Within this cultural milieu of conversations about consent, entertainment media have framed this blurry line in the sexual expression of consent.

For example, the TV series *Bridgerton* included an original rape scene that evidenced changes from its original appearance in the writing in *The Duke and I*, such that the scene is "less explicitly non-consensual," and the narrative moved quickly. However, critics argued that, "although it's framed as a serious violation of trust between consenting parties, it passes without any explicit acknowledgment on the show's part that what just occurred was a deeply disturbing violation of consent" (Romano, 2020, n.p.). Whether and how audiences consider this encounter within a popular program that generally demonstrates concern for informed sexual consent is an interesting question to consider. When reflecting on the future of popular culture and health communication, we should consider the ways in which the framing of the discourse influences how individuals think about expressing consent (or not) in real situations, and how such constructions of consent (or non-consent) may be learned through film, music lyrics, television series, and the extension of video, images, audio, and textual communication through shared social media.

News, Popular and Social Media Help Inform Publics and Diffuse Knowledge

News is a well-understood resource for health information and context. As one case in point, the diffusion of knowledge about medication treatment for opioid use disorder was supported by news media reporting amid the opioid epidemic (Kennedy-Hendricks et al., 2019). Media coverage of certain health and well-being issues draws public attention to disease and health issues; whereas, a lack of representation of other health and well-being issues leads to less attention and focus. Literature, film, journalism, and other forms of popular media reflect and shape public perceptions of health and wellness, which, in turn, can influence public acceptance, stigmatization, or support of solutions and understandings of public health problems. However, mediated popular culture extends the personal relevance of news information for audience interpretations of social reality.

For the public to understand opioid addiction as a treatable illness, they require information about the social origins of the opioid crisis and the range of policy changes and treatments available to combat it. For example, Keefe's (2017) initial *New Yorker* investigative report, "The Family that Built an Empire of Pain," detailed the Sackler family's pharmaceutical empire that relentlessly marketed painkillers to health care providers, generating billions of dollars for their company at the expense of millions of addicts. Similarly, a Pulitzer Prize-winning *New York Times* investigation led to the book, *Pain Killer: An Empire of Deceit and the Origin of America's Opioid Crisis*, (Meier, 2018) that was adapted into a Netflix series, *Painkiller*. These stories captivated the attention of the American public around failed government policy and followed other book projects, such as *Dreamland: The True Tale of America's Opiate Epidemic*, which focused on telling the story of how small rural towns such as Portsmouth, Ohio, and suburbs alike have been devastated by the twin opioid crises of prescription pain medications and an influx of cheap, black tar heroin from Mexico (Quinones, 2016). The 2023 *Painkiller* series presented a comprehensive, current understanding of the crisis, including its impact on first responders, and it built on the work of Netflix's 2017 documentary *Heroin(e)* to depict the opioid epidemic and the potential and limitations of Naloxone as an antidote to save lives in the epidemic. These two examples of popular culture texts both provide an account of the relationship between the rise of Purdue Pharma and others' efforts to expand profits by increasing prescriptions of OxyContin and other opioids that harmed the public ("In case you haven't heard … " 2023). These reports intersperse first-person accounts from people who lost loved ones to the opioid epidemic with facts and commentary to demonstrate the failed regulatory environment that allowed this crisis to develop. In this way, beyond news, popular cultural texts convey personal relevance and context for health-related content and information.

In the same way that a metaphor helps improve understanding of concepts, a theoretical frame of reference can provide specific information, contexts, successes, and knowledge of resources and constraints affecting health and wellness. Promotion of and access to #healthrecipes, for example, on TikTok or other social media, can influence public health attitudes and behaviors. Sandberg et al. (2022)'s thematic analysis of the top 150 #healthyrecipes videos on TikTok revealed the moral, approachability, and appropriation/wellness cultural rhetoric, and characterization of weight norms provided a platform for shaping perceptions of health and healthy food (see also Chapter 4, this volume). Focusing on one aspect of nutrition or healthy recipes (or illness or disease) and presenting it to audiences through mediated popular culture helps to construct a reality for viewers. The salience of making certain aspects of individuals' mediated lived experience (or more healthful recipes, as the case may be) more salient than others fosters viewer reliance on or use of this frame of information to interpret subsequent information (Carter, 2013).

Scholars who take a more rhetorical approach to understanding the influence of popular culture explore the ways in which the audience is constituted by the rhetoric and the situation that it hails (Russell et al., 2008). For example, Simon-Roberts and Hawkins' (2023) study of how COVID-19 vaccination information entered popular discourse revealed the ways that celebrities, such as former

First Lady Michelle Obama, received their vaccines and posted captioned images across social media to help constitute an audience. Simon-Roberts and Hawkins identified how Obama used her social position as First Lady and as a Black woman to hail the Black community and encourage vaccination uptake. Public rhetorical endorsements from trusted leaders – including announcements by former Presidents Bill Clinton, George W. Bush, and Barack Obama of their intention to get vaccinated for COVID-19 – exemplified a national strategy to leverage mediated public culture to enhance demand for vaccination (Volpp et al., 2021; see also Chapter 15, this volume).

Alternatively, micro-bloggers, bots, and other sources of misinformation on social media spread coronavirus conspiracies from a variety of sources (Greve et al., 2022). Greve et al.'s event-history analysis of the COVID-19 pandemic on Twitter revealed how "individuals tweet[ed] new conspiracy theories, and tweet[ed] inconsistent theories simultaneously, when they face[d] a threat posed by a rising COVID-19 case rate and receive[d] attention from others via retweets," operating differently from bots that were less responsive to changes in the environment (e.g., rising case rates), but whose messages are recirculated through retweeting by others (p. 919). Whether and how audiences sort through this sea of misinformation, disinformation, and malinformation in the context of novel or emerging health information (e.g., COVID-19 vaccines) through repeated information exposures constitutes an area for future theoretical development (see also Chapter 11, this volume).

Social media platforms now offer distributed networks of mediated content. The role of social media in promoting health and wellness has evolved from understandings of emerging media as a mass, shared co-experience via virtual communities to considerations of the ways algorithms and platforms drive personalized, engaged experiences influencing health (Engle et al., 2024; Kim, 2024; Triptow et al., 2024). From an advocacy perspective, the method by which diverse social media users access, create, and interpret meaningful and actionable health information merits consideration. For example, the recent proliferation of podcasts and accessibility of podcasting hold the potential to improve health literacy, and it extends audience members' narrative engagement through storytelling (Porter et al., 2022; Shaw et al., 2022).

However, other challenges exist in utilizing social media. Pavlova and Berkers (2020) opined:

> On the one hand, social media can help to bring awareness to stigmatized topics as they give marginalized members of society the possibility to share experiences and voice their discontent. On the other hand, mental health discourse on social media may lead to stigmatization.
> *(para. 1)*

The number of health-promotion-related social media platforms and websites available to the public has grown, providing information with varying degrees of accuracy.

Given the purpose of social media as a network of content creators, interpreters, and community builders, we should note its potential use for shaping and informing health decision-making and reaching a wide range of audiences. Yet, we lack scholarly knowledge with respect to the most effective strategies to harness these tools to scale culturally adapted health promotion activities that are individually relevant and impactful.

Popular Culture Theorizing and Advocating for Changes in Health Behavior and Belief

The second section of the book examines popular culture influences on health behaviors and beliefs. Future work at the intersection of popular culture and health communication may theorize the role of the audience, especially regarding audience agency. One perspective may envision the audience as an "undiscriminating consumer" or, even worse, "victims" of distorted popular health and scientific information. An alternative perspective might imagine audiences as active participants who rely on and draw from popular culture as a resource to engage with complex health and scientific topics.

Media as Storytellers to Influence Social Norms and Behavior Change

Popular culture, itself, also shapes and influences health behaviors and beliefs and changes over time. When looking to the future of popular culture, one must imagine the ways in which future narrators and storytellers of popular culture might define health and well-being in similar or different terms from the present time. Broadcast media provide an opportunity for narrative plots to improve discursive or affirming dialogues about pro-social behavior or improved health outcomes. Entertainment education offers the opportunity for popular culture to teach diversity and critical media literacy (Bryant et al., 2023; Tisdell & Thompson, 2007). According to Bryant et al., educational entertainment media enable viewers to understand themselves as well as others different from them (see also Chapter 17, this volume). Popular culture media can also be utilized to reduce stigma and increase positive attitudes, for example, toward transgender and gender-diverse individuals (Taracuk & Koch, 2023; see also Chapter 8, this volume). Unscripted representations through reality television programs also foster diversity of representations; for example, reality television shows have provided varied depictions of female infertility that steer viewers' perceptions of "abnormality" (de Boer et al., 2022; for more work on women's health and popular culture, please see Chapter 7, this volume). Unscripted conversations on popular media offer an alternative modality for diverse perspectives, but reality television entails a filtered mediated representation of what some consider as normative. Certainly, broadcast media have included or excluded diverse sources and perspectives on health and wellness, and today's social media platforms similarly both originate from and constitute audiences for their respective content.

Technological changes and opportunities to extend safety and well-being create opportunities for norms around health and well-being to change, including what comprises healthy or pro-social health behavior. Perhaps one of the clearest examples can be seen in the normative adoption of seatbelt wearing in society. The data show that, in the U.S., Americans report buckling up about 85% of the time (Strine et al., 2010). However, it takes time for mediated popular culture to catch up to cultural references that reflect changes in technology, the widespread adoption of seatbelts in vehicles, and public policies requiring seatbelt usage to reduce death and serious injuries from motor vehicle accidents. While seatbelt usage is normative, its appearance in mediated popular culture can be variable and certainly subject to fan conversation.

Medical doctors complained in a 1992 *Journal of the American Medical Association* article about how the then-popular *Beverly Hills, 90210* show's actors did not buckle up (Goldhaber & Hamilton, 1992). Since that time, prime-time shows have demonstrated a track record for roughly reflecting norms around seatbelt use. In 2006, when researchers reviewed prime-time U.S. television programs and commercials for a one-month period in 2005, "seatbelt use was depicted in 62% and 86% of individuals in television program and commercial automobile scenes, respectively" (McGwin et al., 2006, p. 400). Yet, the prevalence of seatbelt use in television shows was stronger than in movies. Researchers who studied the "198 top-grossing movies released between 1978 and 1998 found that characters shown driving or riding in vehicles wore seatbelts only 30% of the time" (Martin, 2001, para. 4–5). While it may be understandable that criminals or others in action films and television shows make a fast escape by car without buckling up, the researchers found that even Disney family-friendly movies such as *Space Jam, D2*: *Mighty Ducks*, and *Jungle 2 Jungle* lacked representation of seatbelt use. This lack of seatbelt use on mediated platforms continues to be a concern given that, as of 2021, motor vehicle crash deaths continue to remain one of the leading causes of death among 5–19-year-olds in the United States (West et al., 2021).

In addition to showing seatbelt use, research on media reporting of traffic crashes demonstrates that the words used to describe an injury-involved crash influence people's understanding of what happened. Media describing injury-collisions in terms of a "crash" or "collision" rather than an "accident" can help individuals understand what can be done to prevent the crash. Such mindfulness of word choice has translated into communication strategies for radio-based traffic reporting as well as entertainment education through popular culture. Importantly, over time, as media and modalities for Health Communication interventions change, so do the opportunities to diversify the strategies to intervene to reinforce safe driving behaviors. For example, messages to reach the appropriate target audience have moved from mass media television campaigns to emerging social media strategies, including efforts to use social influencers to reinforce seatbelt use behavior (Drake et al., 2017; Zhang et al., 2020). According to Zhang et al., campaigns to share seatbelt usage selfies (e.g., #SelfieForSafety or #SeatBeltChallenge) on Instagram and Twitter serve as an educational effort to promote seatbelt wearing.

Celebrity Influence in Popular Culture on Health Behavior

Celebrity status influences popular culture in numerous ways, such as endorsements, recommendations, or developed health interventions (for related work, please see Chapter 15, this volume). Examples include the spike in genetic testing for breast cancer after Angelina Jolie wrote a 2013 *New York Times* editorial about her double mastectomy (Desai & Jena, 2016; Evans et al., 2014; Jolie, 2013) and Katie Couric's live broadcasting of her colorectal cancer screening after losing her husband to colorectal cancer, which enhanced public awareness and willingness to get a colonoscopy (Cram et al., 2003). In 2022, Couric also revealed news that she was diagnosed with early-stage, curable breast cancer, once again modeling the benefits of cancer screening behavior and advocating for prevention and treatment (Katie Couric Media, 2023). These research studies demonstrate how celebrity endorsements in popular culture can have a large, positive immediate influence on the use of health services (Cram et al., 2003; Desai & Jena, 2016).

However, celebrity influence can also have a negative effect on popular attitudes toward health behaviors. For example, Jenny McCarthy's claims that vaccines cause autism galvanized an anti-vaccination movement and spearheaded the "Green our Vaccines" movement (Hoffman et al., 2023). Politicians' and other celebrities' vaccination campaigns supporting COVID-19 vaccination during the coronavirus pandemic increased public awareness and confidence in the novel vaccine's safety and efficacy, but other celebrity discourses fostered skepticism about the vaccine and discouraged its use (Beck, 2022). The complexity of discourse over COVID-19 science was clear in popular culture and evident in podcast controversies from Joe Rogan (e.g., presenting COVID-19 vaccine and treatment falsehoods; Bond, 2022), music industry celebrities like Kanye West modeling non-compliance with the recommended COVID-19 vaccine series (BuzzFeed, 2021), or sports figures, such as tennis player Novak Djokovic's refusal to take the COVID-19 vaccine (see also Chapter 14, this volume). With additional amplification of anti-vax-related keywords and hashtags from well-known celebrities adding a layer of complexity, many individuals who positioned themselves as "pro-vaccinations" were accused of being "anti-vax" on Twitter (Honcharov et al., 2023).

Hashtag and Memetic Cultural Influences to Enhance Pro-Social or Anti-Social Behavior

While social media hashtags circulate brief health campaign messages in public culture, we should also examine the ways in which popular culture memes develop to reference pro-social or anti-social health behavior. Memes, which Majmundar et al. (2023, p. 306) defined as "images or videos with text overlay that embody a concept or belief about contemporary society," are popular and widely disseminated via social media platforms. Memes point to popular trends in product preferences and in healthy or unhealthy behavior, and they operate as a cultural referent in shared group communication and for individuals (Kostygina et al., 2020). Emerging evidence suggests that popular culture memes may be used to support health literacy in vulnerable populations, as cultural means make complex health information more accessible (Headley et al., 2022). In fact, Alvelos et al. (2023) argued, "When in Memeland, Speak in Memes" is an adage that can expand the reach and effectiveness of health and scientific information to reach skeptical individuals. Kostygina et al. (para. 1) agreed, asserting that future health communication research may identify how "harnessing cultural elements endemic to social media," such as popular message sources (influencers) and messages (memes), may offer promising opportunities to enhance the reach and effectiveness of health campaigns.

How Transformations of Digital Popular Culture May Be Harnessed for Health

Looking to the future of how popular culture influences behaviors and beliefs requires a consideration of digital temporalities, as changes in telecommunication modalities and the ways in which digital technology and social media afford engagement with health behaviors and beliefs influence culture. A variety of contexts exist where monitoring memes about emerging products (e.g., new vape devices) or pro- or anti-health influencers may facilitate health campaign enhancement strategies on social media to influence attitudes and behaviors. One area for future consideration entails the ways in which influencers utilize promotional tactics and features of pro-health (and anti-health) products to engage audiences. For example, Greene et al. (2022) studied the gendered ways in which influencers promote vape products on social media. Given that e-nicotine and related vaping products comprise a serious public health issue, we should gain a stronger understanding of the influence of social media on initiation and maintenance behaviors. Visual depictions of the use of these devices in popular culture operate as important social cues, increasing use behavior and intentions to quit or abstain (Maloney & Capella, 2016).

Scholars should also take a developmental approach to understanding these types of affordances of technology and media engagement. A recent U.S. Surgeon General's advisory on the use of social media by youth and the influence of social media on the mental health of youth and adolescents contended that what young people do with media, as well as the affordances that it provides them, warrant consideration (Canady, 2023; see also Chapter 24, this volume).

Health Interventions in Popular Culture

The third section of this book considers pro-social health interventions in popular culture, highlighting the many ways in which health interventions continue to change in light of shifts in culture. For example, digital health interventions are growing in prevalence (Weinert et al., 2022). Weinert et al.'s definition of digital health interventions follows that of other researchers to include "efforts to include "eHealth, mHealth, self-tracking, wearable devices, artificial intelligence, and information systems in health care, focusing on health and not technology" to change health outcomes (para. 6). As technology changes, including the evolution of applications such as Zoom and WhatsApp, the affordances of these digital intervention technologies can be leveraged to enhance social interaction and center audience experiences to achieve public health goals (Moschonis et al., 2023; Weinert et al., 2022; Yeshua-Katz et al., 2023).

Although digital culture influences the affordances of communication to improve health outcomes, it also provides a cultural context to buffer against misinformation. Bizzotto et al. (2023) demonstrated the ways that both individual internal factors (e.g., high depression literacy) and external factors (e.g., the context of the online community) may buffer the negative effects of misinformation exposure. Their research also encourages identifying ways that expert community moderators can correct misinformation in online communities as a public health intervention to support outcomes.

Serious interactive games offer another promising digital health context to improve health outcomes. Chen et al. (2023)'s meta-analysis of anti-bullying intervention programs reveals promising effects of interventions that are afforded by the interactive gaming environment and where health interventions include training on both bystander and bully-victim dual roles and coping skills. Game-based digital mental health interventions have the continued potential to bridge health care and entertainment (Drachen, 2023).

Popular media equip users with resources for understanding behaviors and illnesses that affect health (Hoffman, Hoffman, et al., 2023; Hoffman, Sidani, et al., 2023). During the COVID-19 Omicron pandemic with nearly a billion people infected, Chinese individuals used WeChat to share illness narratives and normalize infection symptoms (Cao & Wang, 2023). In this situation, popular social media applications fostered the development of social support and collective narratives about illness and disease. Media also shaped public understanding of pro-social health interventions, such as COVID-19 vaccinations and the effectiveness of early preventive action to arrest infectious disease (Knight et al., 2023).

Media, as resources in popular culture, may assist individual advocacy (Kjærulff et al., 2023). Kjærulff et al. examined how individuals with chronic conditions utilize social media to obtain and share information. The case of the monkeypox outbreak in the United States illustrated how individuals turned to social media to attain information about novel, emerging infectious disease outbreaks (Hong, 2023), reaffirming the view that individuals turn to media as a cultural resource accentuated in the context of stigmatized conditions (Ligami, 2023). Moreover, popular culture provides meaningful sources of support when perceived and experienced stigma and discrimination inhibit their interactions with the healthcare system (Aghaei et al., 2023; see also Chapter 19, this volume).

Popular culture also provides mediated depictions of behavior that affect health and wellness beliefs. Prime time television attention to important public health issues – such as gender-based violence, sexually transmitted infections and condom use, and HIV/AIDS testing through entertainment television – also engages audiences. *MTV Shuga* has exemplified such a drama, following the lives of young African people and serving as a teaching tool globally. In fact, one of the most successful public health interventions – the designated driver campaign – was boosted by features in shows such as *Cheers* and *L.A. Law* in the 1980s (Winsten, 1994).

Virtual communities also offer an opportunity for interpersonal conversations to elaborate on national mass media campaign efforts, for example, the U.S. "How to save a life" campaign to enhance awareness of take-home naloxone and improved overdose knowledge (Sumnall et al., 2023). Virtual communities can also can form via social media. Rohde et al. (2023) described Reddit as a hub for determining the ways in which opinion leadership forms in online communities to discuss vaping. In such established virtual communities, users gain guidance about drug use, misuse, and addiction and benefit from interaction distanced from stigmatized or localized identity (Tullett-Prado et al., 2023).

The opportunity for online influencers to deliver interventions that address stigmatized health conditions or reach marginalized populations also entails an area for future research. Recently, Louik et al. (2023) identified how online interventions show promise for addressing mental health conditions in young Black and Latinx gay and bisexual men and transgender women, who face high levels of mental health-related concerns. Louik et al. established that peer influencers could be an accepted source for delivering mental health support and related sexually transmitted infection (STI) interventions to improve health outcomes.

While media and popular culture representations of health shift over time, so, too, do the health issues in popular culture, given the diverse perspectives and cultural understandings of audience members. Digital media and mobile technologies allow individuals greater autonomy to self-manage their diseases and to interact with the health care system. Mediated popular culture holds much promise for improving awareness, access to resources, and support for a variety of health conditions - from enhancing knowledge about nutrition, promoting healthy relationships, improving individuals' ability to access trustworthy disease-specific information, and encouraging physical activity.

Diversifying Theorizing and Advocacy

The fourth section of this book discusses health issues in popular culture from diverse perspectives. What mechanisms of culture drive the inclusion of perspectives in the media to support health? To what extent do media and platforms provide health information and/or persuasive guidance about health choices? Are audiences agentic, and how? This section strives to theorize inclusively about representation and uses media cases to understand media and health advocacy from diverse perspectives. The essays in this section study the depiction of health issues in popular culture and how they change over time.

For advocates, asking questions about what is depicted, who is responsible, and what health policies may support change fundamentally helps widen public understanding of health issues and discussion of these issues in popular culture. Essays from the book's fourth section explore how mediated representations of health and illness depict diverse populations and perspectives. What is missing, and what needs to change?

For example, digital health applications offer novel application uses for sexual health (Dai, 2023). Studying mediated popular culture also offers a window into how the affordances of technology allow LGBTQI populations to avoid stigma, support dating relationships, and explore sexual health concerns (Brady Robards et al., 2022; see also Chapter 8, this volume).

Of course, the media does not always support positive health outcomes. Diekman et al. (2023) consider how food and nutrition are presented on social media and in popular culture. What we count as nutritious food is an empirical question, but, according to Diekman et al., it also gets addressed by nutritional "gurus" on social media for particular audiences seeking contextual social support from like-minded individuals sharing illness or dietary preferences (see also Chapter 4, this volume). While social comparison in media can be leveraged to promote healthy eating and exercise (Rheu et al., 2023), downward social comparison also results in support groups that promote pro-anorexia and disordered eating (Haas et al., 2010).

Beyond specific examples of how popular culture and media can spotlight attention on minoritized or underserved populations, popular culture also can enhance diversity and inclusion efforts in health care (see also Chapters 22 and 23, this volume). For example, popular culture provides us with pictures of the "best doctors" that we know on television: Heathcliff Huxtable, Doogie Howser, House, J.D. Dorian, Miranda Bailey, Addison Montgomery, among many others. The diversity of these images has changed over time, reflecting the change in access to medical higher education for women and minoritized groups.

The Cosby Show disrupted 1980s race and gender normative representations by documenting the life of Heathcliff and Clair Huxtable as HBCU-educated, black doctor and lawyer, respectively (Barrios, 2008). The show features a woman working outside the home and obstetrician Heathcliff, with a home office, portrayed as a doting husband and engaged father. While Huxtable's medical training was not the focus of the show, McQueeney (2022) analyzed black physicians depicted on CBS's *M*A*S*H*, BBC America's *Copper*, Showtime's *Masters of Sex*, Cinemax's *The Knick*, and PBS's *Mercy Street*. These shows provided entertainment that educated viewers about racism in medical education and the obstacles that African Americans faced as doctors, including racist rejection by patients and peers.

Grey's Anatomy and *Scrubs* exemplify this change, with both shows set in teaching hospitals. Both shows addressed age, race, gender, and sexuality issues that arise during physician training programs and unpacked what constitutes good doctoring (Barrios, 2008; Foss, 2014; Painter et al., 2020). As these popular cultural references change, so, too, does public understanding of the importance of diversity in health positions to meet the needs of an ethnically and racially diverse population (Coronado et al., 2020; Quick, 2009).

Representation of diverse people and perspectives is important for everyone. Such diverse representation widens viewers' perspectives about different cultures and experiences, and it also enables individuals to check the socio-cultural location of their perspectives. When popular television shows represent characters with disabilities, such as Marvel's *Hawkeye* on Disney+ featuring a character who wears hearing aids, or HBO's *The Sex Lives of College Girls*, including a character who uses a wheelchair, it normalizes the lived experiences of those who have experienced hearing loss and allows individuals to relate to components of their identity, health, and well-being (Bahr, 2022).

Understanding health issues in popular culture from the perspective of those who live it, or by taking a community-based perspective, spotlights how local media and popular culture enhance the visibility of indigenous knowledge about health. For example, during the COVID-19 pandemic, Indigenous news maintained a robust and easily accessible online presence for communities connected to Indian country. Carter Olson et al.'s (2022) review of U.S. Indigenous media reported on the variety of strategies that communities used to increase demand for COVID-19 vaccination. Carter Olson et al. detailed how:

> The Muckleshoot Tribe, which is about 30 miles south of Seattle, sent a digital newsletter and held Zoom meetings with members. Tribal Elders received paper copies of the newsletter. The campaign resulted in hundreds of cars lining up for the tribe's first drive-through vaccination clinic.
>
> *(p. 290)*

Though Indigenous communities confront a variety of complex illnesses compounded by cultural isolation (California Health Improvement Network, August 28, 2023), research also links identifying with Indigenous cultures to enhanced self-assessed health and buffering stress from discrimination (Shepherd et al., 2018). In this way, Indigenous media facilitate local understandings of illnesses and disease.

Looking to the Future of Popular Culture and Health Communication

Looking to the future, alternative landscapes of popular mediated culture may offer different affordances to audiences and the ways in which they join, build, and sustain virtual communities and advocacy opportunities through media. Effective Health Communication can be challenging, given competing representations in popular culture. Hudson (2016) asserted:

> Public health professionals face the difficult task of developing effective health communication to encourage healthy lifestyles for an American public distracted by competing demands, such as work obligations and family responsibilities, along with savvy commercial marketing from soft drink makers and fast-food restaurants. Public health educators must do a better job of equipping public health students to meet these challenges.
>
> *(p. 251)*

Individuals navigate health and wellness in multiple cultural arenas and gain insights into what it means to be healthy or well, either as a patient or as part of a broader social community.

Overall, this chapter provided an exploration of the multifaceted relationship between popular culture and Health Communication, highlighting the potential impact on attitudes, beliefs, behaviors, and audience understandings related to health and wellness. It also delved into research examining the influence of popular entertainment media, news, and social media on these outcomes. Looking forward, research at the intersection of Health Communication and popular culture should focus on the role of digital technological change and corresponding implications for audiences considering questions of health and illness.

Technological changes continue to shape the scope, construction, and management of health issues in popular culture. From wearable devices to bringing in health data from mobile applications, individuals now have more access to personalized health data. Many of these devices, imagined from popular television shows such as *The Jetsons* (Rogers-Nelson, 2017) or *Star Trek* (Moschou, 2017), have become a reality as popular culture fiction enabled engineers to imagine health designs for the future. Who could have imagined that a show such as *The Jetsons*, with futuristic scenes about telehealth, virtual exercise classes, etc., would be realized by technological innovations responsive to the 2020 coronavirus pandemic?

Twenty-first century rapid technological changes have given media companies more data on audiences and consumers of popular culture products. Future research may examine the personal privacy and broader ethical implications of wearable health devices that provide companies with greater access to personal data, and who owns these data. Information mined from Google searches or "big data" social media posts can be harvested as credible and reliable information and then quickly transformed by future artificial intelligence interventions. For example, researchers monitoring internet searches after the release of Netflix's *13 Reasons Why* identified that "suicide prevention" and "how to commit suicide" searches increased significantly over historical trends (Ayers et al., 2017). These data suggest an array of futuristic interventions that could develop, ranging from technology companies prompting search retrieval with suicide hotline information numbers to other tailored or targeted interventions embedded in Netflix's content. Whether patients or consumers possess the right to privacy or to be forgotten by these trails of "digital exhaust" or users' applications and devices comprises social issues that warrant future research.

Though artificial intelligence and the advent of chat GPT promise to influence health care, certainly for generations, popular culture has explored the dystopian and utopian opportunities presented by technology and its influence on health. Whether or not the future will blend the vision of humans and machines offered by Eric Topol's (2015) *The Patient Will See You Now* vision remains uncertain. The affordances of technology often shape its cultural influence. For example, Peat et al. (2023) demonstrated how gaming subculture can provide a shared or accepted identity for members and reveal diverse motivations for the ways that popular culture games may support and influence individual beliefs about themselves and health. According to Peat et al., patient participation in video games may allow a more flexible, mediated space for participants to interact with others, irrespective of health or disability status. Augmented and virtual reality games permit researchers to examine how individuals interact and adapt to a platform's unique features for improved gameplay and enhanced interactions to support health outcomes (Tao et al., 2021).

Undoubtedly, popular culture will also help to frame public understanding of the policies that manage privacy, data access, and considerations of law and ethics in relation to health information. Many research questions remain: how will the healthcare industry adapt to these technological opportunities with more personalized, tailored medical and public health interventions, and how will they be mediated in popular culture? How will the healthcare and entertainment industries incorporate technological affordances into their cultural products and media and organizational practices to support health and health communication? How will future digital interventions enhance audience understandings of medical and health information through popular culture products? By considering the role of popular culture in providing resources for understanding these issues, supporting individuals' personal and social advocacy, and representing diverse perspectives, future scholars can explore these and other ethical implications to better understand the multifaceted relationship between popular culture and health communication.

References

Aghaei, A., Sakhaei, A., Khalilimeybodi, A., Qiao, S., & Li, X. (2023). Impact of mass media on HIV/AIDS stigma reduction: A systematic review and meta-analysis. *AIDS and Behavior, 27*(10), 3414–3429

Alexopoulos, C., Taylor, L. D., Roberts, L. (2022). Media messages depicting partner abundance increase intention to commit infidelity. *Sexuality & Culture, 26*(6), 2242–2252. https://doi.org/10.1007/s12119-022-09995-1
Alvelos, H., Pereira, J. B., Chatterjee, A., Barreto, S., Alves da Veiga, P., Lima, C. R., & Penedos-Santiago, E. (2023, December 1). When in memeland, speak in memes: Contributions of design towards the betterment of online behavior regarding public health. In N. Martins & D. Brandão (Eds.), *Advances in design and digital communication IV* (pp. 470–486). Springer Series in Design and Innovation. https://doi.org/10.1007/978-3-031-47281-7_39
Ayers, J. W., Althouse, B. M., Leas, E. C., Dredze, M., & Allem, J. (2017). Internet searches for suicide following the release of *13 Reasons Why*. *JAMA Internal Medicine, 177*(10), 1527–1529. https://doi.org/10.1001/jamainternmed.2017.3333
Bahr, S. (2022, July 25). Study shows disability representation onscreen is increasing, but still falls short. *The New York Times,* https://www.nytimes.com/2022/07/26/arts/television/disability-representation-tv-movies-study.html?unlocked_article_code=1.Yk0.TgQF.YtnHEp8JpSv0&smid=url-share
Ball-Rokeach, S. J. (1998). A theory of media power and a theory of media use: Different stories, questions, and ways of thinking. *Mass Communication and Society, 1*, 5–40. https://doi.org/10.1080/15205436.1998.9676398
Bandura, A. (1977). *Social learning theory*. Prentice-Hall.
Barrios, D. (2008). A dissection of Grey's Anatomy. *California Sociology Forum, 1,* 58–63.
Beck (2022*). Celebrity in the time of Covid: Fandom and the influence of pandemic messaging*. McFarland.
Bizzotto, N., De Bruijn, G.-J., & Schulz, P. J. (2023). Buffering against exposure to mental health misinformation in online communities on Facebook: The interplay of depression literacy and expert moderation. *BioMed Central Public Health, [s. l.], 23*(1), 1–12. https://doi.org/10.1186/s12889-023-16404-1
Bond, S. (2022, January 21). What the Joe Rogan podcast controversy says about the online misinformation ecosystem. *NPR*. https://www.npr.org/2022/01/21/1074442185/joe-rogan-doctor-covid-podcast-spotify-misinformation
Brady Robards, P. B., Byron, P., & D'Souza, S. (2022). LGBTQ+ communities and digital media. In D. A. Rohlinger & S. Sobieraj, (Eds.), *The Oxford handbook of digital media sociology* (online ed., pp. 339–361). Oxford Academic. https://doi.org/10.1093/oxfordhb/9780197510636.013.22
Bryant, J. V., Carcioppolo, N., Lun, D., & Potter, J. (2023). Entertainment-education to reduce internalized stigma, increase intimate partner status disclosure intentions, and increase antiretroviral medical adherence intentions: A randomized controlled trial targeting black women living with HIV in the Southern US. *Social Science & Medicine, 327*, 115945. https://doi.org/10.1016/j.socscimed.2023.115945
BuzzFeed. (2021, November 5). Sigh, Kanye West only received one shot of the COVID-19 vaccine — so he isn't fully vaccinated. https://sports.yahoo.com/kanye-west-isnt-fully-vaccinated-210050802.html
California Improvement Network. (2023, August 28). Understanding indigenous communities to support their health needs. California Health Care Foundation. https://www.chcf.org/publication/understanding-indigenous-communities-to-support-their-health-needs/
Canady, V. A. (2023). Field responds to advisory on use of social media and impact on youth MH. *Mental Health Weekly, 33*(22), 1–4. https://doi.org/10.1002/mhw.33663
Carter, M. J. (2013). The hermeneutics of frames and framing: An examination of the media's construction of reality. *SAGE Open, 3*(2). https://doi.org/10.1177/2158244013487915
Carter Olson, C. S., LaPoe, B., LaPoe, V., Azocar, C. L., & Hazarika, B. (2022). "Mothers are Medicine:" U.S. indigenous media emphasizing indigenous women's roles in COVID-19 coverage. *Journal of Communication Inquiry, 46*(3), 289–310. https://doi.org/10.1177/01968599221083239. PMCID: PMC8907872
Cao, B., & Wang, L. (2023). When epidemic outbreaks meet social media: Collective illness narratives on WeChat during COVID-19 omicron infection in China. *Health Communication* (advance online). https://doi.org/10.1080/10410236.2023.2259695
Chen, Q., Chan, K. L., Guo, S., Chen, M., Lo, C. K. M., & Ip, P. (2023). Effectiveness of digital health interventions in reducing bullying and cyberbullying: A meta-analysis. *Trauma, Violence, & Abuse, 24*(3), 1986–2002.
Coronado, F., Beck, A. J., Shah, G., Young, J. L., Sellers, K., & Leider, J. P. (2020). Understanding the dynamics of diversity in the public health workforce. *Journal of Public Health Management Practice, 26*(4), 389–392. https://doi.org/10.1097/PHH.0000000000001075
Cram, P., Fendrick, A. M., Inadomi, J., Cowen, M. E., Carpenter, D., & Vijan, S. (2003). The impact of a celebrity promotional campaign on the use of colon cancer screening: The Katie Couric effect. *Archives of Internal Medicine, 163*(13), 1601–1605.
Coyne, S. M., Ward, L. M., Krof, S. L., Davis, E. J., Holmgren, H. G., Jensen, A. C., & Essig, L. W. (2019). Contributions of mainstream sexual media exposure to sexual attitudes, perceived peer norms, and sexual behavior: A meta-analysis. *Journal of Adolescent Health, 64*(4), 430–436. https://doi.org/10.1016/j.jadohealth.2018.11.016

Dai, M. (2023). Examine the associations between smartphone hookup application uses and sexual health and relationship outcomes among college students. *Journal of American College Health, 71*(2), 554–561.
Darke, P. (2004). The changing face of representations of disability in the media. *Disabling Barriers-enabling Environments, 12*, 100–105.
de Boer, M. L., Archetti, C., & Solbraekke, K. N. (2022). In/Fertile monsters: The emancipatory significance of representations of women on infertility reality TV. *Journal of Medical Humanities, [s. l.], 43*(1), 11–26. https://doi.org/10.1007/s10912-019-09555-z
Desai, S., & Jena, A. B. (2016, December 14). Do celebrity endorsements matter? Observational study of BRCA gene testing and mastectomy rates after Angelina Jolie's *New York Times* editorial. *British Medical Journal [BMJ], 355*, i6357. https://doi.org/10.1136/bmj.i6357. PMID: 27974323; PMCID: PMC5156611
Diekman, C., Ryan, C. D., & Oliver, T. L. (2023). Misinformation and disinformation in food science and nutrition: Impact on practice. *The Journal of Nutrition, 153*(1), 3–9.
Drachen, A. (2023). Debate: Games-based collaboration as a driver for massive-scale mental health research. *Child and Adolescent Mental Health, 28*(1), 148–149.
Drake, S. A., Zhang, N., Applewhite, C., Fowler, K., & Holcomb, J. B. (2017). A social media program to increase adolescent seat belt use. *Public Health Nursing, 34*(5), 500–504.
Engel, E., Gell, S., Heiss, R., & Karsay, K. (2024). Social media influencers and adolescents' health: A scoping review of the research field. *Social Science & Medicine, 340*, N.PAG. https://doi.org/10.1016/j.socscimed.2023.116387
Evans, D. G. R., Barwell, J., Eccles, D. M., Collins, A., Izatt, L., Jacobs, C., Donaldson, A., Brady, A. F., Cuthbert, A., Harrison, R., & Thomas, S. (2014). The Angelina Jolie effect: How high celebrity profile can have a major impact on provision of cancer related services. *Breast Cancer Research, 16*(5), 1–6.
Fardouly, J., & Vartanian, L. R. (2015). Negative comparisons about one's appearance mediate the relationship between Facebook usage and body image concerns. *Body Image, 12*, 82–88. https://doi.org/10.1016/j.bodyim.2014.10.004
Ferguson, C. J., Munoz, M. E., Garza, A., & Galindo, M. (2014). Concurrent and prospective analyses of peer, television and social media influences on body dissatisfaction, eating disorder symptoms and life satisfaction in adolescent girls. *Journal of Youth and Adolescence, 43*(1), 1–14. https://doi.org/10.1007/s10964-012-9898-9
Foss, K. A. (2014). From Welby to McDreamy: What TV teaches us about doctors, patients, and the health care system. In D. Macey, K. M. Ryan, & N. J. Springer (Eds.). *How television shapes our worldview: Media representations of social trends and change* (pp. 227–246). Lexington Books.
Goldhaber, S. Z., & Hamilton, M. A. (1992). 'Beverly Hills, 90210': The lap belts don't show on TV. *JAMA, 268*(2), 200. https://doi.org/10.1001/jama.1992.03490020044027
Greene, A. K., Carr, S., & Jia, H. (2022). Tech, sex, and e-cigarettes: The gendering of vape promotion on Instagram. *Journal of Health Communication, 27*(9), 682–695. https://doi.org/10.1080/10810730.2022.2150336
Greve, H. R., Rao, H., Vicinanza, P., & Zhou, E. Y. (2022). Online conspiracy groups: Micro-bloggers, bots, and coronavirus conspiracy talk on Twitter. *American Sociological Review, 87*(6), 919–949. https://doi.org/10.1177/00031224221125937
Haas, S. M., Irr, M. E., Jennings, N. A., & Wagner, L. M. (2010). Communicating thin: A grounded model of online negative enabling support groups in the pro-anorexia movement. *New Media & Society, 13*(1), 40–57. https://doi.org/10.1177/1461444810363910
Headley, S. A., Jones, T., Kanekar, A., & Vogelzang, J. (2022). Using memes to increase health literacy in vulnerable populations. *American Journal of Health Education, 53*(1), 11–15.
Hoffman, B. L., Hoffman, R., VonVille, H. M., Sidani, J. E., Manganello, J. A., Chu, K. H., Felter, E. M., Miller, E., & Burke, J. G. (2023). Characterizing the influence of television health entertainment narratives in lay populations: A scoping review. *American Journal of Health Promotion, 37*(5), 685–697.
Hoffman, B. L., Sidani, J. E., Burke, J. G., Chu, K. H., & Felter, E. M. (2023). Vaccine misinformation on social media: Historical contexts, lessons learned, and paths forward. In T. Ginossar, S. Shah, & D. Weiss (Eds.), *Vaccine communication online: Counteracting misinformation, rumors and lies* (pp. 11–33). Springer International Publishing.
Honcharov, V., Li, J., Sierra, M., Rivadeneira, N., Olazo, K., Nguyen, T., Mackey, T., & Sarkar, U. (2023). Public figure vaccination rhetoric and vaccine hesitancy: Retrospective Twitter analysis. *JMIR Infodemiology*, 3, e40575. https://infodemiology.jmir.org/2023/1/e40575 https://doi.org/10.2196/40575
Hong, C. (2023). Mpox on *Reddit*: A thematic analysis of online posts on Mpox on a social media platform among key populations. *Journal of Urban Health, 100*(6), 1–10. https://doi.org/10.1007/s11524-023-00773-4
Huang, Q., Peng, W., & Ahn, S. (2021). When media become the mirror: A meta-analysis on media and body image. *Media Psychology, 24*(4), 437–489. https://doi.org/10.1080/15213269.2020.1737545

Hudson, D. L. (2016). Popular culture and public health. *Pedagogy in Health Promotion, 2*(4), 251–255.
In case you haven't heard… (2023). *Alcoholism & Drug Abuse Weekly, 35*, 8–8. https://doi-org/ 10.1002/adaw.33866
Jolie, A. (2013, May 14). My medical choice. *The New York Times*. https://www.nytimes.com/2013/05/14/opinion/my-medical-choice.html
Katie Couric Media. (2023, October 26). Katie Couric answers your burning questions about her breast cancer journey. https://katiecouric.com/health/cancer/katie-couric-breast-cancer-update/
Keefe, P. R., (2017, October 23). The family that built an empire of pain. *The New Yorker*. https://www-newyorker-com/magazine/2017/10/30/the-family-that-built-an-empire-of-pain
Kennedy-Hendricks, A., Levin, J., Stone, E., McGinty, E. E., Gollust, S. E., & Barry, C. L. (2019). News media reporting on medication treatment for opioid use disorder amid the opioid epidemic. *Health Affairs, 38*(4), 643–651. https://doi.org/10.1377/hlthaff.2018.05075
Kim, J. (2024). The value of a shared experience: Relationships between co-experience and identification with other audiences and audience engagement behaviors on social media. *Computers in Human Behavior, 152*, 108050 https://doi.org/10.1016/j.chb.2023.108050
Kjærulff, E. M., Andersen, T. H., Kingod, N., & Nexø, M. A. (2023). When people with chronic conditions turn to peers on social media to obtain and share information: Systematic review of the implications for relationships with health care professionals. *Journal of Medical Internet Research, 25*, e41156.
Knight, H., Jia, R., Ayling, K., Blake, H., Morling, J. R., Villalon, A. M., ... & Vedhara, K. (2023). The changing vaccine landscape: Rates of COVID-19 vaccine acceptance and hesitancy in young adults during vaccine rollout. *Perspectives in Public Health, 143*(4), 220–224.
Kostygina, G., Tran, H., Binns, S., Szczypka, G., Emery, S., Vallone, D., & Hair, E. (2020). Boosting health campaign reach and engagement through use of social media influencers and memes. *Social Media+ Society, 6*(2). https://doi.org/10.1177/20563051209124
Ligami, C. (2023). Social media helping younger adults combat HIV stigma. *The Lancet HIV, 10*(5), e280–e281.
Lin, W. H., Liu, C. H., & Yi, C. C. (2020). Exposure to sexually explicit media in early adolescence is related to risky sexual behavior in emerging adulthood. *PLOS ONE, 15*(4), e0230242. https://doi.org/10.1371/journal.pone.0230242
Louik, J. L., Horvath, K. J., Golub, S. A., Gutierrez, R. A., Rivera, S., Arnsten, J. J., & Patel, V. (2023). Feasibility and acceptability of a peer influencer delivered social media based intervention to promote mental health awareness for young Black and Latinx gay and bisexual men and transgender women. *Journal of Gay & Lesbian Mental Health*, (s. l.), 1–17. https://doi.org /10.1080/19359705.2023.2239730
Majmundar, A., Pérez, C., Huerta, M., Unger, J. B., & Allem, J.-P. (2023). Describing memes referencing vaping: Thematic analysis. *Substance Use & Misuse, 58*(2), 306–310. https://doi.org/10.1080/10826084.2022.2161316
Maloney, E. K., & Cappella, J. N. (2016). Does vaping in e-cigarette advertisements affect tobacco smoking urge, intentions, and perceptions in daily, intermittent, and former smokers? *Health Communication, 31*(1), 129–138. https://doi.org/10.1080/10410236.2014.993496
Martin, H. (2001, October 9). Films steer us wrong on seat belts, study says. *Los Angeles Times*. https://www.latimes.com/archives/la-xpm-2001-oct-09-me-55032-story.html#:~:text=Researchers%20watched%20198%20top%2Dgrossing,about%2070%25%20of%20the%20time
McGwin, G. Jr., Modjarrad, K., Reiland, A., Tanner, S., & Rue, L. W. (2006). Prevalence of transportation safety measures portrayed in primetime US television programs and commercials. *Injury Prevention, 12*(6), 400–403. https://doi.org/10.1136/ip.2006.012237
McQueeney, L. (2022). The Black doctor on the historical small screen: African American physicians in television period dramas. In K. Bryne, J. A. Taddeo, & J. Leggott, (Eds.), *Diagnosing history: Medicine in television period drama* (pp. 100–114). Manchester University Press.
Meier, B. (2018). *Pain killer: An empire of deceit and the origin of America's opioid epidemic*. Penguin Random House.
Moschou, D., & The Conversation U.S. (2017, June 16). How close are we to a real *Star Trek*-style medical tricorder? *Scientific American*. https://www.scientificamerican.com/article/how-close-are-we-to-a-real-star-trek-style-medical-tricorder/
Moschonis, G., Siopis, G., Jung, J., Eweka, E., Willems, R., Kwasnicka, D., Asare, B. Y. A., Kodithuwakku, V., Verhaeghe, N., Vedanthan, R., & Annemans, L. (2023). Effectiveness, reach, uptake, and feasibility of digital health interventions for adults with type 2 diabetes: A systematic review and meta-analysis of randomised controlled trials. *The Lancet Digital Health, 5*(3), e125–e143.
Oliver, M. B., & Raney, A. A. (2023). Media effects research in *Journalism & Mass Communication Quarterly*. *Journalism & Mass Communication Quarterly, 100*(4), 793–807. https://doi.org/10.1177/10776990231203539

Painter, D. L., Kubala, A., & Parsloe, S. (2020). Playing doctor on TV: Physician portrayals and interactions on medical drama, comedy, and reality shows. *Atlantic Journal of Communication, 28*(5), 322–336.

Pavlova, A., & Berkers, P. (2020). Mental health discourse and social media: Which mechanisms of cultural power drive discourse on Twitter. *Social Science & Medicine, 263*, 113250. https://doi.org/10.1016/j.socscimed.2020.113250

Peat, G., Rodriguez, A., & Smith, J. (2023). "It is easier to not allow them to see your disability straight away, to see you as a person:" An interpretative phenomenological analysis of video gaming from the perspectives of men with Duchenne Muscular Dystrophy. *Palliative Medicine, 37*(7), 1016–1024. https://doi.org/10.1177/02692163231172246

Popova, M. (2019). *Sexual consent*. MIT Press.

Porter, A. W., Cooper, S. C., Palmedo, P. C., Wojtowicz, N., Chong, J., & Maddalon, M. (2022). Podcasts and their potential to improve sexual health literacy in adolescents and young adults. *American Journal of Sexuality Education, 17* (1), 125–136. https://doi.org/10.1080/15546128.2021.1987365

Quick, B. L. (2009). The effects of viewing Grey's Anatomy on perceptions of doctors and patient satisfaction. *Journal of Broadcasting & Electronic Media, 53*(1), 38–55.

Quinones, S. (2016). *Dreamland: The true tale of America's opiate epidemic*. Bloomsbury Publishing.

Rheu, M., Peng, W., & Haung, K. T. (2023). Leveraging upward social comparison in social media to promote healthy parenting. *Health Communication, 38*(2), 205–215.

Robertson, M. (2018). *Growing up queer: Kids and the remaking of LGBTQ identity* (Vol. 3). NYU Press.

Rogers-Nelson, K. (2017, June 19). 7 gadgets from 'The Jetsons' that have become a reality. https://www.rismedia.com/2017/06/19/gadgets-jetsons-that-have-become-reality/

Rohde, J. A., Liu, J., & Rees, V. V. (2023). Community and opinion leadership effects on vaping discourse: A network analysis of online reddit threads. *Journal of Health Communication, 28*(8), 487–497. https://doi.org/10.1080/10810730.2023.2225447

Romano, A. (2020, December 26). Bridgerton has a rape scene, but it's not treated like one. *Vox*. https://www.vox.com/22194033/bridgerton-netflix-rape-scene-novel

Rosen, D. (2022). (Ed.). *The social media debate: Unpacking the social, psychological, and cultural effects of social media.* Routledge.

Rubin, A. M., & Windahl, S. (1986). The uses and dependency model of mass communication, *Critical Studies in Mass Communication, 3*(2), 184–199. https://doi.org/10.1080/15295039609366643

Russell, J., Greenhalgh, T., Byrne, E., & McDonnell, J. (2008). Recognizing rhetoric in health care policy analysis. *Journal of Health Services Research & Policy, 13*(1), 40–46. https://doi-org.ezp3.lib.umn.edu/10.1258/jhsrp.2007.006029

Sandberg, K., Banerjee, O., Harris, C., & Averill, M. (2022). P160 Healthy food, as told by TikTok: A thematic analysis of the most liked #healthyrecipes on TikTok. *Journal of Nutrition Education and Behavior, 54*(7S), S94.

Shaw, P. A., Sumner, A. L., Halton, C., Bailey, S. C., Wolf, M. S., Andrews, E., & Cartwright, T. (2022). "You're more engaged when you're listening to somebody tell their story": A qualitative exploration into the mechanisms of the podcast 'menopause: unmuted' for communicating health information. *Patient Education & Counseling, 105*(12), 3494–3500. https://doi.org/10.1016/j.pec.2022.09.003

Shepherd, S. M., Delgado, R. H., Sherwood, J., & Paradies, Y. (2018). The impact of indigenous cultural identity and cultural engagement on violent offending. *Biomedical Central Public Health, 18*(50), 1–7. https://doi.org/10.1186/s12889-017-4603-2

Simon-Roberts, S., & Hawkins, D. S. (2023). Health messaging and the black community: Analysis of rhetoric in Michelle Obama's social media's posts announcing her COVID-19 vaccination status. *Howard Journal of Communications, 34*(3), 315–336. https://doi.org/10.1080/10646175.2023.2174391

Strine, T. W., Beck, L. F., Bolen, J., Okoro, C., Dhingra, S., & Balluz, L. (2010). Geographic and sociodemographic variation in self-reported seat belt use in the United States. *Accident Analysis & Prevention, 42*(4), 1066–1071. https://doi.org/10.1016/j.aap.2009.12.014

Sumnall, H. R., Atkinson, A. M., Anderson, M., McAuley, A., & Trayner, K. M. A. (2023). How to save a life: Public awareness of a national mass media take home naloxone campaign, and effects of exposure to campaign components on overdose knowledge and responses. *International Journal of Drug Policy,* 104111. https://doi.org/10.1016/j.drugpo.2023.104111

Taracuk, M. D., & Koch, J. M. (2023). Use of a media intervention to increase positive attitudes toward transgender and gender diverse individuals. *International Journal of Transgender Health, 24*(1), 86–98.

Tao, G., Garrett, B., Taverner, T., Cordingley, E., & Sun, C. (2021). Immersive virtual reality health games: A narrative review of game design. *Journal of NeuroEngineering and Rehabilitation, 18*, 1–21.

Tisdell, E. J., & Thompson, P. M. (2007). "Seeing from a different angle:" The role of pop culture in teaching for diversity and critical media literacy in adult education. *International Journal of Lifelong Education, 26*(1), 651–673. https://doi.org/10.1080/02601370701711349

Topol, E. (2015). *The patient will see you now: The future of medicine is in your hands.* Basic Books.

Triptow, C., Freeman, J., Lee, P., & Robinson, T. (2024). #HealthyLifestyle: A Q methodology analysis of why young adults like to use social media to access health information. *Journal of Health Psychology, 29*(2), 123–136. https://doi-org.ezp3.lib.umn.edu/10.1177/13591053231200690

Tullett-Prado, D., Stavropoulos, V., Gomez, R., & Doley, J. (2023). Social media use and abuse: Different profiles of users and their associations with addictive behaviours. *Addictive Behaviors Reports, 17*, 100479. https://doi.org/10.1016/j.abrep.2023.100479

Volpp, K. G., Loewenstein, G., & Buttenheim, A. M. (2021). Behaviorally informed strategies for a national COVID-19 vaccine promotion program. *Journal of the American Medical Association, 325*(2), 125–126. https://doi.org/10.1001/jama.2020.24036

Wahl, O. F. (1992). Mass media images of mental illness: A review of the literature. *Journal of Community Psychology, 20*(4), 343–352.

Ward, L. M. (2003). Understanding the role of entertainment media in the sexual socialization of American youth: A review of empirical research. *Developmental Review, 23*, 347–388. https://doi.org/10.1016/s0273-2297(03)00013-3

Wienert, J., Jahnel, T., & Maaß, L. (2022, June 28). What are digital public health interventions? First steps toward a definition and an intervention classification framework. *Journal of Medical Internet Research, 24*(6), e31921. https://doi.org/10.2196/31921

West, B. A., Rudd, R. A., Sauber-Schatz, E. K., & Ballesteros, M. F. (2021). Unintentional injury deaths in children and youth, 2010-2019. *Journal of Safety Research, 78*, 322–330. https://doi.org/10.1016/j/jsr/2021/07.001

Winsten, J. A. (1994). Promoting designated drivers: The Harvard alcohol project. *American Journal of Preventive Medicine, 10*(3), 11–14.

Yeshua-Katz, D., Shapira, S., Aharonson-Daniel, L., Clarfield, A. M., & Sarid, O. (2023). Matching digital intervention affordances with tasks: The case of a zoom and WhatsApp mental health intervention for seniors during the COVID-19 pandemic. *Health Communication, 38*(3), 499–511.

Zhang, N., Drake, S. A., & Ding, K. (2020). Message appeals on an Instagram account promoting seat belt use that attract adolescents and young adults: Elaboration-likelihood perspective study. *JMIR Formative Research, 4*(9), e16800. https://doi.org/10.2196/16800

INDEX